COMPLICATIONS IN REGIONAL ANESTHESIA AND PAIN MEDICINE

Second Edition

COMPLICATIONS IN REGIONAL ANESTHESIA AND PAIN MEDICINE

Second Edition

Joseph M. Neal, MD
Department of Anesthesiology
Virginia Mason Medical Center
Clinical Professor of Anesthesiology
University of Washington
Seattle, Washington

James P. Rathmell, MD
Vice Chair and Chief
Division of Pain Medicine
Department of Anesthesia, Critical Care and Pain Medicine
Massachusetts General Hospital
Professor of Anaesthesia
Harvard Medical School
Boston, Massachusetts

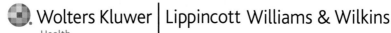
Wolters Kluwer | Lippincott Williams & Wilkins
Health

Philadelphia • Baltimore • New York • London
Buenos Aires • Hong Kong • Sydney • Tokyo

Acquisitions Editor: Brian Brown
Product Manager: Nicole Dernoski
Production Manager: Keith Donnellan
Senior Manufacturing Manager: Benjamin Rivera
Marketing Manager: Lisa Lawrence
Design Coordinator: Holly McLaughlin
Production Service: SPi Global

Library of Congress Cataloging-in-Publication Data
Complications in regional anesthesia and pain medicine / [edited by] Joseph M. Neal, James P. Rathmell. — 2nd ed.
     p. ; cm.
  Includes bibliographical references and index.
  ISBN 978-1-4511-0978-8
 I. Neal, Joseph M. II. Rathmell, James P.
  [DNLM: 1. Anesthesia, Conduction—adverse effects. 2. Analgesia—adverse effects. 3. Pain Management—adverse effects. WO 300]
  617.9'64—dc23

2011049173

To purchase additional copies of this book, call our customer service department at (800) 638-3030 or fax orders to (301) 223-2320. International customers should call (301) 223-2300.

Visit Lippincott Williams & Wilkins on the Internet: at LWW.com. Lippincott Williams & Wilkins customer service representatives are available from 8:30 am to 6 pm, EST.

10 9 8 7 6 5 4 3 2 1

We dedicate this book to the well-being of our patients, to the education of our residents and fellows, and to the collegiality of our colleagues.
Most of all, we offer our heartfelt gratitude to our families.
Without their love and support, nothing would be possible—
Kay, Erin, and Pete Neal
Bobbi, Lauren, James, and Cara Rathmell

In memory of Christopher M. Bernards, MD
Scholar, Scientist, Teacher, Clinician ... Renaissance Man and most of all, Friend
"Don't believe everything you think"

Preface

This text arose from the close collaboration of two physicians who have spent a significant part of their careers fascinated with just how we might improve the safety of the techniques we use in the operating room and the pain clinic. We have both published on topics ranging from how to perform a "test dose" during the conduct of regional anesthesia to detailing the probable mechanism underlying catastrophic neural injuries that have been reported during cervical transforaminal and interlaminar epidural injections.

Over the past decade, we have worked closely in performing the editorial work of the journal *Regional Anesthesia and Pain Medicine*, and in our roles serving the journal we have fielded many case reports detailing new and unexpected complications. The American Society of Regional Anesthesia and Pain Medicine, an organization dedicated to training physicians to safely and effectively conduct regional anesthesia and pain treatment techniques, has expended much effort on assembling guidelines for the safe conduct of these techniques. Indeed, a number of these practice advisories have become the standard references for guiding the conduct of neural blockade in settings where the risk of adverse events is elevated, such as in the administration of anticoagulants to patients, in the recognition and treatment of local anesthetic systemic toxicity, or in the prevention and management of infectious or neurologic complications associated with regional anesthesia and pain treatment.

During one of our frequent discussions, the idea of compiling a single text that would detail what was known about the occurrence, recognition, treatment, and prevention of complications took root and grew into the first edition of this text. When we set out to create a book focusing on the complications associated with regional anesthesia and pain medicine practice, we had just two goals: to compile in a single volume the current best knowledge regarding complications specific to our subspecialties and to seek that knowledge from authors who would be recognized worldwide for their expertise on the chosen topic. While these two goals have not changed since the first edition's 2007 publication, the intervening 5 years have significantly advanced our understanding of many complications. These advancements are wide-ranging and include new imaging modalities (particularly ultrasound guidance), new therapeutic options (such as lipid rescue of local anesthetic systemic toxicity, or increasingly powerful anticoagulants), and new systems-based initiatives (including procedural pauses and standardization of external setup). At the same time, our understanding of the mechanisms underlying specific injuries has been clarified (catastrophic neural injury associated with intra-arterial injection of particulate steroid), and updated techniques for improving safety have arisen (use of cineangiography and digital subtraction technology). Based on these changes, we thought it worthwhile to pursue a second edition of the book.

The book's content is organized into distinct sections. The section on regional anesthesia is somewhat artificially separated from the section on pain medicine; we realize that many complications span both subspecialties. The first, and largest, portion is dedicated to discussing the complications that have been reported with specific techniques or agents, complications both common and uncommon. The last part attempts to clarify issues of informed consent and liability.

We have once again been honored by the willingness of highly respected friends and colleagues to devote their time and expertise to the creation of detailed chapters that were subject to rigorous editing. We believe that any knowledgeable practitioner is likely to recognize these authors as leading experts in the specific complications on which they have written. Our editorial goals were to ensure a consistent framework for how each chapter was organized, to require the authors to be as evidence based as possible, and to provide readers with visually appealing figures and boxes that would facilitate their understanding of each topic.

We could not have produced this book without the valued expertise of others. The spectacular, and now colorized, original artwork is by Gary Nelson, an indefatigable medical illustrator from the University of Vermont. Working with him is almost pleasurable enough to search for yet another book project. No book would ever come to fruition without a dedicated and supportive publishing team. To this end, we offer our sincere thanks to Brian Brown, Nicole Dernoski, Tom Conville, and Keith Donnellan of Wolters Kluwer/Lippincott Williams & Wilkins and to Deepika Bhardwaj of SPi Global. And last but not least, we thank all of those who found value in the first edition of *Complications of Regional Anesthesia and Pain Medicine* and who, through their use of the book and their words of encouragement, have made creating the second edition a stimulating and rewarding enterprise.

If one accepts the Hippocratic dictum "first, do no harm," preventing complications or effectively treating them becomes of paramount importance to practitioners of regional anesthesia and pain medicine and for the patients we serve.

Joseph M. Neal, MD
Seattle, Washington

James P. Rathmell, MD
Boston, Massachusetts

Contributors

Stephen E. Abram, MD
Professor of Anesthesiology
Department of Anesthesiology
Medical College of Wisconsin
Milwaukee, Wisconsin

José Aguirre, MD, MSc, DESRA
Consultant Anesthetist
Balgrist University Hospital
Zürich, Switzerland

Yves Auroy, MD, PhD
Professor, École du Val-de-Grace
Chief, Departement of Anesthesiology
    and ICU,
Hôpital d'Instruction des Armées du
    Val-de-Grâce
Paris, France

Jane C. Ballantyne, MD, FRCA
UW Medicine Professor of Education
    and Research
Department of Anesthesiology and
    Pain Medicine
University of Washington
Seattle, Washington

Dan Benhamou, MD
Professor of Anesthesia and Intensive
    Care
Chairman
Département d'Anesthésie-
    Réanimation
Université Paris-Sud, Hôpital Bicêtre,
Le Kremlin-Bicêtre cedex, France

Honorio T. Benzon, MD
Professor
Department of Anesthesiology
Associate Chair of Academic Affairs
    and Promotions
Northwestern University Feinberg
    School of Medicine
Attending Staff
Department of Anesthesiology
Northwestern Memorial Hospital
Chicago, Illinois

Christopher M. Bernards, MD[‡]
Anesthesiology Faculty
Virginia Mason Medical Center
Clinical Professor of Anesthesiology
University of Washington
Seattle, Washington

**Nikolai Bogduk, BSc(Med), MBBS,
PhD, MD, DSc, Mmed, Dip Anat.**
Professor of Pain Medicine
University of Newcastle
Department of Clinical Research
Newcastle Bone and Joint Institute
Royal Newcastle Centre
Newcastle, New South Wales,
    Australia

Alain Borgeat, MD
Professor and Head of the Division of
    Anesthesiology
Balgrist University Hospital
Zurich, Switzerland

David L. Brown, MD
Professor and Chair
Department of Anesthesiology
Cleveland Clinic
Lerner College of Medicine
Chair
Anesthesiology Institute
Cleveland Clinic
Cleveland, Ohio

John F. Butterworth, MD
Professor and Chair
Department of Anesthesiology
Virginia Commonwealth University
    School of Medicine
Richmond, Virginia

Kenneth D. Candido, MD
Chairman
Department of Anesthesiology
Advocate Illinois Masonic Medical
    Center
Clinical Professor of Anesthesiology
University of Illinois-Chicago
Chicago, Illinois

Adam J. Carinci, MD
Department of Anesthesia, Critical
    Care and Pain Medicine
Massachusetts General Hospital
Instructor in Anaesthesia
Harvard Medical School
Boston, Massachusetts

John D. Cassidy, Esq.
Partner
Ficksman & Conley, LLP
Boston, Massachusetts

Matthew T. Charous, MD
Regional Anesthesiology Fellow
Department of Anesthesiology
University of California
    San Diego
San Diego, California

Steven P. Cohen, MD
Professor
Department of Anesthesiology
Uniformed Services University of the
    Health Sciences
Director of Chronic Pain
    Research
Walter Reed National Military
    Medical Center
Bethesda, Maryland
Associate Professor
Johns Hopkins School of
    Medicine
Baltimore, Maryland

Oscar A. de Leon-Casasola, MD
Professor of Anesthesiology and
    Medicine
Vice-Chair for Clinical
    Affairs
University at Buffalo
Chief
Division of Pain Medicine and
    Professor of Oncology
Roswell Park Cancer Institute
Buffalo, New York

‡Deceased

Timothy R. Deer, MD
Clinical Professor
Anesthesiology Department
West Virginia University School of
    Medicine
President and CEO
The Center for Pain Relief, Inc.
Charleston, West Virginia

Karen B. Domino, MD, MPH
Professor
Department of Anesthesiology and
    Pain Medicine
University of Washington
Seattle, Washington

Kenneth Drasner, MD
Professor of Anesthesia and
    Perioperative Care
University of California
San Francisco, California

Michael A. Erdek, MD
Assistant Professor
Anesthesiology, Critical Care
    Medicine, and Oncology
Johns Hopkins University
Baltimore, Maryland

F. Michael Ferrante
Director
UCLA Pain Management Center
Professor of Clinical Anesthesiology
    and Medicine
David Geffen School of Medicine at
    UCLA
Los Angeles, California

Dermot R. Fitzgibbon, MD
Professor
Department of Anesthesiology and
    Pain Medicine
University of Washington
Seattle, Washington

Halena M. Gazelka, MD
Senior Associate Consultant
Department of Anesthesiology and
    Pain Medicine
Mayo Clinic College of
    Medicine
Rochester, Minnesota

Brian E. Harrington, MD
Staff Anesthesiologist
Billings Clinic Hospital
Billings, Montana

**James E. Heavner, DVM, PhD,
FIPP(Hon)**
Professor and Research Director
Department of Anesthesiology and
    Cell Physiology and Molecular
    Biophysics
Texas Tech University Health Sciences
    Center
Lubbock, Texas

James R. Hebl, MD
Associate Professor of Anesthesiology
Mayo Clinic College of Medicine
Rochester, Minnesota

James M. Hitt, MD, PhD
Associate Professor
Department of Anesthesiology
University at Buffalo
Staff Physician
Department of Anesthesiology
Roswell Park Cancer Institute
Buffalo, New York

Diane E. Hoffmann, JD, MS
Professor of Law
School of Law
University of Maryland
Baltimore, Maryland

Quinn H. Hogan, MD
Professor of Anesthesiology
Director of Pain Research
Anesthesiology Research
Medical College of Wisconsin
Milwaukee, Wisconsin

Terese T. Horlocker, MD
Professor of Anesthesiology and
    Orthopaedics
Department of Anesthesiology
Mayo Clinic
Rochester, Minnesota

Karlo Houra, MD, PhD
Neurosurgeon
Orthopedics, Surgery, Neurology,
    and Physical Medicine and
    Rehabilitation
St. Catherine Specialty Hospital
Zabok, Croatia

Marc A. Huntoon, MD
Professor of Anesthesiology
Chief
Division of Pain Medicine
Vanderbilt University
Nashville, Tennessee

Brian M. Ilfeld, MD, MS
Associate Professor in Residence
Department of Anesthesiology
University of California
San Diego, California

Leonardo Kapural, MD, PhD
Director
Pain Medicine Center
Wake Forest University Baptist Health
Carolinas Pain Institute
Professor of Anesthesiology
Wake Forest University, School of
    Medicine
Winston-Salem, North Carolina

Farooq Khan, MD
Fellow
Pain Medicine
Northwestern University Feinberg
    School of Medicine
Chicago, Illinois

Lorri A. Lee, MD
Associate Professor
Department of Anesthesiology and
    Pain Medicine
University of Washington
Seattle, Washington

Gregory A. Liguori, MD
Anesthesiologist-in-Chief
Hospital for Special Surgery
Clinical Associate Professor in
    Anesthesiology
Weill Medical College of Cornell
    University
New York, New York

Smith C. Manion, MD
Assistant Professor
Department of Anesthesiology
University of Kansas Medical Center
Kansas City, Missouri

Joseph M. Neal, MD
Department of Anesthesiology
Virginia Mason Medical Center
Clinical Professor of Anesthesiology
University of Washington
Seattle, Washington

Adam D. Niesen, MD
Instructor
Department of Anesthesiology
Mayo Clinic College of Medicine
Rochester, Minnesota

Jean-Pierre P. Ouanes, DO
Assistant Professor
Anesthesia and Critical
    Care Medicine
Johns Hopkins University
Anesthesiologist
Anesthesia and Critical
    Care Medicine
The Johns Hopkins Hospital
Baltimore, Maryland

Mehmet S. Ozcan, MD, FCCP
Assistant Professor of Anesthesiology
Department of Anesthesiology
Divisions of Critical Care Medicine
    and Neuroanesthesia
University of Illinois College of
    Medicine at Chicago
Chicago, Illinois

Julia E. Pollock, MD
Chief of Anesthesiology
Virginia Mason Medical Center
Seattle, Washington

Jason E. Pope, MD
Napa Pain Institute
Napa, California
Assistant Professor of
    Anesthesiology
Vanderbilt University Medical
    Center
Nashville, Tennessee

Gabor B. Racz, MD, FIPP
Professor and Chairman Emeritus of
    Anesthesiology
Department of Anesthesiology
Texas Tech University Health Sciences
    Center
Lubbock, Texas

Andrej Radic, MD
Orthopaedic Surgeon
Orthopaedics, Surgery, Neurology
    and Physical Medicine and
    Rehabilitation
St. Catherine Specialty Hospital
Zabok, Croatia

James P. Rathmell, MD
Vice Chair and Chief
Division of Pain Medicine
Department of Anesthesia, Critical
    Care and Pain Medicine
Massachusetts General Hospital
Professor of Anaesthesia
Harvard Medical School
Boston, Massachusetts

Richard L. Rauck, MD
Executive Medical Director
Carolinas Pain Institute
Pain Fellowship Director
Wake Forest University Health
    Sciences
Center for Clinical Research
Winston-Salem, North Carolina

Richard Rosenquist, MD
Chairman
Pain Management Department
Cleveland Clinic
Cleveland, Ohio

John C. Rowlingson, MD
Cosmo A. DiFazio Professor of
    Anesthesiology
Department of Anesthesiology
University of Virginia Health School
    of Medicine and Health System
Charlottesville, Virginia

Stephen M. Rupp, MD
Medical Director
Perioperative Services
Department of Anesthesiology
Virginia Mason Medical Center
Seattle, Washington

Thomas H. Scott, MD
Fellow
Pain Medicine
Department of Anesthesia and Critical
    Care
University of Pennsylvania and
    Hospital of the University of
    Pennsylvania
Philadelphia, Pennsylvania

Linda S. Stephens, PhD
Research Scientist/Engineer
Department of Anesthesiology and
    Pain Medicine
University of Washington
Seattle, Washington

William F. Urmey, MD
Clinical Associate Professor of
    Anesthesiology
Weill Medical College of Cornell
    University
Attending Anesthesiologist Hospital
    for Special Surgery
New York, New York

Denise J. Wedel, MD
Professor
Department of Anesthesiology
Mayo Clinic College of Medicine
Rochester, Minnesota

Guy Weinberg, MD
Professor of Anesthesiology
University of Illinois and Jesse Brown
    VA Medical Center
Chicago, Illinois

M. Kate Welti, RN, JD
Associate
Ficksman & Conley, LLP
Boston, Massachusetts

Indy M. Wilkinson, MD
Department of Anesthesiology
Walter Reed National Military
    Medical Center
Bethesda, Maryland

Christopher L. Wu, MD
Professor
Department of Anesthesiology
The Johns Hopkins University
Chief
Division of Obstetrics and Regional
    Anesthesia and Acute Pain
Department of Anesthesiology
The Johns Hopkins Hospital
Baltimore, Maryland

Contents

An Overview of Risk Analysis

David L. Brown

▶ SOME BACKGROUND ON RISK

A more complete understanding of risk necessarily flows from the development of an accurate definition of the term risk. One dictionary definition of risk is "possibility of suffering harm or loss (danger), a factor, course or element involving uncertain danger (hazard)".[1] To increase our knowledge of this area of medicine, we must first explore society's understanding of risk. Ultimately, the anesthesiologist can then define risk effectively as it pertains to the practice of the specialty (see Box 1-1).

▶ RISK CONCEPTS

We live in a society that struggles with balancing risks. When one takes a step back from risk analysis, it becomes clearer that risk analysis is, in fact, decision analysis. The decision imparts action to balancing the risk involved. For example, many people worry a great deal about flying, despite an outstanding safety record in commercial air travel. Many of these same travelers continue to smoke and to overeat, and it is statistically clear that an individual is more at risk from chronic health conditions than from a commercial air accident.[2] Nevertheless, many in our society worry more about an aviation accident than they do about the risks of smoking or overeating.

It is worthwhile to clarify the difference between "risk" and "hazard." Many people consider these terms to be synonymous, yet they are not. Risk expresses not only the potential for an undesired consequence but the probability that such a consequence will occur. In contrast, hazard expresses the potential for an undesired consequence but without an estimate of how likely it is to occur.[3] Most of us, believing we are reflecting on risk, are really focused on the hazard. As an example, the authors of *Freakonomics* outline that when considering the risks of a school-age girl playing at the home of friends, whose parents own either a swimming pool or a handgun, most parents believe the risk is lower if the girl plays in the home whose parents own a swimming pool.[4] Even with this example, risk analysis is often further confounded. To produce a more accurate analysis, the emotional aspect of risk needs to be understood. Sandman identifies that the outrage principle is operative when people contemplate outrage as part of their risk analysis.[5]

I believe this understanding—or perception of understanding (really a quality of caring)—is quite important for our patients and yet is executed poorly by many physicians. Morgan outlined clearly that any risk analysis needs to place the risk in question on a grid stratified by two important concepts that affect an individual's response to risk decision making. As shown in Figure 1-1, the two axes are controllable/uncontrollable and observable/not observable. These two concepts provide further insight into how an individual responds to risk.[6] As an example, when we explore a common fear (risk) in today's culture (such as terrorism), most of us dread it. We cannot control the events surrounding a terrorist act, and we know little about it, which places it in the upper right-hand (fearful) quadrant of the risk grid (Fig. 1-1). When we consider regional anesthesia risks, we must keep in mind that many patients and their families dread needles and surgery and often do not understand regional anesthesia.

BOX 1-1 The Anesthesiologist and Risk: Essential Concepts

- Balancing patient benefit to anesthetic risk
- Understanding emotional aspects of risk
- Caring for the patient in a comprehensive manner
- Understanding risk analysis

Thus, it is not difficult to imagine one of our poorly communicating colleagues carrying out regional anesthesia in an anxious patient and thereby relating to the individual in the upper right-hand (fearful) quadrant of the risk grid. It is also not difficult to imagine one of our chronic pain patients experiencing an uncontrollable fear of their pain state and being in the upper right-hand quadrant of the risk grid, in that chronic pain is largely unobservable.

If we go back in time for another perspective on risk analysis, de Gondi (an early French statesman) likely said it best. He articulated the essence of all risk analysis as[7] "That which is necessary is never a risk." During any risk (decision) analysis, the real issue is to come to agreement on what is "necessary," what specific risks (hazard plus the incidence) accompany the prescribed technique, and any alternatives that

should be considered. As a result of increased subspecialization in medicine in Western countries, the balance of risk and benefit continues to be perplexing. Increasingly, subspecialists have only a few of the facts available for a specific patient's risk/benefit question, making a patient-focused risk analysis difficult. I believe this is a fundamental issue as anesthesiologists seek to balance risk and benefit for patients (Fig. 1-2).

For this reason, as anesthesiologists interested in subspecialty areas of anesthesia, we must remain engaged in all of medicine, not just the technical features of our subspecialty. For example, becoming technical experts in regional blocks and ultrasound and limiting our understanding of the whole of medical practice is a seductive trap we must avoid. Avoiding this trap is not a unique idea. Rather, it has been expostulated by many, including the late Roy Vandam during his 1979 Rovenstine lecture in San Francisco at the American Society of Anesthesiologists' annual meeting. Dr. Vandam reflected on Dr. Rovenstine and stated[8]: "Rovenstine was truly a clinician who cared for patients in a total manner, considering all of the ramifications, because that is what treatment of pain is all about." Pain management is not the only area of practice that demands our continued clinical experience. Regional anesthesia application in surgical patients also requires this comprehensive knowledge. We as physicians are skilled at making decisions, and this ability in its most developed form is the end result of truly understanding risk (Fig. 1-2).

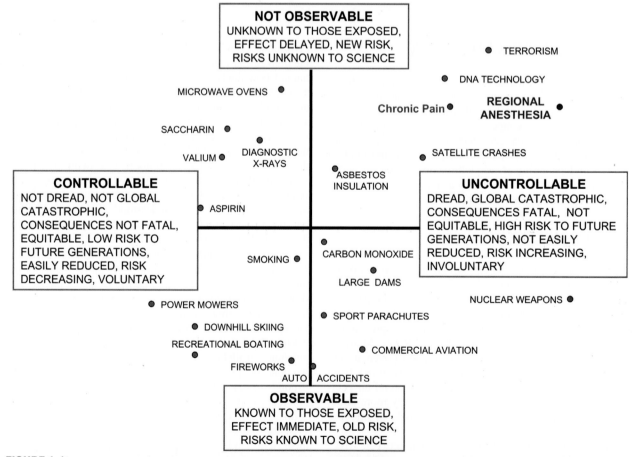

FIGURE 1-1. **Risk space has axes that correspond roughly to a hazard's "dreadfulness" and to the degree to which it is understood.** Risks in the upper right-hand quadrant of this space are most likely to provoke calls for government regulation. (Modified after Morgan MG. Risk analysis and management. *Sci Am* 1993;269:32–41.)

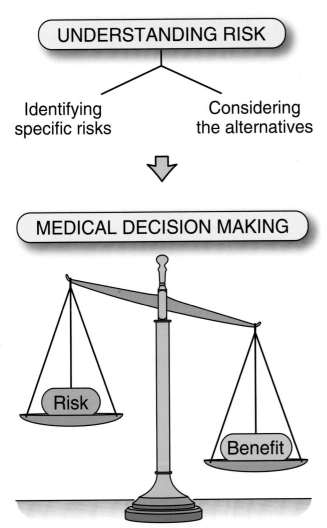

FIGURE 1-2. Understanding risk improves medical decision making. By considering the specific components of risk and determining if the proposed procedure is necessary, we can thereby optimize medical decision making.

Returning to the dilemma of increased subspecialization within medicine and reflecting on the decision analysis used to guide a judgment to operate, the risk/benefit judgment for a surgical procedure has typically already been made by a surgical colleague prior to the anesthesiologist examining the patient and assessing that patient's anesthetic risks. This confounds a real balancing of risk and benefit for the patient, unless the anesthesiologist maintains a true interaction and open communication with the surgical colleague. Thus, anesthesiologists must determine which anesthetic should be prescribed for the patient, most often without a complete understanding of expected surgical benefit. The dilemma of risk/benefit analysis "cuts both ways": from surgeon to anesthesiologist and anesthesiologist to surgeon.

An even more interesting modifying influence on our risk analysis is observed as we consider a concept termed risk homeostasis. A Canadian psychologist, Gerald Wilde, developed the concept of societal risk homeostasis after investigating data on traumatic injury and death during the last century.[9] He and others postulate that as activities become safer in some area of our life, we extend risk in other areas and keep the overall risk (mortality in their studies) at approximately the same level.[10] Teleologically, it is as if we are endowed with a hypothalamic risk feedback loop that keeps our overall risk of traumatic mortality at a specific set point.

For example: "It was in 1987 that Daimler-Benz showed off microprocessor-controlled brakes on a Detroit parking lot that had been soaped on one side and not on the other. The cars stopped beautifully on the soaped parking lot without swerving, and it is reported that the automotive reporters went away convinced that the new anti-lock brakes were the best automotive idea since safety glass. Customers were also impressed, and today most cars carry anti-lock brakes, adding about $500 per car".[10] It appears from National Highway Traffic Safety Administration data that antilock braking system-equipped cars showed a decline in some accidents, yet the overall accident rate went up. Thus, no overall benefit to automobile drivers and passengers resulted from this technological advance.[11] Another example is Wilde's opinion that as downhill skiing has seen safety advances (helmets) added to the sport, deaths have not decreased due to skiers embracing behavior that keeps the risk at a steady level.[12]

This concept makes me wonder what intraoperative, perioperative, and chronic pain care risk behavior we and our surgical colleagues have embraced with the advent of ever more sophisticated monitors such as pulse oximetry and end-tidal carbon dioxide monitors, "safer" intraoperative anesthetic regimens, our increasing use of continuous neuraxial infusions of local anesthetics via sophisticated continuous-flow pumps, and invasive neuraxial instrumentation in our chronic pain patients. Are we impacted by the concept of risk homeostasis in our anesthetic practice? For example, could it be that our postoperative evaluation of motor and sensory block of patients receiving continuous analgesia regimens is less vigorous than it was when the techniques were more difficult to carry out and hence less common? It is my belief that opportunities for effective clinical intervention (rescue) from epidural hematomas have been missed due to the attribution of motor weakness during the first postoperative night to the "epidural running," even in a setting with the infusion containing only opioid. Another example of risk homeostasis might be anesthesiologists being less prepared to treat local anesthetic systemic toxicity than in the past, in that patients are increasingly outpatients and simply do not demand everything our typically more compromised inpatients require. Could it be that even with advantages of lipid rescue from local anesthetic toxicity, the solution is often "too far" from the patient care area to be ideal?[13] I believe we all need to consider the possibility that risk homeostasis does affect our anesthetic and pain practices (see Box 1-2).

I believe the real challenge for regional anesthesia enthusiasts and postoperative analgesia teams today is to establish the advantage of interventional postoperative analgesia. It is

---

BOX 1-2 Risk Homeostasis

As we decrease risk and consequently make one part of our practice safer, we frequently extend risk in other facets of patient management. Overall, risk remains unchanged.

not enough to show that a continuous local anesthetic infusion can be carried out in a hospital and then in the home setting, but rather that there are real (quantifiable) advantages to such therapy for both patients and society. Cost and benefit must be part of the analysis. We so often seem to fall into the trap of technological imperative when we carry out our investigations, and this ultimately diminishes our effectiveness as investigators. We need to take a view of the entire comprehensive patient care experience, not just the analgesic experience.

▶ RISKS IN REGIONAL ANESTHESIA AND PAIN MEDICINE

Rare-event Analysis

The evolution of medical care delivery has important considerations for anesthesia risk analysis. Our patients are increasingly seen only moments before the operation and are often discharged from our care shortly after the operation is complete. This limits the ability of an anesthesiologist (or any physician involved in the patient's care) to fully understand what our patients are experiencing perioperatively. Again, the convergence of advanced monitoring using peripheral oxygen saturation and end-tidal carbon dioxide along with the use of short-acting anesthetics such as propofol suggests that the intraoperative period has become safer. It does not seem too bold to state that except in unusual and unique patient settings, no one will be able to definitively prove general anesthesia or regional anesthesia is safer in the isolated intraoperative period.

Another concept that needs clarification is the understanding of rare events and their impact on our decision analysis, both in society and for an individual patient. So often during my tenure as the editor in chief of *Regional Anesthesia and Pain Medicine*, a manuscript would be submitted for publication with the claim that the new technique described in the report was safer than an alternative because in the 50 patients studied there were no significant complications. It was often difficult for the investigators to appreciate that zero adverse events out of 50 patients might mean a serious complication rate of 1 out of 16 when using a 95% confidence interval methodology (Fig. 1-3). This was reemphasized in a special article in *Regional Anesthesia and Pain Medicine*, and I believe that those of us who are enthusiasts of regional anesthesia need to remember what zero of 50 really means[14] (Box 1-3).

Rare-event analysis may be approached from a different perspective. When mortality of a procedure or anesthetic is known, and one is determining how many patients need to be studied to demonstrate a significant difference between randomization groups, the numbers are also necessarily large. If, for example, one wanted to randomize carotid endarterectomy patients (using a hypothetical mortality of 1%) to a variation in regional anesthetic technique that reduced mortality from 1% to 0.5%, approximately 7,400 patients would have to be studied if a very liberal statistical approach was used: the alpha set at 0.1 and the power at 80%.[15]

Another perspective on rare-event analysis is emphasized when analyzing individual physicians' anesthesia

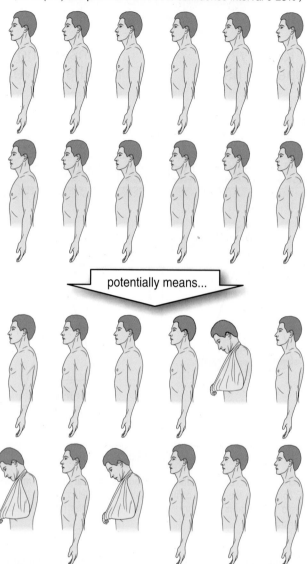

"No complications in 12 patients"

(0/12 (0%) complications with 95% confidence interval 0-25%)

potentially means...

FIGURE 1-3. The true incidence of complications in a study that reports "no complications in 12 patients" could be as high as 1 in 4 patients (25%) when calculated as the upper limit of a 95% confidence interval. Note that 12 patients are illustrated for convenience. The 3/*n* rule is most accurate when *n* >30.

care. If another physician suggested that your administration of anesthesia carried twice the risk of death to your patients as his or hers, given the very "generous" risk of anesthesia-related death of 1:2,000, how many patients would have to be studied to prove the point? If a more traditional statistical methodology was used—the alpha set at 0.05 and the power at 95%—there would have to be 77,935 patients in each group. Given that it is difficult for an individual to perform more than 1,000 anesthetic procedures per year, it would take two professional lifetimes for each anesthesiologist to prove that point. When the magnitude of these numbers is considered, it becomes clear that the only way to amass the data required is to perform multi-institutional studies, or to use a measure short

BOX 1-3 What Does "Zero Out of *n*" Really Mean?: The Upper 95% Confidence Interval

95% CI = 3/n*

*n = Number of trials (for n > 30)

of mortality that allows for interpretation of improvements in anesthetic technique (Tremper KT, *personal communication*, 2010).[16]

It seems to this observer of anesthetic outcome analyses that we have clearly come to the point in the development of anesthetic care at which we need to consider the entire perioperative course for the impact of our regional anesthetic and analgesic prescriptions. Is it not our role as physicians to take a comprehensive view of medical (patient) care and to look at what happens both to the individual patient and to the population of patients over time? Only then will we be able to more accurately balance risk and benefit for patients undergoing surgery, anesthesia, and chronic pain care.

The Cult or Curse of the Needle, Stimulator, and Ultrasound Guidance

Another key element in contemporary anesthetic risk analysis seems to be the cult or curse of the needle (as injury agent) and the peripheral nerve stimulator and ultrasound guidance (as prevention tools). Far too often, an unfortunate perioperative patient outcome is quickly blamed on the use of regional anesthesia, with a reflex assumption that if neural dysfunction develops postoperatively and a needle was used, the needle was causative. During many reviews of records chronicling these events, it often seems that thinking stops when documentation of a needle's use is located within the medical record. Turning back to the anesthesia risk grid, could it be that it is because so many patients and their families find themselves in the upper right-hand quadrant (dreading and not understanding) of the grid? It also may be that some of our anesthesiology colleagues who proclaim themselves experts are really inexperienced in regional anesthesia and are willing to make claims about the inappropriateness of a technique without sufficient personal experience to guide their judgment. This is not a problem just for regional anesthesia cases but for all of medicine when these discussions move into the negligence arena.

We know that no specific needle type or technique is certain to minimize injury, including the addition of a stimulator and ultrasound guidance. Conversely, we understand that no specific needle type or technique is certain to increase injury. Data are available suggesting that both blunted and more highly beveled needles minimize nerve injury.[17–19] This anesthesiologist believes that both claims are likely true, but only for the given conditions represented in the experiment being conducted. The key variable in the use of needles near peripheral nerves, in my opinion, is the operator. Gentleness of needle manipulation and the needle's redirection seems central to minimizing risk, although this must remain speculative in that it is based primarily on my own observations.

The idea that the use of a nerve stimulator or ultrasound guidance minimizes the opportunity for neural injury during regional anesthesia is also a "truism" in need of clarification. It is not uncommon to hear, "Nerve injury could not have developed because I was using a nerve stimulator or ultrasound guidance." Again, similar to the myth that has developed around needle bevel design, there are no definitive investigations available in my review of the literature that clarify the relationship between nerve stimulator use and ultrasound guidance and neural injury. Indeed, analysis of what data do exist on the topic suggests that the frequency of postoperative neurologic symptoms is no different with ultrasound guidance than it was a decade earlier using peripheral nerve stimulation.[20]

Procedural Pain Care

Another area of practice that demands our attention is balancing risks in pain medicine care. Our ability to prescribe invasive and more risky procedures to our chronic pain patients grows yearly. Much of this growth in technical advances has benefited our patients, although there are few randomized controlled trials documenting the benefit. For example, we know that in selected patients the implantation of an intrathecal catheter connected to an implanted opioid reservoir benefits an individual patient, yet we lack large-scale randomized controlled trials documenting which of our patients benefits most and how to balance the cost/benefit ratio most accurately.[21,22] We also need to better understand how to most effectively use the advance in bone stabilization possible with interventional percutaneous vertebroplasty, a technically demanding procedure that needs risk analysis to be sure we understand which patients most benefit.[23,24] Another example is the wider use of opioids in a variety of patient groups. This demands that we understand more completely which patient regimens optimize the risk/benefit ratio for both an individual patient and society.[25]

▶ MINIMIZING RISK FOR OUR PATIENTS

Finally, we need to turn to what we can do to minimize the risks of regional anesthesia and pain medicine practice (Box 1-4). Most important is to educate anesthesiologists about both areas of practice. Far too often it seems we view regional anesthesia as a technical event, rather than as an anesthetic technique to be incorporated into the complete patient care continuum. As part of this education, we need to have our research teams ask big questions about the patient

BOX 1-4 Strategies for Decreasing Risk

- Adopt a comprehensive view of the patient when prescribing specialty-specific interventions.
- Focus research on those big questions that best define populations in which the benefit of an intervention outweighs its risk.
- Educate our nonanesthesiologist colleagues and our patients not only to the benefits but to the risks of our procedures.

care continuum and how regional anesthesia or our analgesia care benefits patients.

Also important is the education of other physicians and allied health workers (nurses, for example) about the analgesia techniques currently being used in our medical centers. Far too often, patients with numb lower extremities receiving a pure opioid epidural infusion are watched over a 12- to 24-hour interval by nonanesthesiologists, all the while with weak lower extremities rather than being appropriately evaluated for potential neuraxial lesions. This education will be more difficult than that for our anesthesiology colleagues because it demands that we clarify our expectations and plans in the busy perioperative period.

The last group demanding our education is our patients. We need to do a better job in preoperative clinics in explaining what regional anesthesia adds to their care. In our risk-averse society, where at least part of our culture expects our birth to retirement to death continuum to be a consistently smooth course, we need to do a better job as physicians in highlighting risks associated with anesthesia and surgery. This education should not be used as a club, but rather as a gentle guide. This concept also needs to be implemented in our chronic pain practices, in that the technological imperative of trying everything in these patients "because we can" needs rethinking so that we have resources available to us to optimize all of our patients' care.

Acknowledgment

This chapter was originally adapted from an earlier manuscript published in *Regional Anesthesia and Pain Medicine*: Brown DL (2004). Labat lecture 2004: Regional anesthesia risks from Labat to tort reform. Reg Anesth Pain Med 29:116–124. We thank the American Society of Regional Anesthesia and Pain Medicine for permission to use portions of the material for this work.

References

1. Webster. *Webster's II: New Riverside University Dictionary*. Boston, MA: Houghton Mifflin Company, 1984.
2. Urquhart J, Heilmann K. *Risk Watch: The Odds of Life*. Munich, Germany: Kindler Verlag, 1984.
3. Glickman TS, Gough M. *Readings in Risk*. Washington, DC: Resources for the Future, 1990.
4. Levitt SD, Dubner SJ. *Freakonoics: A Rogue Economist Explores the Hidden Side of Everything*. New York, NY: Haper-Perennial, 2009:147–179.
5. Sandman PM. *Responding to Community Outrage: Strategies for Effective Risk Communication*. Fairfax, VA: AIHA Press, 1993.
6. Morgan MG. Risk analysis and management. *Sci Am* 1993;269:32–41.
7. de Gondi P. Seventeenth century French statesman and prelate. In: Seldes G, ed. *The Great Thoughts*. New York, NY: Ballantine Books, 1985:399.
8. Vandam LD. Rovenstine lecture: anesthesiologists as clinicians. *Anesthesiology* 1980;53:40–48.
9. Ward NJ, Wilde GJ. Field observation of advanced warning/advisory signage for passive railway crossings with restricted lateral sightline visibility: an experimental investigation. *Accid Anal Prev* 1995;27:185–197.
10. Peterson S, Hoffer G, Millner E. Are drivers of air-bag-equipped cars more aggressive? A test of the offsetting behavior hypothesis. *J Law Econ* 1995;38:251–264.
11. Ross PE. Safety may be hazardous to your health. *Forbes* 1999;164:172–173.
12. Shealy JE, Ettlinger CF, Johnson RJ. How fast do winter sports participants travel on Alpine slopes? *J ASTM Int* 2005;2:59–66.
13. Rowlingson JC. Lipid rescue: a step forward in patient safety? Likely so! *Anesth Analg* 2008;106:1333–1336.
14. Ho AMH, Dion PW, Karmaker MK, et al. Estimating with confidence the risk of rare adverse events, including those with observed rates of zero. *Reg Anesth Pain Med* 2002;27:207–210.
15. Pocock SJ. *Clinical Trials*. London, England: John Wiley & Sons, 1983:125–135.
16. Vitez T. Quality assurance. In: Benumof JL, Saidman LJ, eds. *Anesthesia and Perioperative Complications*. St. Louis, MO: Mosby Year Book, 1992:634–647.
17. Selander D, Dhuner KG, Lundborg G. Peripheral nerve injury due to injection needles used for regional anesthesia: an experimental study of the acute effects of needle point trauma. *Acta Anaesthesiol Scand* 1977;21(3):182–188.
18. Maruyama M. Long-tapered double needle used to reduce needle stick nerve injury. *Reg Anesth* 1997;22:157–160.
19. Rice AS, McMahon SB. Peripheral nerve injury caused by injection needles used in regional anaesthesia: influence of bevel configuration, studied in a rat model. *Br J Anaesth* 1992;69:433–438.
20. Neal JM. Ultrasound-guided regional anesthesia and patient safety. An evidence-based analysis. *Reg Anesth Pain Med* 2010;35:S59–S67.
21. Baker L, Lee M, Regnard C, et al. Tyneside Spinals Group: evolving spinal analgesia practice in palliative care. *Palliat Med* 2004;18:507–515.
22. Burton AW, Rajagopal A, Shah HN, et al. Epidural and intrathecal analgesia is effective in treating refractory cancer pain. *Pain Med* 2004;5:239–247.
23. Hide IG, Gangi A. Percutaneous vertebroplasty: history, technique and current perspectives. *Clin Radiol* 2004;59:461–467.
24. Diamond TH, Champion B, Clark WA. Management of acute osteoporotic vertebral fractures: a nonrandomized trial comparing percutaneous vertebroplasty with conservative therapy. *Am J Med* 2003;114:257–265.
25. Bartleson JD. Evidence for and against the use of opioid analgesics for chronic nonmalignant low back pain: a review. *Pain Med* 2002;3:260–271.

SECTION I

Regional Anesthesia

COMPLICATIONS OF REGIONAL ANESTHESIA

2

Overview of Regional Anesthesia Complications

Dan Benhamou and Yves Auroy

Regional anesthesia (RA) is no longer in a pioneering phase. It is now a well-established technique of anesthesia, and its use has increased significantly during the last 25 years. Valid information describing how anesthesia is performed is not available in many countries, but some useful data became available at the turn of century. In France, a 20-fold increase in the use of spinal anesthesia and peripheral nerve blocks (PNBs) and a 10-fold increase in the use of epidural block for labor analgesia were observed between 1980 and 1996.[1,2] Data in the United States (US) show similar trends, while in the United Kingdom (UK), although the epidural rate remained around 20% to 25% during the same period

of time, RA became the standard practice for cesarean delivery.[3,4]

An additional reason for this increase in the use of RA is related to the increase in the surgical procedures that are well suited for being performed with RA. The best and traditional example is the dramatic increase in the rate of cesarean delivery. Not only is RA safer (as compared to general anesthesia) in this setting, but the rate of cesarean delivery has also increased worldwide to be >20% in many countries. Because the population is aging and has an increased body weight, patients are more in need of orthopedic surgery, especially nonaxial procedures that are good indications for PNBs.

Memsoudis et al.,[5] using data from the National Survey of Ambulatory Surgery for the years 1996 and 2006, have shown that ligamentoplasties, meniscectomies, and shoulder arthroscopies have increased by 66%, 51%, and 349%, respectively. At the same time, the use of PNBs increased from 0.6% to 9.8% for meniscectomies, from 1.5% to 13.7% for ligamentoplasties, and from 11.5% to 24% for shoulder arthrospcopies. Interestingly, in this survey, the overall place of RA (and hence the place of general anesthesia) have changed little, implying a change in the type of RA used rather than an increased use of RA. In other words, after an increase in the use of RA in the 1980s and 1990s, we now face a change in the techniques used, especially an increasing use of PNB techniques.

The goal of this chapter is to provide an overview of how complications are measured and reported, and in particular hopes to educate the reader as to the inherent difficulties involved in studying medically related complications. This overview intends to provide a perspective for the detailed discussions of specific complications that follow in subsequent chapters throughout this book.

▶ HISTORICAL OVERVIEW

Since RA was introduced at the turn of the 20th century, its use has been subject to large waves of enthusiastic and supported practice, followed by periods of declining support, again followed by periods of increased practice. Each change was mainly related to either technical improvements (associated with a decreased rate of complications) or to widely advertised complications, leading to near abandonment of the technique. In 1920, Sherwood-Dunn[6] stated that "Since the concentrated solutions of cocaine have been replaced by less toxic agents … death from local or RA has disappeared from surgical practice …." Thirty years later, Foster Kennedy,[7] an eminent New York neurologist, stated that "… paralysis below the waist is too large a price to pay in order that the surgeon should have a fine relaxed field, and that the method should be rigidly reserved for those patients unable to accept a local or general anesthetic." Although one unfortunate aspect of Dr. Kennedy's article was the deficiency in anesthetic details, its conclusions were at that time unchallenged.

The Wooley and Roe case, which occurred almost at the same time,[8] was generously described in the lay press and led to the near abandonment of RA in the UK and to the supremacy of GA that persisted for many years. In this judgment, it was concluded that permanent paraplegia, which occurred in two patients, resulted from the contamination of the anesthetic solution by the phenol solution in which the ampules were stored for sterilization. By chance, several experts who strongly believed that RA can play a significant role in anesthesia and pain management maintained its use and continued to develop new and better techniques.

A major change occurred at the turn of the 1980s when spinal cord opioid receptors were discovered and led to the development of postoperative analgesic techniques using intrathecal and epidural administration of opioids.[9] Rapidly, however, it became clear that epidural and spinal anesthesia were not specific enough to cover every analgesic or anesthetic need, and PNBs were used more widely. The development and wide application of catheter techniques recently contributed to the large application of PNB, improving the

outcome of major orthopedic surgery,[10] including its use in ambulatory patients who can now leave the hospital earlier with their catheter connected to an analgesic reservoir which distributes the drug for several days, allowing for more stressful surgery being performed in ambulatory conditions.[11,12]

The Wooley and Roe case also reminds us that the near disappearance of RA was not the result of its poor efficacy but rather as a consequence of high-risk complications. These complications were the consequence of the drugs used which had a low therapeutic index and were also related to needles and catheters that were not sophisticated enough and could by themselves create trauma at the site of puncture. Although the categories of risk that are seen now are similar (drug and technique related), it would be expected that their incidence has decreased significantly due to major improvements in both the pharmacology of drugs and industrial and technical refinements of the equipment. It is, however, not well demonstrated that the incidence and severity of complications related to RA has decreased. This could be related to methodologic bias, as discussed later on in this chapter. It is, however, also possible that one set of complications has decreased through our efforts to improve patient care but that another set of complications has arisen. A part of this may be from new clinical situations (e.g., neuraxial anesthesia and concomitant anticoagulation) and a part may be due to patient factors (i.e., older and less healthy patients).

Early reports described only the complications of spinal and epidural anesthesia and generally stated that RA-induced complications were "rare."[13,14] Coincident with the recent increase in the use of PNBs, three series, including a significant number of PNBs, have now been reported describing the complications, frequency, and outcomes.[15–17] A new step has been taken as the relevant question today is to know if modern techniques (such as ultrasound guidance) reduce the risk as compared to traditional ones (such as nerve stimulation or paresthesia seeking). There is a general impression that ultrasound guidance will be a major advance toward reducing the rate of complications (Chapter 17). However, concrete evidence is still lacking for reasons that are mainly related to methodologic factors as described below.

▶ MEASURING COMPLICATIONS

Our practice of anesthesiology and of RA in particular is not safe, when the rate of complications is compared with the level of safety that has been obtained in some high-reliabilty organizations.[18] Reducing the rate of complications and controlling the risks of RA include many well-known strategies such as improved training, use of safer devices and drugs, technologic innovation, and use of quality-improvement programs. Monitoring the rate of complications can be useful but requires a large database, generally including several hospitals, or sometimes needs to be performed at a national level to provide comprehensive results. However, when the overall complication rate is low, traditional methods to assess the level of risk often fail. In a single institution, for example, and even if the volume of procedures is high, the risk of complication is so low that epidemiologic assessment and surveys cannot show if more complications have occurred when comparing two periods of time. When safety has been improved to such a high level that events occur very infrequently, database reporting is no longer efficient. Incident reporting is, by contrast, a useful method to explore the context of a given complication. Organizing a sentinel event system and detecting relevant precursors in near misses are probably the core of the most comprehensive strategy for continuous improvement.[19] The rarer the event, the greater the need for in-depth and professional analysis of the few existing cases to capture relevant precursors. At another level, but providing interesting information on a single patient, case reports can be a window on the health care system and journals should facilitate publication of clinical incidents that describe the chain of events and the contributory factors because these reports would have high educational value. Behind the outcome is the process of care and we have to move from "what happened?" to "why did it happen?" Changing the question, however, requires us to change the investigation tools. According to James Reason,[20] patent failures are those committed by actors working in direct contact with patients while latent failures represent the consequences of structural, technical, or organizational characteristics often related to management decisions. Root-cause analysis used by the Joint Commission in the US[21] or the systems analysis used by Vincent et al.[22] in London are typical examples of innovative methods to study the system errors. It is obviously an added value to share not only the result (i.e., the incidence) but also the very content of the case analysis with a large number of practitioners. Because the level of risk associated with RA can be considered either high or low depending on the comparator used, both traditional and innovative strategies of risk control should be implemented (Chapter 1).

▶ REPORTING COMPLICATIONS

Complications are frequently not reported or reported inaccurately. This stems from a variety of factors that are described below (Box 2-1).

BOX 2-1 Difficulties Measuring and Reporting Medical Complications

The frequency of unusual or rare complications is difficult to measure. Individual case reports lack a denominator, whereas large studies of adequate numbers of subjects are difficult to perform.

The reporting of medical complications can be problematic. For example:

- The anesthesiologists providing care may or may not be expert in the techniques being studied.
- How the complication is reported may be influenced by the nature of the study. For instance, a voluntary reporting of complications versus controlled reporting in a randomized clinical trial.
- The timeframe under which the study is conducted may not be suitable to identify all complications.
- Publication bias may be present on the part of journal editors. For instance, there may be a reluctance to publish a single case report of a previously described complication.

Practitioner Bias

It is basically difficult to study rare events, and RA-induced complications belong to this category. The incidence can be estimated through surveys and large series. Well-performed studies including sufficient numbers of cases are rare. Moreover, most studies come from institutions where RA is well accepted and where physicians who perform the blocks are highly trained, and this may not reflect the true rate of complications. We indeed now know that training is associated with increased performance and a reduced rate of complications. In the rare large-scale studies reporting data from both specialized and nonspecialized centers (i.e., where physicians perform a high or low number of procedures), the incidence of complications appears to be much greater than in high-volume institutions. In a study reporting neuraxial anesthesia-induced infectious epidural abscess from all institutions in Denmark (i.e., including both high- and low-volume centers and thus including a nonselected population of physicians), the incidence was much higher than in other studies.[23]

Reporting Bias

Uncertainty regarding the true incidence may also arise from the quality of data reporting: incidence may increase as a result of better reporting or a better collecting method. In two classic studies, each assessing a large number of spinal blocks, Dripps and Vandam[13] assessed the risk associated with the use of procaine and tetracaine in 10,098 patients, while Phillips et al.[14] monitored 10,440 patients after lidocaine spinal anesthesia. The incidence of complications was monitored prospectively by directly questioning all patients on the day after surgery. A zero incidence of severe complications was described, and these studies started an optimistic period during which the development of RA was rapid as the technique was perceived to be safer than general anesthesia. In one of these studies, the quality of postoperative monitoring and patients' interviews was so good that the authors were able to describe "complaints confined in lumbar and sacral areas of the body which generally lasted few days" and the complaints were described as "numbness, tingling, heaviness or burning and of minor significance in the lives of the individuals affected."[24] The authors had probably described what we now call transient neurologic symptoms (TNS), but these symptoms were dismissed probably because these complications were so minor that they were felt to be clinically insignificant. Although such a prospective design should have guaranteed an excellent quality of data reporting, only a few questions were asked to each patient, that is, "have you had any problems related to the anesthesia…" and "would you recommend spinal anesthesia"[24] which is obviously too simple to ensure adequate reporting. Obstetric patients were the core of these studies, and we now know that the incidence of some complications (i.e., hearing loss and TNS) may be different in this category of patients.[25,26]

Reporting bias can also occur because of the retrospective nature of many past large surveys or absence of detail. Fine analysis of individual cases can often only be found in prospectively reported cases or in cases that have been associated with litigation. In the first survey performed in France,[16] cases were counted prospectively, but details of complications were collected at the end of the 6-month period of the study. It appeared that the information was not as accurate as expected initially. In the American Society of Anesthesiologists Closed Claims project, detailed description of cases was also available as they were extracted from insurance claim files which typically include narrative statements from the personnel involved, medical records, expert and peer reviews, deposition summaries, outcome reports, and the cost of settlement or jury award.[27]

Timing Bias

Moreover, as some complications become apparent only several days after the block, a questionnaire study based on a single interview performed the day after surgery may have missed some complications. The timing at which complications become apparent is indeed variable. Although some patients complain of paresthesia, pain, or motor disturbances within hours after surgery, in other cases, the neurologic complications may only become apparent after several days. This is obviously the case after postoperative continuous infusion of local anesthetic, which precludes any neurologic evaluation before the block has worn off. In this situation, although continuous infusion has advantages, namely absence of any pain during the first days, it does also lead to complete anesthesia and sometimes complete motor block during the same period of time, precluding any neurologic assessment. This suggests that analgesic techniques which allow for some partial recovery at (regular) intervals (i.e., catheter techniques linked to a patient-controlled analgesia (PCA) device or intermittent bolus infusion) may have advantages over the continuous infusion of local anesthetic drugs alone. In patients receiving epidural analgesia, addition of an opioid clearly reduces the dose of local anesthetic needed and thus the motor block, thereby facilitating monitoring of the block. Regular and adequate monitoring and early diagnosis of neurologic complications is important as early detection may allow for rapid recovery (and sometimes lead to early therapeutic actions) while late discovery of a complication may lead to definitive neurologic sequelae. In our experience with SOS-Regional Anesthesia (SOS-RA) Hotline Service over the past 12 years, we have often seen neurologic complications arising in institutions where anesthesiologists were highly trained and where surgeons had a high confidence in RA but where monitoring and nurse training were not adequately organized to allow for rapid diagnosis of complications. Physicians do place a greater emphasis on performing the block than on organizing the postoperative surveillance.

Publication Bias

Large series have taught us much about RA-induced complications, but case reports also have largely contributed to our knowledge. However, even large series may not accurately report rare complications. Looking at the SOS-RA series,[17] one may believe that neuraxial blocks are not associated with a risk of major neurologic event (as none occurred during the 6-month period of the study), while it is obvious that this complication can occur and is a major threat for patients.

Although they are often considered as being minor scientific contributions, case reports have sometimes had a greater impact on our clinical practice than most randomized trials.

Albright's description of a small series of cardiac deaths after bupivacaine administration,[28] Schneider et al.'s[29] description of TNSs after lidocaine spinal administration, cases of cardiac arrests following large dose of ropivacaine,[30,31] and the recovery after cardiac arrest following bupivcacaine toxicity using "lipid rescue"[32] are only four examples of how case reports can strongly impact on the thinking of a whole medical specialty.

One should also consider the tendency of journals to accept a first or second case report of a rare complication, but then not accept subsequent reports. However, since the complication is rare, the next step often cannot be taken (i.e., reporting large case series or doing randomized controlled trials).

▶ PREVENTING COMPLICATIONS

Society's View

Society's expectations of complications are frequently at odds with the medicine's view of complications (Fig. 2-1). Society may be much more likely to expect perfection from physicians who realize that perfection is a worthy ideal which may rarely be attainable. A zero complication rate is not even attained in high-reliability organizations that are considered ultra-safe because they are associated with a 1/10,000,000 rate of complications. "Six-sigma" strategies that have proven their efficacy in the industrialized world are being implemented in medicine today with the hope that they will help reaching this ultra-low level of danger, but initial data in patient-related processes do not show as excellent results as expected.[33]

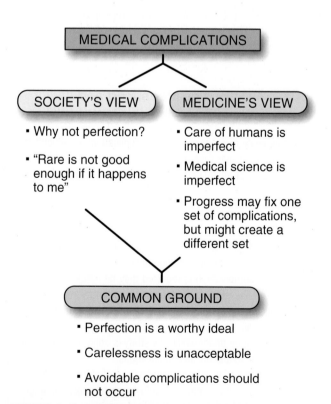

FIGURE 2-1. Medical complications: the conflict between society's view of risk and medicine's view of risk.

Many complications that physicians consider minor because they do not lead to long-term sequelae (such as hoarseness after an interscalene block, or a meningeal puncture headache that resolves) are considered major complications to those who suffer from them. Such complaints mainly occur in minor procedures where patients' expectations of complete and rapid recovery are not met or in situations in which the anesthesiologist has convinced the patient that regional anestheia is a better choice than general anesthesia.

Medicine's View

Scientific Limitations to Understanding Complications: The Meaning of Paresthesia

It is only recently that series including a significant number of PNBs have been reported to describe their complications, frequency, and outcome.[15–17] These reports came from European institutions where the use of nerve stimulation was already accepted and had introduced a relatively new debate relating to the significance of paresthesia occurring during puncture; some experts searching deliberately for a paresthesia to block the nerve while others felt that a paresthesia is associated with an increased rate of complications. This debate is far from being closed as contradictory information exists. Complications apparently related to the regional block can occur even though a gentle technique has been applied and no paresthesia has occurred, while by contrast it has been shown that immediately after a paresthesia has occurred, nerve stimulation can fail, suggesting that the nerve is not as close to the needle as expected or that paresthesia may have different meanings.[34–36] Experts using ultrasound guidance have also recently reported several cases in which the needle makes physical contact with a nerve, but no paresthesia is felt by the patient.

Diagnosing and Treating Complications

One significant problem is the difficulty attributing a given complication to RA (i.e., to determine if RA is the cause of the neurologic injury) when surgery, positioning, or a preexisting disease might have caused the complication. Two clinically significant and frequent situations are obstetrical nerve injuries and neurologic complications after hip replacement. RA is often blamed first, whereas the relative incidences of complications related to the procedure versus to RA should lead us to first blame the delivery or surgery and not RA. Postpartum nerve injuries occur 5- to 10-fold more often as the direct consequence of vaginal delivery than as caused by RA.[37–39] Vaginal birth of a large newborn after a long labor and using instrumental delivery are traditional risk factors, but these situations often accompany highly painful labor for which epidural analgesia will be requested more often by the parturient.[40]

A similar situation is seen after hip surgery in which the intrinsic rate of sciatic nerve injury (i.e., in the absence of any other contributory factor such as PNB) ranges between 0.5% and 3%.[41,42] However, RA is often blamed by surgeons and patients, and anesthesiologists need to make major efforts to correct the diagnosis. As for obstetric nerve palsies, surgery itself causes nerve injury much more often than RA, and this should be emphasized. Female patients and patients operated for hip dysplasia appear to have a higher risk of neurologic injury. Also, the risk of neurologic injury following total hip arthroplasty appears to be higher with revisions/reoperations and with an inexperienced surgeon or with a misplaced retractor. Nerve injury can also occur postoperatively and be caused by cement migration. To prevent the occurrence of intraoperative nerve injury, somatosensory evoked potentials have been used, but the efficacy of this technique has not been demonstrated in total hip arthroplasty. Other experts have also chosen to avoid using sciatic nerve block in patients at high risk of postoperative nerve injury to minimize conflicts and litigation. Note also that sciatic nerve block may interfere with intraoperative neurologic monitoring. We agree with Ben-David et al.[43] that "with the expansion of regional anesthetic techniques in acute pain management, the finding of a new postoperative deficit must be jointly investigated by both anesthesiologists and surgeons. Timely and open communication between services is critical because rapid intervention may be essential to achieving full recovery of an affected nerve." Adequate follow-up and evaluation using a systematic method involving experts is extremely important when deciding if the complication is or is not related to RA. Early examination by a neurologist is extremely useful to precisely define the clinical picture and help localize the nerve lesion. The neurologist is not asked to make any firm assumption on the mechanism of the nerve injury. In many situations, it is recommended to perform ultrasound or computed tomography scanning to search for an hematoma or migrated cement. This can lead to early reoperation and rapid recovery of the nerve injury.

Electrodiagnostic techniques are extremely useful, and the first examination should be done as early as possible (within the first 48 hours) because abnormal findings at this stage strongly support the role of a preexisting neurologic disease. They will be repeated within 3 to 4 weeks where more definitive information can be obtained about the site, nature, and severity, all factors that can guide prognostication.[44] Electromyography provides findings suggestive of denervation (i.e., fibrillation potentials and abnormal muscle unit recruitment) while nerve conduction studies provide an estimate of the number of axon loss by analysis of the size of the muscle response. Of crucial importance, it provides some information on the site of the injury which is often the cause of debate between the surgeon and the anesthesiologist. Separating the role of RA and surgery respectively is sometimes easy (e.g., sciatic injury at the popliteal level during knee replacement in a patient who has undergone femoral and sciatic block at the hip), but this is not always the case when the block and the surgical location are situated in the same nerve segment. In this latter case, indirect arguments are useful, such as relative risk of injury and patient history. In our experience, anesthesiologists often need some help, and this is a daily role for SOS-RA experts to provide some guidance on the diagnostic tools to be used and their timing, but also to discuss arguments that can help in separating the role of RA from other causes (surgery, positioning, and patient history). Whatever the cause, anesthesiologists are also often asked to follow these patients and manage neuropathic pain, which can be difficult to treat, and advice on management is often provided.

Training Issues

In experienced hands, the complication rate is logically lower than when trainees are studied. This emphasizes the role of adequate supervision during the training period and the methods to ensure a rapid learning curve. Although it is out of the scope of this chapter to overview all aspects of safe, efficacious, and ethical training, RA is, as surgery, a field in which the period of learning is critical. It is still too often that physicians try for the first time in their next patient a new block technique that was described (as being easy to do, safe, and with a high rate of success) by an enthusiastic speaker in a meeting. Excellent knowledge of anatomy is critical and should be learned precisely before puncturing any patient. Simulators now exist (manikins or computer programs), which may play a key role in rapid training. Although studies show that a mean number of blocks (often found to be around 50) is necessary to ensure adequate training,[45] every trainee should be followed individually as the learning curve is likely to be different, some being rapidly proficient in the technique while others need more time to reach a minimum success rate. It should be noted also that the minimal number of blocks performed does not guarantee a 100% success rate or avoid the occurrence of complications, thus requiring the trainee to maintain his/her vigilance and perform the blocks with gentleness and attention to continue learning from each new experience.

▶ TRENDS IN RA COMPLICATIONS

Major versus Minor Complications

It is also difficult to compare the early studies and the more recent ones as definitions of complications vary and preclude any good comparison. While some studies aim at reporting all complications and thus provide an overview of the risks associated with RA, others have chosen to report only major complications to avoid difficulties in analysis and to facilitate the understanding of the topic. Cardiac arrest has a clearer definition than "minor" neurologic complication for which the threshold line between major and minor is more difficult to draw. Moreover, many minor complications are only transient and have only a small impact on patients' lives. Major complications are however less frequent and may thus be difficult to study. By contrast, minor complications may be more common and may be surrogate endpoints that can lead to an interesting analysis while being easier to study. Moreover, minor complications are easier to discuss because they carry less emotional weight as the patient outcome is not endangered. In voluntary incident reporting systems, the risk of underreporting is reduced with minor complications because these incidents do not lead to negative comments regarding competence and are easy to discuss between peers. By contrast, minor complications that are by nature less important may easily be omitted in these voluntary reporting systems. Although reporting only major complications such as cardiac arrest should make it easy to compare incidences between studies (and thus show whether or not the risk associated with RA has decreased), other factors increase the complexity.

Systemic Local Anesthetic Toxicity

Systemic local anesthetic toxicity during RA can lead to death. Apart from early implementation of the traditional test dose, consistent efforts have been made to reduce this risk (Chapter 7). The commercial release of drugs with lower cardiac toxicity (ropivacaine and levobupivacaine) has certainly played a role. Indeed, in the Auroy et al.[16] survey describing data obtained in 1998 to 1999, the authors suggested that they had observed a decreased rate of local anesthetic-induced systemic toxicity when compared to their previous survey. The beneficial effect of these drugs has been demonstrated in many preclinical studies, but case reports appearing increasingly in the clinical literature have confirmed a less toxic profile. What seems for example a major safety advance is the fact that almost all ropivacaine-induced cardiac arrests are easily resuscitated, and to our knowledge ropivacaine induced-death is an extremely rare event.[46] Levobupivacaine can sometimes cause convulsions or cardiac arrest, but to our knowledge, in no case has the event has been terminated by patient death.

Another significant advance has been the introduction of the "lipid rescue" technique. From the pioneering experimental work of Weinberg,[47] we have learned that using an infusion of a lipid emulsion, the life-threatening events associated with bupivacaine infusion can be reversed. More recently, several case reports have described the reversal of cardiac arrhythmias and neurologic involvement both in adults and children. We however only rely on case reports since clinical studies cannot be performed in this context. Although at least one case report has described the failure of lipid rescue, most published cases describe an impressive effect with almost immediate reversal of toxicity.

Even practitioners with limited experience have rapidly discovered that using ultrasound guidance, nerves can be easily surrounded with only a very small amount of the local anesthetic solution. Studies have rapidly confirmed this notion. Marhofer et al.[48] have indeed shown that a fourfold reduction in the amount of local anesthetic can provide an effective axillary plexus block (from 0.4 to 0.11 mL/mm^2 cross-sectional area). The trend toward reduced doses has culminated with the work of O'Donnell and Iohom[49] who have reported a successful axillary brachial plexus block with as little as 1 mL of 2% lidocaine per nerve. Even if these volumes reflect these authors' extraordinary expertise, we now confidently use smaller volumes in our everyday practice. As the total dose administered is one major cause of systemic toxicity, ultrasound guidance is expected to decrease the rate of cardiac and neurologic complications due to high plasma concentrations. Cases of local anesthetic systemic toxicity continue, however, to be reported in patients in whom the block was performed using ultrasound, suggesting that this technique may not completely protect against the occurrence of this complication (Chapter 17). From the data available today, the incidence of complications related to systemic toxicity has not yet decreased consistently. This may reflect that all team members are not still perfectly trained and that increasing experience will decrease the ratio. Visualization of the needle tip is not always easy during an ultrasound-guided procedure and vessel puncture remains possible, thus leading to direct intravascular injection and signs of toxicity.

Cardiac Arrest

We discuss in this chapter only cardiac arrest caused by hemodynamic disturbances, as systemic toxicity of local anesthetics has been reviewed above. When looking at studies describing cardiac arrest during the last 50 years, no significant decrease in the incidence of this complication can really be observed. Old studies reported cardiac arrest and death as a rare complication of spinal anesthesia (1/10,440)[13] (0.3/10,000),[50] while in 1995, Scott and Tunstall[51] reported two cardiac arrests in 122,989 obstetric patients who had received epidural or spinal anesthesia, that is a very low incidence as well. These results should be compared with those obtained for spinal anesthesia-induced cardiac arrests in nonobstetric studies. Auroy et al.[17] showed that spinal anesthesia was associated with a 2.7/10,000 rate of cardiac arrest in nonobstetric patients, a much higher incidence than in the studies mentioned above. Obstetric patients are overall young and healthy and have a lower risk of complications than other patients who are receiving RA. In the Auroy et al.'s[16,17] study, the authors demonstrated that patients who died from cardiac arrest after spinal anesthesia were much older, had an increased ASA score, and underwent hip surgery more often than those who survived.

Neurologic Injury after Neuraxial Blocks

Spinal hematoma after neuraxial blocks are more frequent after orthopedic surgery than after obstetric anesthesia, and this can be explained by the role of thromboprophylaxis and by enlarged osteoporotic vertebrae which narrow the spinal canal and increase the risk that a small hematoma causes a clinically significant complication[46] (Chapter 4). In their review of neurologic complications after neuraxial blocks in Sweden, Moen et al.[52] emphasized the role of spinal stenosis, which was associated with an increase in the incidence of spinal hematoma and cauda equina syndrome. Since this problem was highlighted by Moen et al., several recent reports have confirmed the role spinal stenosis may play as aggravating the risk of neurologic complications after neuraxial anesthesia.[53,54]

Spinal hematoma has been largely related to the use of anticoagulants. In his excellent 1981 review, Kane[55] emphasized the role of anticoagulants in the occurrence of this complication. In the 1980s, the drug most widely used was unfractionated heparin. We have progressively learned how to use unfractionated heparin in the context of RA, and we have succeeded in mastering the rate of complications associated with it. Disappointingly, an epidemic of spinal hematoma following the use of high prophylactic doses of low-molecular-weight heparin occurred in the US nearly 20 years later,[56] mainly associated with an excessive dosage and uncontrolled timing of injections. Analysis of these cases led to new guidelines emphasizing a more restrictive approach,[57] and the current feeling is that the risk of low-molecular-weight heparin–associated spinal hematoma is well controlled. Should we however be frightened by the massive arrival in our patients' prescriptions of antiplatelet therapy (often prescribed as dual treatment)? Although the present recommendations are wise, it remains possible that complications may increase since a recent report suggests that RA may be safely performed in patients receiving clopidogrel.[58] In a slightly different context, a recent review article analyzing the risk of spinal hematoma following neuraxial anaesthesia or lumbar puncture in thrombocytopenic individuals states that based on the current litterature, a platelet count of 80,000/L is a "safe" count for placing an epidural or spinal anesthetic and 40,000/L is a "safe" count for lumbar puncture.[59] They further state that "For patients with platelet counts of 50,000–80,000/L requiring epidural or spinal anesthesia and patients with a platelet count 20,000–40,000/L requiring a lumbar puncture, an individual decision based on assessment of risks and benefits should be made." Although these investigators may be right, such statements may lead to more liberal practice, and there is a strong need to monitor closely what happens with these new guidelines to see if the complication rate rises again.

At the other end of the spectrum, by contrast, TNS are a clinical situation for which our understanding has rapidly increased through a combination of clinical and experimental studies which have precisely defined the incidence and the potential mechanisms including the role of drugs, namely lidocaine. Our knowledge on lidocaine-induced neurotoxicity has increased very rapidly and is such now that evidence exists that apoptosis is the main effect through which lidocaine may produce direct nerve injury.[60] Studies are also underway to demonstrate the benificial effect of mitogen-activated protein kinase inhibitors to reduce the cytotoxic effects of lidocaine.[61]

Neurologic Complications after PNB

Suggested etiologies include mechanical trauma from the needle, nerve edema and/or hematoma, pressure effects of the local anesthetic injectate, and neurotoxicity of the injected compounds, both local anesthetics and adjuvants (e.g., epinephrine) (Chapters 8 and 14). A renewed interest in these complications has arisen because of the increased use of these techniques and the improved knowledge that has been gained by the use of ultrasound technique. Sonography has indeed highlighted the frequency with which the needle tip penetrates in the nerve and produces intraneural injection (identified by nerve swelling). We have also learned that despite this high frequency, related complications are rare, leading to the idea that only intraneural, intrafascicular injection is dangerous. Robards et al.[62] reported that in 83% of patients, a motor response (using current intensity of 0.2 to 0.5 mA) could only be obtained on the entry of the needle into the nerve. Again, despite the high frequency of intraneural injection, no patient developed postoperative neurologic dysfunction.

These studies are extremely useful as they suggest some preventive measures: the minimal current intensity should probably not be diminished below 0.5 mA, injection should be stopped (and the needle slightly withdrawn) when nerve swelling occurs, and injection pressure should be controlled. These precautions are aimed at avoiding any form of intraneural injection. Because intraneural extrafascicular injection, however, seems safe and is often associated with a more rapid onset of the block, some authors suggest that intraepineural injection should be evaluated as a worthy replacement of the traditional extraneural technique[63] (Chapter 17).

Although ultrasound guidance has helped us to better understand anatomy and procedure-related complications, epidemiologic data do not yet show a clear benefit as the largest studies today do not suggest a reduced rate of neurologic complications. Brull et al.[64] have published a nice study which can be considered as providing an estimate of the neurologic risk before the introduction of ultrasound guidance. When comparing the risk provided by Brull et al., the studies by Fredrickson et al.[65] and by Barrington et al.[66] do not show a convincing reduction. The reason why the difference is not obvious is unclear. It might be that contrary to our thoughts, ultrasound really has no effect on the risk level. Alternatively, this may be because of lack of statistical power or because physicians were not completely trained at the time these studies were performed. It is our premise that ultrasound will reduce the rate of severe neurologic injury as some surrogate endpoints that are easier to evaluate are already different. Liu et al.,[67] for example, has indeed shown that ultrasound reduces the number of needle passes needed to perform interscalene block as compared to a nerve stimulation technique.

Continuous Peripheral Catheters

As techniques of PNB improve and their indications increase, the need to use catheter techniques also becomes obvious to prolong the duration of analgesia. Capdevila et al.[68] have reported a series of 1,416 PNBs with a catheter maintained for postoperative analgesia during 2 to 3 days. Although they described only three cases of neurologic complication (which all resolved within weeks or months), the incidence was 0.21%. In a similar study performed on 405 axillary catheters used for postoperative analgesia, new neurologic complications occurred at a rate of 0.5%, and the authors concluded that the risk is similar to that of single-shot techniques.[69] These incidence figures are not, however, low and require attention and future studies. The apparently high incidence of complications in this setting may be related to various factors. Although new local anesthetics are inherently safer than older ones, prolonged contact with the nerve sheath may be dangerous. Our knowledge and optimization of catheter use are becoming progressively refined. Stimulating catheters provide an advantage compared with nonstimulating catheters at various block locations as a recent semiquantitative systematic review of 11 randomized studies concluded that there is evidence of improved efficacy as measured by local anesthetic volume required, rescue analgesics, and complete surgical block compared with nonstimulating catheters.[70] Ilfeld et al.[71] compared administration of ropivacaine for 24 or 96 hours after knee arthroplasty and concluded that a 4-day ambulatory continuous femoral nerve block was beneficial as regards to both discharge criteria and pain relief. These studies are useful as they help define better how to use these perineural catheters, and by optimizing their use the incidence of complications might be reduced. Technique-related characteristics also need to be explored as trauma from the catheter may also lead to neurologic complication. Mariano et al.[72] recently showed that for popliteal-sciatic perineural catheters, ultrasound guidance takes less time and results in fewer placement failures compared with stimulating catheters, suggesting a potentially reduced risk of complications.

Another interesting lesson from the work by Capdevila et al.[68] is that catheter cultures were positive in 29% of cases, inflammatory local signs were seen in 3% of their cases,

and one patient developed a severe psoas abscess. Although infectious complications can occur with single-shot PNB techniques, it seems obvious that perineural catheter techniques are more prone to be associated with infection. Diabetic patients are highly sensitive to infection, and *Staphylococcus aureus* was found in three of the four cases published. Local inflammatory signs were frequent. These data suggest that excellent antiseptic preparation is mandatory, and catheter management should be as rigorous as with central venous catheters.

New Concerns

In the previous paragraphs, we have presented a overall optimistic view supported by many articles which show that novel techniques, drugs, and practices do have a positive effect on minimizing the rate of RA-induced complications. While this is the major tendency, some alarm signals suggest that we have not completely defined the scope of the question and that unknown (or poorly identified complications) can represent a significant threat to our patients and require greater attention in the near future.

Local anesthetic induced chondrolysis is one example of a complication that was virtually unknown 5 years ago. With the development of "pain pumps" which provide direct intra-articular infusion of a local anesthetic in a joint after surgery, several authors have observed a devastating complication termed postarthroscopic glenohumeral chondrolysis because the vast majority of these complications have occurred after shoulder surgery in young and previously healthy patients (athletes). Joint destruction is often rapid and severe, and there is no easy treatment available. Case series have identified that chondrolysis occurs mainly in patients receiving an intraarticular infusion of bupivacaine[73] with increased toxicity when using larger concentrations. Addition of epinephrine may increase the toxic effect.[74] Other local anesthetic drugs also possess chondrolytic properties but to a lesser degree. A long (i.e., ≥1 day) contact duration is needed for the effect to become severe. The effect may be linked to a proapoptotic effect and mitochondrial dysfunction induced by bupivacaine.[75] This complication was not anticipated when the use of intra-articular infusion increased rapidly some years ago, suggesting that every new usage should be submitted to intense monitoring, even for drugs that are thought to be very well known.

Another devastating complication for which interest has recently increased is the occccurrence of ischemic cerebral complications after shoulder surgery (Chapter 6). This complication, although exceptional,[76] should be known by all anesthesiologists who perform surgery in sitting (beach chair) position.[77] At least two main mechanisms can lead to cerebral ischemia. The sitting position is associated with venous pooling in the lower limbs and reduces venous return to the heart, leading to bradycardia and hypotension. Moreover, because the arterial pressure cuff is placed on the upper limb, the blood pressure measured does not take into account the pressure gradient and the blood pressure is overestimated by nearly 20 mm Hg. When the pressure cuff is placed on the calf (often as a request from the surgeon), then overestimation may be ≥50 mm Hg (Figure 6-4). Hypotension is thus not detected and cerebral ischemia may occur. Adding an interscalene block may also increase the risk as this regional technique may further activate the Bezold-Jarisch reflex.[78] Apart from limiting the indications of beach chair positioning, prevention relies mainly on integrating the blood pressure difference in the value seen on the screen to avoid prolonged hypotension. Murphy et al.[79] have also shown recently that cerebral ischemia can be detected by continuous monitoring of cerebral near-infrared spectroscopy.

In recent years, a significant focus has been made on human factors that may contribute to errors (Chapter 3). Medication errors are among the most common causes and can occur at any time during the process, that is during delivery from the pharmacy, preparation of the solution, or during administration. The different strategies that are aimed at decreasing the rate (and severity) of medication errors are well described and not mutually exclusive.[80,81]

When RA is considered, general causes of errors can occur, but it has been shown that spinal administration of toxic drugs (not intended for spinal use) can have devastating consequences. Interestingly, in the UK, the National Patient Safety Agency has issued a Patient Safety Alert, with the aim of eliminating Luer connectors from equipment for lumbar puncture and subarachnoid injections by April 1, 2011, to reduce drug errors by using a mistake-proofing technique and avoiding Luer connections for all devices related to neuraxial anesthesia. The deadline has been recently updated to April 1, 2012, because technical solutions are not yet perfect.[82] Whatever the need for update, the agency should be commended for this decisive action, which had not been taken by any other country before.

► SUMMARY

The number of RA procedures has increased significantly since the turn of the 20th century, not only in relation with the increased number of surgical procedures but also as an increased proportion of anesthetic procedures. All types of regional anesthetic techniques are being more widely used, including the traditional (spinal and epidural) and more modern ones (PNB as single-shot or continuous techniques). In contrast with this increased use, which suggests an increased safety of these techniques, data from large-scale surveys do not yet show a decrease in the overall rate of complications. The unchanged incidence could be related to methodologic bias, but it is likely that overall safety has improved. Many strategies such as improved training, use of safer devices and drugs, technologic innovation, and the use of quality-improvement programs have indeed been implemented to control the risks of RA. This probably explains why severe complications are now very rare in healthy patients (e.g., obstetric patients). It is however possible that, in contrast to the general decrease in the rate of traditional complications, the trend might be reversed by the negative anatomical or physiologic effect of ageing which is also associated with an increased use of concomitant anticoagulation. Apart from these complications, our recent experience has seen the occurrence of new complications. Fortunately, because these new complications have been rapidly identified, it is to be expected that they will not have any significant effect on the overall slope. Complications related to anesthesia and especially those related to RA are often poorly accepted by patients because RA is viewed as a technique safer than general anesthesia and used in clinical conditions associated with comfort and pain control. If we wish that RA not undergo a new wave of blaming and litigation, major efforts to improve safety remain to be done. Improvement in techniques and training is mandatory but are not enough. Procedures should be better defined, and applied and system errors should be cured if one wants RA to become an ultra-safe technique.

References

1. Clergue F, Auroy Y, Pequignot F, et al. French survey of anesthesia in 1996. *Anesthesiology* 1999;91:1509–1520.
2. Auroy Y, Laxenaire MC, Clergue F, et al. Anesthetics in obstetrics. *Ann Fr Anesth Reanim* 1997;17:1342–1346.
3. Burnstein R, Buckland R, Pickett JA. A survey of epidural analgesia for labour in the United Kingdom. *Anaesthesia* 1999;54:634–640.
4. Shibli KU, Russell IF. A survey of anaesthetic techniques used for caesarean section in the UK in 1997. *Int J Obstet Anesth* 2000;9:160–167.
5. Memsoudis SG, Kuo C, Edwards AM, et al. Changes in anesthesia related factors in ambulatory knee and shoulder surgery: United States 1996–2006. *Reg Anesth Pain Med* 2011;36:327–331.
6. Fox MAL, Webb RK, Singleton RJ, et al. Problems with regional anaesthesia: an analysis of 2000 incident reports. *Anaesth Intensive Care* 1993;21: 646–649.
7. Kennedy F, Effron AS, Perry G. The grave spinal cord paralyses caused by spinal anesthesia. *Surg Gynecol Obstet* 1950;91:385–398.
8. Cope RW. The Wooley and Roe case. *Anaesthesia* 1954;9:249–270.
9. Cousins MJ, Mather LE. Intrathecal and epidural administration of opioids. *Anesthesiology* 1984;61:276–310.
10. Capdevila X, Barthelet Y, Biboulet P, et al. Effects of perioperative analgesic technique on the surgical outcome and duration of rehabilitation after major knee surgery. *Anesthesiology* 1999;91:8–15.
11. Ilfeld BM, Enneking FK. Continuous peripheral nerve blocks at home: a review. *Anesth Analg* 2005;100:1822–1833.
12. Hadzic A, Williams BA, Karaca PE, et al. For outpatient rotator cuff surgery, nerve block anesthesia provides superior same-day recovery over general anesthesia. *Anesthesiology* 2005;102:1001–1007.
13. Dripps RD, Vandam LD. Long-term follow-up of patients who received 10,098 spinal anesthetics: failure to discover major neurological sequelae. *JAMA* 1954;156:1486–1491.
14. Phillips OC, Ebner H, Nelson AT, et al. Neurologic complications following spinal anesthesia with lidocaine: a prospective review of 10,440 cases. *Anesthesiology* 1969;30:284–289.
15. Borgeat A, Ekatodramis G, Kalberer F, et al. Acute and nonacute complications associated with interscalene block and shoulder surgery: a prospective study. *Anesthesiology* 2001;95:875–880.
16. Auroy Y, Narchi P, Messiah A, et al. Serious complications related to regional anesthesia: results of a prospective survey in France. *Anesthesiology* 1997;87:479–486.
17. Auroy Y, Benhamou D, Bargues L, et al. Major complications of regional anesthesia in France: the SOS Regional Anesthesia Hotline Service. *Anesthesiology* 2002;97:1274–1280.
18. Gaba D. Safety first: ensuring quality care in the intensely productive environment—the HRO model. *APSF Newsletter*. Spring, 2003.
19. Auroy Y, Benhamou D, Amaberti R. Risk assessment and control require analysis of both outcomes and process of care. *Anesthesiology* 2004;101:815–817.
20. Reason J. Human error: models and management. *BMJ* 2000;320:768–770.
21. Aviation Safety Reporting System. Available at: http://asrs.arc.nasa.gov. Accessed July 14, 2004.
22. Vincent C, Taylor-Adams S, Stanhope N. Framework for analysing risk and safety in clinical medicine. *BMJ* 1998;316:1154–1157.

23. Wang LP, Hauerberg J, Schmidt JF. Incidence of spinal epidural abscess after epidural analgesia: a national 1-year survey. *Anesthesiology* 1999;91:1928–1936.

24. Vandam LD, Dripps RD. A long-term follow-up of 10,098 spinal anesthetics. II. Incidence and analysis of minor sensory neurological defects. *Surgery* 1955;38:463–469.

25. Finegold H, Mandell G, Vallejo M, et al. Does spinal anesthesia cause hearing loss in the obstetric population? *Anesth Analg* 2002;95:198–203.

26. Wong CA, Slavenas P. The incidence of transient radicular irritation after spinal anesthesia in obstetric patients. *Reg Anesth Pain Med* 1999;24:55–58.

27. Caplan RA, Posner KL, Ward RJ, et al. Adverse respiratory events in anesthesia: a closed claims analysis. *Anesthesiology* 1990;72:828–833.

28. Albright GA. Cardiac arrest following regional anesthesia with etidocaine or bupivacaine. *Anesthesiology* 1979;51:285–287.

29. Schneider MC, Hampl KF, Kaufmann M. Transient neurologic toxicity after subarachnoid anesthesia with hyperbaric 5% lidocaine. *Anesth Analg* 1994;79:610.

30. Chazalon P, Tourtier JP, Villevielle T, et al. Ropivacaine-induced cardiac arrest after peripheral nerve block: successful resuscitation. *Anesthesiology* 2003;99:1449–1451.

31. Huet O, Eyrolle LJ, Mazoit JX, et al. Cardiac arrest after injection of ropivacaine for posterior lumbar plexus blockade. *Anesthesiology* 2003;99:1451–1453.

32. Rosenblatt MA, Abel M, Fischer GW, et al. Successful use of a 20% lipid emulsion to resuscitate a patient after a presumed bupivacaine-related cardiac arrest. *Anesthesiology* 2006;105:217–218.

33. Frankel HL, Crede WB, Topal JE, et al. Use of corporate six sigma performance-improvement strategies to reduce incidence of catheter-related bloodstream infections in a surgical ICU. *J Am Coll Surg* 2005;201:349–358.

34. Bollini CA, Urmey WF, Vascello L, et al. Relationship between evoked motor response and sensory paresthesia in interscalene brachial plexus block. *Reg Anesth Pain Med* 2003;28:384–388.

35. Karaca P, Hadzic A, Yufa M, et al. Painful paresthesiae are infrequent during brachial plexus localization using low-current peripheral nerve stimulation. *Reg Anesth Pain Med* 2003;28:380–383.

36. Hogan Q. Finding nerves is not simple. *Reg Anesth Pain Med* 2003;28:367–371.

37. Holdcroft A, Gibberd FB, Hargrove RL, et al. Neurological complications associated with pregnancy. *Br J Anaesth* 1995;75:522–526.

38. Wong CA. Neurologic deficits and labor analgesia. *Reg Anesth Pain Med* 2004;29:341–351.

39. Wong CA, Scavone BM, Dugan S, et al. Incidence of postpartum lumbosacral spine and lower extremity nerve injuries. *Obstet Gynecol* 2003;101:279–288.

40. Alexander JM, Sharma SK, McIntire DD, et al. Intensity of labor pain and cesarean delivery. *Anesth Analg* 2001;92:1524–1528.

41. Nercessian OA, Macaulay W, Stinchfield FE. Peripheral neuropathies following total hip arthroplasty. *J Arthroplasty* 1994;9:645–651.

42. DeHart MM, Riley Jr LH. Nerve injuries in total hip arthroplasty. *J Am Acad Orthop Surg* 1999;7:101–111.

43. Ben-David B, Joshi R, Chelly JE. Sciatic nerve palsy after total hip arthroplasty in a patient receiving continuous lumbar plexus block. *Anesth Analg* 2003;97:1180–1182.

44. Aminoff MJ. Electrophysiologic testing for the diagnosis of peripheral nerve injuries. *Anesthesiology* 2004;100:1298–1303.

45. Kopacz DJ, Neal JM, Pollock JE. The regional anesthesia "learning curve." What is the minimum number of epidural and spinal blocks to reach consistency? *Reg Anesth* 1996;21:182–190.

46. Lascarrou JB, Thibaut F, Malinovsky JM. Cardiac arrest after axillary plexic anaesthesia with ropivacaine in a chronic kidney failure dialysis patient. *Ann Fr Anesth Reanim* 2008;27:495–498.

47. Weinberg GL, Ripper R, Murphy P, et al. Lipid infusion accelerates removal of bupivacaine and recovery from bupivacaine toxicity in the isolated rat heart. *Reg Anesth Pain Med* 2006;31:296–303.

48. Marhofer P, Eichenberger U, Stöckli S, et al. Ultrasonographic guided axillary plexus blocks with low volumes of local anaesthetics: a crossover volunteer study. *Anaesthesia* 2010;65:266–271.

49. O'Donnell BD, Iohom G. An estimation of the minimum effective anesthetic volume of 2% lidocaine in ultrasound-guided axillary brachial plexus block. *Anesthesiology* 2009;111:25–29.

50. Noble AB, Murray JG. A review of the complications of spinal anaesthesia with experience in canadian teaching hopsitals from 1959 to 1969. *Can Anaesth Soc J* 1971;18:5–17.

51. Scott DB, Tunstall ME. Serious complications associated with epidural/spinal blockade in obstetrics: a two-year prospective study. *Int J Obstet Anesth* 1995;4:133–139.

52. Moen V, Dahlgren N, Irestedt L. Severe neurological complications after central neuraxial blockades in Sweden 1990–1999. *Anesthesiology* 2004;101:950–959.

53. Hebl JR, Horlocker TT, Kopp SL, et al. Neuraxial blockade in patients with preexisting spinal stenosis, lumbar disk disease, or prior spine surgery: efficacy and neurologic complications. *Anesth Analg* 2010;111:1511–1519.

54. de Sèze MP, Sztark F, Janvier G, et al. Severe and long-lasting complications of the nerve root and spinal cord after central neuraxial blockade. *Anesth Analg* 2007;104:975–979.

55. Kane RE. Neurologic deficits following epidural or spinal anesthesia. *Anesth Analg* 1981;60:150–161.

56. Wysowski DK, Talarico L, Bacsanyi J, et al. Spinal and epidural hematoma and low-molecular-weight heparin. *N Engl J Med* 1998;338:1774–1775.

57. Horlocker TT, Wedel DJ, Rowlingson JC, et al. Executive summary: regional anesthesia in the patient receiving antithrombotic or thrombolytic therapy: American Society of Regional Anesthesia and Pain Medicine Evidence-Based Guidelines (Third Edition). *Reg Anesth Pain Med* 2010;35:102–105.

58. Osta WA, Akbary H, Fuleihan SF. Epidural analgesia in vascular surgery patients actively taking clopidogrel. *Br J Anaesth* 2010;104:429–432.

59. van Veen JJ, Nokes TJ, Makris M. The risk of spinal haematoma following neuraxial anaesthesia or lumbar puncture in thrombocytopenic individuals. *Br J Haematol* 2010;148:15–25.

60. Johnson ME, Uhl CB, Spittler KH, et al. Mitochondrial injury and caspase activation by the local anesthetic lidocaine. *Anesthesiology* 2004;101:1184–1194.

61. Myers RR, Sekiguchi Y, Kikuchi S, et al. Inhibition of p38 MAP kinase activity enhances axonal regeneration. *Exp Neurol* 2003;184:606–614.

62. Robards C, Hadzic A, Somasundaram L, et al. Intraneural injection with low-current stimulation during popliteal sciatic nerve block. *Anesth Analg* 2009;109:673–677.

63. Hadzic A, Dewaele S, Gandhi K, et al. Volume and dose of local anesthetic necessary to block the axillary brachial plexus using ultrasound guidance. *Anesthesiology* 2009;111:8–9.

64. Brull R, McCartney CJ, Chan VW, et al. Neurological complications after regional anesthesia: contemporary estimates of risk. *Anesth Analg* 2007;104:965–974.

65. Fredrickson MJ, Kilfoyle DH. Neurological complication analysis of 1000 ultrasound guided peripheral nerve blocks for elective orthopaedic surgery: a prospective study. *Anaesthesia* 2009;64:836–844.

66. Barrington MJ, Watts SA, Gledhill SR, et al. Preliminary results of the Australasian Regional Anaesthesia Collaboration: a prospective audit of more than 7000 peripheral nerve and plexus blocks for neurologic and other complications. *Reg Anesth Pain Med* 2009;34:534–541.

67. Liu SS, Zayas VM, Gordon MA, et al. A prospective, randomized, controlled trial comparing ultrasound versus nerve stimulator guidance for interscalene block for ambulatory shoulder surgery for postoperative neurological symptoms. *Anesth Analg* 2009;109:265–271.

68. Capdevila X, Pirat P, Bringuier S, et al. Continuous peripheral nerve blocks on hospital wards after orthopedic surgery: a multicenter pro-

spective analysis of the quality of postoperative analgesia and complications in 1,416 patients. *Anesthesiology* 2005;103:1035–1045.

69. Bergman BD, Hebl JR, Kent J, et al. Neurologic complications of 405 consecutive continuous axillary catheters. *Anesth Analg* 2003;96:247–252.

70. Morin AM, Kranke P, Wulf H, et al. The effect of stimulating versus nonstimulating catheter techniques for continuous regional anesthesia: a semiquantitative systematic review. *Reg Anesth Pain Med* 2010;35:194–199.

71. Ilfeld BM, Mariano ER, Girard PJ, et al. A multicenter, randomized, triple-masked, placebo-controlled trial of the effect of ambulatory continuous femoral nerve blocks on discharge-readiness following total knee arthroplasty in patients on general orthopaedic wards. *Pain* 2010;150:477–484.

72. Mariano ER, Loland VJ, Sandhu NS, et al. Comparative efficacy of ultrasound-guided and stimulating popliteal-sciatic perineural catheters for postoperative analgesia. *Can J Anesth* 2010;57:919–926.

73. Anderson SL, Buchko JZ, Taillon MR, et al. Chondrolysis of the glenohumeral joint after infusion of bupivacaine through an intra-articular pain pump catheter: a report of 18 cases. *Arthroscopy* 2010;26:451–461.

74. Dragoo JL, Korotkova T, Kanwar R, et al. The effect of local anesthetics administered via pain pump on chondrocyte viability. *Am J Sports Med* 2008;36:1484–1488.

75. Grishko V, Xu M, Wilson G, et al. Apoptosis and mitochondrial dysfunction in human chondrocytes following exposure to lidocaine, bupivacaine, and ropivacaine. *J Bone Joint Surg Am* 2010;92:609–618.

76. Friedman DJ, Parnes NZ, Zimmer Z, et al. Prevalence of cerebrovascular events during shoulder surgery and association with patient position. *Orthopedics* 2009;32: 256.

77. Pohl A, Cullen DJ. Cerebral ischemia during shoulder surgery in the upright position: a case series. *J Clin Anesth* 2005;17: 463–469.

78. D'Alessio JG, Weller RS, Rosenblum M. Activation of the Bezold-Jarisch reflex in the sitting position for shoulder arthroscopy using interscalene block. *Anesth Analg* 1995;80: 1158–1162.

79. Murphy GS, Szokol JW, Marymony JH, et al. Cerebral oxygen desaturation events assessed by near-infrared spectroscopy during shoulder arthroscopy in the beach chair and lateral decubitus positions. *Anesth Analg* 2010;111: 496–505.

80. Jensen LS, Merry AF, Webster CS, et al. Evidence based strategies for preventing drug errors during anaesthesia. *Anaesthesia* 2004;59: 493–504.

81. National Patient Safety Agency. Seven steps to patient safety: the full reference guide. 2004;11. Available from http://www.nrls.npsa.nhs.uk/resources/collections/seven-steps-to-patient-safety/. Accessed January 23, 2011.

82. Cook TM, Payne S, Skryabina E, et al. A simulation-based evaluation of two proposed alternatives to Luer devices for use in neuraxial anaesthesia. *Anaesthesia* 2010;65:1069–1079.

3

An Overview of Strategies to Reduce Risk

Stephen M. Rupp

Let's face it. Regional anesthesia is fun for the practitioner and usually beneficial for the patient. The completion of a successful block usually results in an appreciative patient and surgeon. The practitioner gets immediate gratification related to the technical performance of the block and satisfaction in avoidance or mitigation of the side effects of deep general anesthesia. The transition from the operating room (OR) to recovery is smooth and typically pain free. A deep sense of professional accomplishment can be gained from mastery of regional anesthesia techniques. Unfortunately, things do not always go well. Misadventures range from failed blocks requiring general anesthesia all the way to death of the patient. This chapter is devoted to understanding the sources and causes of error and how a regional anesthesia (RA) practice can be set up to prevent and treat complications of RA. The chapter is focused on mistake-proofing the block once the anesthesiologist and patient have agreed to proceed. Absolute and relative contraindications to the choice of regional anesthesia are handled in other parts of this book.

ERRORS, DEFECTS, AND MISTAKE-PROOFING

In manufacturing, the concept of quality includes the making of a product that performs as expected and has zero defects.[1] This concept can be applied to the practice of medicine.[2] A defect is a poor-quality result that cannot be undone. Examples of defects in the practice of regional anesthesia are wrong-sided block, wrong-medication injection, seizure due to undetected intravascular injection of local anesthetic, and total spinal anesthesia. Errors are precursors to defects. Examples of errors that might lead to the defects noted above include an incorrect consent form, a mislabeled drug, a needle entering the vascular system, or an epidural needle entering the subarachnoid space. It is critical to quality that errors are either prevented at the source from occurring or detected and corrected immediately before they become defects.[1]

Thus, three major strategies are used in manufacturing and medicine to prevent errors from becoming defects: physically making it impossible to create the error; checking at the source for error (also known as self-check); and checking for error just prior to the next step in a process (sequential check).[1] Examples of these strategies in regional anesthesia include respectively removing a dangerous drug from the hospital formulary, reading the label of a syringe prior to injection, and watching carefully for a change in heart rate while injecting a local anesthetic that contains an epinephrine test dose during a block.

SOURCE OF ERRORS

Any human system has a built-in error rate due to the limitations of human performance. Errors include slips, lapses, and mistakes.[3,4] A slip is when the action conducted is not what was intended. A lapse is a forgotten or missed action. A mistake is when the planned action was wrong.[3] Since we are all human, there is a baseline rate of errors that will occur in any system we create. It is important for any system to not only recognize and accept this, but to build in checks to discover and correct these errors before they become defects.

The practice of regional anesthesia represents the interface of humans, knowledge, and technology. Technology includes the space, lighting, equipment, supplies, and drugs we use. Knowledge includes information about the patient's history, medical condition, surgical objectives, and our knowledge of techniques and drugs. Traditional medical education focuses on the information and some of the technical aspects predominantly. However, recent efforts to improve safety have turned attention to the human conditions that compromise performance (Box 3-1).[4–6] Human factors such as fatigue, interruptions, interpersonal conflict, and distractions have drawn significant attention and must be addressed and eliminated or reduced for best performance.[4,7] The culture of medicine can create danger when a hierarchical environment creates fear of speaking up in members of the team.[5,6,8] Everyone needs to feel free to ask a question for a clarification about the intention or potential safety

issue. Leadership, openness, accountability, and intentional planning are required to change the culture.[9,10]

Production pressure is pressure to perform care delivery in less time. It is present in the modern health care delivery system.[11] Unfortunately, this "hurry-up" mentality results too often in cutting corners and speeding up tasks to the point where mistakes and safety risks occur. Later in this chapter, we address the appropriate response to production pressure.

THE EFFECT OF VARIATION ON QUALITY AND SAFETY

Process engineers in industry understand the devastating effect of variation on quality. Eliminating variation for the sake of creating a consistent product is one of the foundational principles of manufacturing.[1,12,13] Thus, standards are created for parts and supplies to ensure performance within a predictable and acceptable range. Similarly, standard work is created for each job at the interface between product, machines, supplies, and humans.[13] Specific job training was a foundational element that allowed women to take over jobs traditionally performed by men in the United States during World War II.[14] Unfortunately, the lack of standard work in medicine has hampered our ability to provide a reliable product for our patients. The cry of "No Anesthesia by Cookbook" is a common phrase.[15] However, physicians and nurses should understand that all our work is not the complex "organic" decision-making type.[16] Some of our work is routine and easily subjected to standards that drive out variation and risk and improve quality. Large variation in the tools of regional anesthesia, for example, the number and types of needles to perform a single kind of block, results in variations in practice, unfamiliarity with equipment, difficulty in acquisition and stocking, and ultimately more risk of error or failure.

EVIDENCE-BASED MEDICINE AND THE HUMAN CONDITION

Traditional medical training emphasizes the importance of evidence-based medicine. Physicians are expected to use evidence-based medicine in their practice. Still, the Institute of Medicine reported that it can take up to 15 to 20 years before proven practices become routine.[17,18] Execution of well-accepted clinical guidelines remains a major challenge. Not following evidence-based guidelines has resulted in external regulatory bodies instituting public reporting and incentive payment strategies. Why is delivering evidence-based medicine so difficult? Is it because the studies are too complex? Or are we practitioners too busy to read? Is there just too much to know? Do we expect too much of ourselves to be able to read, assimilate, and create the pathways that will provide such care? Why is my memory failing me? The level of complexity and speed of modern health care creates a sense of challenge that can be fulfilling but too commonly results in burnout, despair, and self-doubt.[19,20] Perhaps we are too self-reliant. Perhaps we expect too much of ourselves.

With this background, the rest of this chapter is devoted to practical examples of system design that will allow mistake-proofing regional anesthesia.

BOX 3-1 Sources of Errors in Regional Anesthesia Practice

- Human Factors: fatigue, interruptions, personal conflicts
- Fear of speaking up: not identifying a defect for fear of being low on the hierarchy
- Variation: nonstandard approaches to patients undergoing the same operation or multiple versions of epidural anesthesia trays
- Individual approaches to the same procedure: rather than a common approach based on guidelines, scientific evidence, or departmental consensus

THE THEMATIC SOLUTION: A CULTURE OF SAFETY WITH FOCUS ON THE PATIENT AND CONTINUOUS IMPROVEMENT

The acceptance that we all are fallible and need help is present in a culture of safety. Teamwork and communication is maximized. The expectation that errors do and will occur is critical to fostering the requisite self-check and sequential check to detect errors. The culture of safety allows teammates to question and speak up when they sense or detect an error.[4,21] Acquisition of appropriate knowledge of anatomy, pharmacology, techniques, and potential complications prior to applying this knowledge to patients is an appropriate goal. The learner is closely supervised and progressively advanced. Understanding the requisite repetitions to mastery is important in training.[22] Dry laboratory and simulation scenarios can help train the novice and help prepare the expert for dealing with the unexpected or the extremely rare event.[4,23] The workplace is studied scientifically with measures of cycle time, distances traveled, error rates, and defect rates, all of which in turn are systematically and repetitively improved.[2] Patients, families, and providers are involved in the improvement of the workplace and the work flow. Continuous improvement allows successive approximations toward the ultimate goal of perfection.[2,13] Carelessness is unacceptable. Avoidable complications should not occur. Knowing and meeting external regulatory requirements ensures corporate integrity and builds confidence in the team, the patients, and the public.

THE WORKPLACE

The patient experience is foremost in mind, and their experience is actively managed.[2,17] Patients come informed, know what to expect, and arrive on time. The environment is quiet, comforting, and supportive. Waiting is minimized.

Standardization of the workplace drugs and supply system eases the workflow (Box 3-2). A standardized cart with all the supplies needed for a block can be created so that it

can be drawn to the bedside. The drawers are labeled and organized in a manner that allows learning where things belong and ease of routine access. The concept of "just-in-time" supply means that the practitioner has what he/she needs, when he/she needs it, in the amount he/she needs.[13,24] If not, the waste of time in walking, searching, and returning will prolong the time it takes for the block and ultimately tire the provider toward the end of the day and frustrate the surgeon during the day.[2] Accordingly, distances traveled for patients, providers, drugs, supplies, equipment, and information should be minimized as much as possible.[2]

VISUAL SYSTEMS: REMOVING AMBIGUITY AND MISTAKES

One only needs to visit a new environment to appreciate how much ambiguity there is in the activity going on around them. Visual system design is critical to signaling and removing ambiguity.[2,13,24] Patient-tracking systems showing where they are in the process is critical to coordination of care and anticipating next steps. Medication errors due to look-alike bottles and labels have had catastrophic results. The safety improvement from clear to consistent labels is obvious. The Institute for Safe Medication Practice has recommended abandoning color-coded labels as practitioners can unintentionally reach for a "color" in a class of drugs and commit a syringe-swap error.[25] Black printing on white labels leaves only one way to determine what drug and concentration is in the syringe: read the label. Sterile preprinted labels can be produced to allow consistent, efficient, and easy use every time. An example of sterile preprinted labels in a peel-pack for epidural block is included in Figure 3-1. A standard block tray setup can improve supply and drug recognition and the flow of a block (Fig. 3-2). Everyone should know the agreement about the layout. This can reduce mistakes and needle-stick injuries. The standard layout allows easy finding of supplies and drugs, should a learner need help from a more experienced practitioner.

BOX 3-2 Improving the Regional Anesthesia Workplace

- Optimize the human aspect of work: teamwork, communication, effective, and ongoing training
- Standardize the workplace: drugs, supplies
- Optimize workflow: organize supplies, minimize travel distances, send for the patient based on a time predetermined to be adequate for block placement
- Optimize visual systems: patient tracking, clear labeling of drugs and supply sources
- Develop, then periodically reevaluate clinical pathways
- Embrace checklists
- Optimize external setup—preoperative exams, patient consent, standard block trays
- Secure skilled assistance when performing the block

SIMPLIFY, STANDARDIZE, CREATE PATHWAYS AND CHECKLISTS

As mentioned earlier, the complexity of the practice of medicine is a challenge. How to treat each patient individually with a well-tailored, evidence-based approach is daunting. Here is where a systematic review of the literature and then creation of care pathways or protocols can improve care.[17] These protocols can be developed for the highest volume cases in an OR. For example, evidence-based medicine can be applied to create a multimodal analgesic care pathway for total knee arthroplasty that utilizes regional anesthesia, peripheral nerve catheters, and oral analgesics to minimize reliance on parenteral narcotics.[26–28] The department's anesthesiologists review the evidence and draft, revise, and ultimately accept the protocol. Unnecessary complexity is removed from protocols to allow simplicity and ease of application. Still, each patient who presents is evaluated for

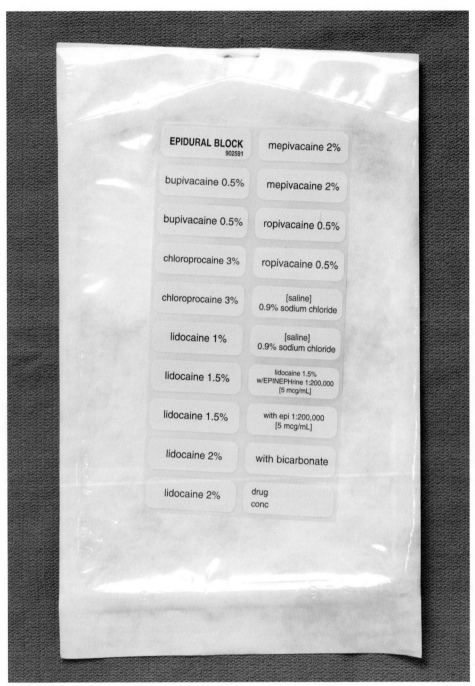

FIGURE 3-1. **A preprinted label set in a sterile peel-pack that can be opened onto a sterile epidural block tray field.** The labels allow quick labeling of all syringes and basins. Separate label sets for spinal block and peripheral nerve block can be created.

entry into the protocol according to their medical condition. Necessary adjustments to the individual patient's condition in the application of the protocol are made. Quickly, the anesthetic product line of the department is improved. Quality outcome measures are reported such as postoperative IV narcotic use, quality of sleep, pain control, nausea/vomiting, as well as the time of successful completion of physical therapy milestones. Assessment of quality outcomes allows rapid adjustment of the protocol within the institution.[29,30] Some of the improvement is simply driving out variation; some comes from allowing the practitioner to focus on the critical issues that vary with each patient while allowing them to fall into a routine pathway. There is a transition from a system hugely reliant on the performance of a single anesthesiologist to the performance of the team. Since everyone knows the pathway, others can more easily help to set up. Finally, checklists can be created to ensure that certain critical tasks are not omitted due to stress or memory failure should the unusual occur.[31] Safety is maximized. The anesthesiologist's enjoyment and confidence in their practice is enhanced. Measures of patient confidence and satisfaction increase.

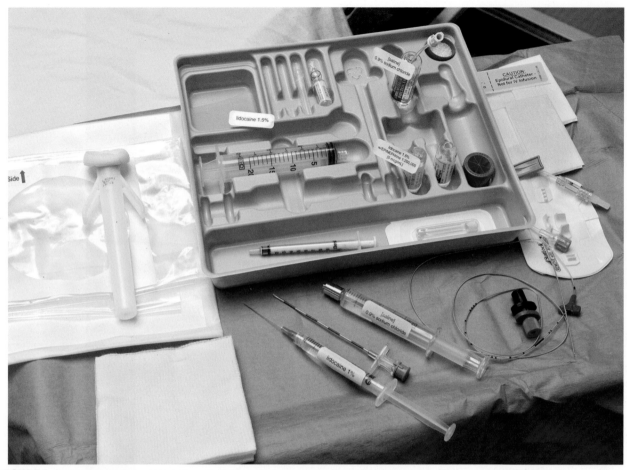

FIGURE 3-2. **A standard epidural block tray setup is pictured.** The tray is thematically set up like a book that reads from left to right. The items for prep and drape are on the left, the syringes and needles are arranged from left to right in their order of use. The catheter and fixation supplies are at the right. All drugs and basins are labeled. This standard setup allows others to know exactly what is needed in a setup, and this facilitates training and safety. When the actual block commences, steps can proceed without fumbling. Accidental needle sticks due to stray sharps can be minimized.

▶ NOT RUSHING CREATES SAFETY

It is critical to address production pressure by understanding the sources of waste in a process and eliminating them. Additionally, it is important to know the cycle time of a block, for example, the time it takes to perform an epidural catheter placement, and use that knowledge to pull the patient at the appropriate time to the block area. Timing of the start of the block should allow the normal cycle time to occur external to the internal clock of the OR. This means that if the block cannot be performed within the time allowed during normal OR turnover, additional external setup of prep, supplies, and providers needs to occur (see below). Rushing or cutting corners due to time constraints should not be allowed.

▶ EXTERNAL SETUP

Setup is the assembly and arrangement of tools and apparatus required for the performance of an operation.[32] If the setup must be performed in the OR just prior to the operation, for example, final draping prior to incision, it is referred to as "internal setup."[2] If the setup can be performed at some

time prior to the time the operation occurs, for example, daily anesthesia machine safety check, it is called "external setup." One of the keys to eliminating rushing is adequate external setup. Examples of opportunities for external setup in regional anesthesia include creating the expectation in the patient for a block, informed consent, gathering and positioning equipment such as the ultrasound machine, positioning the patient, application of monitors, and provision of supplemental oxygen. Standard block tray setup allows someone else to prepare the block tray according to a pre-agreed standard while the anesthesiologist makes the final compact with the patient about the agreed-to plan (see Fig. 3-2). Due to sterile precautions best practice, the final block tray setup should occur just prior to the performance of the block.

▶ INFORMED CONSENT: KNOWING THE PATIENT'S AND SURGEON'S INTENTIONS

The anesthesia workup and plan for anesthesia are discussed with the patient. Confirmation of accurate name and second identifier on the patient's armband is an important routine.[33] Confirmation with the patient of the intended surgery including site and side is performed. Matching the written and signed consent to the patient's understanding of the plan is a key step and should not be delegated. Agreement on the anesthetic plan is reached. All questions are answered. Ensure that the surgeon marks the operative site (with the patient involved if possible) using the agreed-upon organizational mark ("yes" or surgeon initials). The site of a sided block is also marked with a different mark. For our hospital, "yes" marks the surgical site while the anesthesiologist's initials mark the site of a block. "X" is not approved by the Joint Commission due to its ambiguity of meaning.[33]

▶ ROLES DURING A BLOCK

The fact that the anesthesiologist is wearing sterile gloves and mask and is working in a sterile field makes it very difficult to attend to patient needs (like fine-tuning sedation, ensuring appropriate positioning, etc.) Accordingly, safety is served if at least one provider is not sterile and can help. This person could be a nurse (who could help with sedation) or a technician (who in most states cannot help with sedation). They can enhance safety by providing an additional "set of eyes" to be a safety inspector, for example, participating in the time-out. Other duties include the ability to fetch a needed supply that might have accidentally fallen or position and operate equipment (e.g., ultrasound).

▶ FINAL PREPARATION PRIOR TO BLOCK

The patient is positioned for the block. Appropriate monitors are applied (ECG, pulse oximeter, blood pressure cuff). Supplemental oxygen is provided as a precaution, and the patient is sedated to reduce anxiety and pain while ensuring that the patient is responsive to participate in the time-out but also alert the practitioner to severe pain or alterations in sensorium that might indicate an unintended intraneural needle placement or intravascular injection of local anesthetic. The choice of a local anesthetic depends on the type of block, the expected duration of surgery, and the desired length of analgesia after the operation. A drug with the highest therapeutic index for the clinical situation makes the most sense.[34,35] The addition of epinephrine to anesthetic solutions intended for the epidural space should contain epinephrine 1/200,000 (5 μg/mL) to adequately perform a test for intravascular injection.[36–38] Local anesthetic solutions intended for peripheral nerve block should contain epinephrine 1/400,000 (2.5 μg/mL).[40]

The consensus guidelines from the American Society of Regional Anesthesia and Pain Medicine (ASRA) based on best evidence and expert opinion recommends the following sterile precautions: operator and assistant washing their hands prior to the procedure, removing jewelry, chlorhexidine skin prep, sterile drape, sterile gloves, mask (covering nose and mouth), and absence of dangling objects from the neck.[41,42] A time-out according to the universal protocol created by the Joint Commission is performed just prior to the block.[33] This serves as a final sequential check that all agree that the block that is about to occur is being done on the correct patient, for the correct indication, and on the correct site and side, with all drugs and supplies ready and labeled, and that there are no safety concerns from anyone (including the patient).

▶ PERFORMANCE OF THE BLOCK

The resolution of the controversy on the best regional anesthesia technique among the use of paresthesia-seeking, nerve stimulator, or ultrasound-guided techniques is beyond the scope of this chapter (Chapter 17). While the evidence continues to be gathered about enhancements in safety, one can accept that the introduction and widespread application of ultrasound has allowed the practice of regional anesthesia to grow.[43] The use of ultrasound shortens the performance time of most blocks, reduces the amount of local anesthetic required for some blocks (theoretically increasing safety), and enhances the onset time (thus improving work flow).[43] To this author, an appealing aspect of ultrasound-guided regional anesthesia is the ability to visualize the nerves and blood vessels beneath the skin. This allows one to steer away from undesirable anatomic locations. Accordingly, the incidence of vascular puncture is reduced.[43] Additionally, the target of the needle can be *next* to the nerve rather than *the nerve itself*.

The applications of the "test dose" to detect intravascular or subarachnoid injection and "incremental injection" with intermittent aspiration for blood have become routine safety steps in regional anesthesia.[37,38] For neuraxial block such as epidural, the operator checks for the absence of a 10% change in heart rate after an epinephrine 15 micrograms test dose.[37,38]

Knowing potential complications and awareness of signs and symptoms of their onset is an aspect of the vigilant practitioner. Thus, supraclavicular block could have the following complications that could be detected by the associated signs or symptoms: an intravascular injection (increase in the heart rate or blood pressure), severe pain on injection (possible intraneural injection), and cough (if the needle enters the pleural space). Readiness and watchfulness for complications is the key.

▶ PREPARATION FOR THE UNEXPECTED

The system should be ready to provide resuscitation equipment, supplies, and drugs immediately. Sources of oxygen, suction, positive pressure ventilation by mask, and endotracheal intubation should be at hand. The code cart should be within easy reach and in a standard location.[38] Simulation of rescue can help build readiness and teamwork.[39] Availability of a lipid emulsion rescue kit with a checklist for guidance in use is important.[38] The value of a checklist has been proven in aviation and has recently grown in popularity in medicine as a way to ensure that during a rare and stressful event, easy and potentially life-saving steps are correctly followed and not forgotten.[31] An example of a local anesthetic systemic toxicity rescue checklist is shown in Figure 3-3.

▶ MONITORING AFTER THE BLOCK

After the performance of a block, the sterile prep and drape are taken down and equipment and supplies are removed from the bedside. It is important to provide for continuous monitoring of the patient in case a delayed adverse reaction occurs (e.g., hypotension due to neuraxial block or delayed local anesthetic toxicity due to systemic absorption). For neuraxial blocks, a qualified anesthesia provider should be

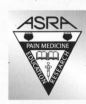

AMERICAN SOCIETY OF REGIONAL ANESTHESIA AND PAIN MEDICINE

Checklist for Treatment of Local Anesthetic Systemic Toxicity

The Pharmacologic Treatment of Local Anesthetic Systemic Toxicity (LAST) is Different from Other Cardiac Arrest Scenarios

❑ **Get Help**

❑ **Initial Focus**

    ❑ **Airway management:** ventilate with 100% oxygen

    ❑ **Seizure suppression:** benzodiazepines are preferred; **AVOID propofol** in patients having signs of cardiovascular instability

    ❑ **Alert** the nearest facility having **cardiopulmonary bypass** capability

❑ **Management of Cardiac Arrhythmias**

    ❑ **Basic and Advanced Cardiac Life Support (ACLS)** will require adjustment of medications and perhaps prolonged effort

    ❑ **AVOID vasopressin, calcium channel blockers, beta blockers, or local anesthetic**

    ❑ **REDUCE epinephrine dose to <1 mcg/kg**

❑ **Lipid Emulsion (20%) Therapy** (values in parenthesis are for 70kg patient)

    ❑ **Bolus 1.5 mL/kg** (lean body mass) intravenously over 1 minute (~100mL)

    ❑ **Continuous infusion 0.25 mL/kg/min** (~18 mL/min; adjust by roller clamp)

    ❑ Repeat bolus once or twice for persistent cardiovascular collapse

    ❑ **Double the infusion rate** to 0.5 mL/kg/min if blood pressure remains low

    ❑ **Continue infusion** for at least10 minutes after attaining circulatory stability

    ❑ Recommended upper limit: Approximately 10 mL/kg lipid emulsion over the first 30 minutes

❑ **Post LAST events at** www.lipidrescue.org and report use of lipid to www.lipidregistry.org

FIGURE 3-3. **Emergency checklist of the American Society of Regional Anesthesia and Pain Medicine (ASRA).**[38] This checklist can be printed and kept with an emergency cache of sterile lipid emulsion in the regional block area. Should signs or symptoms of local anesthetic systemic toxicity occur, the kit can be brought to the bedside. The checklist provides an easy guide to the safety steps that can be followed accurately and without memory lapse. (Reprinted with permission of ASRA. PDF copies of this checklist are available free of charge at www.asra.com.)

continuously present. For peripheral nerve blocks, a protocol for monitoring should be in place if there will be a delay prior to the beginning of surgery. This protocol should be site specific and involve nursing and immediate availability of qualified anesthesia personnel.

▶ PATIENT FOLLOW-UP, ONGOING OUTCOME, AND QUALITY ASSESSMENT

The postprocedure follow-up with the patient is important for the assessment of patient satisfaction and complications. If a patient has a complaint, service recovery can occur. Additionally, if there is a possibility of nerve injury, appropriate evaluation and involvement of the surgeon and expert consultants such as a neurologist can be obtained.

Electrodiagnostic studies performed in the early postoperative period can help localize the site of the injury.[44] As mentioned earlier, obtaining an ongoing set of quality metrics can allow evaluation and changes to institutional protocols, which can improve quality.[29] A sentinel event system to internally report and analyze errors, defects, and near misses is important to recognize and improve systems so that chance of repetition of a defect is mitigated.[45,46]

▶ CONCLUSION

Mistake-proofing blocks is a journey. It requires leadership, teamwork, communication, and dedication. The acceptance of the human fallibilities of the regional anesthesia practitioner is critical. Making the performance of the blocks easy is important. Removing ambiguities and dangers created by unnecessary variation allows one to focus on the critical aspects of a patient's care. Department-based roles, routines, and protocols allow everyone to meet a baseline level of safe practice. Everyone knows the protocol and performs their role. The experts in the department pave the way for improvement and remove obstacles for the others. Incorporating the best new evidence-based practices is critical to quality and safety. Continuous improvement, training, readiness, and practice for the unexpected are the sine qua non of a successful and rewarding environment.

References

1. Shingo S. *Zero Quality Control: Source Inspection and the Poke-Yoke System*. Portland, OR: Productivity Press, 1986.
2. Kenney C. *Transforming Health Care. Virginia Mason Medical Center's Pursuit of the Perfect Patient Experience*. New York, NY: Productivity Press, 2011.
3. Reason J. *Human Error*. Cambridge, UK: Cambridge University Press, 1990.
4. Institute of Medicine. *To Err is Human. Building a safer health system*. Washington, DC: National Academy Press, 2000.
5. Leonard M, Graham S, Bonacum D. The human factor: the critical importance of effective teamwork and communication in providing safe care. *Quality Saf Health Care* 2004;13:i85–i90.
6. Carthey J, de Leval, Reason JT. The human factor in cardiac surgery: errors and near misses in a high technology surgical domain. *Ann Thorac Surg* 2001;72:300–305.
7. Sexton JB, Thomas EJ, Helmreich RL. Error, stress, and teamwork in medicine and aviation: cross sectional surveys. *BMJ* 2000;320:745–749.

8. Gaiser RR. Teaching professionalism during residency: why it is failing and a suggestion to improve its success. *Anes Analg* 2009;108:948–954.
9. Timmel J, Kent PS, Holzmueller CG, et al. Impact of the Comprehensive Unit-based Safety Program (CUSP) on safety culture in a surgical inpatient unit. *Jt Comm J Qual Patient Saf* 2010;36:252–260.
10. Goeschel CA, Holzmueller CG, Berenholtz SM, et al. Executive/Senior Leader Checklist to improve culture and reduce central line-associated bloodstream infections. *Jt Comm J Qual Patient Saf* 2010;36:519–524.
11. Gaba DM, Howard SK, Jump B. Production pressure in the work environment. California anesthesiologists' attitudes and experiences. *Anesthesiology* 1994;81:488–500.
12. Tennant G. *Six Sigma SPC and TQM in manufacturing and services*. Surrey: Gower, 2001.
13. Ohno T. *Toyota Production System. Beyond Large-Scale Production*. Portland, OR: Productivity Press, 1988.
14. Graupp P, Wrona RJ. *The TWI Workbook: Essential Skills of Supervisors*. New York, NY: Taylor & Francis, 2006.
15. Savarese JJ, Lowenstein E. The name of the game: no anesthesia by cookbook. *Anesthesiology* 1985;62:703–705.
16. Liker JK, Meier DP. *Toyota Talent. Developing your people the Toyota way*. New York, NY: McGraw-Hill, 2007.
17. Institute of Medicine. Crossing the quality chasm: a new health system for the 21st Century. Washington, DC: National Academy Press, 2001.
18. Balas EA, Weingarten S, Garb CT, et al. Improving preventive care by prompting physicians. *Arch Int Med* 2000;160:301–308.
19. Hyman SA, Michaels DR, Berry JM, et al. Risk of burnout in perioperative clinicians. A survey study and literature review. *Anesthesiology* 2011;114:194–204.
20. Shanafelt T. Burnout in anesthesiology: a call to action. *Anesthesiology* 2011;114:1–2.
21. Kohn LT, Corrigan JM, Donaldson MS, eds. *To err is human: building a safer health system. A report of the Committee on Quality of Health Care in America, Institute of Medicine*. Washington, DC: National Academy Press, 2000.
22. Kopacz D, Neal J, Pollock J. The regional anesthesia "learning curve": what is the minimum number of epidural and spinal blocks to reach consistency? *Reg Anesth* 1996;21:182–190.
23. Sexton JB, Marsch SC, Helmreich RL, et al. Jumpseating in the operating room. In: Henson L, Lee A, Basford A, eds. *Simulators in anesthesiology education*. New York, NY: Plenum, 1998:107–108.
24. Womack JP, Jones DT. *Lean Thinking*. New York, NY: Simon & Shuster, 1996.
25. Institute for Safe Medication Practices: Principles of designing a medication label for injectable syringes for patient specific, inpatient use. http://www.ismp.org/tools/guidelines/labelFormats/Piggyback.asp. Accessed January 9, 2011.
26. Horlocker TT, Kopp SL, Pagnano MW, et al. Analgesia for total hip and knee arthroplasty: a multimodal pathway featuring peripheral nerve block. *J Am Acad Orthop Surg* 2006;14:126–135.
27. Hebl JR, Kopp SL, Ali MH, et al. A comprehensive anesthesia protocol that emphasizes peripheral nerve blockade for total knee and total hip arthroplasty. *J Bone Joint Surg Am* 2005;87(Suppl 2):63–70.
28. Hebl JR, Dilger JA, Byer DE, et al. A pre-emptive multimodal pathway featuring peripheral nerve block improves perioperative outcomes after major orthopedic surgery. *Reg Anesth Pain Med* 2008;33:510–517.
29. Speroff T, James BC, Nelson EC, et al. Guidelines for appraisal and publication of PDSA quality improvement. *Qual Manag Health Care* 2004;13:33–39.
30. Davidoff F, Batalden P, Stevens D, et al. Squire Publication Guidelines for Improvement Studies in Health Care: Evolution of the SQUIRE project. *Ann Int Med* 2008;149:670–676.

31. Gawande A. *The checklist manifesto. How to get things right.* New York, NY: Henry Holt and Company, 2009.

32. Mirriam-Webster On-line dictionary. http://www.merriam-webster.com/dictionary/set-up?show=0&t=1294611200. Accessed January 9, 2011.

33. Joint Commission: National Patient Safety Goals 2011. http://www.jointcommission.org/assets/1/6/2011_NPSGs_HAP.pdf. Accessed January 9, 2011.

34. Chazalon P, Tourtier JP, Villevielle T, et al. Ropivacaine-induced cardiac arrest after peripheral nerve block: successful resuscitation. *Anesthesiology* 2003;99:1449–1451.

35. Huet O, Eyrolle LJ, Mazoit JX, et al. Cardiac arrest after injection of ropivacaine for posterior lumbar plexus blockade. *Anesthesiology* 2003;99:1451–1453.

36. Moore DC, Batra MS. The components of an effective test dose prior to epidural block. *Anesthesiology* 1981;55:693–696.

37. Mulroy MF, Hejtmanek MR. Prevention of local anesthetic systemic toxicity. *Reg Anesth Pain Med* 2010;35:177–180.

38. Neal JM, Bernards CM, Butterworth JF, et al. ASRA practice advisory on local anesthetic systemic toxicity. *Reg Anesth Pain Med* 2010;35:152–161.

39. Neal JM, Hsiung RL, Mulroy MF, et al. ASRA checklist improves trainee performance during a simulated episode of local anesthetic systemic toxicity. *Reg Anesth Pain Med* 2012;37:8–15.

40. Neal JM. Effects of epinephrine in local anesthetics on the central and peripheral nervous systems: neurotoxicity and neural blood flow. *Reg Anesth Pain Med* 2003;28(2):124–134.

41. Hebl JR. The importance and implications of aseptic techniques during regional anesthesia. *Reg Anesth Pain Med* 2006;31:311–323.

42. Horlocker TT, Birnbach DJ, Connis RT, et al. Practice advisory for the prevention, diagnosis, and management of infectious complications associated with neuraxial techniques: a report by the American Society of Anesthesiologists Task Force on infectious complications associated with neuraxial techniques. *Anesthesiology* 2010;112:530–545.

43. Neal JM, Brull R, Chan VWS, et al. The ASRA evidence-based medicine assessment of ultrasound-guided regional anesthesia and pain medicine: Executive Summary. *Reg Anesth Pain Med* 2010;35:S1–S9.

44. Sorenson, EJ. Neurological injuries associated with regional anesthesia. *Reg Anesth Pain Med* 2008;33:442–448.

45. Auroy Y, Benhamou D, Amaberti R. Risk assessment and control require analysis of both outcomes and process of care. *Anesthesiology* 2004;101:815–817.

46. Reason J. Human error: models and management. *BMJ* 2000;320:768–770.

4

Bleeding Complications

Terese T. Horlocker and Denise J. Wedel

Spinal hematoma, defined as symptomatic bleeding within the spinal neuraxis, is a rare and potentially catastrophic complication of spinal or epidural anesthesia. Although hemorrhagic complications can occur after virtually all regional anesthetic techniques, bleeding into the spinal canal is perhaps the most serious hemorrhagic complication associated with regional anesthesia (RA) because the spinal canal is a concealed and nonexpandable space. Spinal cord compression from expanding hematoma may result in neurologic ischemia and paraplegia.

Within 10 years of the first spinal anesthetic, administered by Bier in 1898, the first spinal hematoma following neuraxial blockade was reported in a 36-year-old male after unsuccessful spinal anesthesia for excision of a pilonidal cyst.[1] Repeated lumbar punctures yielded blood-tinged cerebrospinal fluid with each attempt. The procedure was eventually performed under local infiltration. Ten days later, the patient complained of paresthesias and weakness of his lower extremities. Lumbar radiograph demonstrated spina bifida occulta. Dilated spinal veins consistent with a vascular tumor were noted during decompressive laminectomy, and neurologic recovery was poor. There was no evidence for a preexisting coagulopathy. However, spina bifida occulta and vertebral column vascular abnormalities were subsequently regarded as contraindications to spinal or epidural anesthesia.

The first spinal hematoma in a patient with altered hemostasis was noted by Bonica in 1953.[2] The patient complained of signs consistent with cauda equina syndrome 4 days after bloody spinal puncture. Exploratory laminectomy revealed extensive clots within the subarachnoid space, which were compressing the conus medullaris. Hemostasis was difficult due to continued intrathecal bleeding. The wound was packed, exacerbating neurologic ischemia, and the patient sustained irreversible neurologic injury.

Although patients with preexisting coagulopathies were considered at increased risk for hemorrhagic complications following neuraxial blockade, the clinical introduction of heparin in 1937, and coumarin derivatives in 1941, heralded new concerns regarding the regional anesthetic management of perioperatively anticoagulated patients. These concerns were further amplified as medical standards for the prevention of perioperative venous thromboembolism were established and potent antithrombotic and antiplatelet drugs, such as low-molecular-weight heparin (LMWH), clopidogrel, and dabigatran, were introduced.[3] Health care organizations are increasingly required to comply with outcome and process measures to receive reimbursement for patient care. Quality measures established by both the Centers for Medicare and Medicaid Services (CMS; http://www.cms.hhs.gov) and the Joint Commission (http://www.jointcommission.org) require standardized processes for accessing the risk of thromboembolism, ordering appropriate therapy and reducing the likelihood of harm in patients receiving antithrombotic therapy.

▶ SCOPE OF THE PROBLEM

The actual incidence of neurologic dysfunction resulting from hemorrhagic complications associated with central neural blockade is unknown. In an extensive review of the literature, Tryba[4] identified 13 cases of spinal hematoma following 850,000 epidural anesthetics and 7 cases among 650,000 spinal techniques. Based on these observations, the calculated incidence was approximated to be <1 in 150,000 epidural and <1 in 220,000 spinal anesthetics. Since these estimates represented the upper limit of the 95% confidence interval (CI), the *overall* frequency would presumably be much less. However, this estimation was performed in 1994, before the implementation of routine perioperative thromboprophylaxis. A more recent survey involving 1,710,000 neuraxial epidural blocks performed in Sweden over a 10-year period between 1990 and 1999 reported 33 spinal hematomas, for an overall frequency of 1.9 per 100,000 neuraxial anesthetics (95% CI 1.3–2.7 per 100,000).[5] This epidemiologic study as well as other case series suggests a substantial increase in the frequency over the last two decades.[5–7] Patient characteristics and anesthetic variables also modify the risk of spinal bleeding[8] (Table 4-1). Although it is useful to identify patient populations at risk, even more crucial are management techniques that facilitate the detection and evaluation of new perioperative neurologic deficits, since neurologic outcome is dependent on timely intervention. Finally, improved perioperative outcomes associated with peripheral/plexus blocks have lead to an increased popularity of these techniques. However, it is important to note that serious hemorrhagic complications have also occurred with peripheral and plexus blockade.[9–11]

TABLE 4-1 Risk Factors and Estimated Incidence for Spinal Hematoma Associated with Neuraxial Anesthesia

	RELATIVE RISK OF SPINAL HEMATOMA	ESTIMATED INCIDENCE FOR EPIDURAL ANESTHESIA	ESTIMATED INCIDENCE FOR SPINAL ANESTHESIA
No heparin			
Atraumatic	1.00	1:220,000	1:320,000
Traumatic	11.2	1:20,000	1:29,000
With aspirin	2.54	1:150,000	1:220,000
Heparin anticoagulation following neuraxial procedure			
Atraumatic	3.16	1:70,000	1:100,000
Traumatic	112	1:2,000	1:2,900
Heparin >1 h after puncture	2.18	1:100,000	1:150,000
Heparin <1 h after puncture	25.2	1:8,700	1:13,000
With aspirin	26	1:8,500	1:12,000

Data from Stafford-Smith M. Impaired haemostasis and regional anaesthesia. *Can J Anaesth* 1996;43:R129–R141. With permission.

► PATHOPHYSIOLOGY

The majority of spinal hematomas occur in the epidural space because of the prominent venous plexus.[12] However, the actual source of the bleeding (arterial vs. venous) is controversial. Bleeding from an arterial source should accumulate rapidly and cause neural ischemia soon after vessel trauma. However, most spinal hematomas become symptomatic several days after needle/catheter placement, *not* immediately postoperatively, suggesting the bleeding is not arterial. On the other hand, a venous source would accumulate more slowly but theoretically would tamponade prior to overcoming spinal cord perfusion pressure. Thus, neither model entirely represents the clinical scenario. The volume of blood required to cause cord ischemia also varies and is affected by the site of bleeding (the cauda equina is relatively resistant, while the watershed areas of the cord are more easily compromised), the presence of vertebral column abnormalities, and the rapidity with which the blood accumulates. It is interesting to note that several of the LMWH hematomas involved less blood than that typically injected during the performance of an epidural blood patch.[13]

Of special interest to the anesthesiologist are those spinal hematomas that have occurred *spontaneously* in the patient receiving antithrombotic or antiplatelet therapy.[14] Risk factors include the intensity of the anticoagulant effect, increased age, female gender, history of gastrointestinal bleeding, concomitant aspirin use, and length of therapy.[15] During warfarin therapy, an international normalized ratio (INR) of 2.0 to 3.0 is associated with a low risk of bleeding: <3% during a 3-month treatment period. Higher intensity regimens (INR > 4) are associated with a significantly greater risk of bleeding (7%). The incidence of hemorrhagic complications during therapeutic anticoagulation with standard heparin, as well as LMWH, is <3%. Thrombolytic therapy represents the greatest risk of bleeding between 6% and 30% of patients.[15]

► RISK FACTORS

An understanding of the mechanisms of blood coagulation, the pharmacologic properties of the anticoagulant and antiplatelet medications, and also the clinical studies involving patients undergoing central neural blockade while receiving these medications is paramount in reducing the risk of spinal hematoma in patients undergoing neuraxial blockade (Table 4-2). In a review of the literature between 1906 and

TABLE 4-2 Pharmacologic Activities of Anticoagulants, Antiplatelet Agents, and Thrombolytics

AGENT	EFFECT ON COAGULATION VARIABLES		TIME TO PEAK EFFECT	TIME TO NORMAL HEMOSTASIS AFTER DISCONTINUATION
	PT	APTT		
Intravenous heparin	↑	↑↑↑	Minutes	4–6 h
Subcutaneous heparin	—	↑	40–50 min	4–6 h
Low-molecular-weight heparin	—	—	3–5 h	12–24 h
Warfarin	↑↑↑	↑	4–6 d (less with loading dose)	4–6 d
Dabigatran	↑	↑↑	2 h	4–7 d
Antiplatelet agents				
Aspirin	—	—	Hours	5–8 d
Other NSAIDs			Hours	1–3 d
Ticlopidine, clopidogrel, prasugrel			Hours	1–2 wk
Platelet glycoprotein IIb/IIIa receptor inhibitors			Minutes	8–48 h
Fibrinolytics	↑	↑↑	Minutes	24–36 h

PT, prothrombin time; aPTT, activated partial thromboplastin time; ↑, clinically insignificant increase; ↑↑, possibly clinically significant increase; ↑↑↑, clinically significant increase; NSAID, nonsteroidal antiinflammatory drug.

1994, Vandermeulen et al.[12] reported 61 cases of spinal hematoma associated with epidural or spinal anesthesia. Included were five parturients and four patients with anatomic abnormalities of the spine, such as spina bifida occulta, spinal ependymoma, and spinal angioma. A spinal anesthetic was performed in 15 cases, the remaining 46 received an epidural technique. Of the 32 patients who underwent continuous epidural block, the hematoma occurred immediately at the time of catheter removal, suggesting that coagulation status at the time of catheter removal as well as placement should be considered.

In 42 of the 61 patients (68%), the spinal hematoma occurred in patients with evidence of hemostatic abnormality. Twenty-five patients had received intravenous heparin (18 patients), subcutaneous heparin (3 patients), or LMWH (4 patients), while an additional five patients presumably received heparin during a vascular surgical procedure. In addition, 12 patients had evidence of coagulopathy or thrombocytopenia or were treated with antiplatelet medications (aspirin, indomethacin, ticlopidine), oral anticoagulants (phenprocoumone), thrombolytics (urokinase), or dextran 70 immediately before or after the neuraxial anesthetic. Needle placement was reported as difficult in 25% of patients and/or bloody in 25% of patients. Multiple punctures were reported in 20% of patients. Therefore, in 87% of patients, a hemostatic abnormality or traumatic/difficult needle placement was present. More than one risk factor was present in 20 of 61 cases.

Neurologic compromise presented as progression of sensory or motor block (68% of patients) or bowel/bladder dysfunction (8% of patients), not as severe radicular back pain. Importantly, although only 38% of patients had partial or good neurologic recovery, spinal cord ischemia tended to be reversible in patients who underwent laminectomy within 8 hours of onset of neurologic dysfunction.

The need for prompt diagnosis and intervention in the event of a spinal hematoma was also demonstrated in a review of the American Society of Anesthesiologists (ASA) Closed Claims database which noted that spinal cord injuries were the leading cause of claims in the 1990s.[16] Spinal hematomas accounted for nearly half of the spinal cord injuries. Risk factors for spinal hematoma included epidural anesthesia in the presence of intravenous heparin during a vascular surgical or diagnostic procedure. Importantly, the presence of postoperative numbness or weakness was typically attributed to local anesthetic effect rather than spinal cord ischemia, which delayed the diagnosis. Patient care was rarely judged to have met standards (1 of 13 cases) and the median payment was very high.

It is impossible to conclusively determine the risk factors for the development of spinal hematoma in patients undergoing neuraxial blockade solely through review of the case series, which represent only patients with the complication and do not define those who underwent uneventful neuraxial analgesia. However, large inclusive surveys which evaluate the frequencies of complications (including spinal hematoma), as well as identify subgroups of patients with higher or lower risk, enhance risk stratification. Moen et al.[5] investigated serious neurologic complications among 1,260,000 spinal and 450,000 epidural blocks performed in Sweden over a 10-year period. Among the 33 spinal hematomas, 24 occurred in females; 25 were associated with an epidural technique. A coagulopathy (existing or acquired) was present in 11 patients; two of these patients were parturients with hemolysis, elevated liver enzymes, and low platelet (HELLP) syndrome. Spinal pathology was present in six patients. The presenting complaint was typically lower extremity weakness. Only 5 of the 33 patients recovered neurologically (due to delay in the diagnosis/intervention). These demographics, risk factors, and outcomes confirmed those of previous series. However, the methodology allowed for calculation of the frequency of spinal hematoma among patient populations. For example, the risk associated with epidural analgesia in women undergoing childbirth was significantly less (1 in 200,000) than that in elderly women undergoing knee arthroplasty (1 in 3,600, $p < .0001$). Likewise, women undergoing hip fracture surgery under spinal anesthesia had a statistically increased risk of spinal hematoma (1 in 22,000) compared to all patients undergoing spinal anesthesia (1 in 480,000).

Overall, these series report that the risk of clinically significant bleeding varies with age (and associated abnormalities of the spinal cord or vertebral column), the presence of an underlying coagulopathy, difficulty during needle placement, and an indwelling neuraxial catheter during sustained anticoagulation (particularly with standard heparin or LMWH), perhaps in a multifactorial manner. They also consistently demonstrate the need for prompt diagnosis and intervention.

Patient Risk Factors

Patient factors are not "controllable," but should be considered when selecting a regional technique and the intensity of neurologic monitoring perioperatively. The patient factors for spinal hematoma are similar to those for spontaneous bleeding with antithrombotic therapy—increased age, female gender, and concomitant hepatic or renal disease (which exaggerate the anticoagulant response).[5,13,15] In a series of 40 spinal hematomas associated with LMWH thromboprophylaxis, 75% of the patients were elderly women.[13] Similarly, Moen et al. noted that 70% of patients with spinal hematoma were females and often had preexisting spinal stenosis due to osteoporosis.[5] The increased frequency among elderly women may be due to increased sensitivity to thromboprophylactic medications and/or changes in the vertebral column with age.

Since pregnancy and the immediate postpartum interval are associated with a hypercoagulable state, it is often assumed that parturients are not at risk for spinal hematoma. However, in the series by Vandermeulen et al.[12] 5 of 61 spinal hematomas involved parturients. In two cases, a clotting disorder (thrombocytopenia, preeclampsia) was present. One parturient had a previously undiagnosed epidural ependymoma. No risk factors were reported in the remaining two patients. The two parturients in the series by Moen et al.[5] occurred in the presence of severe coagulopathy. To date, there have been no published spinal hematomas associated with peripartum antithrombotic therapy. However, there is no large series documenting the safety of neuraxial block in the presence of the therapeutic levels of anticoagulation required among this patient population. Therefore, the relative risk is unknown.

Anesthetic Risk Factors

Anesthetic variables that may affect the risk of spinal hematoma include needle/catheter gauge, the trauma incurred during needle/catheter insertion, and the placement of an indwelling neuraxial catheter. Although the presence of blood during neuraxial block does not portend spinal hematoma, traumatic needle or catheter placement has often been described in case reports of spinal hematoma.[12,13,17,18] In addition, larger gauge needles and the insertion of an epidural or spinal catheter increase the likelihood of traumatic needle placement,[17,19] and nearly three-fourths of spinal hematomas are associated with a continuous catheter technique.[5,12,13] Several studies have verified that the placement of an indwelling intrathecal or epidural catheter increased the risk of minor (clinically insignificant) spinal bleeding.[17,19] Horlocker et al.[17] reported that blood was present during the placement of 18 of 46 (39%) intrathecal or 138 of 575 (24%) epidural catheters. This was significantly higher than the frequency associated with single-dose spinal anesthesia, 64 of 362 (18%). Patients with blood present during needle and catheter placement were more likely to have blood present in the catheter at the time of removal. These investigations demonstrate that indwelling neuraxial catheters result in trauma to spinal vasculature. The presence of anticoagulation theoretically increases the chance that bleeding will be increased and may become clinically significant, particularly when the catheter is removed during altered hemostasis.[12,16]

Pharmacologic Actions and Interactions

Patients react with different sensitivities to anticoagulants. Highly sensitive patients will exhibit a greater increase in the degree of anticoagulation and prolonged effect after discontinuation of the medication. A single dose (3–5 mg) of warfarin resulted in the prolongation of the prothrombin time (PT) in approximately 20% of patients.[20] Conversely, in resistant patients, the anticoagulant effects will be decreased and short-lived. For example, patients with acute thromboembolic disease exhibit heparin resistance secondary to a reduction in anti-thrombin III. A number of factors affect a patient's sensitivity to heparin and warfarin including overall medical condition, diet, renal function, and liver disease (Box 4-1). Finally, the anticoagulant effects may be potentiated by the administration of concomitant medications, such as nonsteroidal antiinflammatory medications or dextran. Therefore, it is imperative that the clinician be knowledgeable of the patient's preexisting medical conditions, the anticipated method and the level of perioperative anticoagulation, and the potential for drug interactions. In addition, anticoagulant activity should be closely monitored, particularly in patients with indwelling catheters.

Preoperative Anticoagulation

Patients who require chronic anticoagulant therapy, such as those with a history of atrial fibrillation or cardiac valve replacement, are not ideal candidates for neuraxial techniques. Often the anticoagulant effect is only partially reversed to avoid thrombotic complications and/or they are aggressively anticoagulated postoperatively. Normal hemostasis for needle/catheter placement is present only for a

---

BOX 4-1 Summary of Patient Characteristics Associated with Enhanced Prothrombin Time Response to Warfarin

- Age >65 years
- Female gender
- Weight <100 lbs
- Excessive surgical blood loss
- Liver, cardiac, renal disease
- Oriental race
- CYP2C9 and/or VKORC1 genetic variation

---

short interval and may not be maintained (making catheter removal problematic).

Unanticipated Anticoagulation or Thrombolysis

Patients who have recently undergone neuraxial anesthesia and require emergent anticoagulation for limb ischemia, acute coronary syndrome, or deep-venous thrombosis/pulmonary embolism represent a conundrum for the anesthesiologist. Ideally, the patient should be queried prior to antithrombotic or thrombolytic therapy for a recent history of lumbar puncture, spinal or epidural anesthesia, or epidural steroid injection to allow appropriate management and monitoring. The decision to maintain or remove an existing neuraxial catheter is based on the degree/duration of antithrombotic therapy. Since combination therapy (antiplatelet medications with heparin and/or thrombolytics) represents a greater risk of bleeding, treatment options with the least impact on coagulation should be considered.[15] Unfortunately, while the anesthesia community is well aware of the potential for spinal bleeding in this patient population, other specialties have only recently become cognizant of the risk.[21] As a result, the anesthesiologist may not be notified until after the establishment of therapeutic anticoagulation. Under these circumstances, a consensus on when hemostasis may be restored to allow catheter removal must be achieved, balancing the relative risks of hemorrhage and thrombosis. Complete reversal of the anticoagulant effect may *not* be feasible due to the risk of thromboembolic complications. Most importantly, ongoing efforts to educate clinicians responsible for administering hemostasis-altering medications are critical.

▶ GUIDELINES FOR ANTITHROMBOTIC THERAPY

In 2008, the American College of Chest Physicians (ACCP) released the proceedings of the Eighth Conference on Antithrombotic and Thrombolytic Therapy[3] (Table 4-3). These recommendations represent new challenges in the management of patients undergoing neuraxial (and invasive/noncompressible peripheral) blockade. In general, higher degrees of thromboprophylaxis for extended intervals are recommended (Box 4-2). An acceptable alternative to

TABLE 4-3 Pharmacological Venous Thromboembolism Prophylaxis and Treatment Regimens	
Total Hip or Knee Arthroplasty and Hip Fracture Surgery	
Fondaparinux	2.5 mg SC qd started 6–8 h after surgery
LMWH[a]	5,000 U SC qd started 12 h before surgery, *or* 2,500 U SC given 4–6 h after surgery, then 5,000 U SC daily, *or* 30 mg U SC 8–10 h after surgery, then 30 mg q12h
Warfarin	Started the night before or immediately after surgery and adjusted to prolong the INR = 2.0–3.0
Minor General Surgery, Spine, Vascular, and Arthroscopic Procedures (with NO additional risk factors present)[b]	
Early mobilization	
No pharmacologic thromboprophylaxis	
Minor General Surgery, Vascular or Spine Surgery (*with* additional risk factors present) and	
Major General or Gynecologic Surgery (*without* additional risk factors present)	
Unfractionated heparin	5,000 U SC q12h, started 2 h before surgery
LMWH	≤3,400 U SC qd, started 1–2 h before surgery
Major General or Gynecologic Surgery and Open Urologic Procedures (*with* additional risk factors present)	
Unfractionated heparin	5,000 U SC q8h, started 2 h before surgery
LMWH	>3,400 U SC qd, started 1–2 h before surgery
Acute Coronary Syndrome and Venous Thromboembolism Therapy	
LMWH	120 U/kg SC q12h or 200 U/kg SC qd (non-q-wave MI)

SC, subcutaneous; LMWH, low-molecular-weight heparin; INR, international normalized ratio.
[a]LMWH formulations available in North America are enoxaparin and dalteparin.
[b]The risk factors for thromboembolism include trauma, immobility/paresis, malignancy, previous thromboembolism, increasing age (over 40 years), pregnancy, estrogen therapy, obesity, smoking history, varicose veins, and inherited or congenital thrombophilia. Based on recommendations from Geerts WH, Bergqvist D, Pineo GF, et al. Prevention of venous thromboembolism: American College of Chest Physicians Evidence-Based Clinical Practice Guidelines (8th Edition). *Chest* 2008;133:381S–453S. With permission.

the ACCP guidelines are those developed by the Surgical Care Improvement Project (SCIP, www.qualitynet.org). In addition, it is important to note that in response to ongoing concerns regarding surgical bleeding associated with thromboprophylaxis, the American Academy of Orthopaedic Surgeons (AAOS) also published guidelines in 2007 for the prevention of symptomatic pulmonary embolism (rather than deep-venous thrombosis) in patients undergoing total joint replacement (www.aaos.org/guidelines.pdf). In general, the AAOS guidelines are more conservative and recommend routine mechanical prophylaxis and aggressive chemoprophylaxis for higher risk patients only.

Intravenous and Subcutaneous Standard Heparin

Complete systemic heparinization is usually reserved for the most high-risk patients, typically patients with an acute thromboembolism. However, intraoperative admin-istration of a modest intravenous dose is occasionally performed during vascular or orthopedic procedures. In a study involving over 4,000 patients, Rao and El-Etr[22] demonstrated the safety of indwelling spinal and epidural catheters during systemic heparinization. However, the heparin activity was closely monitored, the indwelling catheters were removed at a time when circulating heparin levels were relatively low, and patients with a preexisting coagulation disorder were excluded. A subsequent study in the neurologic literature by Ruff and Dougherty[18] reported spinal hematomas in 7 of 342 patients (2%) who underwent a diagnostic lumbar puncture and subsequent heparinization. Traumatic needle placement, initiation of anticoagulation within 1 hour of lumbar puncture, or concomitant aspirin therapy were identified as risk factors in the development of spinal hematoma in anticoagulated patients (Table 4-1). Overall, large published series and extensive clinical experience suggests that the use of regional techniques during systemic heparinization does

BOX 4-2 Trends in Thromboprophylaxis That May Increase the Risk of Spinal Hematoma

- Thromboprophylaxis (e.g., standard and LMWH for patients undergoing general surgery) is often administered in close proximity to surgery. Unfortunately, early postoperative dosing is associated with surgical (and often anesthesia-related) bleeding.
- Fondaparinux is recommended as an anti-thrombotic agent following major orthopedic surgery. The extended half-life (~ 20 h) impedes safe catheter removal.
- LMWH and dabigatran are dependent on renal metabolism. Dose adjustment for decreased weight and/or renal function is not performed routinely and may result in an exaggerated and prolonged effect.
- The duration of prophylaxis has been extended to include "postdismissal" administration. It has been demonstrated that the risk of bleeding complications is increased with the duration of anticoagulant therapy.
- Newly released and investigational antithrombotic agents are associated with prolonged half-lives, are not routinely monitored for anticoagulant effect, and do not have pharmacologic antidotes.

not appear to represent a significant risk. However, the cases of paralysis relating to spinal hematoma in the ASA Closed Claims database suggest that these events continue to occur and that extreme vigilance is necessary to diagnose and intervene as early as possible, should spinal hematoma be suspected.[16]

Since the publication of the initial American Society of Regional Anesthesia and Pain Medicine (ASRA) guidelines in 1998,[23] there have been continued discussions regarding the relative risk (and benefit) of neuraxial anesthesia and analgesia in the patient undergoing heparinization for cardiopulmonary bypass. Further reports of small series have appeared, again with no reported complications. To date, there is a single case of spinal hematoma following the full heparinization associated with cardiopulmonary bypass.[24] However, there are confounding variables in that the patient was *initially* neurologically intact, but developed paraplegia after anticoagulation/thrombolysis on the second day. Thus, this analgesic technique remains controversial in that the risk appears too great for the perceived benefits. A review has recommended certain precautions to be taken to minimize the risk[25]:

1. Neuraxial blocks should be avoided in a patient with known coagulopathy from any cause,
2. Surgery should be delayed 24 hours in the event of a traumatic tap,
3. Time from instrumentation to systemic heparinization should exceed 60 minutes,
4. Heparin effect and reversal should be tightly controlled (smallest amount of heparin for the shortest duration compatible with therapeutic objectives),

5. Epidural catheters should be removed when normal coagulation is restored, and patients should be closely monitored postoperatively for signs and symptoms of hematoma formation.

Furthermore, Ho et al. calculated the risk of hematoma using a complex mathematical analysis of the probability of predicting a rare event that has not occurred yet; they estimate the probability of a spinal hematoma (based on the totals of 4,583 epidural and 10,840 spinal anesthetics reported without complications) to be in the neighborhood of 1:1,528 for epidural and 1:3,610 for spinal technique.[26] The theoretically increased risk of spinal hematoma and lack of substantial improvement in morbidity and mortality associated with neuraxial techniques among patients undergoing cardiopulmonary bypass warrants caution in this approach.[27]

Administration of 5,000 units of heparin subcutaneously every 12 hours has been used extensively and effectively for prophylaxis against deep-venous thrombosis. There is often no detectable change in the clotting parameters, as measured by the aPTT. There is a minority of patients, perhaps up to 15%, who may develop measurable changes in coagulation, although the aPTT rarely exceeds 1.5 times the normal level.[28] There is a smaller subset (2%–4%) of patients who may become therapeutically anticoagulated during subcutaneous heparin therapy. With therapy >5 days, there is a subset of patients who will develop a decrease in the platelet count.[29]

The widespread use of subcutaneous heparin and paucity of complications suggests that there is little risk of spinal hematoma associated with this therapy. There are nine published series totaling over 9,000 patients who have received this therapy without complications,[23] as well as extensive experience in both Europe and United States without a significant frequency of complications. There are only five case reports of neuraxial hematomas, four epidural,[12,30] and one subarachnoid,[31] during neuraxial block with the use of subcutaneous heparin.

The relative safety of higher doses (e.g., thrice daily dosing) of subcutaneous heparin is unknown. The clinician is currently faced with a decision to proceed with epidural analgesia, as there are no data of concern, or to take a more anticipatory approach of caution, awaiting adverse reports such as may appear in the ASA closed claims database. A review of relevant literature shows that there are reports that document an increased risk of minor and major bleeding in surgical and in nonsurgical patients receiving thrice daily subcutaneous UFH.[32,33] Until more information is provided, a somewhat more cautious approach is suggested, such as enhanced neurologic monitoring and avoidance of additional hemostasis-altering drugs in these patients.

Low-Molecular-Weight Heparin

Prior to the introduction of LMWH for thromboprophylaxis following major orthopedic surgery, spinal hematoma was rarely reported. However, a total of 30 cases of spinal hematoma in patients undergoing spinal or epidural anesthesia while receiving LMWH perioperatively were reported between May 1993 and November 1997 through the MedWatch system.[13] An FDA Health Advisory was issued in

December 1997, and the manufacturers of all LMWH and heparinoids were requested to revise the labeling of their respective products and place a "black box warning."

The majority of spinal hematomas were associated with an epidural technique. Early postoperative (or intraoperative) LMWH administration and concomitant antiplatelet therapy have been identified as risk factors for both increased surgical and anesthetic related bleeding complications[5,6,13] (Box 4-3). The risk of spinal hematoma in patients receiving LMWH was estimated to be approximately 1 in 3,000 continuous epidural anesthetics compared to 1 in 40,000 spinal anesthetics.[7] However, this was most likely an underestimation—there were a number of spinal hematomas that had occurred but had not been reported (and therefore included in the calculations). In total, nearly 60 spinal hematomas were tallied by the FDA between 1993 and 1998.[34] This is noteworthy in that Vandermeulen et al.[12] had identified a total of 61 spinal hematomas in the first 100 years of neuraxial blockade. Although it initially appeared that once daily dosing of LMWH allowed for safe maintenance of indwelling neuraxial catheters, new information from Sweden and Germany suggests that the risk may be nearly as high as that associated with twice daily dosing.[5,35]

The indications and labeled uses for LMWH continue to evolve. Indications for thromboprophylaxis as well as treatment of thromboembolism and acute coronary syndrome have been introduced[3,36] (Table 4-3). In addition, several off-label applications of LMWH are of special interest to the anesthesiologist. LMWH has been demonstrated to be efficacious as a "bridge therapy" for patients chronically anticoagulated with warfarin, including parturients, patients with prosthetic cardiac valves, a history of atrial fibrillation, or preexisting hypercoagulable condition.[37] The doses of LMWH are those associated with thromboembolism treatment, not prophylaxis, and are much higher. The antithrombotic effect may be present for 24 hours following administration.

Oral Anticoagulants

Anesthetic management of patients anticoagulated perioperatively with warfarin is dependent on the dosage and timing of initiation of therapy. The PT and INR of patients on chronic oral anticoagulation will require 3 to 5 days to normalize after discontinuation of the anticoagulant therapy.[37] Theoretically, since the PT and INR reflect predominantly factor VII activity (and factor VII has only a 6- to 8-hour half-life), there may be an interval during which the PT and INR approach normal values, yet factors II and X levels may not be adequate for hemostasis. Adequate levels of *all* vitamin K-dependent factors are typically present when the INR is in the normal range. Therefore, it is recommended that documentation of the patient's normal coagulation status be achieved prior to the implementation of neuraxial block.[10] It is important to note that patients who have only recently normalized their PT/INR following discontinuation of warfarin will have an accelerated response to postoperative warfarin therapy because of residual (subclinical) effect.

Upon initiation of warfarin therapy, the effects are not apparent until a significant amount of biologically inactive factors are synthesized and are dependent on factor half-life:

FACTOR	HALF-LIFE (HOURS)
Factor VII	6–8
Factor IX	24
Factor X	25–60
Factor II	50–80

An understanding of the correlation between the various vitamin K-dependent factor levels and the INR is critical to regional anesthetic management. Clinical experience with patients who congenitally are deficient in factors II, IX, or X suggests that a factor activity level of 40% for *each* factor is adequate for normal or near-normal hemostasis. Bleeding may occur if the level of any clotting factor is decreased to 20% to 40% of baseline. The PT and INR are most sensitive to the activities of factors VII and X and are relatively insensitive to factor II. Since factor VII has a relatively short half-life, prolongation of the PT and INR may occur in 24 to 36 hours. Prolongation of the INR (INR >1.2) occurs when factor VII activity is reduced to approximately 55% of baseline, while an INR = 1.5 is associated with a factor VII activity of 40%. Thus, an INR <1.5 should be associated with normal hemostasis. A recent analysis of factor VII activity levels and PT/INR supported this, but also reported that patients with prolonged PT/INR may have factor VII activity levels that range from normal to markedly decreased. This suggests that a normal PT/INR is reassuring for neuraxial catheterization, but interpretation of a *prolonged* PT/INR and factor VII

BOX 4-3 Patient, Anesthetic, and Low-Molecular-Weight Heparin (LMWH) Dosing Variables Associated with Spinal Hematoma

Patient factors
    Female gender
    Increased age
    Spinal stenosis or ankylosing spondylitis
    Impaired renal function
Anesthetic factors
    Traumatic needle/catheter placement
    Epidural (compared to spinal) technique
    Indwelling epidural catheter during LMWH administration
LMWH dosing factors
    Immediate preoperative or intraoperative LMWH administration
    Early postoperative administration
    Twice daily dosing
    Concomitant antiplatelet or anticoagulant medications

Adapted from Horlocker TT, Wedel DJ, Benzon H, et al. Regional anesthesia in the anticoagulated patient: defining the risks (the second ASRA Consensus Conference on Neuraxial Anesthesia and Anticoagulation). *Reg Anesth Pain Med* 2003;28:172–197. With permission.

activity is difficult and may result in early (and unnecessary) removal of an epidural in approximately 10% of patients.[38]

Management of patients receiving warfarin is based on the pharmacology of the drug, the levels of vitamin K dependent factors required for adequate hemostasis in the surgical setting, and the cases of reported spinal hematoma. Few data exist regarding the risk of spinal hematoma in patients with indwelling epidural catheters who are anticoagulated with warfarin. The optimal duration of an indwelling catheter and the timing of its removal also remain controversial. To date, only three studies, with a combined total of nearly 1,700 patients, have evaluated the risk of spinal hematoma in patients with indwelling spinal or epidural catheters who receive oral anticoagulants perioperatively.[39–41] These investigations noted that patients respond with great variability to warfarin, although the mean PT may not increase outside the normal range until 48 hours after the initiation of therapy; a substantial number of patients will have prolongation after a single dose. Larger doses (greater than warfarin 5 mg) may exaggerate these findings. As a result, it is important to monitor the PT daily to avoid excessive prolongation.[10]

Antiplatelet Medications

Antiplatelet medications are increasingly used as primary agents of thromboprophylaxis. In addition, many orthopedic patients report the chronic use of one or more antiplatelet drugs.[17] Although Vandermeulen et al.[12] implicated antiplatelet therapy in 3 of the 61 cases of spinal hematoma occurring after spinal or epidural anesthesia, several large studies have demonstrated the relative safety of neuraxial blockade in both obstetric, surgical, and pain clinic patients receiving these medications.[17,42,43] In a prospective study involving 1,000 patients, Horlocker et al.[17] reported that preoperative antiplatelet therapy did not increase the incidence of blood present at the time of needle/catheter placement *or* removal, suggesting that trauma incurred during needle or catheter placement is neither increased nor sustained by these medications. The clinician should be aware of the possible increased risk of spinal hematoma in patients receiving antiplatelet medications who undergo subsequent heparinization with a standard or LMWH.[13]

Ticlopidine and clopidogrel, thienopyridines, are also platelet aggregation inhibitors. These agents interfere with platelet-fibrinogen binding and subsequent platelet-platelet interactions. The effect is irreversible for the life of the platelet. Ticlopidine and clopidogrel have no effect on platelet cyclooxygenase and act synergistically with aspirin. Platelet dysfunction is present for 5 to 7 days after discontinuation of clopidogrel and 10 to 14 days with ticlopidine. Serious bleeding complications have been reported after both neuraxial and peripheral (psoas compartment and lumbar sympathetic) techniques in patients receiving ticlopidine or clopidogrel.[9,21] Prasugrel is a new thienopyridine that inhibits platelets more rapidly, more consistently, and to a greater extent than do standard and higher doses of clopidogrel. In the United States, the only labeled indication is for acute coronary syndrome in patients intended to undergo percutaneous coronary intervention. After a single oral dose, 50% of platelets are irreversibly inhibited, with maximum effect 2 hours after administration. Platelet aggregation normalizes in 7 to 9 days after discontinuation of therapy. The labeling

recommends that the drug "be discontinued at least 7 days prior to any surgery."

Platelet glycoprotein (GP) IIb/IIIa receptor antagonists, including abciximab (Reopro), eptifibatide (Integrilin), and tirofiban (Aggrastat), inhibit platelet aggregation by interfering with platelet-fibrinogen binding and subsequent platelet-platelet interactions. Time to normal platelet aggregation following discontinuation of therapy ranges from 8 hours (eptifibatide, tirofiban) to 48 hours (abciximab).

There are no large series of patients who have undergone neuraxial block in combination with the potent antiplatelet agents. However, increased perioperative *surgical* bleeding in patients undergoing cardiac and vascular surgery after receiving ticlopidine, clopidogrel, and GP IIb/IIIa antagonists has been reported.[44] Thus, the risk is likely to be relatively increased. The absolute risk remains undetermined.

Herbal Medications

There is a widespread use of herbal medications in surgical patients. Such complications include bleeding from garlic, ginkgo, and ginseng and potential interaction between ginseng and warfarin. For example, garlic inhibits *in vivo* platelet aggregation in a dose-dependent fashion. The effect of one of its constituents, ajoene, appears to be irreversible and may potentiate the effect of other platelet inhibitors such as prostacyclin, forskolin, indomethacin, and dipyridamole. Although these effects have not been consistently demonstrated in volunteers, there is one case in the literature of an octagenarian who developed a spontaneous epidural hematoma that was attributed to heavy garlic use.[45] Ginkgo also inhibits platelet-activating factor. Clinical trials in a small number of patients have not demonstrated bleeding complications, but four reported cases of spontaneous intracranial bleeding and one case of spontaneous hyphema have been associated with ginkgo use. Based upon the pharmacokinetic data, normalization of coagulation occurs 36 hours after discontinuation of ginkgo.[46] Finally, ginseng inhibits platelet aggregation *in vitro* and prolong both thrombin time (TT) and activated partial thromboplastin time in rats. These findings await confirmation in humans. Although ginseng may inhibit the coagulation cascade, ginseng use was associated with a significant decrease in warfarin anticoagulation in one reported case.[47] The pharmacokinetics of ginsenosides suggest that 24 hours is required to allow resolution of ginseng's effect on hemostasis.

The risk of perioperative (surgical or anesthetic related) bleeding in patients who use herbal medications has not been previously investigated. Likewise, data on the combination of herbal therapy with other forms of anticoagulation/thromboprophylaxis are lacking.

Thrombolytic and Fibrinolytic Therapy

Thrombolytic agents actively dissolve fibrin clots that have already formed. Exogenous plasminogen activators, such as streptokinase and urokinase, not only dissolve thrombus but also affect circulating plasminogen as well, leading to decreased levels of both plasminogen and fibrin. Recombinant tissue-type plasminogen activator (rt-PA), an endogenous agent, is more fibrin selective and has less effect on circulating plasminogen levels. Clot lysis leads to the elevation of fibrin degradation products which themselves have an anticoagulant effect by inhibiting platelet aggregation. Hemostasis remains altered for approximately 1 day after administration of a thrombolytic drug. Fibrinogen is the last factor to recover.

In addition to the fibrinolytic agent, these patients frequently receive intravenous heparin to maintain an aPTT of 1.5 to 2 times normal and clopidogrel/aspirin. No controlled studies have examined the risk. Several cases of spinal hematoma in patients with indwelling epidural catheters who received thrombolytic agents have been reported in the literature and through the MedWatch system.[34]

Guidelines detailing original contraindications for thrombolytic drugs suggest avoidance of these drugs within 10 days of puncture of noncompressible vessels. Data are not available to clearly outline the length of time neuraxial puncture should be avoided after discontinuation of these drugs.

Fondaparinux

Fondaparinux, a synthetic pentasaccharide, was approved in December 2001. The FDA released fondaparinux (Arixtra) with a black box warning similar to that of the LMWHs and heparinoids. Fondaparinux produces its antithrombotic effect through factor Xa inhibition. The plasma half-life of fondaparinux is 21 hours, allowing for single daily dosing, with the first dose administered 6 hours postoperatively. Investigators reported a spinal hematoma among the initial dose-ranging study (at a dose that was subsequently determined to be twice required for thromboprophylaxis).[48,49] No additional spinal hematomas were reported in the combined series of 3,600 patients who underwent spinal or epidural anesthesia in combination with fondaparinux thromboprophylaxis. However, the conditions for performance of neuraxial block were strictly controlled. Patients were included in subsequent clinical trials only if needle placement was atraumatic and accomplished on the first attempt. In addition, indwelling epidural catheters were removed 2 hours prior to fondaparinux administration.[49] These practice guidelines may not be feasible in clinical practice. For example, in a prospective series, <40% of neuraxial blocks were successful with one pass.[17] A recent series of 1,631 patients undergoing continuous neuraxial or deep peripheral block reported no serious hemorrhagic complications. However, the catheters were removed 36 hours after the last dose of fondaparinux, and subsequent dosing was delayed for 12 hours after catheter removal.[50] While these results are reassuring, the deviation from the manufacturer's suggested dosing guidelines is of concern. Although the actual risk of spinal hematoma with fondaparinux is unknown, extreme caution is warranted given the sustained antithrombotic effect, early postoperative dosing, and "irreversibility."

Dabigatran

Dabigatran etexilate is a prodrug that specifically and reversibly inhibits both free and clot-bound thrombin. The drug is absorbed from the gastrointestinal tract with a bioavailability of 5%.[51] Once absorbed, it is converted by esterases into its active metabolite, dabigatran. Plasma levels peak at 2 hours. The half-life is 8 hours after a single dose and up to 17 hours after multiple doses. It is likely that once daily dosing will be possible for some indications because of the prolonged half-life. Because 80% of the drug is excreted unchanged by the kidneys, it is contraindicated in patients with renal

failure.[52] Dabigatran prolongs the aPTT, but its effect is not linear and reaches a plateau at higher doses. *However, the ecarin clotting time (ECT) and thrombin time (TT) are particularly sensitive and display a linear dose response at therapeutic concentrations.* Reversal of anticoagulant effect is theoretically possible through the administration of recombinant factor VIIa, although this has not been attempted clinically.[52] Indeed, product labeling suggests that dialysis may be considered for patients with significant bleeding due to dabigatran.

Clinical trials comparing dabigatran (150 mg or 220 mg, with the first dose administered one to four hours postoperatively) with enoxaparin (40 mg daily with the first dose 12 hours preoperatively) noted little difference in efficacy or bleeding.[53–55] Among published series, there has been no attempt to randomize patients with respect to anesthetic technique nor impose exclusion criteria based on the performance of neuraxial block, including the presence of an indwelling epidural catheter or traumatic needle/catheter placement.[53–55] While there have been no reported spinal hematomas, the lack of information regarding the specifics of block performance and the prolonged half-life warrants a cautious approach. Currently, the only labeled indication is for patients with nonvalvular atrial fibrillation. Fortunately, suspension of anticoagulation therapy in these patients does not place them at significant risk of thromboembolism. Thus, an early discontinuation to allow complete resolution of drug effect (5–7 days, depending on renal function) in anticipation of surgery as well as delayed resumption of dabigatran postoperatively is reasonable.

Rivaroxaban

Rivaroxaban is a potent selective and reversible oral activated factor Xa inhibitor, with an oral bioavailability of 80%. Phase III clinical trials have been completed in the United States. After administration, the maximum inhibitory effect occurs one to four hours; however, inhibition is maintained for 12 hours. The antithrombotic effect may be monitored with the PT, aPTT, and Heptest, all of which demonstrate linear dose effects. Rivaroxaban is cleared by the kidneys and gut. The terminal elimination half-life is 9 hours in healthy volunteers and may be prolonged to 13 hours in the elderly due to a decline in renal function (hence a need for dose adjustment in patients with renal insufficiency and contraindicated in patients with severe liver disease).

Overall, clinical trials comparing rivaroxaban (5–40 mg daily, with the first dose 6 to 8 hours after surgery) with enoxaparin (40 mg, beginning 12 hours before surgery) demonstrate similar rates of bleeding and a comparable efficacy.[49,56–58] While a "regional anesthetic" was performed in over half of the patients included in the clinical trials, no information regarding needle placement or catheter management was included. Although there have been no reported spinal hematomas, the lack of information regarding the specifics of block performance and the prolonged half-life warrants a cautious approach.

Peripheral Techniques

Although spinal hematoma is the most significant hemorrhagic complication of regional anesthesia due to the catastrophic nature of bleeding into a fixed and noncompressible space, the associated risk following plexus and peripheral techniques remains undefined. There are no investigations that examine the frequency and severity of hemorrhagic complications following plexus or peripheral blockade in anticoagulated patients. However, few reports of serious complications following neurovascular sheath cannulation for surgical, radiological, or cardiac indications have been reported. Overall, there have been 26 cases of hemorrhagic complications in patients reported following plexus/peripheral techniques; in 13 cases, the patient had altered hemostasis. The cases of major bleeding were likely to occur following psoas compartment or lumbar sympathetic blockade and/or in the presence of anticoagulants or antiplatelet agents. Neurologic compromise was not always reported.[9,10,59,60]

These cases suggest that significant blood loss (resulting in transfusion or even death), rather than neural deficits, may be the most serious complication of non-neuraxial regional techniques in the anticoagulated patient. Given the paucity of information, it is impossible to make definitive recommendations. Conservatively, the Consensus Statements on Neuraxial Anesthesia and Anticoagulation may be applied to plexus and peripheral techniques.[10] However, this may be more restrictive than necessary for techniques involving superficial and compressible vasculature.

▶ DIAGNOSIS

The differential diagnosis of new or progressive postoperative neurologic symptoms includes surgical neuropraxia, prolonged/exaggerated neuraxial block, anterior spinal artery syndrome, exacerbation of a preexisting neurologic disorder, and presentation of a previously undiagnosed neurologic condition, as well as spinal hematoma. The onset of symptoms immediately postoperatively is uncommon; it is rare for a spinal hematoma to present as a "prolonged" neuraxial block.[5,6,12] The time interval between needle placement/initiation of thromboprophylaxis and neurologic dysfunction is typically on the order of days.[6,12] Once new neurologic deficits are noted, complete paralysis develops over 10 to 15 hours.

▶ PREVENTION

Recommendations are based on the proceedings of the American Society of Regional Anesthesia and Pain Medicine Third Consensus Conference on Regional Anesthesia and Anticoagulation[10] (Table 4-4). The consensus statements and the supporting document are available on the Society's website, asra.com.

Standard Heparin

- Regional anesthesia and intravenous heparinization for patients undergoing vascular surgery is acceptable with the following recommendations (Grade 1A):
  - Delay intravenous heparin administration for 1 hour after needle/catheter placement.
  - Prolonged anticoagulation appears to increase the risk of spinal hematoma formation, especially if combined with other anticoagulants or thrombolytics. If systematic anticoagulation therapy is begun with an epidural catheter in

place, delay catheter removal for 2 to 4 hours following heparin discontinuation and after evaluation of coagulation status.
  - Remove indwelling catheters 1 hour before a subsequent heparin administration.
- There is no contradiction to the use of neuraxial techniques during subcutaneous standard heparin at total doses <10,000 units daily. The risk of spinal hematoma with larger daily subcutaneous doses is unclear; assess on an individual basis and implement more aggressive neurologic monitoring (Grade 2C).
- A platelet count is indicated for patients receiving subcutaneous heparin for >5 days (Grade B).

Low-Molecular-Weight Heparin

- Concomitant antiplatelet or oral anticoagulant medications administered in combination with LMWH is not recommended (Grade 1A).

Preoperative LMWH

- Perform neuraxial techniques at least 10 to 12 hours after a thromboprophylaxis dose and 24 hours after a "treatment" dose of LMWH (Grade 1C).
- Avoid neuraxial techniques in patients who have received a dose of LMWH 2 hours preoperatively (general surgery patients), as needle placement would occur during peak anticoagulant activity (Grade 1A).

Postoperative LMWH

- With twice daily dosing, administer the first dose of LMWH no earlier than 24 hours postoperatively, regardless of anesthetic technique, and only in the presence of adequate hemostasis (Grade 1C).
  - Remove indwelling catheters prior to the initiation of LMWH thromboprophylaxis.
  - The first dose of LMWH administered 2 hours after catheter removal and 24 hours after needle/catheter placement, whichever is later.
- Once daily dosing requires 6 to 8 hours between needle/catheter placement and the first dose of LMWH. Subsequent dosing should occur no sooner than 24 hours later (Grade 1C).

Oral Anticoagulants

- Discontinue oral anticoagulation and verify PT normalization prior to neuraxial block (Grade 1B).
- Monitor the PT and INR daily (Grade 2C).
- Remove indwelling neuraxial catheters when the INR <1.5 in order to ensure adequate levels of all vitamin K-dependent factors are present (Grade 2C).
- There is no definitive recommendation for facilitating the removal of neuraxial catheters in patients with and INR >1.5 but <3.0. Removal of neuraxial catheters should be done with caution and neurologic status assessed until the INR has stabilized (Grade 1C).
- In patients with an INR >3, warfarin should be held. No definitive recommendation can be made regarding the management to facilitate removal of neuraxial catheters (e.g., partial or complete reversal of anticoagulant effect vs. discontinuation of warfarin therapy with spontaneous recovery of hemostasis). Individual factor levels may be helpful (Grade 2C).

TABLE 4-4 Recommendations for Management of Patients Receiving Neuraxial Blockade and Anticoagulant Drugs

Warfarin	Discontinue chronic warfarin therapy 4–5 d before spinal procedure and evaluate INR. INR should be within the normal range at time of procedure to ensure adequate levels of all vitamin K-dependent factors. Postoperatively, daily INR assessment with catheter removal occurring with INR<1.5.
Antiplatelet medications	No contraindications with aspirin or other NSAIDs. Thienopyridine derivatives (clopidogrel and prasugrel) should be discontinued 7 d and ticlopidine 14 d prior to procedure. GP IIb/IIIa inhibitors should be discontinued to allow recovery of platelet function prior to procedure (8 h for tirofiban and eptifibatide, 24–48 h for abciximab).
Thrombolytics/fibrinolytics	There are no available data to suggest a safe interval between procedure and initiation or discontinuation of these medications. Follow fibrinogen level and observe for signs of neural compression.
LMWH	Delay procedure at least 12 h from the last dose of thromboprophylaxis LMWH dose. For "treatment" dosing of LMWH, at least 24 h should elapse prior to the procedure. LMWH should not be administered within 24 h after the procedure. Indwelling epidural catheters should be maintained only with once daily dosing of LMWH and strict avoidance of additional hemostasis-altering medications, including ketorolac.
Unfractionated SQ heparin	There are no contraindications to neuraxial procedure if total daily dose is <10,000 units. For higher dosing regimens, increase neurologic monitoring and cautiously co-administer antiplatelet medications.
Unfractionated IV heparin	Delay needle/catheter placement 2–4 h after the last dose, document normal aPTT. Heparin may be restarted 1 h following procedure. Sustained heparinization with an indwelling neuraxial catheter associated with increased risk; monitor neurologic status aggressively.
Dabigatran	Discontinue 7 d prior to procedure; for shorter time periods, document normal TT. First postoperative dose 24 h after needle placement and 2 h postcatheter removal (whichever is later).

NSAIDs, nonsteroidal antiinflammatory drugs; GP IIb/IIIa, platelet glycoprotein receptor IIb/IIIa inhibitors; INR, international normalized ratio; LMWH, low-molecular-weight heparin; aPTT, activated partial thromboplastin time; TT, thrombin time.
Recommendations from Horlocker TT, Wedel DJ, Rowlingson JC, et al. Regional anesthesia in the patient receiving antithrombotic or thrombolytic therapy: American Society of Regional Anesthesia and Pain Medicine Evidence-Based Guidelines (Third Edition). *Reg Anesth Pain Med* 2010;35:64–101.

Antiplatelet Medications

- The concurrent use of medications that affect other components of the clotting mechanisms, such as oral anticoagulants, standard heparin, and LMWH, increases the risk of bleeding complications for patients receiving antiplatelet agents (Grade 2C).
- NSAIDs, by themselves, represent no significant risk for the development of spinal hematoma in patients having epidural or spinal anesthesia (Grade 1A).
- Allow platelet function to recover prior to neuraxial block after the administration of ticlopidine, clopidogrel, and platelet GP IIb/IIIa receptor antagonists. The time to normal platelet aggregation following discontinuation of therapy is 14 days for ticlopidine, 5 to 7 days for clopidogrel, and 7 to 10 days for prasugrel. For the platelet GP IIb/IIIa inhibitors, the duration ranges from 8 hours for eptifibatide and tirofiban to 48 hours following abciximab administration (Grade 1C).

Herbal Therapy

- Herbal drugs do not add significant risk for the development of spinal hematoma in patients having epidural or spinal anesthesia and may be safely administered in combination (Grade 1C).

Thrombolytics and Fibrinolytics

- Patients receiving fibrinolytic and thrombolytic drugs should be cautioned against receiving spinal or epidural anesthetics except in highly unusual circumstances (Grade 1A).
- There is no definitive recommendation for the removal of neuraxial catheters in patients who unexpectedly receive fibrinolytic and thrombolytic therapy during a neuraxial catheter infusion. The measurement of fibrinogen may be helpful in making a decision about catheter removal or maintenance (Grade 2C).

Fondaparinux

• Until additional clinical information is obtained, perform neuraxial techniques under conditions utilized in clinical trials (single-needle pass, atraumatic needle placement, avoidance of indwelling neuraxial catheters). If this is not feasible, an alternate method of prophylaxis should be utilized (Grade 2C).

Dabigatran

• Given the irreversibility of dabigtran, the prolonged half-life and the uncertainty of an individual patient's renal function, dabigatran should be discontinued 7 days prior to neuraxial block. If a shorter time interval is desired, reversal of anticoagulant effect should be documented by the assessment of TT. Neuraxial catheters should be removed at least 2 hours prior to the initiation of dabigatran therapy (Grade 2C).

Anesthetic Management of the Patient Undergoing Plexus or Peripheral Block

For patients undergoing deep plexus or deep peripheral block, recommendations regarding neuraxial techniques should be similarly applied (Grade 1C).

▶ TREATMENT

Evaluation is focused on the identification of reversible/treatable causes. Therefore, any new or progressive neurologic symptoms occurring in the presence of epidural analgesia warrant immediate discontinuation of the infusion (with the catheter left *in situ*) to rule out any contribution from the local anesthetic or volume effect. If the epidural is the etiology of the deficits, a prompt return of function should be noted. Since neurologic outcome is linked to early diagnosis and intervention, it is critical to obtain radiographic imaging, preferably magnetic resonance imaging (MRI), as soon as possible. Consultation with a neurosurgeon should also occur as soon as possible to determine the urgency of surgery. Interestingly, not all spinal hematomas are treated with emergency laminectomy; spontaneous resolution of deficits has been reported.[5,12,13] However, the decision to observe versus surgically intervene is a neurosurgical one.

In all series, the neurologic outcome is poor for the majority of patients.[5,12,13] In addition, it was noted that if more than 8 hours was allowed to elapse between the development of paralysis and surgical intervention, complete neurologic recovery was unlikely.[12]

▶ FUTURE DIRECTIONS

Finally, new antithrombotic drugs that target various steps in the hemostatic system, such as inhibiting platelet aggregation, blocking coagulation factors, or enhancing fibrinolysis, are continually under development. The most extensively studied are antagonists of specific platelet receptors and direct thrombin inhibitors. Many of these antithrombotic agents have prolonged half-lives and bleeding is difficult (or impossible) to reverse even with the administration of blood components.

It will probably not be possible to evaluate the risk of spinal hematoma based on data from the Phase II and III clinical trials of new agents. Pharmaceutical companies and the Food and Drug Administration (FDA) construct methodologies to minimize the potential for this catastrophic complication. Until a large body of literature is available to document the safety of neuraxial techniques in patients treated with antithrombotic medications such as fondaparinux, the decision to perform neuraxial blockade should consider the frequency and severity of surgical bleeding (as a surrogate for spinal bleeding), the conditions under which neuraxial block was performed during the clinical trials, and the risk of alternative anesthetic techniques. Importantly, the prolonged effect of the investigational antithrombotic agents will make it difficult to remove indwelling catheters during normal hemostasis. As a result, it is likely that indwelling neuraxial catheters will be removed prior to the initiation of thromboprophylaxis.

▶ SUMMARY

Recognition of the risk associated with spinal and epidural blockade and anticoagulation, continued surveillance and evaluation of the current information, and education are all crucial to averting future cases of spinal hematoma. Ultimately, this will require the combined efforts of the FDA, health care providers, and the industry. The introduction of new anticoagulants and antiplatelet agents, the complexity of balancing thromboembolic with hemorrhagic complications, and the evolving indications for regional anesthesia/analgesia necessitate an individualized approach. Thus, the decision to perform spinal or epidural anesthesia/analgesia and the timing of catheter removal in a patient receiving antithrombotic therapy should be made on an individual basis, weighing the small, though definite risk of spinal hematoma with the benefits of regional anesthesia for a specific patient. Alternative anesthetic and analgesic techniques exist for patients considered an unacceptable risk. The patient's coagulation status should be optimized at the time of spinal or epidural needle/catheter placement, and the level of anticoagulation must be carefully monitored during the period of epidural catheterization. Indwelling catheters should not be removed in the presence of therapeutic anticoagulation, as this appears to significantly increase the risk of spinal hematoma. It must also be remembered that identification of risk factors and establishment of guidelines will not completely eliminate the complication of spinal hematoma. In Vandermeulen et al.'s[12] series, although 87% of patients had a hemostatic abnormality or difficulty with needle puncture, 13% had no identifiable risk factor. Vigilance in monitoring is critical to allow early evaluation of neurologic dysfunction and prompt intervention. We must focus not only on the prevention of spinal hematoma, but also on the optimization of neurologic outcome.

References

1. Usubiaga JE. Neurologic complications following epidural anesthesia. *Int Anesthesiol Clin* 1975;13:1–153.

2. Bonica JJ. *The Management of Pain (First Edition)*. Philadelphia, PA: Lea and Febiger, 1953.
3. Geerts WH, Bergqvist D, Pineo GF, et al. Prevention of venous thromboembolism: American College of Chest Physicians Evidence-Based Clinical Practice Guidelines (8th Edition). *Chest* 2008;133:381S–453S.
4. Tryba M. Epidural regional anesthesia and low molecular heparin: Pro. *Anasthesiol Intensivmed Notfallmed Schmerzther* 1993;28:179–181.
5. Moen V, Dahlgren N, Irestedt L. Severe neurological complications after central neuraxial blockades in Sweden 1990–1999. *Anesthesiology* 2004;101:950–959.
6. Horlocker TT, Wedel DJ. Anticoagulation and neuraxial blockade: historical perspective, anesthetic implications, and risk management. *Reg Anesth Pain Med* 1998;23:129–134.
7. Schroeder DR. Statistics: detecting a rare adverse drug reaction using spontaneous reports. *Reg Anesth Pain Med* 1998;23:183–189.
8. Stafford-Smith M. Impaired haemostasis and regional anaesthesia. *Can J Anaesth* 1996;43:R129–R141.
9. Maier C, Gleim M, Weiss T, et al. Severe bleeding following lumbar sympathetic blockade in two patients under medication with irreversible platelet aggregation inhibitors. *Anesthesiology* 2002;97:740–743.
10. Horlocker TT, Wedel DJ, Rowlingson JC, et al. Regional anesthesia in the patient receiving antithrombotic or thrombolytic therapy: American Society of Regional Anesthesia and Pain Medicine Evidence-Based Guidelines (Third Edition). *Reg Anesth Pain Med* 2010;35:64–101.
11. Weller RS, Gerancher JC, Crews JC, et al. Extensive retroperitoneal hematoma without neurologic deficit in two patients who underwent lumbar plexus block and were later anticoagulated. *Anesthesiology* 2003;98:581–585.
12. Vandermeulen EP, Van Aken H, Vermylen J. Anticoagulants and spinal-epidural anesthesia. *Anesth Analg* 1994;79:1165–1177.
13. Horlocker TT, Wedel DJ. Neuraxial block and low-molecular-weight heparin: balancing perioperative analgesia and thromboprophylaxis. *Reg Anesth Pain Med* 1998;23:164–177.
14. Groen RJ, van Alphen HA. Operative treatment of spontaneous spinal epidural hematomas: a study of the factors determining postoperative outcome. *Neurosurgery* 1996;39:494–508;discussion 508–509.
15. Schulman S, Beyth RJ, Kearon C, et al. Hemorrhagic complications of anticoagulant and thrombolytic treatment: American College of Chest Physicians Evidence-Based Clinical Practice Guidelines (8th Edition). *Chest* 2008;133:257S–298S.
16. Cheney FW, Domino KB, Caplan RA, et al. Nerve injury associated with anesthesia: a closed claims analysis. *Anesthesiology* 1999;90:1062–1069.
17. Horlocker TT, Wedel DJ, Schroeder DR, et al. Preoperative antiplatelet therapy does not increase the risk of spinal hematoma associated with regional anesthesia. *Anesth Analg* 1995;80:303–309.
18. Ruff RL, Dougherty JH Jr. Complications of lumbar puncture followed by anticoagulation. *Stroke* 1981;12:879–881.
19. Lindgren L, Silvanto M, Scheinin B, et al. Erythrocyte counts in the cerebrospinal fluid associated with continuous spinal anaesthesia. *Acta Anaesthesiol Scand* 1995;39:396–400.
20. Horlocker TT, Wedel DJ, Schlichting JL. Postoperative epidural analgesia and oral anticoagulant therapy. *Anesth Analg* 1994;79:89–93.
21. Layton KF, Kallmes DF, Horlocker TT. Recommendations for anticoagulated patients undergoing image-guided spinal procedures. *AJNR Am J Neuroradiol* 2006;27:468–470.
22. Rao TL, El-Etr AA. Anticoagulation following placement of epidural and subarachnoid catheters: an evaluation of neurologic sequelae. *Anesthesiology* 1981;55:618–620.
23. Liu SS, Mulroy MF. Neuraxial anesthesia and analgesia in the presence of standard heparin. *Reg Anesth Pain Med* 1998;23:157–163.
24. Rosen DA, Hawkinberry DW 2nd, Rosen KR, et al. An epidural hematoma in an adolescent patient after cardiac surgery. *Anesth Analg* 2004;98:966–969.
25. Chaney MA. Intrathecal and epidural anesthesia and analgesia for cardiac surgery. *Anesth Analg* 1997;84:1211–1221.
26. Ho AM, Chung DC, Joynt GM. Neuraxial blockade and hematoma in cardiac surgery: estimating the risk of a rare adverse event that has not (yet) occurred. *Chest* 2000;117:551–555.
27. Liu SS, Block BM, Wu CL. Effects of perioperative central neuraxial analgesia on outcome after coronary artery bypass surgery: a meta-analysis. *Anesthesiology* 2004;101:153–161.
28. Gallus AS, Hirsh J, Tutle RJ, et al. Small subcutaneous doses of heparin in prevention of venous thrombosis. *N Engl J Med* 1973;288:545–551.
29. Hirsh J, Bauer KA, Donati MB, et al. Parenteral anticoagulants: American College of Chest Physicians Evidence-Based Practice Guidelines (8th Edition). *Chest* 2008;133:141S–159S.
30. Sandhu H, Morley-Forster P, Spadafora S. Epidural hematoma following epidural analgesia in a patient receiving unfractionated heparin for thromboprophylaxis. *Reg Anesth Pain Med* 2000;25:72–75.
31. Greaves JD. Serious spinal cord injury due to haematomyelia caused by spinal anaesthesia in a patient treated with low-dose heparin. *Anaesthesia* 1997;52:150–154.
32. King CS, Holley AB, Jackson JL, et al. Twice vs three times daily heparin dosing for thromboembolism prophylaxis in the general medical population: a metaanalysis. *Chest* 2007;131:507–516.
33. Leonardi MJ, McGory ML, Ko CY. The rate of bleeding complications after pharmacologic deep venous thrombosis prophylaxis: a systematic review of 33 randomized controlled trials. *Arch Surg* 2006;141:790–797.
34. Horlocker TT, Wedel DJ, Benzon H, et al. Regional anesthesia in the anticoagulated patient: defining the risks (the second ASRA Consensus Conference on Neuraxial Anesthesia and Anticoagulation). *Reg Anesth Pain Med* 2003;28:172–197.
35. Litz RJ, Gottschlich B, Stehr SN. Spinal epidural hematoma after spinal anesthesia in a patient treated with clopidogrel and enoxaparin. *Anesthesiology* 2004;101:1467–1470.
36. Douketis JD, Berger PB, Dunn AS, et al. The perioperative management of antithrombotic therapy: American College of Chest Physicians Evidence-Based Clinical Practice Guidelines (8th Edition). *Chest* 2008;133:299S–339S.
37. Heit JA. Perioperative management of the chronically anticoagulated patient. *J Thromb Thrombolysis* 2001;12:81–87.
38. Benzon HT, Avram MJ, Benzon HA, et al. Factor VII levels and international normalized ratios in the early phase of warfarin therapy. *Anesthesiology* 2010;112:298–304.
39. Horlocker TT, Cabanela ME, Wedel DJ. Does postoperative epidural analgesia increase the risk of peroneal nerve palsy after total knee arthroplasty? *Anesth Analg* 1994;79:495–500.
40. Odoom JA, Sih IL. Epidural analgesia and anticoagulant therapy. Experience with one thousand cases of continuous epidurals. *Anaesthesia* 1983;38:254–259.
41. Wu CL, Perkins FM. Oral anticoagulant prophylaxis and epidural catheter removal. *Reg Anesth* 1996;21:517–524.
42. CLASP: a randomised trial of low-dose aspirin for the prevention and treatment of pre-eclampsia among 9364 pregnant women. CLASP (Collaborative Low-dose Aspirin Study in Pregnancy) Collaborative Group. *Lancet* 1994;343:619–629.
43. Horlocker TT, Bajwa ZH, Ashraf Z, et al. Risk assessment of hemorrhagic complications associated with nonsteroidal antiinflammatory medications in ambulatory pain clinic patients undergoing epidural steroid injection. *Anesth Analg* 2002;95:1691–1697.
44. Kovesi T, Royston D. Is there a bleeding problem with platelet-active drugs? *Br J Anaesth* 2002;88:159–163.
45. Rose KD, Croissant PD, Parliament CF, et al. Spontaneous spinal epidural hematoma with associated platelet dysfunction from excessive garlic ingestion: a case report. *Neurosurgery* 1990;26:880–882.

46. Chung KF, Dent G, McCusker M, et al. Effect of a ginkgolide mixture (BN 52063) in antagonising skin and platelet responses to platelet activating factor in man. *Lancet* 1987;1:248–251.

47. Janetzky K, Morreale AP. Probable interaction between warfarin and ginseng. *Am J Health Syst Pharm* 1997;54:692–693.

48. Landow L. A synthetic pentasaccharide for the prevention of deep-vein thrombosis. *N Engl J Med* 2001;345:291–292.

49. Turpie AG, Fisher WD, Bauer KA, et al. BAY 59–7939: an oral, direct factor Xa inhibitor for the prevention of venous thromboembolism in patients after total knee replacement. A phase II dose-ranging study. *J Thromb Haemost* 2005;3:2479–2486.

50. Singelyn FJ, Verheyen CC, Piovella F, et al. The safety and efficacy of extended thromboprophylaxis with fondaparinux after major orthopedic surgery of the lower limb with or without a neuraxial or deep peripheral nerve catheter: the EXPERT Study. *Anesth Analg* 2007;105:1540–1547.

51. Weitz JI, Hirsh J, Samama MM. New antithrombotic drugs: American College of Chest Physicians Evidence-Based Clinical Practice Guidelines (8th Edition). *Chest* 2008;133:234S–256S.

52. Eriksson BI, Quinlan DJ, Weitz JI. Comparative pharmacodynamics and pharmacokinetics of oral direct thrombin and factor xa inhibitors in development. *Clin Pharmacokinet* 2009;48:1–22.

53. Eriksson BI, Dahl OE, Buller HR, et al. A new oral direct thrombin inhibitor, dabigatran etexilate, compared with enoxaparin for prevention of thromboembolic events following total hip or knee replacement: the BISTRO II randomized trial. *J Thromb Haemost* 2005;3:103–111.

54. Eriksson BI, Dahl OE, Rosencher N, et al. Oral dabigatran etexilate vs. subcutaneous enoxaparin for the prevention of venous thromboembolism after total knee replacement: the RE-MODEL randomized trial. *J Thromb Haemost* 2007;5:2178–2185.

55. Eriksson BI, Dahl OE, Rosencher N, et al. Dabigatran etexilate versus enoxaparin for prevention of venous thromboembolism after total hip replacement: a randomised, double-blind, non-inferiority trial. *Lancet* 2007;370:949–956.

56. Fisher WD, Eriksson BI, Bauer KA, et al. Rivaroxaban for thromboprophylaxis after orthopaedic surgery: pooled analysis of two studies. *Thromb Haemost* 2007;97:931–937.

57. Lassen MR, Ageno W, Borris LC, et al. Rivaroxaban versus enoxaparin for thromboprophylaxis after total knee arthroplasty. *N Engl J Med* 2008;358:2776–2786.

58. Eriksson BI, Borris LC, Dahl OE, et al. A once-daily, oral, direct Factor Xa inhibitor, rivaroxaban (BAY 59–7939), for thromboprophylaxis after total hip replacement. *Circulation* 2006;114:2374–2381.

59. Klein SM, D'Ercole F, Greengrass RA, et al. Enoxaparin associated with psoas hematoma and lumbar plexopathy after lumbar plexus block. *Anesthesiology* 1997;87:1576–1579.

60. Weller R, Rosenblum M, Conard P, et al. Comparison of epidural and patient-controlled intravenous morphine following joint replacement surgery. *Canad J Anaesth* 1991;38:582–586.

5

Infectious Complications

Adam D. Niesen, Denise J. Wedel, and Terese T. Horlocker

Although infectious complications are rarely associated with regional anesthetic or pain-management techniques, they can range from minor colonization of indwelling devices to major medical emergencies associated with meningitis or epidural abscess. This chapter explores the infectious complications of neuraxial and peripheral nerve blockade.

▶ DEFINITION

Infectious complications may occur after any regional anesthetic technique but are of greatest concern if the infection occurs near or within the neuraxis. The possible risk factors include underlying sepsis, diabetes, depressed immune status, steroid therapy, localized bacterial colonization or infection, and prolonged catheter duration. Bacterial infection within the neuraxis may present either as meningitis or with cord compression secondary to abscess formation. The infectious source may be exogenous (as from contaminated equipment or medication) or endogenous (seeding from a bacterial source to the needle or catheter site). Microorganisms can also be transmitted via a break in aseptic technique, and indwelling catheters may be colonized from superficial

skin pathogens, which subsequently spread to the epidural or intrathecal space. Peripheral nerve blocks, with or without catheter placement, may also rarely be associated with infectious sequelae.

▶ SCOPE

Although individual cases have been reported, serious neuraxial infections such as meningitis and abscess following spinal or epidural anesthesia are fortunately rare (Table 5-1). Infectious complications following peripheral nerve blockade are even less common. In the early 1980s, a combined series of more than 65,000 spinal anesthetics reported only three cases of meningitis and failed to disclose a single epidural or intrathecal infection in approximately 50,000 epidural anesthetics.[1] In 1997, a French multicenter prospective study by Auroy et al. that included 40,640 spinal and 30,413 epidural anesthetics reported no infectious complications.[2] Several recent large Scandinavian studies have attempted to define the risk in their populations by reviewing large databases with known denominators. Aromaa et al.[3] reported eight cases of bacterial infections in Finnish

TABLE 5-1 **Infectious Complications Following Neuraxial Anesthesia**

AUTHOR, YEAR	NUMBER OF PATIENTS	POPULATION	REGIONAL TECHNIQUES	ANTIBIOTIC PROPHYLAXIS	DURATION OF INDWELLING CATHETER	COMPLICATIONS
Kane, 1981[1]	115,000	Surgical and obstetric	65,000 spinal 50,000 epidural	Unknown	Unknown	Three meningitis (all after spinal anesthesia)
DuPen, 1990[28]	350	Cancer and AIDS patients	Permanent (tunneled) epidural analgesia	No	4–1,460 d	30 insertion site infections, 19 deep-track or epidural space infections. Treated with antibiotics and epidural removal. Fifteen uneventfully replaced.
Scott, 1990[10]	505,000	Obstetrics	Epidural	Unknown	Unknown	One epidural abscess, partial recovery after laminectomy
Bader, 1992[24]	319	Parturients with chorioamnionitis	224 epidural 29 spinal 50 local anesthesia (26 general anesthesia)	Yes, in 13%	Surgery only	None
Strafford, 1995[27]	1,620	Pediatric surgical	Epidural analgesia	No	2.4 d median	Three positive epidural catheter tip cultures One candida colonization of epidural space (also with necrotic tumor)
Goodman, 1996[25]	531	Parturients with chorioamnionitis	15 spinal 517 epidural anesthesia and analgesia	Yes, in 23%	>24 h in 64 patients	None
Dahlgren, 1995[20]	18,000	All indications and ages	8,768 spinal 9,232 epidural	Unknown	Unknown	None
Kindler, 1996[21]	13,000	4,000 obstetrics 9,000 surgical	Epidural	Unknown	Unknown	Two epidural abscess, both required laminectomy
Auroy, 1997[2]	71,053	Surgical	40,640 spinal 30,413 epidural	Unknown	Unknown	None
Aromaa, 1997[3]	720,000	Surgical	170,000 epidural 550,000 spinal	Unknown	Unknown	Four meningitis Two epidural abscess Two discitis Two superficial skin infection

(Continued)

TABLE 5-1   Infectious Complications Following Neuraxial Anesthesia (Continued)

AUTHOR, YEAR	NUMBER OF PATIENTS	POPULATION	REGIONAL TECHNIQUES	ANTIBIOTIC PROPHYLAXIS	DURATION OF INDWELLING CATHETER	COMPLICATIONS
Wang, 1999[4]	17,372	Perioperative, cancer, and trauma pain	Epidural	Unknown	11 d mean 6 d median	Nine epidural abscesses Two subcutaneous infections
Moen, 2004[5]	1,710,000	Pain, surgical, and parturients (200,000)	1,260,000 spinal 450,000 epidural	Unknown	2 d–5 wk	29 meningitis 13 epidural abscess
Cameron, 2007[6]	8,210	Postoperative pain	Epidural	Unknown	2.8 d mean	Six epidural abscess, one required laminectomy; all recovered 184 epidural insertion site infection
Christie, 2007[8]	8,100	Postoperative pain	Epidural	Unknown	5.5 d median for epidural abscess 4 d median for meningitis	Six epidural abscess Three meningitis
The Third National Audit Project of The Royal College of Anaesthetists, 2009[9]	707,425	Perioperative, obstetric, chronic pain, and pediatric	324,950 spinal 293,050 epidural 41,875 combined spinal-epidural 47,550 caudal	Unknown		15 epidural abscess Three meningitis
Green, 2010[7]	9,482	Obstetric	Epidural			Two epidural abscess Two paraspinal abscess

patients undergoing 170,000 epidural and 550,000 spinal anesthetics (1.1:100,000 blocks). A matter of concern is that Wang et al's.[4] Danish survey estimated the incidence of epidural abscess following epidural catheter to be 1:1,930 cases. Finally, Moen et al.[5] reviewed the Swedish experience from 1990 to 1999, reporting a low incidence of epidural abscess but an alarming association of postspinal block meningitis with alpha-hemolytic streptococcal cultures, suggesting a nosocomial origin.

More recent data from multiple reports worldwide confirm the infrequent incidence of major infectious complications following neuraxial blockade, but echo this wide variability in frequency. In Australia, epidural abscesses were identified at a rate of 1:1,368 in patients receiving epidural analgesia for acute postoperative pain,[6] and 1:4,742 in women who received an epidural for labor and delivery.[7] A United Kingdom (UK) 5-year retrospective review of epidural catheters placed for postoperative analgesia in a cohort of 8,100 patients reported six cases of epidural abscess (1:1,350) and three cases of meningitis (1:2,700).[8] A subsequent nationwide audit of major complications after epidural, subarachnoid, caudal, and combined spinal/epidural techniques in the UK was performed. Fifteen cases of epidural abscess and three cases of meningitis were identified in an estimated 707,425 procedures annually (1:39,301).[9] Of note, epidural analgesia was found to have a significantly higher risk of infectious complications when compared to spinal anesthesia.

The obstetrical patient group is an interesting subset, with epidural-related infections being extremely rare. Scott and Hibbard[10] reported only a single epidural abscess in 505,000 epidurals for obstetrical analgesia and anesthesia over a 4-year period in the UK. Moen et al.[5] also noted a significantly lower incidence of infectious complications following epidural anesthesia in the obstetrical population (1:25,000) compared to the nonobstetrical population (1:3,600). A more recent retrospective chart review of 9,482 epidural placements in obstetric patients by Green and Paech[7] from a major teaching hospital in Australia reported two epidural abscesses (1:4,741). There was no comparison to nonobstetric epidural catheter placement in this study. Relatively short catheter durations and lack of immunocompromise in this generally healthy population are factors that may contribute to the apparently lower incidence of infectious complications.

▶ PATHOPHYSIOLOGY

Meningitis

Meningeal puncture has long been considered a risk factor in the pathogenesis of meningitis (Table 5-2). Exactly how microbes cross from the bloodstream into the spinal fluid is unknown. The suggested mechanisms include the introduction of blood into the intrathecal space during needle placement and/or the disruption of the protection provided by the blood-brain barrier. However, lumbar puncture is often performed in patients with fever or infection of unknown origin. If dural puncture during bacteremia results in meningitis, definite clinical data should exist. In fact, clinical studies are sparse and often outdated.

Early laboratory and clinical investigations date back to the early 1900s (Table 5-1), when Weed et al.[11] demonstrated in an animal model that lumbar or cisternal puncture performed during septicemia (produced by lethal doses of IV-administered gram-negative bacillus) invariably resulted in a fatal meningitis. In the same year, Wegeforth and Latham[12] reported their clinical observations on 93 patients with suspected meningitis who received a diagnostic lumbar puncture. Blood cultures were taken simultaneously. The diagnosis of meningitis was confirmed in 38 patients. The remaining 55 patients had normal cerebrospinal fluid (CSF). However, 6 of these 55 patients were bacteremic at the time of lumbar puncture, and 5 of the 6 patients subsequently developed meningitis. It was implied, but not stated, that patients with both sterile blood and CSF cultures at the time of puncture did not develop meningitis. Unfortunately, these lumbar punctures were performed during two epidemics of meningitis at a military installation, and it is possible that some (or all) of these patients may have developed meningitis without lumbar puncture. These two historical studies provided support for the claim that lumbar puncture during bacteremia was a risk factor for meningitis. Subsequent clinical studies reported conflicting results. In two studies of bacteremic patients undergoing diagnostic lumbar puncture, the incidence of meningitis was no greater among patients subjected to lumbar puncture than those who were not[13]; and there was also no difference in the incidence of postlumbar puncture meningitis compared to spontaneous meningitis.[14] The authors concluded: "If lumbar puncture induced meningitis does occur, it is rare enough to be clinically insignificant."[14] In contrast, a review of meningitis associated with serial lumbar punctures to treat posthemorrhagic hydrocephalus in premature infants implicated bacteremia (typically associated with central venous or umbilical artery catheterization) as a risk factor for developing meningitis.[15] Results regarding the relative risk of repeated dural punctures, difficult or traumatic procedures, and the use of antibiotics around the time of the lumbar puncture are mixed and likely affected by treatment bias.[15,16]

Although the prevention of lumbar puncture-induced meningitis with antibiotic therapy seems intuitively possible, there are limited clinically applicable data in the literature. In a more modern version of the animal study performed in the early 1900s, 12 of 40 rats subjected to cisternal puncture during *Escherichia coli* bacteremia subsequently developed meningitis.[17] Meningitis occurred only in animals with blood cultures documenting >50 colony-forming units/mL at the time of dural puncture, a circulating bacterial count observed in patients with infective endocarditis. However, bacteremic rats treated with a single dose of gentamicin immediately prior to cisternal puncture did not develop meningitis. Unfortunately, this study did not include a group of animals that were treated with antibiotics *after* dural puncture, which would more closely mirror the timing of prophylactic antibiotic administration in a typical operating room. In addition, although *E. coli* is a common cause of bacteremia, it is an uncommon cause of meningitis in humans. Also, the authors knew the sensitivity of the bacteria injected, allowing for appropriate antibiotic coverage. Although these results may apply to the performance of spinal anesthesia in the bacteremic patient, they do not apply to administration of epidural anesthesia in the febrile patient, which is associated with a higher incidence of infectious complications. While bacteremia may well be a factor in the development of meningitis following lumbar puncture, it is difficult to quantify the

TABLE 5-2   Meningitis After Dural Puncture

AUTHOR, YEAR	NUMBER OF PATIENTS	POPULATION	MICROORGANISM(S)	PATIENTS WITH SPONTANEOUS MENINGITIS	PATIENTS WITH DURAL PUNCTURE-INDUCED MENINGITIS	COMMENTS
Wegeforth, 1919[12]	93	Military personnel	*Neisseria meningitidis Streptococcus pneumoniae*	38/93 (41%)	5/93 (5.4%), including five of six bacteremic patients	Lumbar punctures performed during meningitis epidemics
Pray, 1941[13]	416	Pediatric patients with bacteremia	*Streptococcus pneumoniae*	86/386 (22%)	8/30 (27%)	80% of patients with meningitis were <2 y of age
Eng, 1981[14]	1,089	Adults with bacteremia	*Atypical and typical bacteria*	30/919 (3.3%)	3/170 (1.8%)	Atypical organisms responsible for lumbar puncture-induced meningitis
Teele, 1981[16]	271	Pediatric patients with bacteremia	*Streptococcus pneumoniae Neisseria meningitidis Haemophilus influenzae*	2/31 (8.7%)	7/46 (15%)[a]	All cases of meningitis occurred in children <1 y of age; antibiotic therapy reduced risk
Smith, 1986[15]	11	Preterm infants with neonatal sepsis		0%	0%	
Centers for Disease Control and Prevention, 2010[81]	5	Parturients	*Streptococcus salivarius*	0%	100%	Anesthesiologist not wearing mask during spinal placement in two cases, visitors not wearing mask during spinal placement in three cases; four patients recovered, one died

[a]Significant association (*p* < .001).
Spontaneous meningitis = concurrent bacteremia and meningitis (without a preceding lumbar puncture).
Lumbar puncture-induced meningitis = positive blood culture with sterile CSF on initial exam; subsequent positive CSF culture (same organism present in the blood).

specific risk. Multiple factors, including the type of infectious organism, the timing and choice of concurrent antibiotic therapy, and patient immune status all contribute to the individual patient's unique risk profile.

Epidural Abscess

The incidence of epidural abscess was historically reported to be extremely low. However, several recent studies have shown alarming incidence rates near 1:1,350,[4,6–8] while others suggest that the occurrence is rare.[5,9] Differences in patient selection, local practices, study design, and statistical analysis may contribute to this variation. Because of this, a true risk estimate for each individual patient may be difficult to ascertain.

Several studies have specifically examined the risk of epidural abscess in patients receiving epidural anesthesia and/ or analgesia (Box 5-1). In a historical large retrospective review, epidural abscess from *all causes* accounted for 0.2 to 1.2 cases per 10,000 admissions to tertiary hospitals.[18] Of the 39 cases of epidural abscess occurring over a 30-year period from 1947 to 1974, *Staphylococcus aureus* (57%), streptococci (18%), and gram-negative bacilli (13%) were the most common pathogens. The source of infection was most often due to osteomyelitis (38%), bacteremia (26%), and postoperative infection (16%). Only 1 of the 39 cases was related to an epidural catheter. In a more recent review, 4 of 10 cases of epidural abscess reported from a Scandanavian database were associated with neuraxial procedures, including repeated lumbar punctures in the presence of meningitis (two cases), epidural catheter placement (one case), and a paravertebral anesthetic injection (one case).[19] As with the meningitis data, variability in the incidence of this devastating complication was observed in the recent literature. Retrospective reviews reporting a low incidence of epidural abscess include a Swedish study reporting 0 in 9,232 epidurals[20] and a German report of 2 cases in 13,000 procedures.[21] However, these reassuring studies notwithstanding, Wang et al.[4] present a differing view in the results of their 1-year prospective survey of Danish anesthesiologists. Seventy-eight percent of anesthesia departments participated, performing 17,372 epidural anesthetics. Twelve possible epidural abscesses were reported; nine were subsequently determined to be spinal-epidural abscesses, two were subcutaneous infections, and one was a misplaced catheter. The nine abscesses represented an incidence of 1:1,930 catheters and differed between university (1:5,661) and nonuniversity community hospitals (1:796). The epidural catheters in the affected cases were *in situ* for a mean of 11 days. Five of the nine involved thoracic catheters, and 67% were placed for perioperative pain management. The majority (67%) had received low–molecular-weight heparin (LMWH) as thromboprophylaxis before epidural catheter placement, and all but one patient were deemed immunocompromised. *S. aureus* was the pathogen in six of the nine cases (two patients had no bacterial growth). Several common factors, with undetermined significance, were noted in the affected patients: longer mean catheter times, immunocompromised patients with chronic disease states, and perioperative antithrombotic agents were administered in the majority. The authors also pointed out that the overall neurological outcome in these patients was grave, perhaps due to the insidious progression of symptoms and often late intervention (Box 5-2). The diagnosis of epidural abscess is more difficult and often delayed in patients with chronic epidural abscesses because these patients are less likely to be febrile or have elevated leukocyte counts compared to patients with acute abscesses. However, rapid neurologic deterioration may still occur in either group. In addition, earlier diagnosis and treatment improves the neurologic outcome. Steroid administration and increased neurologic impairment at the time of surgery adversely affects the outcome.[22]

Although infection has long been a concern in epidural anesthesia and analgesia, most cases of epidural catheter-induced spinal epidural abscess or meningitis appear as individual case reports or in retrospective reviews.[3,5,18,19,23] Although epidural catheters frequently show positive cultures, clinical signs of epidural infection at the time of catheter removal or during follow-up are rare. Most epidural abscesses are not due to contamination during the placement of indwelling catheters, but appear to be related to preexisting infections of the skin, soft tissue, or spine, or hematogenous spread to the epidural space. Longer catheter duration for postoperative pain management, immunocompromised host, and concurrent anticoagulation seem likely to be contributors to a higher observed incidence in some studies.

BOX 5-1 Clinical Challenges and Considerations in Immunocompromised Patients

- The range of microorganisms causing invasive infection in the compromised host is much broader than that affecting the general population.
- The altered inflammatory response within the compromised patient may mute the clinical signs and symptoms often associated with infection, delaying diagnosis, and treatment.
- A major factor in determining the prognosis and outcome of immunocompromised patients is the institution of early and effective therapy.
- Prolonged therapy is often required because of persistent and ongoing host defense abnormalities.
- Prevention of infection should be the goal in managing immunocompromised patients.

BOX 5-2 Factors That May Increase the Risk for Neuraxial Infection

- Prolonged catheter *in situ*
- Immunocompromised patient
- Thromboprophylaxis
- Chronically ill patient
- Breaks in aseptic technique
- Preexisting infection of skin, soft tissues, or spine at the insertion site
- Epidural placement (versus spinal)

Obstetrics

Once again the obstetric patient presents a unique challenge. The anesthesiologist is frequently faced with the management of the parturient with suspected chorioamnionitis, approximately 8% of whom are bacteremic.[24,25] These data are derived from two seminal studies in the literature describing the outcome of epidural catheter placement in bacteremic parturients with and without antibiotic treatment. Bader et al.[24] investigated the use of regional anesthesia in women with chorioamnionitis. Three hundred nineteen women were identified from a total of 10,047 deliveries. Of the 319 women, 100 had blood cultures taken on the day of delivery. Eight of these had blood cultures consistent with bacteremia. Two hundred ninety three of the 319 patients received a regional anesthetic (in 43 patients, antibiotics were administered prior to needle or catheter placement). Goodman et al.[25] also retrospectively reviewed the hospital records of 531 parturients who received epidural or spinal anesthesia and were subsequently diagnosed with chorioamnionitis. Blood cultures were drawn in 146 patients (13 were positive). Antibiotics were administered before the regional block was placed in only 123 patients, whereas nearly one-third of patients did not receive antibiotic therapy in the entire peripartum period. As with the study by Bader et al.[24], leukocytosis, fever, abdominal tenderness, or foul-smelling discharge were not predictors of positive blood cultures. No patient in either study, including those with documented bacteremias, had infectious complications. The authors concluded that administering spinal and epidural anesthesia in patients with suspected chorioamnionitis was acceptable because the potential benefits of regional anesthesia outweighed the small theoretical risk of infectious complications. However, the relatively small number of patients with documented bacteremias in both studies precludes a definitive statement regarding the risk of CNS infections in patients suspected of chorioamnionitis undergoing regional anesthetic techniques.

Pediatrics

Studies focusing on pediatric patients report similar findings to those in adults. Specifically, longer catheter duration and placement for treatment of chronic pain (3.2%) rather than acute postoperative pain (0.057%) are risk factors for developing neuraxial infection.[26,27] Vigilant monitoring for early signs of infection and early intervention to avoid serious neurologic sequelae are critical to a good outcome.

Technical issues during neuraxial blockade have been implicated as sources of infection. The catheter hub, catheter insertion site, and hematogenous spread are three major routes of entry for microorganisms into the epidural space, with the catheter hub accounting for nearly half of the sources (Fig. 5-1).[28–30] A bacterial filter placed at the catheter hub acts as a physical barrier to bacteria present in the infusing solution and should theoretically reduce the incidence of epidural colonization. However, studies of epidural catheter tip cultures have reported mixed results, and cases of epidural infection following hub colonization despite the use of filters have been reported.[28,29,31] Possible explanations for hub-related epidural infections in patients with bacterial filters include a reduced antimicrobial effectiveness with prolonged use and direct contamination of the hub during filter-changing techniques. A positive trend

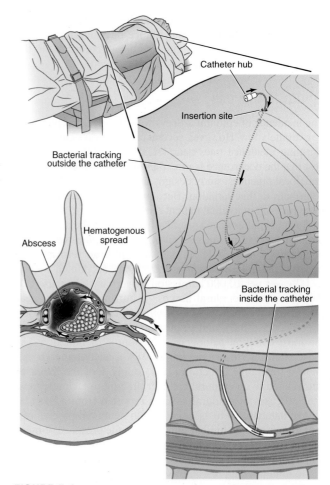

FIGURE 5-1. Bacteria may gain access to the epidural space through the catheter hub, the catheter insertion site, or via hematogenous spread.

between the number of filter changes and the rate of positive hub cultures has been reported.[32] These data suggest that continued close attention to aseptic technique is warranted throughout the period of epidural catheterization and that the use of bacteriologic filters alone is unlikely to be efficacious in preventing epidural colonization and infection.[33] Overall, epidural abscess following neuraxial anesthetic procedures is uncommon, with the most commonly reported incidence near 1:40,000, and tends to arise from the introduction of nosocomial organisms during the procedure itself or via the contamination of an indwelling catheter.

▶ RISK FACTORS

Meningitis after spinal anesthesia has been only rarely reported. In an older study evaluating the frequency of meningitis in patients undergoing spinal anesthesia, Kilpatrick and Girgis[34] retrospectively reviewed the records of all patients admitted to the meningitis ward in Cairo, Egypt. During a 5-year period from 1975 to 1980, 17 of 1,429 patients admitted with a diagnosis of meningitis had a history of recent spinal anesthesia. Ten of the 17 had positive CSF cultures: eight were *Pseudomonas aeruginosa*, one was *S. aureus*, and one was *S. mitis*. These organisms were not cultured from patients who had not undergone spinal anesthesia. Two additional patients with a history of recent spinal anesthesia demonstrated evidence of tuberculous meningitis. These results suggest that meningitis occurring in patients with a history of recent spinal anesthesia is often due to unusual or nosocomial organisms. Few data suggest that spinal or epidural anesthesia during bacteremia are risk factors for neuraxial infection. In the previously cited large studies, the number of patients who were febrile during the administration of the spinal or epidural anesthetic was not reported. A significant number of the patients in these studies underwent obstetric or urologic procedures, and it is therefore likely that at least some patients were bacteremic after (and perhaps during) needle or catheter placement. In a retrospective review by Horlocker et al.[35] of 4,767 consecutive spinal anesthetics, there were two infectious complications noted. One patient, who developed a disc space infection following spinal anesthesia, was noted to have had a recent untreated episode of urosepsis. The second patient developed a paraspinal abscess 11 days following spinal anesthesia, performed after unsuccessful attempts at caudal blockade for suspected rectal fistula. Despite the apparent low risk of central nervous system infection following regional anesthesia, anesthesiologists have long considered sepsis to be a relative contraindication to the administration of spinal or epidural anesthesia. This impression is based largely on anecdotal reports and conflicting laboratory and clinical investigations.

Several studies have evaluated the risk factors for the development of epidural space infections in patients with indwelling epidural catheters. Darchy et al.[36] studied 75 patients in an intensive care unit who were receiving epidural analgesia (median 4 days). Nine patients had local (catheter insertion site) infections, including four patients with epidural catheter (local inflammation with positive epidural catheter culture) infections, representing a frequency of 2.7 local (catheter insertion site) infections and 1.2 epidural infections per 100 days of epidural catheterization. *Staphylococcus epidermidis* was the most frequently cultured microorganism. All catheters were removed upon the appearance of discharge at the catheter insertion site, and antibiotic therapy was not specifically prescribed. The presence of both local erythema and discharge was associated with positive epidural catheter cultures. Concomitant infection at other sites, antibiotic therapy, and duration of indwelling epidural catheter were not significant risk factors for epidural infections. The authors recommended a meticulous daily inspection of the catheter insertion site and an immediate removal of the catheter if both erythema and local discharge are present. This recommendation precludes the use of dressings that obscure the catheter insertion site preventing inspection for signs of infection.

Controversy exists regarding the conditions under which a disconnected epidural catheter can be safely reconnected. In an *in vitro* investigation, epidural catheters containing a 5 µg/mL fentanyl solution were inoculated with *S. aureus*, *E. coli*, or *P. aeruginosa*[37]. Eight hours after catheter contamination, provided the fluid in the catheter remained static, no bacteria were detected more than 20 cm from the contaminated catheter hub. Vertical or horizontal positioning of the catheter during incubation did not affect bacterial advancement along the catheter, as long as the fluid was displaced distally <20 cm. However, if the fentanyl solution was allowed to

drain and advance 33 cm, bacteria were found at the epidural end of the catheter 88 cm away. The advancement of bacteria by fluid displacement is clinically significant. In more than two-thirds of patients, fluid will drain by gravity into the epidural space in <1 hour after the discontinuation of an epidural infusion. The authors concluded that the interior of a disconnected epidural catheter would remain sterile for at least 8 hours if the fluid in the catheter remains static, and the catheter may be aseptically reconnected after the removal of the contaminated section. In addition, the presence of a meniscus >20 to 25 cm from the free end of a disconnected catheter may indicate the contamination of the catheter tip in the epidural space, and immediate catheter removal was recommended. Unfortunately, the authors did not evaluate the advancement of bacteria in epidural catheters filled with local anesthetic solutions or investigate the effect of a local anesthetic injected after bacterial inoculation and incubation.

Immunocompromise, due to either injection of epidural steroids or underlying disease processes, theoretically increases the risk of infection.[38,39] In a case report, Strong[39] described a 71-year-old man who developed *S. aureus* epidural abscess following the administration of methylprednisolone via thoracic epidural catheter (Fig. 5-2). An emergency decompressive laminectomy and antibiotic

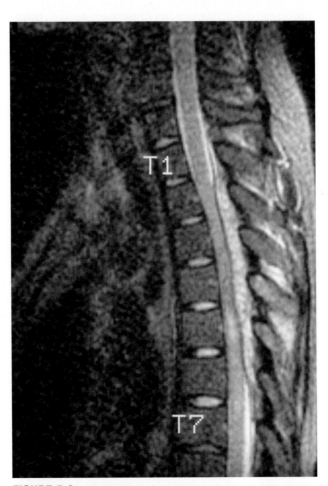

FIGURE 5-2. A thoracic epidural abscess is demonstrated on a magnetic resonance image in a patient who underwent thoracic epidural placement for the management of herpetic neuralgia. (From Finucane BT, ed. *Complications of Regional Anesthesia.* New York, NY: Churchill Livingstone, 1999:178, with permission.)

treatment resulted in a good outcome. Factors contributing to this patient's epidural infection included an immunocompromised host (as suggested by the activation of a latent herpes infection), multiple catheter placements, and decreased immunologic response secondary to steroid administration. The use of an epidural in the presence of localized infection is somewhat controversial. Jakobsen et al.[40] examined the records of 69 patients with localized infections who had a total of 120 epidural catheters placed, undergoing on average four epidural anesthetics with catheters left in place for a mean of 9 days. On 12 occasions, the catheter was removed due to local infection, no specific therapy was instituted, and the infection was resolved. There was one case of spondylitis, which was not apparently related to epidural catheterization. The retrospective nature of this study and the small number of patients limit the conclusions but suggest that placing an epidural catheter in a chronically infected patient may not be associated with a high risk of epidural infection.

Patients with measurable alterations in either natural or acquired immunity may be at constant risk of life-threatening infections. In general, patient classification of immunocompromised states include: (i) patients with congenital immunodeficiencies (i.e., severe combined immunodeficiency disease, SCID), (ii) patients with acquired immunodeficiency syndrome (i.e., AIDS), and (iii) patients with acquired deficits secondary to disease states (i.e., hematologic malignancies) or more commonly to related therapy (i.e., posttransplant therapy). Acute and chronic illness, the stress of trauma or major surgical intervention, and the potential for associated malnutrition during the perioperative period all increase the risk of immunosuppression. It has been suggested that many of the complications associated with regional anesthetic techniques (infection, bleeding, postoperative neuropathies, and cerebral herniation) may be more apt to occur in immunocompromised patients when compared to healthy individuals.

Chronic epidural catheterization in patients who are immunocompromised at baseline is also a potential risk for epidural infection. In patients with HIV and cancer who received permanent (tunneled) epidural catheters, the rate of epidural and deep-track catheter-related infections was 1 in every 1,702 days of catheter use in the 19 patients who developed deep-track (8) or epidural (15) infections.[28] Four of the 19 patients had both deep-track and epidural involvement; bacteria cultured were most frequently skin flora. All 19 patients with deep infections were treated with catheter removal and antibiotics. None required surgical decompression or debridement. Catheters were replaced in 15 of the 19 patients who requested them after treatment with no recurrent infections. The authors state recommendations similar to Strafford et al.,[27] specifically that long-term epidural catheterization in chronically immunocompromised patients is safe when patients are carefully monitored for signs of infection and receive prompt treatment when the diagnosis is established.

Importantly, the clinical management of patients suffering from immunocompromising disease states requires careful assessment and thoughtful consideration of a variety of factors (Box 5-1). The low frequency of significant epidural infection associated with epidural catheter placement (one to two cases per 10,000 hospital admissions[18]) is particularly notable when compared to the frequency of intra-

venous catheter-related septicemia, which approaches 1% (or >50,000 cases) annually. Several factors may contribute to the low incidence of epidural space infections, including meticulous attention to aseptic technique, careful monitoring of catheter insertion site, antibiotic prophylaxis, and the use of bacterial filters. However, because these interventions are also commonly initiated in patients with indwelling central venous catheters, additional factors unique to epidural anesthesia and analgesia (such as the bacteriostatic effect of local anesthetic solutions) may also contribute significantly. Bupivacaine and lidocaine have been shown to inhibit the growth of a variety of microorganisms in culture.[41] Unfortunately, the bacteriostatic effect decreases significantly with concentrations of local anesthetic typically used to provide analgesia. Opioid-only solutions exhibit no ability to inhibit bacterial growth. In addition, the growth of S. aureus and coagulase-negative Staphylococcus (the most commonly identified pathogens in epidural infections) is inhibited only at higher concentrations of local anesthetic, such as solutions of 2% lidocaine and 0.5% bupivacaine. Levobupivacaine, ropivacaine, clonidine, and epinephrine do not exhibit significant bacteriostatic properties at clinically relevant concentrations.[42] Therefore, although it appears that local anesthetic solutions are unlikely to prevent epidural infections in most patients receiving epidural analgesia, it is possible that in immunocompromised patients, bupivacaine may inhibit the growth of more fastidious organisms even at low concentrations. Further clinical studies are needed to investigate the *in vivo* bacteriostatic effects of dilute local anesthetic solutions. In addition, solutions intended for neuraxial or peripheral nerve catheter infusion may be contaminated during preparation.[43]

Conservatively, all patients with an established local or systemic infection should be considered at risk for developing infection of the CNS. Patients should be observed carefully for signs of infection when a continuous epidural catheter is left in place for prolonged periods (more than 4–5 days). In addition, injection of local anesthetic or insertion of a catheter in an area at high risk for bacterial contamination (such as the sacral hiatus) may also increase the risk for abscess formation, emphasizing the importance of meticulous aseptic technique.

▶ DIAGNOSIS

A delay in the diagnosis and treatment of major CNS infections of even a few hours significantly worsens neurologic outcome. Bacterial meningitis is a medical emergency. Mortality is approximately 30%, even with antibiotic therapy. Meningitis presents most often with fever, severe headache, altered level of consciousness, and meningismus. The diagnosis is confirmed with a lumbar puncture; however, this procedure should not be performed if epidural abscess is suspected, as contamination of the intrathecal space may result. CSF examination in the patient with meningitis reveals leukocytosis, a glucose level of <30 mg/dL, and a protein level of >150 mg/dL. The CSF and blood should also be cultured to aid in the identification of the pathogen(s) and sensitivity to antimicrobials. The anesthesiologist should consider atypical organisms in patients suspected of meningitis following spinal anesthesia. Even when meningitis occurs temporally after spinal anesthesia, it is often difficult to establish a cause-and-effect relationship between spinal anesthesia and meningitis. The clinical course of epidural abscess progresses from spinal ache and root pain to weakness (including bowel and bladder symptoms) and eventually paralysis[22,44] (see Chapter 10). There may also be associated fever and leukocytosis (Table 5-2). The initial back pain and radicular symptoms may remain stable for hours to weeks. However, the onset of weakness often progresses to complete paralysis within 24 hours. Although the diagnosis was historically made with myelogram, magnetic resonance imaging is currently recommended, as it is the most sensitive modality for evaluation of the spine when infection is suspected[45–47] (Fig. 5-2). If MRI is unable to be performed, computed tomography scanning is recommended. Surgical intervention, if needed, should be within 12 hours of symptom onset to achieve the best chance of neurological recovery. As with spinal hematoma, neurologic recovery is dependent on the duration of the deficit and the severity of neurologic impairment before treatment.[22]

▶ TREATMENT

Initial therapy for meningitis is typically broad-spectrum antibiotics and supportive care. Initiation of antibiotics should not be delayed during the diagnostic workup. Patients may exhibit signs of septic shock, requiring rapid fluid resuscitation and pharmacologic hemodynamic support. Tracheal intubation and mechanical ventilation may be required, particularly in patients with altered mentation.

Abscess formation following epidural or spinal anesthesia can be superficial, requiring limited surgical drainage and IV antibiotics, or can occur deep in the epidural space with associated cord compression (Fig. 10-4). The latter is fortunately a rare complication, but it requires aggressive and early (<12 hours) surgical management in combination with initial broad-spectrum antibiotic therapy in order to avoid permanent neurological compromise. When the infectious organism(s) and sensitivities to specific antibiotics are identified, antibiotic coverage may be narrowed. Superficial infections present with local tissue swelling, erythema, and drainage, often associated with fever but rarely causing neurologic problems unless left untreated.

▶ PREVENTION

Despite the report by Kilpatrick and Girgis,[34] most cases of meningitis associated with spinal anesthesia are reported as single cases or small case series (Table 5-2). Older case reports often reported an association of meningitis with a break in sterilization techniques affecting patient preparation or the use of reusable equipment.[48] Disposable kits have reduced this risk; however nosocomial contamination is still a concern. In 2006, the American Society of Regional Anesthesia and Pain Medicine recommended that surgical masks be worn during the performance of regional anesthesia and pain-management procedures in an effort to reduce infectious complications.[49] The Centers for Disease Control and Prevention[50] and American Society of Anesthesiologists[51] subsequently made similar recommendations. However,

breaches of aseptic technique continue to generate infections and case reports. In 2010, a series of *Klebsiella pneumoniae* and *Enterobacter aerogenes* bacteremia associated with an interventional pain clinic in New York City were reported by Wong and colleagues from the New York Department of Health and Mental Hygiene.[52] There were four laboratory confirmed and five suspected cases of bacteremia in nine patients treated over a 3-day span. All nine patients underwent procedures at the same pain clinic, performed by the same physician and allied health assistant. Lapses in aseptic technique included lack of hand hygiene, not donning a surgical mask for interventional procedures, poor aseptic cleansing, and use of single-dose medication vials for more than one patient. It is difficult to pinpoint which of these breaks in aseptic technique was most responsible for the outbreak; it is likely that multiple factors acted synergistically to play a role. The plethora of case reports in the literature of neuraxial infections, some fatal, related to breaches in aseptic technique suggest that the reports from New York City were not isolated incidents.[34,48,53–56] This suggests that improving aseptic technique is something that every provider should consider in everyday practice. This includes simple measures such as performing appropriate hand hygiene; removing rings and watches; and donning of a surgical cap, mask, and sterile gloves prior to neuraxial anesthetic procedures[49]. The use of antiseptic solutions is also instrumental in preventing infectious complications when performing neuraxial procedures. Chlorhexidine products have been shown to have a more effective, rapid, and longer-lasting bactericidal effect than povidone iodine; the addition of isopropyl alcohol to chlorhexidine accelerates this effect.[49,57–66] Nearly, all bacteria and nosocomial fungi are susceptible to chlorhexidine; resistance is exceedingly rare. Its efficacy is maintained even in the presence of organic compounds, such as blood. It is important to note that the United States Food and Drug Administration has not formally approved chlorhexidine for skin preparation prior to neuraxial preparation. This is due to a lack of animal studies studying the potential for neurotoxic effects of chlorhexidine, not due to any reported human cases of nerve injury. In fact, there are no confirmed cases of nerve injury with either chlorhexidine or isopropyl alcohol. Hence, alcohol-based chlorhexidine solutions are recommended by the American Society of Regional Anesthesia and Pain Medicine, American Society of Anesthesiologists, and Royal College of Anaesthetists as the skin antiseptic of choice prior to neuraxial anesthetic procedures.[9,49,51]

Preparation of an infusion in an inappropriate manner can lead to contamination and infection. In an effort to standardize and improve the practice of compounding sterile preparations, the United States Pharmacopeia (USP) and The National Formulary published Chapter 797 in 2004.[67] USP Chapter 797 is the national standard for sterile compounding, including the preparation of local anesthetics. This regulation is enforceable by the Food and Drug Administration, the State Boards of Pharmacy, and the State Boards of Health. Importantly, full compliance with USP Chapter 797 became a requirement of the Joint Commission on Accreditation of Healthcare Organizations in 2008. Specifically, preparations (including local anesthetics) intended to be infused over several days are recommended to be prepared by pharmacy personnel in an International Standards Organization (ISO) Class 5 laminar flow workbench, within an ISO Class 7 buffer room.[68] When local anesthetic solutions are prepared according to these standards, infusions may remain microbiologically stable well beyond 72 hours.[69–71] However, any breaks within the sterile circuit (e.g., solution bag changes, local anesthetic boluses, catheter-hub disconnects) may significantly increase the risk of contamination and subsequent localized or systemic infection.[32,72,73]

SUMMARY OF NEURAXIAL INFECTIOUS COMPLICATIONS

Meningitis or epidural abscess following neuraxial blockade is an uncommon occurrence. Based on the most current, largest studies, the incidence is most likely around 1:40,000, with epidurals more likely to result in an infectious complication.[5,9] Individual patient and specific practice factors may affect this value. Risk factors that increase the chances of neuraxial infection include longer duration of catheter *in situ*, immunocompromised patients, critically ill patients, and the use of pharmocologic thromboprophylaxis (Box 5-2). However, as with all clinical judgments, the decision to perform a regional anesthetic technique must be made on an individual basis considering the anesthetic alternatives, the benefits of regional anesthesia, and the risk of CNS infection, which may theoretically occur in any patient.

Although patient selection is important, close attention to aseptic technique remains the most effective means of preventing infection related to neuraxial regional anesthesia. This includes hand washing; removing rings and wristwatches; skin preparation with an alcohol-based chlorhexidine solution; donning of a surgical hat, mask, and sterile gloves; and maintenance of an adequate procedural field with sterile drapes. Additionally, any regional anesthetic solution intended for multiple-day infusion should be prepared by pharmacy personnel in accordance with USP 797 guidelines.

Numerous clinical and laboratory studies have suggested an association between dural puncture during bacteremia and meningitis. The data are equivocal, however. The clinical studies are limited to pediatric patients, who are historically at high risk for meningitis. Many of the original animal studies utilized bacterial counts that were far in excess of those noted in humans in early sepsis, making CNS contamination more likely.[11,74] Despite these conflicting results, many experts suggest that except in the most extraordinary circumstances, neuraxial block should not be performed in patients with untreated systemic infection.

Available data suggest that patients with evidence of systemic infection may safely undergo spinal anesthesia, provided appropriate antibiotic therapy is initiated prior to dural puncture and the patient has demonstrated a response to therapy such as a decrease in fever.[17,75] Although few data exist on the administration of epidural anesthesia in the patient with a treated systemic infection, the existing literature is reassuring.[24,25] Placement of an indwelling epidural (or intrathecal) catheter in this group of patients remains controversial.

Available data suggest that spinal anesthesia may be safely performed in patients at risk for low-grade transient bacteremia after dural puncture. Once again, little information exists concerning the risk of epidural anesthesia in patients suspected of developing an intraoperative transient bacteremia (such as during a urologic procedure). However, short-term epidural catheterization is most likely safe, as suggested by large retrospective reviews that included a significant number of obstetric and urologic patients (Box 5-3).[1,2]

INFECTIOUS COMPLICATIONS OF PERIPHERAL NERVE BLOCKADE

Scope

The use of peripheral nerve blockade, including continuous peripheral nerve blockade, has expanded greatly in recent years. Despite increased clinical use, there are few investigations regarding the incidence of infectious complications with these techniques. Of the investigations in the literature, none approach the sample size of the large studies involving complications of neuraxial blockade. In the current literature, 23% to 57% of peripheral nerve catheters may become colonized, with 0% to 3% resulting in localized infection and a proven systemic infection associated with the catheter occurring in 0% to 0.9% (Table 5-3).[76] The

---

BOX 5-3 Recommendations for Management of Neuraxial Infections

- Serious neuraxial infections such as arachnoiditis, meningitis, and abscess after spinal or epidural anesthesia are rare.
- The decision to perform a regional anesthetic technique must be made on an individual basis considering the anesthetic alternatives, the benefits of regional anesthesia, and the risk of CNS infection (which may theoretically occur in any bacteremic patient).
- Despite conflicting results, many experts suggest that, except in the most extraordinary circumstances, neuraxial block should not be performed in patients with untreated systemic infection.
- Available data suggest that patients with evidence of systemic infection may safely undergo spinal anesthesia, provided

appropriate antibiotic therapy is initiated prior to dural puncture and the patient has demonstrated a response to therapy such as a decrease in fever (placement of an indwelling epidural, or intrathecal, catheter in this group of patients remains controversial).
- Available data suggest that spinal anesthesia may be safely performed in patients at risk for low-grade transient bacteremia after dural puncture.
- Injection of epidural steroids and underlying disease processes resulting in immunocompromise theoretically increase the risk of infection.
- A delay in diagnosis and treatment of major CNS infections of even a few hours significantly worsens neurologic outcome.

TABLE 5-3 Infectious Complications Following Peripheral Blockade

AUTHOR, YEAR	NUMBER OF PATIENTS	POPULATION	REGIONAL TECHNIQUES	ANTIBIOTIC PROPHYLAXIS	DURATION OF INDWELLING CATHETER	COMPLICATIONS
Bergman, 2003[82]	405	Surgical	Axillary catheter	Unknown	Mean 55 h	One localized skin infection, treated with catheter removal and a course of antibiotics
Capdevila, 2005[78]	1,416	Surgical	256 interscalene, 126 axillary, 20 posterior lumbar plexus, 683 femoral, 94 fascia iliaca, 32 proximal sciatic, 167 popliteal, and 38 distal median and ulnar catheters	Yes, in some	Mean 56 h	28.7% of catheters colonized One psoas abscess following femoral nerve block, treated with antibiotics
Capdevila, 2008[43]	1	Surgical	Interscalene catheter	Yes	39 h	Acute neck cellulitis, interscalene and sternocleidomastoid abscess, mediastinitis requiring surgical debridement, and prolonged antibiotic therapy
Neuburger, 2007[79]	2,285	Surgical	600 axillary, 303 interscalene, 92 infraclavicular, 65 psoas compartment, 574 femoral, 296 sciatic, and 355 popliteal catheters	97% received perioperative single dose after catheter placement and before surgery	Median 4 d	96 local inflammation 73 local infection 20 infections requiring surgical drainage
Nseir, 2004[77]	1	Surgical	Axillary block, single injection	No	None	Fatal necrotizing fasciitis, provider did not wear mask during block
Wong, 2010[52]	9	Pain management	Sacroiliac joint steroid injection	No	None	Four laboratory-confirmed and five suspected cases of *Klebsiella pneumoniae* and *Enterobacter aerogenes* bacteremia, provider did not adhere to multiple facets of aseptic technique

incidence of infection following single-injection peripheral nerve blocks is even less well defined, with the data limited to a single case report of fatal necrotizing fasciitis following a single-injection axillary block.[77] However, as this case demonstrates, the infections occurring following single-injection techniques can nonetheless be devastating.

Pathophysiology

Catheters are most frequently colonized with the most common skin microorganism, *S. epidermidis.* However, *S. aureus* is the most commonly described organism in cases of localized infection and abscess formation.[78,79] Colonization and infection during peripheral blockade likely occurs in a similar fashion as with neuraxial blockade. In particular, breaks in aseptic technique, localized infection at the skin puncture site, contamination of the local anesthetic solution, and tracking of organisms along the length of the catheter all are proposed mechanisms. For example, a patient developed acute neck cellulitis, interscalene and sternocleidomastoid abscesses, and mediastinitis following an infusion delivered via an elastomeric pump via an interscalene catheter.[43] The catheter was placed under strict aseptic conditions and dressed with a sterile dressing. However, the elastomeric pump was filled outside of the pharmacy by a member of the anesthesia team who did not wear sterile gloves and performed multiple manipulations of the infusion line. This patient required surgical debridement and prolonged intravenous antibiotics.

Risk Factors

Important risk factors for developing a peripheral nerve catheter-associated infection are reported as a stay in the intensive care unit: odds ratio (95% confidence interval) (5.07 [0.33–18.1]), duration of catheter use over 48 hours (4.61 [1.57–15.9]), absence of antibiotic prophylaxis (1.92 [1.03–3.9]), axillary or femoral location (3.39 [1.48–7.79]), and frequent dressing changes (2.12 [1.37–3.29]) (Box 5-4).[76] Additional factors that may play a role, but that the authors felt were unproven, were male gender, diabetes mellitus, absence of tunneling the peripheral nerve catheter, placement of the catheter at sites where it could be affected by motion of the head and neck, and placement of catheters with suboptimal sterile technique. Although single-injection peripheral nerve blocks might have a lower risk of infectious

---

complications than continuous catheter techniques,[80] this assumption has not been proven. Breaches in aseptic technique can put patients at risk for infection as well. In the previously mentioned case of fatal necrotizing fasciitis following single-injection axillary block, the provider performing the block was not wearing a mask.[77] The risk associated with peripheral nerve block in the immunocompromised or bacteremic patient is unclear.

Diagnosis/treatment

Infections related to peripheral nerve blockade typically present as erythema and/or tenderness at the block site and can usually be diagnosed with history and physical examination. Occasionally, this may progress to cellulitis or abscess formation, and radiologic imaging with ultrasound, computed tomography, or magnetic resonance imaging may be required to define the extent of the abscess. Laboratory evaluation of the blood may reveal an elevated leukocyte count. Most localized infections can be treated with no more than catheter removal, with the occasional need for antibiotic therapy, and rarely surgical drainage.[80]

Prevention

Strict adherence to aseptic technique is a cornerstone of preventing infectious complications in peripheral regional anesthesia. As with neuraxial techniques, the American Society of Regional Anesthesia and Pain Medicine, The Centers for Disease Control and Prevention, and American Society of Anesthesiologists recommend that surgical masks be worn during the performance of peripheral blocks.[49–51] Donning a hat, removal of rings and wristwatches, performing hand hygiene prior to donning sterile gloves, and skin preparation with an alcohol-based chlorhexidine solution are also recommended.[49] In addition, solutions intended for multiple-day infusion via peripheral nerve catheters should be prepared by pharmacy personnel according to USP 797 guidelines.[68] Prophylactic antibiotics may be protective, but adequate data are not available to support this concept.

References

1. Kane RE. Neurologic deficits following epidural or spinal anesthesia. *Anesth Analg* 1981;60(3):150–161.
2. Auroy Y, et al. Serious complications related to regional anesthesia: results of a prospective survey in France. *Anesthesiology* 1997;87(3):479–486.
3. Aromaa U, Lahdensuu M, Cozanitis DA. Severe complications associated with epidural and spinal anaesthesias in Finland 1987–1993. A study based on patient insurance claims. *Acta Anaesthesiologica Scandinavica* 1997;41(4):445–452.
4. Wang LP, Hauerberg J, Schmidt JF. Incidence of spinal epidural abscess after epidural analgesia: a national 1-year survey. *Anesthesiology* 1999;91(6):1928–1936.
5. Moen V, Dahlgren N, Irestedt L. Severe neurological complications after central neuraxial blockades in Sweden 1990–1999. *Anesthesiology* 2004;101(4):950–959.
6. Cameron CM, et al. A review of neuraxial epidural morbidity: experience of more than 8,000 cases at a single teaching hospital. *Anesthesiology* 2007;106(5):997–1002.
7. Green LK, Paech MJ. Obstetric epidural catheter-related infections at a major teaching hospital: a retrospective case series. *Int J Obstet Anesth* 2010;19(1):38–43.

BOX 5-4 Factors That May Increase the Risk for Infection Following Peripheral Nerve Block

- Intensive care unit stay
- Prolonged catheter *in situ* (>48 h)
- Absence of antibiotic prophylaxis
- Axillary or femoral location
- Breaks in aseptic technique
- Preexisting infection of skin, soft tissues, or spine at the insertion site
- Frequent dressing change

8. Christie IW, McCabe S. Major complications of epidural analgesia after surgery: results of a six-year survey. *Anaesthesia* 2007;62(4):335–341.

9. The 3rd National Audit Project of The Royal College of Anaesthetists: Major Complications of Central Neuraxial Block in the United Kingdom. 2009; Available from: http://www.rcoa.ac.uk/docs/NAP3_web-large.pdf.

10. Scott DB, Hibbard BM. Serious non-fatal complications associated with extradural block in obstetric practice. *Br J Anaesth* 1990;64(5):537–541.

11. Weed LH, et al. The production of meningitis by release of cerebrospinal fluid during an experimental septicemia. *JAMA* 1919;72:190–193.

12. Wegeforth P, Latham JR. Lumbar puncture as a factor in the causation of meningitis. *Am J Med Sci* 1919;148:183–202.

13. Pray LG. Lumbar puncture as a factor in the pathogenesis of meningitis. *Am J Dis Child* 1941;295:62–68.

14. Eng RHK, Seligman SJ. Lumbar puncture-induced meningitis. *JAMA* 1981;245(14):1456–1459.

15. Smith KM, Deddish RB, Ogata ES. Meningitis associated with serial lumbar punctures and post-hemorrhagic hydrocephalus. *J Pediatr* 1986;109(6):1057–1060.

16. Teele DW, et al. Meningitis after lumbar puncture in children with bacteremia. *N Engl J Med* 1981;305(18):1079–1081.

17. Carp H, Bailey S. The association between meningitis and dural puncture in bacteremic rats. *Anesthesiology* 1992;76(5):739–742.

18. Baker AS, et al. Spinal epidural abscess. *N Engl J Med* 1975;293(10):463–468.

19. Ericsson M, Algers G, Schliamser SE. Spinal epidural abscesses in adults: review and report of iatrogenic cases. *Scand J Infect Dis* 1990;22(3):249–257.

20. Dahlgren N, Tornebrandt K. Neurological complications after anaesthesia. A follow-up of 18,000 spinal and epidural anaesthetics performed over three years. *Acta Anaesthesiologica Scandinavica* 1995;39(7):872–880.

21. Kindler C, et al. Extradural abscess complicating lumbar extradural anaesthesia and analgesia in an obstetric patient. *Acta Anaesthesiologica Scandinavica* 1996;40(7):858–861.

22. Danner RL, Hartman BJ. Update on spinal epidural abscess: 35 cases and review of the literature. *Rev Infect Dis* 1987;9(2):265–274.

23. Ready LB, Helfer D. Bacterial meningitis in parturients after epidural anesthesia. *Anesthesiology* 1989;71(6):988–990.

24. Bader AM, et al. Regional anesthesia in women with Chorioamnionitis. *Reg Anesth* 1992;17(2):84–86.

25. Goodman EJ, Dehorta E, Taguiam JM. Safety of spinal and epidural anesthesia in parturients with chorioamnionitis. *Reg Anesth* 1996;21(5):436–441.

26. Sethna NF, et al. Incidence of epidural catheter-associated infections after continuous epidural analgesia in children. *Anesthesiology* 2010;113(1):224–232.

27. Strafford MA, Wilder RT, Berde CB. The risk of infection from epidural analgesia in children: a review of 1620 cases. *Anesth Analg* 1995;80(2):234–238.

28. Du Pen SL, et al. Infection during chronic epidural catheterization: diagnosis and treatment. *Anesthesiology* 1990;73(5):905–909.

29. Hunt JR, Rigor BM Sr, Collins JR. The potential for contamination of continuous epidural catheters. *Anesth Analg* 1977;56(2):222–225.

30. James III FM, et al. Bacteriologic aspects of epidural analgesia. *Anesth Analg* 1976;55(2):187–190.

31. Barreto RS. Bacteriologic culture of indwelling epidural catheters. *Anesthesiology* 1962;23:643–646.

32. De Cicco M, et al. Time-dependent efficacy of bacterial filters and infection risk in long- term epidural catheterization. *Anesthesiology* 1995;82(3):765–771.

33. Abouleish E, Amortegui AJ, Taylor FH. Are bacterial filters needed in continuous epidural analgesia for obstetrics? *Anesthesiology* 1977;46(5):351–354.

34. Kilpatrick ME, Girgis NI. Meningitis–A complication of spinal anesthesia. *Anesth Analg* 1983;62(5):513–515.

35. Horlocker TT, et al. A retrospective review of 4767 consecutive spinal anesthetics: central nervous system complications. *Anesth Analg* 1997;84(3):578–584.

36. Darchy B, et al. Clinical and bacteriologic survey of epidural analgesia in patients in the intensive care unit. *Anesthesiology* 1996;85(5):988–998.

37. Langevin PB, et al. Epidural catheter reconnection: safe and unsafe practice. *Anesthesiology* 1996;85(4):883–888.

38. Mahendru V, Bacon DR, Lema MJ. Multiple epidural abscesses and spinal anesthesia in a diabetic patient: case report. *Reg Anesth* 1994;19(1):66–68.

39. Strong WE. Epidural abscess associated with epidural catheterization: a rare event? Report of two cases with markedly delayed presentation. *Anesthesiology* 1991;74(5):943–946.

40. Jakobsen KB, Christensen MK, Carlsson PS. Extradural anaesthesia for repeated surgical treatment in the presence of infection. *Br J Anaesth* 1995;75(5):536–540.

41. Feldman JM, Chapin-Robertson K, Turner J. Do agents used for epidural analgesia have antimicrobial properties? *Reg Anesth* 1994;19(1):43–47.

42. Coghlan MW, et al. Antibacterial activity of epidural infusions. *Anaesth Intensive Care* 2009;37(1):66–69.

43. Capdevila X, et al. Acute neck cellulitis and mediastinitis complicating a continuous interscalene block. *Anesth Analg* 2008;107(4):1419–1421.

44. Russell NA, Vaughan R, Morley TP. Spinal epidural infection. *Can J Neurol Sci* 1979;6(3):325–328.

45. Del Curling O Jr, Gower DJ, McWhorter JM. Changing concepts in spinal epidural abscess: a report of 29 cases. *Neurosurgery* 1990;27(2):185–192.

46. Mamourian AC, et al. Spinal epidural abscess: three cases following spinal epidural injection demonstrated with magnetic resonance imaging. *Anesthesiology* 1993;78(1):204–207.

47. Shintani S, et al. Iatrogenic acute spinal epidural abscess with septic meningitis: MR findings. *Clin Neurol Neurosurg* 1992;94(3):253–255.

48. Corbett JJ, Rosenstein BJ. Pseudomonas meningitis related to spinal anesthesia. Report of three cases with a common source of infection. *Neurology* 1971;21(9):946–950.

49. Hebl JR. The importance and implications of aseptic techniques during regional Anesthesia. *Reg Anesth Pain Med* 2006;31(4):311–323.

50. Siegel J, et al. 2007 Guidelines for isolation precautions: preventing transmission of infectious agents in healthcare settings. 2007; Available from: http://www.cdc.gov/hicpac/2007IP/2007isolationPrecautions.html.

51. Horlocker TT, et al. Practice advisory for the prevention, diagnosis, and management of infectious complications associated with neuraxial techniques. *Anesthesiology* 2010;112(3):530–545.

52. Wong MR, et al. An outbreak of klebsiella pneumoniae and enterobacter aerogenes bacteremia after interventional pain management procedures, New York City, 2008. *Reg Anesth Pain Med* 2010;35(6):496–499.

53. Berman RS, Eisele JH. Bacteremia, spinal anesthesia, and development of meningitis. *Anesthesiology* 1978;48(5):376–377.

54. Couzigou C, et al. Iatrogenic *Streptococcus salivarius* meningitis after spinal anaesthesia: need for strict application of standard precautions [2]. *J Hosp Infect* 2003;53(4):313–314.

55. Laurila JJ, Kostamovaara PA, Alahuhta S. *Streptococcus salivarius* meningitis after spinal anesthesia. *Anesthesiology* 1998;89(6):1579–1580.

56. Trautmann M, Lepper P, Schmitz FJ. Three cases of bacterial meningitis after spinal and epidural anesthesia. *Eur J Clin Microbiol Infect Dis* 2002;21(1):43–45.

57. Birnbach DJ, et al. Comparison of povidone iodine and duraprep, an iodophor-in-isopropyl alcohol solution, for skin disinfection

prior to epidural catheter insertion in parturients. *Anesthesiology* 2003;98(1):164–169.

58. Gibson KL, et al. Comparison of two pre-surgical skin preparation techniques. *Can J Vet Res* 1997;61(2):154–156.

59. Haley CE, Marling-Cason M, Smith JW. Bactericidal activity of antiseptics against methicillin-resistant *Staphylococcus aureus*. *J Clin Microbiol* 1985;21(6):991–992.

60. Kinirons B, et al. Chlorhexidine versus povidone iodine in preventing colonization of continuous epidural catheters in children: a randomized, controlled trial. *Anesthesiology* 2001;94(2):239–244.

61. Maki DG, Ringer M, Alvarado CJ. Prospective randomised trial of povidone-iodine, alcohol, and chlorhexidine for prevention of infection associated with central venous and arterial catheters. *Lancet* 1991;338(8763):339–343.

62. Mimoz O, et al. Chlorhexidine compared with povidone-iodine as skin preparation before blood culture: a randomized, controlled trial. *Ann Intern Med* 1999;131(11):834–837.

63. Sakuragi T, et al. Skin flora on the human back and disinfection with alcoholic chlorhexidine, povidone iodine, and ethyl alcohol. *Pain Clin* 1986;1(3):183–188.

64. Sakuragi T, Yanagisawa K, Dan K. Bactericidal activity of skin disinfectants on methicillin-resistant *Staphylococcus aureus*. *Anesth Analg* 1995;81(3):555–558.

65. Sato S, Sakuragi T, Dan K. Human skin flora as a potential source of epidural abscess. *Anesthesiology* 1996;85(6):1276–1282.

66. Selwyn S, Ellis H. Skin bacteria and skin disinfection reconsidered. *Br Med J* 1972;1(793):136–140.

67. Kastango ES, Bradshaw BD. USP chapter 797: establishing a practice standard for compounding sterile preparations in pharmacy. *Am J Health-Syst Pharm* 2004;61(18):1928–1938.

68. Head S, Enneking FK. Infusate contamination in regional anesthesia: what every anesthesiologist should know. *Anesth Analg* 2008;107(4):1412–1418.

69. Jappinen A, et al. Stability of sufentanil and levobupivacaine solutions and a mixture in a 0.9% sodium chloride infusion stored in polypropylene syringes. *Eur J Pharm Sci* 2003;19(1):31–36.

70. Sevarino FB, Pizarro CW, Sinatra R. Sterility of epidural solutions–Recommendations for cost-effective use. *Reg Anesth Pain Med* 2000;25(4):368–371.

71. Wulf H, et al. The stability of mixtures of morphine hydrochloride, bupivacaine hydrochloride, and clonidine hydrochloride in portable pump reservoirs for the management of chronic pain syndromes. *Journal of Pain and Symptom Management* 1994;9(5):308–311.

72. Centers for Disease Control and Prevention. Guidelines for the prevention of intravascular catheter-related infections. *MMWR Morb Mortal Wkly Rep* 2002;51(RR-10):1–29.

73. De Cicco M, et al. Source and route of microbial colonisation of parenteral nutrition catheters. *Lancet* 1989;2(8674):1258–1261.

74. Petersdorf RG, Swarner DR, Garcia M. Studies on the pathogenesis of meningitis. II. Development of meningitis during pneumococcal bacteremia. *J Clin Invest* 1962;41:320–327.

75. Chestnut DH. Spinal anesthesia in the febrile patient. *Anesthesiology* 1992;76(5):667–669.

76. Capdevila X, Bringuier S, Borgeat A. Infectious risk of continuous peripheral nerve blocks. *Anesthesiology* 2009;110(1):182–188.

77. Nseir S, et al. Fatal streptococcal necrotizing fasciitis as a complication of axillary brachial plexus block. *Br J Anaesth* 2004; 92(3):427–429.

78. Capdevila X, et al. Continuous peripheral nerve blocks in hospital wards after orthopedic surgery: a multicenter prospective analysis of the quality of postoperative analgesia and complications in 1,416 patients. *Anesthesiology* 2005;103(5): 1035–1045.

79. Neuburger M, et al. Inflammation and infection complications of 2285 perineural catheters: a prospective study. *Acta Anaesthesiologica Scandinavica* 2007;51(1):108–114.

80. Kent CD, Bollag L. Neurological adverse events following regional anesthesia administration. *Local and Regional Anesthesia* 2010;3(1):115–128.

81. Centers for Disease Control and Prevention. Bacterial meningitis after intrapartum spinal anesthesia–New York and Ohio, 2008–2009. *MMWR Morb Mortal Wkly Rep* 2010;59(3):65–69.

82. Bergman BD, et al. Neurologic complications of 405 consecutive continuous axillary catheters. *Anesth Analg* 2003;96(1): 247–252.

6

Hemodynamic Complications

Gregory A. Liguori

The most significant hemodynamic complications associated with regional anesthesia are hypotension and bradycardia. They are the most common physiologic changes associated with neuraxial anesthesia and in certain situations may be associated with peripheral nerve blockade. This chapter considers the pathophysiology of regional anesthesia-associated hypotension and bradycardia, the factors that increase the patient risk for these occurrences, and strategies to prevent and treat these common side effects, which can potentially lead to major adverse events.

▶ DEFINITION

Hypotension is broadly defined as abnormally low blood pressure. Investigators have often developed operational definitions of hypotension for use in individual studies. It is the variations in these operational definitions that often lead to confusion and inconsistencies when comparing different studies. One common operational definition of hypotension is any systolic blood pressure below a predetermined level, usually 80 or 90 mm Hg. Alternatively, a fixed percentage reduction (commonly 30%) in systolic or mean blood pressure from that patient's baseline can also be considered hypotension. Finally, some studies classify hypotension as a rapid rate of decline in blood pressure (such as 30% or 30 mm Hg over 5 minutes) regardless of the absolute value. The mechanisms involved in this latter definition of hypotension may be different from those involved in slower rates of decline. Furthermore, the method by which blood pressure is measured is essential to understanding the occurrence of hypotension in any study. Invasive measurements versus noninvasive measurements should be specified, as well as the level at which the transducer is placed, or the location at which the noninvasive blood pressure cuff is situated. These variables may all impact the interpretation of hypotension.

Bradycardia can be broadly defined as an abnormally low heart rate. This complication can also be described operationally as a heart rate below a fixed level (50 beats per minute, bpm), a percentage reduction from baseline (30%), or a sudden decrease at a predetermined rate. Again, the mechanisms involved in a slow decline in heart rate over the course of a regional anesthetic may be very different from a sudden drop in heart rate over 1 to 2 minutes (Fig. 6-1). Although the complications of hypotension and bradycardia are most often associated with neuraxial anesthesia, these hemodynamic changes have also been described during shoulder arthroscopy in the sitting position under interscalene block.[1] Although it may seem as though this setting has little in common with spinal or epidural anesthesia, some mutual hemodynamic conditions exist that make the pathophysiological origin of these events related.

▶ SCOPE OF THE PROBLEM

The incidence of hypotension and bradycardia in patients undergoing neuraxial anesthesia is quite significant. Several

Panel A

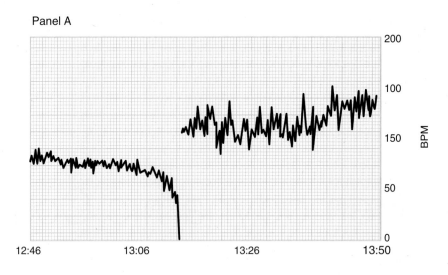

Panel B

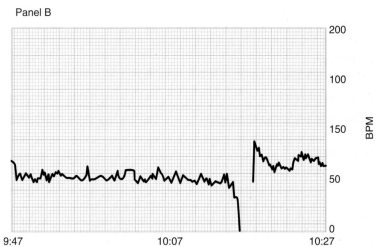

FIGURE 6-1. An example of a slow decline in heart rate (panel A) versus a sudden drop (panel B).

large-scale reports place the incidence of bradycardia between 2% and 13%. The incidence of hypotension in these same studies ranges from 8% to 33% (Table 6-1). Although the incidence of these hemodynamic complications is relatively high, the medical significance of the events is variable. Quite often, these occurrences are ignored or easily treated or in some cases they are desirable hemodynamic conditions[2] for a given operation.

Severe hypotension and bradycardia leading to cardiac arrest may also occur with regional anesthesia. An early case in the anesthesia literature of a cardiac arrest following a regional anesthetic was reported by Wetstone and Wang in 1974.[3] The patient was a healthy 29-year-old male undergoing a minor urologic procedure under spinal anesthesia. The arrest was successfully treated with atropine and closed-chest cardiac massage, with no long-term sequelae. Over a decade later, the issue of sudden unexpected cardiac arrest under spinal anesthesia was again highlighted in the anesthesia literature. Caplan et al.'s closed-claims analysis in 1988[4] described 14 cases of cardiac arrest under spinal anesthesia in healthy patients. Half of the cases were possibly attributable to respiratory events. The remainder were likely of a primary circulatory etiology. The majority of patients in this report had poor outcomes. A subsequent report in 1989[5] described three cardiac arrests during spinal anesthesia that were not respiratory in nature, as evidenced by oxygen saturation

immediately prior to the arrest remaining normal. This finding was confirmed in multiple other case reports involving both spinal[6–10] and epidural[11,12] anesthetics. It is now clear that cardiac arrests may be precipitated primarily by nonhypoxic circulatory conditions during a neuraxial anesthetic.

Several large-scale studies have attempted to determine the incidence of cardiac arrest under regional anesthesia (Table 6-2). Although the rate of occurrence of cardiac arrests during regional anesthesia is low, the mortality associated specifically with spinal anesthesia remains exceedingly high. In one report, cardiac arrest secondary to a neuraxial block accounted for the largest category of malpractice claims associated with death or brain damage.[13]

Sudden severe hypotension and bradycardia have also been noted during shoulder surgery under interscalene block in the sitting position. Several prospective and retrospective studies have confirmed that these events may occur in 13% to 29% of cases (Table 6-3). Although acute hypotension and bradycardia do occur with significant frequency, serious morbidities or mortality have yet to be reported in this scenario.

A related situation that has recently been described is the occurrence of cerebrovascular events during shoulder surgery in the sitting position utilizing *intentional* hypotension to minimize blood loss.[14] Since only case reports are available, the incidence of these events is unknown. Given the likelihood that the incidence of these events is extremely rare,

TABLE 6-1 Reported Incidence of Hypotension and Bradycardia Associated with Neuraxial Anesthesia

AUTHOR AND YEAR OF PUBLICATION	ANESTHETIC	N	INCIDENCE OF HYPOTENSION	INCIDENCE OF BRADYCARDIA
Tarkkila et al. 1991[104]	Spinal	1,881	16.4%[d]	8.9%[a]
Carpenter et al. 1992[87]	Spinal	952	33%[c]	13%[a]
Curatolo et al. 1996[105]	Epidural	1,050	15%[c]	2.3%[b]
Fanelli et al. 1998[106]	Epidural and GA	1,200	31.6%[e]	12.7%[a]
Hartmann et al. 2002[107]	Spinal	3,315	8.2%[e]	N/A
Lesser et al. 2003[86]	Spinal or Epidural	6,663	N/A	10.2%[a]
Klasen et al. 2003[44]	CSE	1,023	10.9%[e]	N/A

[a]HR < 50.
[b]HR < 45.
[c]SBP < 90.
[d]A 30% decrease in SBP from baseline or SBP < 85.
[e]A 30% decrease in SBP from baseline.
GA, general anesthesia; SBP, systolic blood pressure; CSE, combined spinal epidural; and N/A, not applicable.

large-scale studies will be required to evaluate their occurrence. It is clear, however, that the morbidity during these events has the potential to be catestrophic. Using near-infrared spectroscopy, Murphy et al. described an 80% incidence of cerebral desaturation events in the sitting position (compared with 0% in the lateral position) for patients undergoing shoulder arthroscopy.[15] None of these patients, however, developed any significant anesthestic morbidities.

▶ PATHOPHYSIOLOGY

Neuraxial Regional Anesthesia

The primary determinant of hypotension induced by spinal or epidural anesthesia is sympathetic nerve blockade.[16] The greater the extent of sympathetic block achieved, the more hypotensive the patient may become. These sympathetically induced effects on blood pressure are mediated through changes in systemic vascular resistance and cardiac output. By inhibiting sympathetic neuronal output to resistance and capacitance vessels,[17,18] systemic vascular resistance and cardiac output are both decreased. This is mediated through a shift in blood volume from the heart and thorax to the mesentery, kidneys, and lower extremities.[19] The mean arterial pressure, in turn, falls (Fig. 6-2). Interestingly, in one study on elderly patients with cardiac disease, ejection fraction increased significantly during spinal anesthesia,[19] indicating enhanced cardiac performance and contractility in this setting.

Low sensory levels of neuraxial anesthesia (below T5) often result in minimal hemodynamic changes. Vasoconstriction

TABLE 6-2 Incidence of Cardiac Arrests (and Death) Associated with Regional Anesthesia

AUTHOR AND YEAR	N	SPINAL	EPIDURAL	PNB
Auroy et al. 1997[46]	103,730	26 (6)	3 (0)	3 (0)
Olsson et al. 1998[53]	35,000	7 (5)	2 (0)	0 (0)
Biboulet et al. 2001[52]	29,943	5 (4)	0 (0)	0 (0)
Auroy et al. 2002[47]	158,083	10 (3)	0 (0)	1 (0)
Kopp et. al. 2006[48]	77,685	10 (6)	4 (3)	N/A

PNB, peripheral nerve block.

TABLE 6-3 Incidence of Hypotensive/Bradycardic Events Associated with Shoulder Arthroscopy in the Sitting Position Under Interscalene Block

AUTHOR AND YEAR OF PUBLICATION	INCIDENCE OF EVENT (%)
Roch et al. 1991[108]	24[a]
D'Alessio et al. 1995[1]	20[b]
Liguori et al. 1998[60]	28[b]
Kahn et al. 1999[59]	13[b]
Sia et al. 2003[58]	29[b]

Definition of event: A decrease in HR of >30 BPM in <5 min or any decrease to <50 BPM and/or a decrease in SBP of >30 mm Hg in <5 min or any decrease to <90 mm Hg.
[a]Epinephrine added to ISB and beta blocker use not addressed.
[b]Epinephrine added to ISB and no beta blockers given.

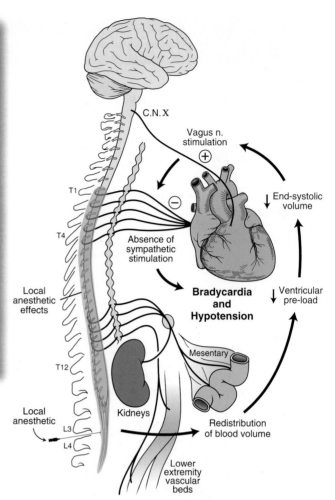

FIGURE 6-2. Pathophysiology of bradycardia and hypotension during neuraxial anesthesia. ⊕ = positive feedback ⊖ = negative feedback.

above the level of the block often compensates for the vasodilatory effects below the level of blockade.[20–23] The measurement of sympathetic level achieved during a neuraxial anesthetic is not straightforward. Several studies[24,25] have attempted to relate the level of sympathetic blockade to the sensory level achieved. It is clear that predicting the degree of sympathetic block does not parallel the sensory or motor block achieved during spinal or epidural anesthesia. Early studies reported that neuraxial anesthesia had little, if any, effect on heart rate if the sensory level was below the fifth thoracic dermatome.[26] This response may be partially influenced by the cardioaccelerator fibers originating from the first through fourth thoracic spinal levels (Fig. 6-2). It is now clear that the heart rate often decreases during neuraxial blockade involving lower dermatomal levels as well. As noted, the sensory level often underestimates the level of sympathetic blockade.[24] Therefore, hemodynamically significant hypotension and bradycardia may occur at any time during the course or resolution of neuraxial anesthesia. Case series have given support to this theory.[12]

Another mechanism that explains how spinal or epidural anesthesia may induce hypotension or bradycardia is via the systemic effects of local anesthetics or vasoactive additives used during the course of an anesthetic. Local anesthetics have direct effects on both the myocardium and smooth muscle of the peripheral vasculature. All local anesthetics cause a dose-dependent negative inotropic effect on cardiac muscle.[26,27] These effects are usually only observed at systemic concentrations that are higher than those attained in normal clinical settings. Furthermore, the more potent local anesthetics (e.g., tetracaine or bupivacaine) cause a greater degree of myocardial depression than less potent drugs (e.g., lidocaine or mepivacaine).[26]

Two common additives to local anesthetics used in regional anesthesia that may affect hemodynamic variables are epinephrine and clonidine. Epinephrine is often added to local anesthetic injections to decrease the rate of vascular absorption, increase the duration of action, or act as an intravascular marker. Absorbed epinephrine has been reported to cause a decrease in blood pressure due to β_2 adrenergic stimulation.[23] However, hypotension seen with epidural injection of local anesthetic and epinephrine may also be secondary to a more profound degree of sympathetic blockade.[26] Clonidine induces hypotension through stimulation of α_2 adrenergic receptors. Neuraxial administration causes hemodynamic effects by systemic absorption to central and peripheral sites, as well as direct effects on the spinal cord. Therefore, the degree of hypotension may be greater with thoracic epidural use compared to lumbar injection, due to the local density of sympathetic preganglionic neurons in the thoracic region. Clonidine also reduces the heart rate by presynaptic inhibition of norepinephrine release and by direct parasympathomimetic effects. These hemodynamic effects occur within 30 minutes and last from 6 to 8 hours.[28]

Decreased cardiac output and systemic vascular resistance caused by sympathetic blockade or direct effects of local anesthetics or additives are reasonable explanations for the slow, progressive decreases in heart rate and blood pressure observed during neuraxial anesthetics. However,

BOX 6-1 Differences in Hypotension and Bradycardia Associated with Regional Anesthesia

Gradual onset caused by sympathetic blockade secondary to:

- Local anesthetic effects
- Epinephrine or clonidine additives

Sudden onset caused by intracardiac reflex secondary to:

- Upright posture (in shoulder surgery patients)
- Reduced preload
- Increased circulating catecholamines leading to vigorous myocardial contractility

sudden acute events require an additional mechanism of action to explain their occurrence (Box 6-1). Nonsurgical patients who experience sudden severe hypotension and bradycardia resulting in syncope can be evaluated by tilt-table testing. This test is based on the observation that syncope is associated with the upright posture and that concentrations of circulating catecholamines increase before the onset of symptoms.[29] Therefore, syncope can be precipitated by placing a patient on a 60-degree upright tilt table and administering exogenous catecholamines.[30] This response has arguably been attributed to the Bezold-Jarisch reflex.[31] Stimulation of this reflex increases parasympathetic activity and inhibits sympathetic activity, resulting in bradycardia, vasodilatation, and hypotension. The hemodynamic conditions required for activation of these reflex events are a poorly filled ventricle (caused by the upright posture)[32,33] and vigorous myocardial contractility (caused by endogenous or exogenous catecholamines), which in turn stimulates mechanoreceptors within the ventricular walls.[32] An intact system of vagal afferent fibers is required for mediation of the reflex.[31]

During the course of a neuraxial anesthetic, a complex redistribution of blood volume occurs between the heart and various circulatory beds.[34] The result of this redistribution of blood volume to the mesentery, kidneys, and lower extremities is a poorly filled ventricle with enhanced contractility.[19] Therefore, the hemodynamic conditions described during tilt-table-inducible syncope are paralleled. This hypothesis was demonstrated in patients developing presyncopal symptoms during epidural anesthesia.[35] Echocardiography performed in these patients confirmed reductions in central blood volume and left ventricular diameters. Furthermore, acute bradycardia and hypotension during spinal anesthesia were associated with a sudden increase in vagal activity as measured by heart rate variability analysis.[36]

Peripheral Regional Anesthesia

Less intuitively, shoulder surgery under interscalene block may also be associated with a decrease in left ventricular volume caused by the upright posture of the sitting position. Furthermore, enhanced cardiac contractility may occur by the addition of epinephrine to the local anesthetic or arthroscopic irrigating solution (Fig. 6-3). These hemodynamic conditions during shoulder surgery have yet to be confirmed by direct measurements in a prospective evaluation.

There is considerable controversy in the literature regarding whether these mechanisms truly explain all vasodepressor-mediated syncope[33,37–39] or the potential relationships to sudden severe hypotension and bradycardia seen with regional anesthesia.[40] One explanation for some of the controversy surrounding this mechanism is that activation of the Bezold-Jarisch reflex may be affected by the relative contributions of central volume depletion to the degree of fractional myocardial shortening. In other words, a vigorously contracting moderately empty ventricle may be as prone to slowing as a normally contracting severely depleted one. Another likely explanation for the contradictions in the cited studies is that this reflex arc is one of many intracardiac reflexes whose final common pathway is sudden severe hypotension and bradycardia.[41,42] In any case, it is clear that a poorly filled vigorously contracting heart with an intact vagal system is prone to sudden severe bradycardia and hypotension.

The pathophysiology of the cases of cerebral ischemia during shoulder surgery in the upright position remains unclear. A proposed mechanism may be a reduction of cerebral blood flow secondary to relative intraoperative postural hypotension.[14] However, each of the four cases reported involved general anesthesia. Therefore, there is no direct relationship between these events and regional anesthesia *per se*. In fact, a recent retrospective review of 4169 shoulder operations performed in the sitting position under interscalene block revealed a zero incidence of overt stroke in the setting of induced hypotension.[43]

▶ RISK FACTORS

Neuraxial Regional Anesthesia

Predicting which patient or anesthetic characteristics may predispose to hypotension or bradycardia during regional anesthesia is a difficult task (Box 6-2). Several large-scale studies have attempted to evaluate various risk factors (Table 6-4). Common themes among the six studies that evaluated the risk of developing hypotension include a higher sensory anesthetic level (five studies), elevated body mass index (three studies), older patients (two studies), and the addition of general anesthesia (two studies). One study noted an increased incidence of hypotension in patients receiving combined spinal-epidural anesthesia compared with spinal anesthesia alone.[44] Interestingly, Smiley et al. found evidence that genetic variations in the beta adrenoreceptor affected the incidence of hypotension during cesarean delivery.[45] The common characteristics among the five studies that attempted to predict the risk factors of bradycardia include higher dermatomal level (two studies), beta-blocker use (two studies), younger patients (two studies), and lower baseline heart rate (two studies). It is clear from this summary that definitive predictive factors for the development of hypotension or bradycardia remain speculative.

Determining risk factors for the development of cardiac arrest under regional anesthesia is even more complex. Three studies found that the incidence of cardiac arrest during spinal anesthesia was significantly increased compared with epidural or peripheral nerve block.[46–48] It is interesting

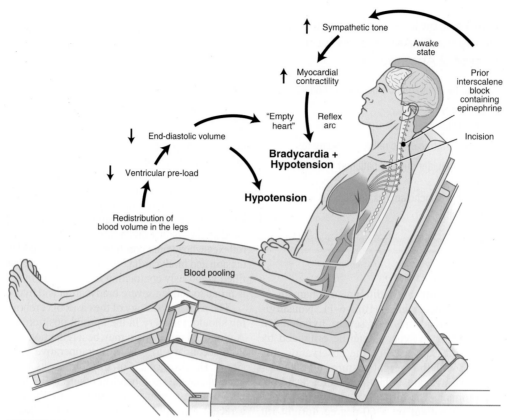

FIGURE 6-3. Pathophysiology of bradycardia and hypotension during shoulder surgery in the sitting position under interscalene block.

to note that in many of the cases, the arrests were preceded by bradycardia. One may speculate that if we can predict and prevent bradycardia, we can predict and prevent cardiac arrest.[49] Gratadour et al. employed a continuous noninvasive technique that measured sympathovagal effects of spinal anesthesia.[42] They found patients who experienced acute bradycardia and hypotension during the course of a spinal anesthetic did not have abnormally high parasympathetic activity prior to the spinal anesthetic. This finding indicates that patients at risk of developing acute bradycardia and hypotension during spinal anesthesia may not be prospectively identified by this technique. Chamchad et al.[50] used heart rate variability analysis in obstetric patients to determine the risk of developing hypotension. They found that by using a baseline point correlation dimension (PD2) of >3.90, hypotension during spinal anesthesia could be accurately predicted. Similarly, Hanss et al.[51] prospectively evaluated the ability to predict hypotension based on low-frequency/high-frequency (LF/HF) ratios of heart rate variability. They determined that this analysis might be suitable for predicting hypotension during spinal anesthesia for cesarean delivery. More research in this area is needed prior to advocating this technology for routine use.

Other common themes for the development of cardiac arrests in several studies[46,47] included hip arthroplasty and advanced age. Two other studies also found spinal anesthesia, hip arthroplasty, and advanced age to be common related factors for intraoperative cardiac arrest during regional anesthesia.[52,53] Clinicians should be extremely vigilant during hip replacement surgery under neuraxial anesthesia in the elderly population. A likely mechanism for this finding is the frequent occurrence of embolic material migrating to the heart and lungs during cemented hip arthroplasty.[54,55] This material (fat, thrombus, bone marrow) causes an acute pulmonary embolism-type hemodynamic response. Low cardiac output secondary to right heart distention and failure may lead to bradycardia and cardiac arrest.[56] Secondary effects on the pulmonary vasculature caused by the release of vasoactive substances may also play a role in the development of cardiac failure. Emboli, as described previously, may predispose to an exaggerated release of these humoral substances and potentiate the mechanical obstructive effects.[57] These humoral and obstructive effects in the setting of spinal or epidural anesthesia may enhance the development of a volume-depleted vigorously contracting left ventricle.

Pollard analyzed three case reports of severe bradycardia or asystole during spinal anesthesia and found that patients who develop these events fit a high-risk profile.[49] Younger patients (<50 years old), healthy patients (ASA 1), and higher sensory level (>T6) were common themes in many of the reports. Kopp et al. observed that many cardiac arrests that occur in association with spinal or epidural anesthesia are in fact caused by surgical, and not anesthetic, factors.[48] It is clear that the development of bradycardia or asystole during regional anesthesia is complex in nature and difficult to predict. However, there are some similarities between risk factors for the development of bradycardia or hypotension and cardiac arrest.

BOX 6-2 Risk Factors for Hypotension, Bradycardia, and Cardiac Arrest Associated with Neuraxial Regional anesthesia

Hypotension
- High sensory block level
- Elevated body mass index
- Elderly patients
- Combined regional/general anesthesia

Bradycardia
- High sensory block level
- Beta blocker use
- Younger patients
- Baseline bradycardia

Cardiac arrest
- Spinal anesthesia more frequent than epidural anesthesia or peripheral nerve block
- Development of bradycardia
- Hip arthroplasty
- Elderly patients

Peripheral Regional Anesthesia

Risk factors for acute bradycardia and hypotension that may occur during shoulder surgery in the sitting position under interscalene block have not been well studied. Several studies evaluated the effect of multiple variables on the development of these events.[1,58-60] Baseline heart rate and blood pressure, level of sedation, amount of intravenous fluid, age, gender, height, weight, and ASA physical status were not risk factors for developing acute bradycardia or hypotension. However, none of the studies were adequately powered to evaluate these variables. One study[58] found that administration of exogenous epinephrine did contribute to the development of hypotension and bradycardia in this setting. This finding is consistent with the previously discussed pathophysiologic mechanisms of these events.

There are not enough data to speculate on the risk factors for cerebral ischemia during shoulder surgery in the upright position. One may speculate that significant decreases in intraoperative blood pressure compared with preoperative values may place a patient at risk for such an event. Central to this concept might be the practitioner's failure to recognize that blood pressure measured at the arm or leg is different from that present at the brain level when the patient is in the sitting position. Such hydrostatic differences might lead to a false sense of security, when in fact perfusion to the brain is at or below threshold values. Again, it needs to be emphasized that the four cases present in the literature[14] all occurred during a general anesthetic. Therefore, it is quite possible that general anesthesia is a risk factor for these events, and the impact of regional anesthesia on perioperative cerebral events in the sitting position is nonexistent.

▶ PREVENTION

The vast majority of the literature on prevention of hypotension occurs in the setting of spinal or epidural anesthesia for caesarian delivery. Early reports indicated that hypotension in this setting can be greatly reduced by "preloading" patients with intravenous fluids.[61-63] More recent studies have shown that volume loading patients prior to spinal anesthesia for cesarean delivery has little or no effect on the incidence of hypotension in this setting.[64-66] Fewer studies have evaluated hypotension during neuraxial anesthesia in nonpregnant patients. Coe et al. found no significant effect of prehydration on the incidence of hypotension in elderly patients undergoing abdominal or orthopedic surgery.[67] These results were confirmed by Buggy et al. in a similar population.[68] Furthermore, Arndt et al. found that prehydration caused a significant reduction in the incidence of hypotension, but only for a brief (15-minute) period of time following spinal anesthesia.[69] Taken as a whole, the literature offers little support for the routine practice of preventing hypotension by prehydration in the obstetric[65,66,70] or nonobstetric[71] populations. The practice of preventing hypotension by prehydration with colloid solutions versus crystalloid solutions is also controversial. Three studies found no benefit of colloid administration versus crystalloid administration in the obstetric population.[72-74] Other reports did find a benefit of a variety of colloids such as albumen[75] or other synthetic volume expanders.[76-80] However, the potential risks of fluid overload must be weighed against the transient benefits of preanesthetic volume expansion as a routine practice in a variety of surgical populations.[81]

The prophylactic use of vasopressor infusions to prevent hemodynamic complications of neuraxial block has also been studied. A prophylactic infusion of ephedrine was found to significantly reduce the incidence of hypotension compared with crystalloid prehydration in a postpartum population.[82] Incidentally, no patients developed hypertension in this report. The prophylactic use of dihydroergotamine[69] or phenylephrine[83] also decreased the incidence of cardiovascular side effects in nonobstetric populations. However, the effect of this therapy was delayed, reducing hypotensive episodes that occurred at least 30 minutes following induction of spinal anesthesia. Ngan Kee et. al.[84] found that a combination of phenylephrine and crystalloid prevented hypotension during spinal anesthesia for cesarean delivery.

Taken as a whole, prophylactic use of crystalloid, colloids, or vasopressors should not be utilized as a routine practice. These therapies should be considered in specific situations depending on the medical condition of the patient, preoperative state of hydration, and surgical procedure.

Due to the infrequent occurrence of cardiac arrests during neuraxial anesthesia, no randomized studies have been performed to evaluate factors that may prevent these events. However, if we assume that the mechanisms responsible for these events are similar to those responsible for acute vasovagal syncope in the nonsurgical populations, several conclusions can be drawn. The theoretical basis for prevention of these acute events is by preventing one of the hemodynamic

TABLE 6-4 Risk Factors for Hypotension and Bradycardia During Neuraxial Anesthesia

AUTHOR AND YEAR OF PUBLICATION	ANESTHETIC TYPE	HYPOTENSION	BRADYCARDIA
Tarkkila 1992[109]	Spinal	Age > 50 Level > T6 BMI > 30 Bupivacaine Opiate pre-med	Age < 50 Level > T6
Carpenter 1992[87]	Spinal	Age > 40 Level > T5 Baseline SBP < 120 L 1/2 or L 2/3 puncture Addition of GA Add phenylephrine to local	Level > T5 ASA PS 1 Baseline HR < 60 Use of beta blocker PR interval > 0.2
Curatolo 1996[105]	Epidural	BMI > 30 Increasing "spread of block" Use of lidocaine Use of epidural fentanyl Not using a tourniquet	Male
Fanelli 1998[106]	Epidural and GA	ASA PS > 2 No pre-op volume loading Addition of GA	ASA PS > 2 Use of epidural clonidine
Hartmann 2002[107]	Spinal	Baseline hypertension Chronic alcohol consumption BMI > 28 Level > T6 Emergency procedure	N/A
Lesser 2003[86]	Spinal or epidural	N/A	Age < 37 male ASA PS 1 or 2 BMI < 30 Baseline HR < 60 h/o diabetes mellitus Use of alpha1 blockers Use of beta blockers Nonemergency surgery
Klasen 2003[44]	CSE	Baseline hypertension Level > T6	N/A

BMI, body mass index; GA, general anesthesia; HR, heart rate; and ASA PS, American Society of Anesthesiologists physical status.

triggering mechanisms from activating reflex vagal output and sympathetic withdrawal. These triggering mechanisms, as noted previously, are a poorly filled ventricle and vigorous myocardial contractility.

Abe et al. concluded that beta blockade significantly reduced the incidence of vasodepressor syncope in patients who tested positive for tilt-table-inducible syncope.[85] This hypothesis was tested during shoulder surgery in the sitting position under interscalene block.[60] Treatment with metoprolol significantly decreased the incidence of acute hypotensive and bradycardic events. Furthermore, Sia et al.[58] found that omitting the use of exogenous epinephrine significantly decreased the incidence of hypotensive bradycardic events

during shoulder surgery in the sitting position under interscalene block, presumably by preventing a state of enhanced myocardial contractility.

No studies to date have attempted to evaluate the effect of beta blockade or epinephrine use on the incidence of cardiac arrest during spinal or epidural anesthesia. Although there may be theoretical benefits to using beta blockers in this situation, several studies[86,87] clearly found that beta blockade is a risk factor for bradycardia during spinal anesthesia. Because asystole and cardiac arrest are often preceded by bradycardia,[49] one may expect beta blockade to increase, not decrease, the incidence of acute events. Furthermore, prophylactic treatment with positive inotropes is often used to prevent acute bradycardia during neuraxial anesthesia.[2] These contradictions can possibly be explained by differing mechanisms responsible for acute reflex events versus a gradual slowing of the heart rate. Further investigations are required in these areas.

Since there is insufficient information to determine the actual etiology of cerebral ischemia during shoulder surgery in the upright position, any clinical pearl on preventing these events remains speculative. It is clear that measuring blood pressure in the sitting position is different from the supine position. Therefore, it is important to correct measured values for the hydrostatic effect of this position. The ratio of cm H_2O pressure to mm Hg pressure is 4:3 (or ~ 1.33 cm H_2O–1 mm Hg). Thus, for every centimeter of distance from the source of blood pressure measurement (arm or leg) to the external auditory meatus, there is a corresponding decrease in blood pressure measured at the brain. These corrections may be even more important in patients with chronic hypertension, cerebrovascular disease, etc. Whether this practice will have any effect on the incidence of these catestrophic events is unknown (Fig. 6-4).

▶ TREATMENT

Mild or moderate hypotension and bradycardia during regional anesthesia do not need to be treated in all patients. The decision to treat often depends on the medical condition of the patient and surgical conditions required (Box 6-3). During severe hypotension or bradycardia, or when the patient's medical condition will not allow for any degree of hemodynamic instability, treatment should be expeditious and definitive. The use of intravenous fluids alone to treat hypotension and bradycardia during regional anesthesia, although theoretically plausible, is often not practical. The response of heart rate and blood pressure to fluid therapy alone requires at least several minutes,[88] which in many cases may not be fast enough. Therefore, vasopressors and anticholinergics are the first-line therapies for cases of hemodynamic instability that require treatment.[16,89]

Many studies have evaluated the role of vasopressors in the treatment of regional anesthesia-induced hypotension. Dopamine,[90] phenylephrine,[91] metaraminol,[92] and epinephrine[91] have all proven to be rapid and efficacious therapeutic options. Ephedrine is a mixed alpha- and beta-adrenergic agonist that acts by both direct and indirect mechanisms. It primarily causes release of norepinephrine and is therefore subject to tachyphylaxis because norepinephrine stores are depleted. The cardiovascular effects are similar to epinephrine, although ephedrine is both longer acting and less potent.[93] It provides effective therapy for all hemodynamic perturbations caused by neuraxial anesthesia. Several studies[17,92,94] and reviews[16,89] have confirmed that ephedrine should be considered a first-line therapy in both the obstetric and nonobstetric populations (Box 6-3). During cases in which ephedrine alone is insufficient to correct the hypotension, other agents can be added. It is also essential to consider the potential deleterious effects of these inotropes and vasopressors on patients with coronary artery disease. Titration to effect is important, as is the particular choice of agent in any given patient.

The treatment of cardiac arrests during regional anesthesia obviously requires immediate therapy to restore blood flow and circulation (Box 6-3). Case reports of cardiac arrests during regional anesthesia[5-10,12] that were treated immediately were uniformly associated with excellent outcomes. Conversely, cases resulting in poor outcomes were associated

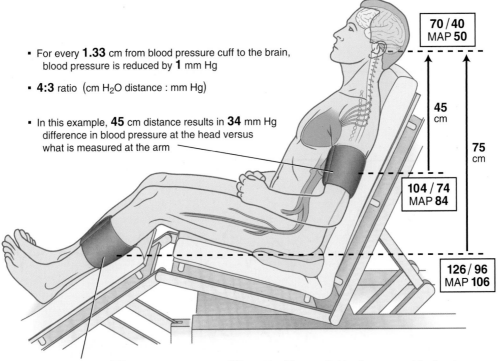

- For every **1.33** cm from blood pressure cuff to the brain, blood pressure is reduced by **1** mm Hg

- **4:3** ratio (cm H_2O distance : mm Hg)

- In this example, **45** cm distance results in **34** mm Hg difference in blood pressure at the head versus what is measured at the arm

70/40 MAP **50**

45 cm

75 cm

104/74 MAP **84**

126/96 MAP **106**

- In this example, **75** cm distance results in **56** mm Hg difference in blood pressure at the head versus what is measured at the leg

FIGURE 6-4. Correction for hydrostatic differences in blood pressure measurement in the sitting position.

therapy. As noted previously, arrests during regional anesthesia are often associated with nonhypoxic conditions. Patients are well oxygenated at the time of the arrest.[5,12] Therefore, if circulation can be immediately restored, airway and ventilatory control can often be avoided. This hypothesis is supported by the many case reports and case series previously referenced. Vigilance of hemodynamic trends and diagnosis within seconds are completely essential.

Several medications have been used to treat severe bradycardia or cardiac arrest in the setting of regional anesthesia. These include ephedrine, atropine, and epinephrine. Combinations of an anticholinergic and a sympathomimetic are often indicated in this setting. Obviously, no prospective human studies have been carried out to assess the most effective options. However, a recent study in a pig model of cardiac arrest in the setting of epidural anesthesia concluded that both epinephrine and vasopressin increased coronary perfusion pressure, but vasopressin may be more desirable.[95] In a single dose, it was longer acting and was associated with less acidosis compared with epinephrine. However, bradycardia was more common with vasopressin, requiring additional treatment with atropine.

In addition to pharmacologic options, the technique of thump pacing has been used with success in a variety of settings.[96–99] This maneuver, consisting of rapid forceful precordial thumps, combined with pharmacologic therapy (as noted previously), has been successful in treating regional anesthesia-induced cardiac arrests (Fig. 6-5).

with delays in resuscitation[4]. Basic and advanced cardiac life support (BCLS/ACLS) protocols are often simplified using the acronym ABC or "airway, breathing, circulation." These protocols were developed for "community" arrests, which are often respiratory in nature and associated with a delay in

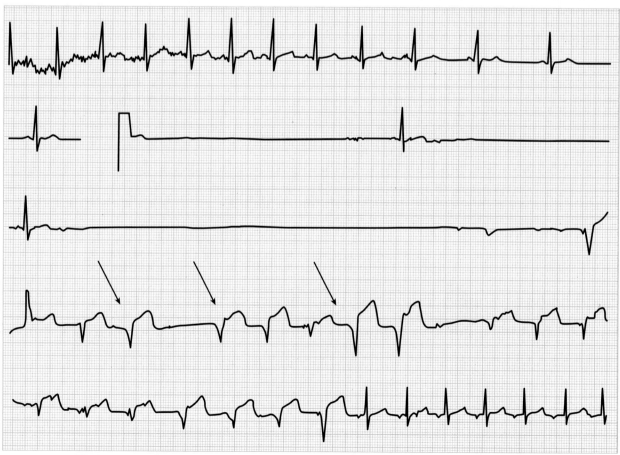

FIGURE 6-5. A real-time recording of an evolving severe bradycardia treated with thump pacing. *Arrows* depict the application of precordial thumps.

If this initial therapy is unsuccessful, however, a full ACLS protocol should be initiated without delay including full ventilatory support. Furthermore, other causes of severe bradycardia or asystole should be considered in the differential diagnoses in these cases. Unfortunately, cases where a cardiac arrest requiring full ACLS protocols occurred in the setting of a neuraxial blockade closed-chest cardiac massage have not enjoyed tremendous success. In a dog model of cardiac arrest after spinal anesthesia, cardiopulmonary resuscitation (CPR) was found to be ineffective in maintaining coronary perfusion.[100] A likely contributory mechanism is impaired release of endogenous catecholamines[101] and vasopressin[102,103] during spinal or epidural anesthesia. The exogenous administration of epinephrine[94,100] or vasopressin[94] improves coronary perfusion, the efficacy of CPR, and ultimate survival. These findings in experimental animal models confirm earlier clinical observations that delaying epinephrine treatment during cardiac arrest and spinal anesthesia contributed to poor survival and patient outcomes.[4] Interestingly, the conclusions of a large, but retrospective, study indicate that cardiac arrests during neuraxial anesthesia were associated with an equal or better likelihood of survival compared with cardiac arrests that occur during general anesthesia.[48] However, due to the variable etiologies of the arrests in this report, no definitive conclusions can be made.

▶ SUMMARY

Hypotension and bradycardia are frequent and often benign complications of regional anesthesia. Severe bradycardia and cardiac arrest also occur, although much less frequently. The mechanisms of these events are complex and usually of a primary circulatory etiology. Fortunately, by understanding the pathophysiology of these events, severe hemodynamic instability with regional anesthesia is potentially preventable. When severe hypotension and bradycardia occur, treatment must be immediate and aggressive in order to achieve the highest success and best long-term outcome.

References

1. D'Alessio JG, Weller RS, Rosenblum M. Activation of the Bezold-Jarisch reflex in the sitting position for shoulder arthroscopy using interscalene block. *Anesth Analg* 1995;80:1158–1162.
2. Sharrock NE, Salvati EA. Hypotensive epidural anesthesia for total hip arthroplasty: a review. *Acta Orthop Scand* 1996;67:91–107.
3. Wetstone DL, Wong KC. Sinus bradycardia and asystole during spinal anesthesia. *Anesthesiology* 1974;41:87–89.
4. Caplan RA, Ward RJ, Posner K, et al. Unexpected cardiac arrest during spinal anesthesia: a closed claims analysis of predisposing factors. *Anesthesiology* 1988;68:5–11.
5. Mackey DC, Carpenter RL, Thompson GE, et al. Bradycardia and asystole during spinal anesthesia: a report of three cases without morbidity. *Anesthesiology* 1989;70:866–868.
6. Lovstad RZ, Granhus G, Hetland S. Bradycardia and asystolic cardiac arrest during spinal anaesthesia: a report of five cases. *Acta Anaesthesiol Scand* 2000;44:48–52.
7. Jordi EM, Marsch SC, Strebel S. Third degree heart block and asystole associated with spinal anesthesia. *Anesthesiology* 1998;89:257–260.
8. McConachie I. Vasovagal asystole during spinal anaesthesia. *Anaesthesia* 1991;46:281–282.
9. Thrush DN, Downs JB. Vagotonia and cardiac arrest during spinal anesthesia. *Anesthesiology* 1999;91:1171–1173.
10. Nishikawa T, Anzai Y, Namiki A. Asystole during spinal anaesthesia after change from Trendelenburg to horizontal position. *Can J Anaesth* 1988;35:406–408.
11. Geffin B, Shapiro L. Sinus bradycardia and asystole during spinal and epidural anesthesia: a report of 13 cases. *J Clin Anesth* 1998;10:278–285.
12. Liguori GA, Sharrock NE. Asystole and severe bradycardia during epidural anesthesia in orthopedic patients. *Anesthesiology* 1997;86:250–257.
13. Lee LA, Posner KL, Domino KB, et al. Injuries associated with regional anesthesia in the 1980s and 1990s: a closed claims analysis. *Anesthesiology* 2004;101:143–152.
14. Pohl A, Cullen D. Cerebral ischemia during shoulder surgery in the upright position: a case series. *J Clin Anesth* 2005;17:463–469.
15. Murphy G, Szokol J, Marymont J, et al. *Anesth Analg* 2010;111:496–505.
16. Mark JB, Steele SM. Cardiovascular effects of spinal anesthesia. *Int Anesthesiol Clin* 1989;27:31–39.
17. Butterworth JFt, Piccione W Jr, Berrizbeitia LD, et al. Augmentation of venous return by adrenergic agonists during spinal anesthesia. *Anesth Analg* 1986;65:612–616.
18. Butterworth JFt, Austin JC, Johnson MD, et al. Effect of total spinal anesthesia on arterial and venous responses to dopamine and dobutamine. *Anesth Analg* 1987;66:209–214.
19. Rooke GA, Freund PR, Jacobson AF. Hemodynamic response and change in organ blood volume during spinal anesthesia in elderly men with cardiac disease. *Anesth Analg* 1997;85:99–105.
20. Kennedy WF Jr, Bonica JJ, Ward RJ, et al. Cardiorespiratory effects of epinephrine when used in regional anesthesia. *Acta Anaesthesiol Scand Suppl* 1966;23:320–333.
21. Kennedy WF Jr, Sawyer TK, Gerbershagen HY, et al. Systemic cardiovascular and renal hemodynamic alterations during peridural anesthesia in normal man. *Anesthesiology* 1969;31:414–421.
22. Shimosato S, Etsten BE. The role of the venous system in cardiocirculatory dynamics during spinal and epidural anesthesia in man. *Anesthesiology* 1969;30:619–628.
23. Bonica JJ, Akamatsu TJ, Berges PU, et al. Circulatory effects of peridural block. II. Effects of epinephrine. *Anesthesiology* 1971;34:514–522.
24. Chamberlain DP, Chamberlain BD. Changes in the skin temperature of the trunk and their relationship to sympathetic blockade during spinal anesthesia. *Anesthesiology* 1986;65:139–143.
25. Malmqvist LA, Bengtsson M, Bjornsson G, et al. Sympathetic activity and haemodynamic variables during spinal analgesia in man. *Acta Anaesthesiol Scand* 1987; 31:467–473.
26. Covino BG. Cardiovascular effects of regional anesthesia. *Effects of Anesthesia* 1985;207–215.
27. Feldman H, Covino B, Sage D. Direct chronotropic and inotropic effects of local anesthetic agents in isolated guinea pig atria. *Reg Anesth* 1982;7:149–156.
28. Eisenach JC, De Kock M, Klimscha W. Alpha(2)-adrenergic agonists for regional anesthesia: a clinical review of clonidine (1984–1995). *Anesthesiology* 1996;85:655–674.
29. Chosy JJ, Graham DT. Catecholamines in vasovagal fainting. *J Psychosom Res* 1965;9:189–194.
30. Almquist A, Goldenberg IF, Milstein S, et al. Provocation of bradycardia and hypotension by isoproterenol and upright posture in patients with unexplained syncope. *N Engl J Med* 1989;320:346–351.
31. Mark AL. The Bezold-Jarisch reflex revisited: clinical implications of inhibitory reflexes originating in the heart. *J Am Coll Cardiol* 1983;1:90–102.
32. Shalev Y, Gal R, Tchou PJ, et al. Echocardiographic demonstration of decreased left ventricular dimensions and vigorous myocardial contraction during syncope induced by head-up tilt. *J Am Coll Cardiol* 1991;18:746–751.
33. Liu JE, Hahn RT, Stein KM, et al. Left ventricular geometry and function preceding neurally mediated syncope. *Circulation* 2000;101:777–783.

34. Arndt JO, Hock A, Stanton-Hicks M, et al. Peridural anesthesia and the distribution of blood in supine humans. *Anesthesiology* 1985;163:616–623.

35. Jacobsen J, Sofelt S, Brocks V, et al. Reduced left ventricular diameters at onset of bradycardia during epidural anaesthesia. *Acta Anaesthesiol Scand* 1992;36:831–836.

36. Critchley LA, Chan S, Tam YH. Spectral analysis of sudden bradycardia during intrathecal meperidine anesthesia. *Reg Anesth Pain Med* 1998;23:506–510.

37. Liu S, Paul GE, Carpenter RL, et al. Prolonged PR interval is a risk factor for bradycardia during spinal anesthesia. *Reg Anesth* 1995;20:41–44.

38. Davrath LR, Gotshall RW, Tucker A, et al. The heart is not necessarily empty at syncope. *Aviat Space Environ Med* 1999;70:213–219.

39. Novak V, Honos G, Schondorf R. Is the heart "empty" at syncope? *J Auton Nerv Syst* 1996;60:83–92.

40. Campagna JA, Carter C. Clinical relevance of the Bezold-Jarisch reflex. *Anesthesiology* 2003;98:1250–1260.

41. Dickinson CJ. Fainting precipitated by collapse-firing of venous baroreceptors. *Lancet* 1993;342:970–972.

42. Gratadour P, Viale JP, Parlow J, et al. Sympathovagal effects of spinal anesthesia assessed by the spontaneous cardiac baroreflex. *Anesthesiology* 1997;87:1359–1367.

43. Yadeau JT, Casciano M, Liu SP, et al. Stroke, regional anesthesia in the sitting position and hypotension: a review of 4169 ambulatory surgery patients. *Reg Anesth Pain Med* 2011;36:430–435.

44. Klasen J, Junger A, Hartmann B, et al. Differing incidences of relevant hypotension with combined spinal-epidural anesthesia and spinal anesthesia. *Anesth Analg* 2003;96:1491–1495.

45. Smiley R, Blouin J, Negron M, Landau R. B2-adrenoreceptor genotype affects vasopressor requirements during spinal anesthesia for cesarean delivery. *Anesthesiology* 2006;104:644–50.

46. Auroy Y, Narchi P, Messiah A, et al. Serious complications related to regional anesthesia: results of a prospective survey in France. *Anesthesiology* 1997;87:479–486.

47. Auroy Y, Benhamou D, Bargues L, et al. Major complications of regional anesthesia in France: The SOS Regional Anesthesia Hotline Service. *Anesthesiology* 2002;97:1274–1280.

48. Kopp S, Horlocker T, Warner M, et. al. Cardiac arrest during neuraxial anesthesia: frequency and predisposing factors associated with survival. *Anesth Analg* 2005;100:855–865.

49. Pollard JB. Cardiac arrest during spinal anesthesia: common mechanisms and strategies for prevention. *Anesth Analg* 2001;92:252–256.

50. Chamchad D, Arkoosh VA, Horrow JC, et al. Using heart rate variability to stratify risk of obstetric patients undergoing spinal anesthesia. *Anesth Analg* 2004;99:1818–1821.

51. Hanss R, Bein B, Ledowski T, et al. Heart rate variability predicts severe hypotension after spinal anesthesia for elective cesarean delivery. *Anesthesiology* 2005;102:1086–1093.

52. Biboulet P, Aubas P, Dubourdieu J, et al. Fatal and non fatal cardiac arrests related to anesthesia. *Can J Anaesth* 2001;48:326–332.

53. Olsson GL, Hallen B. Cardiac arrest during anaesthesia: a computer-aided study in 250,543 anaesthetics. *Acta Anaesthesiol Scand* 1988;32:653–664.

54. Kim YH, Oh SW, Kim JS. Prevalence of fat embolism following bilateral simultaneous and unilateral total hip arthroplasty performed with or without cement: a prospective, randomized clinical study. *J Bone Joint Surg Am* 2002;84-A:1372–1379.

55. Hagio K, Sugano N, Takashina M, et al. Embolic events during total hip arthroplasty: an echocardiographic study. *J Arthroplasty* 2003;18:186–192.

56. Thames MD, Alpert JS, Dalen JE. Syncope in patients with pulmonary embolism. *Jama* 1977;238:2509–2511.

57. Buckley J, Popovich J. Pulmonary Embolism. In: Parrillo J, Dellinger R, eds.*Critical Care Medicine: Principles of Diagnosis and Management in the Adult.* St. Louis: Mosby, 2002:881–885.

58. Sia S, Sarro F, Lepri A, et al. The effect of exogenous epinephrine on the incidence of hypotensive/bradycardic events during shoulder surgery in the sitting position during interscalene block. *Anesth Analg* 2003;97:583–588.

59. Kahn RL, Hargett MJ. Beta-adrenergic blockers and vasovagal episodes during shoulder surgery in the sitting position under interscalene block. *Anesth Analg* 1999;88:378–381.

60. Liguori GA, Kahn RL, Gordon J, et al. The use of metoprolol and glycopyrrolate to prevent hypotensive/bradycardic events during shoulder arthroscopy in the sitting position under interscalene block. *Anesth Analg* 1998;87:1320–1325.

61. Wollman SB, Marx GF. Acute hydration for prevention of hypotension of spinal anesthesia in parturients. *Anesthesiology* 1968;29:374–380.

62. Lewis M, Thomas P, Wilkes RG. Hypotension during epidural analgesia for Caesarean section: arterial and central venous pressure changes after acute intravenous loading with two litres of Hartmann's solution. *Anaesthesia* 1983;38:250–253.

63. Clark RB, Thompson DS, Thompson CH. Prevention of spinal hypotension associated with Cesarean section. *Anesthesiology* 1976;45:670–674.

64. Jackson R, Reid JA, Thorburn J. Volume preloading is not essential to prevent spinal-induced hypotension at caesarean section. *Br J Anaesth* 1995;75:262–265.

65. Rout CC, Akoojee SS, Rocke DA, et al. Rapid administration of crystalloid preload does not decrease the incidence of hypotension after spinal anaesthesia for elective caesarean section. *Br J Anaesth* 1992;68:394–397.

66. Rout CC, Rocke DA, Levin J, et al. A reevaluation of the role of crystalloid preload in the prevention of hypotension associated with spinal anesthesia for elective cesarean section. *Anesthesiology* 1993;79:262–269.

67. Coe AJ, Revanas B. Is crystalloid preloading useful in spinal anaesthesia in the elderly? *Anaesthesia* 1990;45:241–243.

68. Buggy D, Higgins P, Moran C, et al. Prevention of spinal anesthesia-induced hypotension in the elderly: comparison between preanesthetic administration of crystalloids, colloids, and no prehydration. *Anesth Analg* 1997;84:106–110.

69. Arndt JO, Bomer W, Krauth J, et al. Incidence and time course of cardiovascular side effects during spinal anesthesia after prophylactic administration of intravenous fluids or vasoconstrictors. *Anesth Analg* 1998;87:347–354.

70. Rout C, Rocke DA. Spinal hypotension associated with Cesarean section: will preload ever work? *Anesthesiology* 1999;91:1565–1567.

71. McCrae AF, Wildsmith JA. Prevention and treatment of hypotension during central neural block. *Br J Anaesth* 1993;70:672–680.

72. Ramanathan S, Masih A, Rock I, et al. Maternal and fetal effects of prophylactic hydration with crystalloids or colloids before epidural anesthesia. *Anesth Analg* 1983;62:673–678.

73. Murray AM, Morgan M, Whitwam JG. Crystalloid versus colloid for circulatory preload for epidural caesarean section. *Anaesthesia* 1989;44:463–436.

74. Karinen J, Rasanen J, Alahuhta S, et al. Effect of crystalloid and colloid preloading on uteroplacental and maternal haemodynamic state during spinal anaesthesia for caesarean section. *Br J Anaesth* 1995;75:531–535.

75. Mathru M, Rao TL, Kartha RK, et al. Intravenous albumin administration for prevention of spinal hypotension during cesarean section. *Anesth Analg* 1980;59:655–658.

76. Riley ET, Cohen SE, Rubenstein AJ, et al. Prevention of hypotension after spinal anesthesia for cesarean section: six percent hetastarch versus lactated Ringer's solution. *Anesth Analg* 1995;81:838–842.

77. Vercauteren MP, Hoffmann V, Coppejans HC, et al. Hydroxyethylstarch compared with modified gelatin as volume preload before spinal anaesthesia for Caesarean section. *Br J Anaesth* 1996;76:731–733.

78. Baraka AS, Taha SK, Ghabach MB, et al. Intravascular administration of polymerized gelatin versus isotonic saline for prevention of spinal-induced hypotension. *Anesth Analg* 1994;78: 301–305.

79. Sharma SK, Gajraj NM, Sidawi JE. Prevention of hypotension during spinal anesthesia: a comparison of intravascular administration of hetastarch versus lactated Ringer's solution. *Anesth Analg* 1997;84:111–114.

80. Hallworth D, Jellicoe JA, Wilkes RG. Hypotension during epidural anaesthesia for Caesarean section: a comparison of intravenous loading with crystalloid and colloid solutions. *Anaesthesia* 1982;37:53–56.

81. Holte K, Sharrock NE, Kehlet H. Pathophysiology and clinical implications of perioperative fluid excess. *Br J Anaesth* 2002;89: 622–632.

82. Gajraj NM, Victory RA, Pace NA, et al. Comparison of an ephedrine infusion with crystalloid administration for prevention of hypotension during spinal anesthesia. *Anesth Analg* 1993;76:1023–1026.

83. Nishikawa K, Yamakage M, Omote K, et al. Prophylactic IM small-dose phenylephrine blunts spinal anesthesia-induced hypotensive response during surgical repair of hip fracture in the elderly. *Anesth Analg* 2002;95:751–756.

84. Ngan Kee W, Khaw K, Ng F. Prevention of hypotension during spinal anesthesia for cesarean delivery. *Anesthesiology* 2005;103: 744–750.

85. Abe H, Kobayashi H, Nakashima Y, et al. Effects of beta-adrenergic blockade on vasodepressor reaction in patients with vasodepressor syncope. *Am Heart J* 1994;128:911–918.

86. Lesser JB, Sanborn KV, Valskys R, et al. Severe bradycardia during spinal and epidural anesthesia recorded by an anesthesia information management system. *Anesthesiology* 2003;99: 859–866.

87. Carpenter RL, Caplan RA, Brown DL, et al. Incidence and risk factors for side effects of spinal anesthesia. *Anesthesiology* 1992;76:906–916.

88. Critchley LA, Stuart JC, Short TG, et al. Haemodynamic effects of subarachnoid block in elderly patients. *Br J Anaesth* 1994;73: 464–470.

89. Morgan P. The role of vasopressors in the management of hypotension induced by spinal and epidural anaesthesia. *Can J Anaesth* 1994;41:404–413.

90. Lundberg J, Norgren L, Thomson D, et al. Hemodynamic effects of dopamine during thoracic epidural analgesia in man. *Anesthesiology* 1987;66:641–646.

91. Brooker RF, Butterworth JF, Kitzman DW, et al. Treatment of hypotension after hyperbaric tetracaine spinal anesthesia: a randomized, double-blind, cross-over comparison of phenylephrine and epinephrine. *Anesthesiology* 1997;86:797–805.

92. Critchley LA, Short TG, Gin T. Hypotension during subarachnoid anaesthesia: haemodynamic analysis of three treatments. *Br J Anaesth* 1994;72:151–155.

93. Lawson N, Johnson J. Autonomic Nervous System: Physiology and Pharmacology. In: Barash P, Cullen B, and Stoelting R, eds. *Clinical Anesthesia*. Philadelphia: Lippincott, Williams & Wilkins, 2001:298.

94. Taivainen T. Comparison of ephedrine and etilefrine for the treatment of arterial hypotension during spinal anaesthesia in elderly patients. *Acta Anaesthesiol Scand* 1991;35:164–169.

95. Krismer AC, Hogan QH, Wenzel V, et al. The efficacy of epinephrine or vasopressin for resuscitation during epidural anesthesia. *Anesth Analg* 2001;93:734–742.

96. Boni F. Sudden bradycardia and asystole in an obese patient after spinal anaesthesia: successful resuscitation with inadvertent "pacing thumps." *West Afr J Med* 1997;16:50–52.

97. Gibbons JJ, Ditto FF III. Sudden asystole after spinal anesthesia treated with the "pacing thump." *Anesthesiology* 1991;75:705.

98. Chester WL. Spinal anesthesia, complete heart block, and the precordial chest thump: an unusual complication and a unique resuscitation. *Anesthesiology* 1988;69:600–602.

99. Scherf D, Bornemann C. Thumping of the precordium in ventricular standstill. *Am J Cardiol* 1960;5:30–40.

100. Rosenberg JM, Wahr JA, Sung CH, et al. Coronary perfusion pressure during cardiopulmonary resuscitation after spinal anesthesia in dogs. *Anesth Analg* 1996;82:84–87.

101. Rosenberg JM, Wortsman J, Wahr JA, et al. Impaired neuroendocrine response mediates refractoriness to cardiopulmonary resuscitation in spinal anesthesia. *Crit Care Med* 1998;26:533–537.

102. Peters J, Schlaghecke R, Thouet H, et al. Endogenous vasopressin supports blood pressure and prevents severe hypotension during epidural anesthesia in conscious dogs. *Anesthesiology* 1990;73:694–702.

103. Ecoffey C, Edouard A, Pruszczynski W, et al. Effects of epidural anesthesia on catecholamines, renin activity, and vasopressin changes induced by tilt in elderly men. *Anesthesiology* 1985;62:294–297.

104. Tarkkila PJ, Kaukinen S. Complications during spinal anesthesia: a prospective study. *Reg Anesth* 1991;16:101–106.

105. Curatolo M, Scaramozzino P, Venuti FS, et al. Factors associated with hypotension and bradycardia after epidural blockade. *Anesth Analg* 1996;83:1033–1040.

106. Fanelli G, Casati A, Berti M, et al. Incidence of hypotension and bradycardia during integrated epidural/general anaesthesia: an epidemiologic observational study on 1200 consecutive patients. Italian Study Group on Integrated Anaesthesia. *Minerva Anestesiol* 1998;64:313–319.

107. Hartmann B, Junger A, Klasen J, et al. The incidence and risk factors for hypotension after spinal anesthesia induction: an analysis with automated data collection. *Anesth Analg* 2002;94:1521–1529.

108. Roch J, Sharrock NE. Hypotension during shoulder arthroscopy in the sitting position under interscalene block. *Reg Anesth* 1991;16:64.

109. Tarkkila P, Isola J. A regression model for identifying patients at high risk of hypotension, bradycardia and nausea during spinal anesthesia. *Acta Anaesthesiol Scand* 1992;36:554–558.

7

Local Anesthetic Systemic Toxicity

John F. Butterworth, Kenneth D. Candido, Mehmet S. Ozcan, and Guy Weinberg

Local anesthesia was first used by medical doctors in 1884 when Koller and Gartner performed topical cocaine anesthesia of each other's cornea and Halsted injected cocaine into nerves for surgical anesthesia.[1,2] Nevertheless, the medicinal properties of cocaine were well known and widely used by the Incas long before explorers brought the compound back to Europe for its medical properties to be "rediscovered." Once local and regional anesthesia became widely used, local anesthetic (LA) systemic cardiovascular and central nervous system (CNS) toxicity and allergy were recognized. By the 1930s, concerns about lethal cardiovascular reactions led the American Medical Association to assign a panel of physicians to review deaths associated with topical anesthesia for endoscopy. These concerns continued even as the topical anesthetic of choice shifted from cocaine to procaine to tetracaine, prompting further panels of inquiry. Finally, concerns about LA cardiovascular toxicity intensified after 1979 when Albright[3] described patients with cardiac arrest after attempted regional anesthesia with either bupivacaine or etidocaine. This chapter focuses on these various forms of LA systemic toxicity.

▶ DEFINITION OF THE PROBLEM

Local anesthetic systemic toxicity (LAST) may result from unintended intravascular injection of what would have been an appropriate dose of LA (had it been injected in the intended site), or from absorption of LA after peripheral tissue injections (this could arise from unexpectedly rapid absorption of an appropriate dose or absorption at the customary rate of an excessive dose). The end result of all these scenarios is excessive concentrations of LAs at an active site for toxicity. The central nervous and cardiovascular systems (CNS and CVS) are the "toxic" organ targets of increasing LA blood levels. The CNS, being more sensitive to LAST than the CVS, manifests the characteristics of intoxication before the CVS in most circumstances (except in some cases of bupivacaine or etidocaine intoxication).[4,5] CNS toxicity is "classically" expressed in two stages. It may begin with an excitation phase (with a progressive sequence of signs and symptoms including shivering, muscle tremors, tonic-clonic seizure activity) due to depression of central inhibitory pathways (so-called disinhibition), which may progress to a depressant phase—for example, hypoventilation and respiratory arrest—due to more global CNS inhibition. The pathophysiology of LA CVS toxicity has both indirect and direct components. With CNS excitation, sympathetic nervous system activation produces tachycardia and hypertension. However, as blood concentrations increase, direct LA-mediated arrhythmogenic and myocardial depressant actions first blunt, then supersede the sympathetic nervous system effects. The resulting arrhythmias, hypotension, and contractile dysfunction contribute to difficulties with resuscitation, altogether defining the LA toxicity phenotype.

▶ SCOPE OF THE PROBLEM

Since Albright's[3] report of cardiac arrest after bupivacaine and etidocaine, the incidence of LAST appears to have declined, although the data to document this conclusion are sketchy at best. If true, this improvement could be attributed to better regional anesthesia techniques, greater awareness of the problem, earlier recognition of potential LA toxicity, or reduced use of 0.75% bupivacaine. Findings from preclinical laboratory investigations underlie all of these potential etiologies.[6–8] Even so, data from an American Society of Anesthesiology Closed Claims Project show that toxicity from unintentional intravenous (IV) LA injection was the second largest category of regional anesthesia-related claims (behind spinal anesthesia) that resulted in death or brain damage.[9] Currently, the incidence of CNS toxicity (seizure) with epidural anesthesia is estimated at 3/10,000 patients and with peripheral nerve blockade the incidence is estimated at 11/10,000 patients.[10–12] In Brown's[12] retrospective study of nearly 26,000 patients receiving regional anesthesia, the incidence of seizures from brachial plexus anesthesia was 7.9/1,000 with interscalene or supraclavicular blocks and 1.2/1,000 with axillary blocks (the difference likely arises from the nearly mandatory seizure from injection of any amount of LA into the carotid or vertebral arteries during attempted interscalene block). Taken together with the increasing popularity of nerve block anesthesia among anesthesiologists and surgeons, clinicians are obliged to understand the pathophysiology and management of LAST to ensure favorable clinical outcomes.

▶ PATHOPHYSIOLOGY

Mechanisms of LA Action

To understand the mechanisms of LAST, it is helpful to review LA mechanisms of action, specifically, interactions between LAs and voltage-gated sodium (Na_v) channels. Interactions with Na_v channels underlie peripheral nerve block and regional anesthesia. These Na_v channels are integral membrane proteins containing one larger α-subunit and one or two smaller β-subunits. The α-subunit, the site of ion conduction and LA binding, consists of roughly 2,000 amino acids arranged in four homologous domains, each with six α-helical membrane-spanning segments.[13,14]

Na_v channels exist in at least three native conformations: *resting, open,* and *inactivated.* The neuronal Na_v channels

"open" briefly during an action potential, which allows extracellular Na ions to flow into the cell and depolarize the plasma membrane. After only a few milliseconds, Na_v channels "inactivate" (whereupon the Na current ceases). Local anesthesia and antiarrhythmic actions result when LAs bind Na_v channels and inhibit the Na permeability that underlies action potentials in neurons and cardiac myocytes.[15,16] The effects of membrane potential (voltage) on this process are complex: membrane potential influences both Na_v channel conformations and LA affinity. Membrane depolarization favors first "opening" and then inactivation of the channels. LAs have greater affinity for open or inactivated channels than they do for resting Na_v channels. LA inhibition of Na currents increases with repetitive depolarizations, a phenomenon called "use-dependent" or "phasic" block. With successive depolarizations, a declining fraction of Na_v channels remain yet "unbound" by an LA, thus the evoked current decline to a nadir.[15–17]

Aside from Na_v channels, LAs will bind to many different sites, including potassium (K) and calcium (Ca) channels, enzymes, *N*-methyl-D-aspartate receptors, β-adrenergic receptors, and nicotinic acetylcholine receptors. LA binding to these other sites may underlie LA production of toxic side effects,[15,16,18] and it is not necessarily true that LAST reactions arise from a mechanism similar to that underlying local anesthesia.

LA Concentrations, Protein Binding, and Metabolism

The likelihood of systemic toxicity increases as the LA concentration in blood increases. Peak LA concentrations vary widely even when the various nerve block techniques are performed properly. Intercostal blocks consistently produce greater peak LA concentrations (after the same LA dose) than plexus or epidural blocks (Fig. 7-1).[2,19–21] Addition of

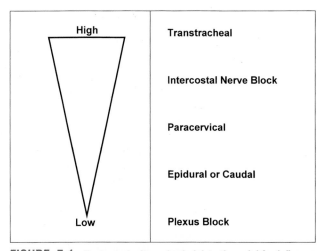

FIGURE 7-1. Route and sites of administration of LAs influence systemic absorption and rate of accumulation. Schematic represents LA plasma concentrations from highest to lowest after the same dose of LA is injected at different sites. (Reprinted from Groban L, Dolinski SY. Differences in cardiac toxicity among ropivacaine, levobupivacaine, bupivacaine, and lidocaine. *Tech Reg Anesth Pain Manag* 2001;5:48–55, with permission.)

epinephrine to LA mixtures will usually reduce peak LA blood concentrations, while the addition of clonidine may increase peak LA blood concentrations. In blood, all LAs are partially protein bound, primarily to α_1-acid glycoprotein (AAG) and secondarily to albumin.[1,2,19] The more potent, more lipid-soluble LAs have a greater extent of protein binding than the less potent, less lipid-soluble agents. The extent of protein binding of a specific LA is influenced by the plasma concentration of AAG. Both protein binding and protein concentration decline during pregnancy.[22] A long-standing assumption in regional anesthesia is that protein binding serves to reduce the potential systemic toxic effects of absorbed or injected LAs. The apparent safety of longer-term epidural infusions of LA and LA-opioid combinations may result in part from progressively increased concentrations of the LA/AAG complexes.[23] Other physiochemical properties that influence systemic toxicity are listed in Table 7-1.[24]

The latency of LAST onset, particularly related to CNS symptoms, depends on the specific regional technique. As noted previously, seizure activity may occur sooner during placement of an interscalene block than during an epidural, reflecting the inherent differences between an unintentional injection of LA into an artery feeding the brain versus an unintended injection in an epidural vein. Additionally, the time to seizure could be delayed up to 30 minutes after a peripheral nerve block when the seizure is the result of systemic absorption after peripheral injection of a large LA dose.[10–12]

LA metabolism may also influence the extent and duration of LAST reactions. In general, LAs with greater rates of elimination will have a greater margin of safety. The archetypical example of an agent with a fast rate of elimination is 2-chloroprocaine, and when given to human volunteers, 2-chloroprocaine-induced CNS symptoms abate rapidly.

2-Chloroprocaine and other esters undergo rapid hydrolysis in blood, catalyzed by pseudocholinesterase.[1,2,19] Thus procaine and benzocaine are rapidly metabolized to para-aminobenzoic acid (PABA), the compound underlying anaphylaxis to these agents.[2] The amides undergo metabolism in the liver.[1,2,19] Prilocaine undergoes hydrolysis to o-toluidine, which causes methemoglobinemia in a dose-dependent manner.[2,23] For this reason, prilocaine is no longer used in large doses in the United States, and in recent studies benzocaine (used for topical anesthesia) was the most common LA associated with medically important methemoglobinemia in American hospitals.[25]

CNS Pathophysiology

While CNS manifestations of LAST have historically been described as occurring along a spectrum of clinical findings culminating in seizures (and possibly in CVS collapse if seizures are not aborted), in reality this stereotypical progression of clinical findings occurs only about 60% of the time following increases in LA blood concentrations.[26] In a case series of 93 incidents of LAST, the presenting signs were referable to the CNS in 45%, to both the CNS and the CVS in 44%, and to the CVS in the remaining 11%.[26]

A general relationship exists between the anesthetic potency and CNS LAST. LAs that are more potent at causing conduction blockade produce seizures at lower blood concentrations and lower doses than less potent LAs. In animal studies, there are also age-related considerations, with younger pigs requiring greater doses to produce convulsions than older ones, in animals receiving lidocaine infusions to create EEG-confirmed seizures.[27] Among the LAs in the pipecoloxylidide family (including mepivacaine, ropivacaine, and bupivacaine), potency at CNS toxicity is 1.5 to 2.5 times greater for the R(+) isomer as compared to the S(−) isomer. In rabbits, the mean convulsive dose of S(−) bupivacaine was nearly double that of R(+) bupivacaine.[6] In sheep, 40 mg R(+) bupivacaine consistently induced convulsions while convulsions never occurred after the same dose of S(−) bupivacaine.[28] These stereospecific dose relationships were confirmed in a study by Denson et al.[29] in which a more profound depression of the firing rate of cells of the nucleus tractus solitarius occurred with R(+) bupivacaine than with S(−) bupivacaine in anesthetized rats. Racemic bupivacaine and ropivacaine have differing potency at inducing CNS toxicity, although in equipotent concentrations in experimentally induced respiratory acidosis in rats, both agents similarly suppress baroreflex sensitivity, believed to be crucial for maintaining CVS stability.[30]

The mean convulsant dose of ropivacaine in sheep was 1.33 times that of bupivacaine.[31] Likewise, human volunteers tolerated 25% larger IV doses of ropivacaine (124 mg)

TABLE 7-1 Physiochemical Properties That Influence Systemic Toxicity

FACTOR	TOXICITY RELEVANCE
pH	Neutral (not protonated) form more readily permeates the cell membrane decreasing systemic absorption, but ionized form more potently interacts with Na_v channels (nerve, brain, cardiac)
Lipophilicity	More lipophilic LAs permeate membranes more readily; they also bind more avidly to other lipid structures (e.g., myelin and meninges), decreasing systemic absorption
Protein binding	Increased protein binding reduces free fraction of LA; more lipid-soluble agents are more highly protein bound (but also more potent)
Ester linkage	Rapid hydrolysis in plasma and rapid elimination (reduces systemic toxicity)
Stereospecificity	R(+) isomer binds more avidly to cardiac Na_v channel than S(−) isomer (increasing propensity for cardiotoxicity)

Adapted from Groban L, Dolinski SY. Differences in cardiac toxicity among ropivacaine, levobupivacaine, bupivacaine, and lidocaine. *Tech Reg Anesth Pain Manag* 2001;5:48–55, with permission.

as compared to bupivacaine (99 mg).[32] Knudsen et al.'s[33] double-blind crossover study in human volunteers demonstrated that the threshold concentration associated with CNS symptoms was approximately 0.6 mg/L for ropivacaine and 0.3 mg/L for bupivacaine and the time to disappearance of all symptoms was significantly shorter for ropivacaine than bupivacaine. Nevertheless, in rats, the same concentration of bupivacaine and ropivacaine (10 μg/mL) inhibited hippocampal field potentials in the CA1 region. These inhibitory effects on hippocampal field potential amplitude and recovery rate following washout *may* represent the underlying mechanism for CNS-related LAST.[34]

There have also been comparisons between S(−) isomers. The relative potency of levobupivacaine and ropivacaine at CNS toxicity varies among species.[35–37] In the anesthetized, ventilated rat, Ohmura et al.[35] showed that cumulative convulsive doses were similar for levobupivacaine and ropivacaine. In conscious sheep, the convulsant dose was slightly greater for ropivacaine than for levobupivacaine.[36,37] When levobupivacaine and ropivacaine were administered to human volunteers in a double-blind randomized crossover trial, early CNS toxic symptoms occurred after equal concentrations, equal milligram doses, and equal infusion rates[38] (Box 7-1).

Cardiovascular Pathophysiology

The CVS is affected at all stages of LA systemic toxicity. In early stages when CNS symptoms dominate the clinical picture, CV toxicity occurs indirectly (due to CNS excitation) rather than a direct effect on myocardium. This is typically observed in situations in which the toxicity is due to an LA with a greater CV/CNS toxicity ratio, for example, lidocaine, or the route of LA administration results in a gradual systemic absorption. Ladd et al.[39] have elegantly demonstrated the actual CV pathophysiology during the CNS excitation phase. In their study, carotid injection of LAs in awake ewes at a dose range that resulted in CNS symptoms (hypertonia, seizures) without arrhythmias or cardiac arrest resulted in hypertension, tachycardia, and a decrease in stroke volume. On the other hand, if the LA being used has a low CV/CNS ratio, signs related to direct cardiac toxicity, for example, arrhythmias and hypotension, might occur first when there is a rapid increase in plasma concentration. This might be a common scenario as a review showed that 55% of cases with LAST presented with CV signs and symptoms (alone or CV and CNS signs together at presentation).[26]

Direct cardiac toxicity is a complex phenomenon at the molecular level.[40] LAs bind and inhibit cardiac Na channels much as they do in neural tissue.[15,41–46] In addition, LAs block

potassium channels on the cell membrane, prolonging action potential and contributing the cardiotoxicty.[43] Calcium channels at the plasma membrane as well as the sarcoplasmic reticulum are also targeted, decreasing the intracellular Ca^{2+} release and thereby depressing contractility.[44–46] Binding and inhibition of the cardiac Ca and K channels by LAs generally occur at concentrations greater than those at which binding to Na channels is maximal.[5,15,47] Prolongation of the action potential via the inhibition of Na and K channels and blockage of Ca^{2+} channels at multiple locations are classically thought to be the major molecular mechanisms behind the major clinical findings of LA-related cardiac toxicity.[48] However, metabotropic cellular signaling systems, for example, beta adrenergic and lysophosphatidyl, also appear to contribute to the phenotype of LA-induced cardiac toxicity. Recent observations suggest that inhibition of mitochondrial metabolism and oxidative phosphorylation might also play a role in severe cardiac toxicity.[49]

Physicochemical properties of the LAs can explain at the molecular level the variation in their potential for causing clinical toxicity. Lipophilicity, anesthetic potency, and the proclivity for protein binding covary with toxicity. For instance, bupivacaine, the canonical cardiotoxic LA, is more lipophilic and more highly protein bound than lidocaine. It also binds more avidly and longer than lidocaine to cardiac Na channels.[50] Stereoselectivity is another important factor in determining toxicity.[51] The R(+) enantiomer of bupivacaine binds cardiac Na channels more avidly than the S(−) enantiomer, and this finding led to the clinical development of the enantiomeric formulations, levobupivacaine, and ropivacaine.[52] As a general rule, LAs inhibit conduction in the heart, with the same rank order of potency as for nerve block.[53–55]

Similarly, LAs bind β-adrenergic receptors and inhibit epinephrine-stimulated cyclic adenosine monophosphate (AMP) formation, with the same rank order as for LA potency at peripheral nerve block sites. Inadequate signaling by cAMP (by either mechanism) could underlie the refractoriness of bupivacaine CV toxicity to standard resuscitation measures.[20,21,56,57] Bupivacaine is also more effective than other less toxic LAs at collapsing the mitochondrial chemiosmotic gradient needed for oxidative phosphorylation. It is also a very potent inhibitor of other enzymes at the inner mitochondrial membrane, such as those necessary for uptake of fatty acids, the heart's preferred fuel under normal aerobic metabolism. A description of the potential sites at which LAs interfere with cardiac function is displayed in Figure 7-2.

Arrhythmogenicity, myocardial contractility, and survivability (ease of resuscitation) are the most commonly used endpoints to investigate LA cardiotoxicity in experimental models using intact animals. Nevertheless, there is a great deal of variability in such laboratory studies with respect to the species used as well as experimental design, metrics, and endpoints. There is no consensus as to which model and design most faithfully represent the cardiovascular toxicity from LAs in humans.[40]

Arrhythmogenicity

The overall *direct* effects of LAs on cardiac rhythm are depression of excitability and delay in conduction.[58] As stated above, when the plasma levels of the LA in question are not sufficiently high, tachyarrhythmias could indirectly

---

BOX 7-1 Factors Influencing the Threshold LA Dose to Induce Convulsions

- Site of injection
- Rate of injection
- Rate at which blood concentrations increase
- Acidosis
- Level of sedation
- Stereospecificity of LA

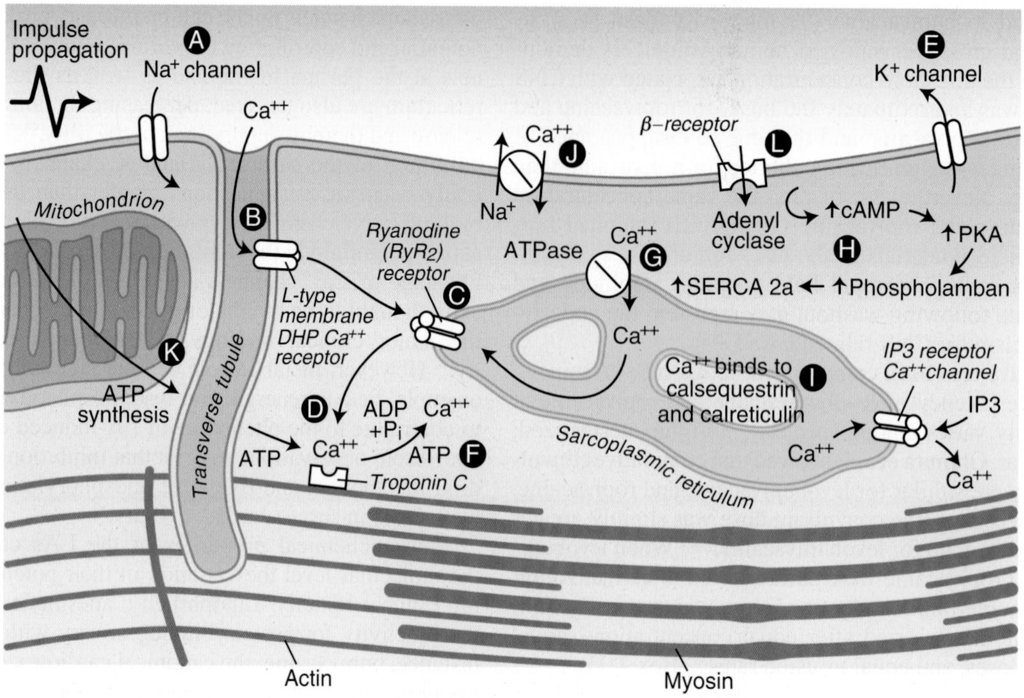

FIGURE 7-2. **Cardiac myocyte transport processes and potential sites of LA-induced cardiac toxicity (A-L).** LAs block cardiac Na⁺ channels **(A)**. Bupivacaine displays fast-in, slow-out kinetics, whereas lidocaine displays fast-in, fast-out kinetics within the Na⁺ channels of the myocardium. The net effect is inhibition of Na⁺ conductance, leading to a slowed conduction block that may be associated with reduced myocardial contractility. At high concentrations, LAs bind and inhibit cardiac K⁺ **(E)** and Ca²⁺ **(B)** channels as well as beta-adrenoreceptors. Blockade of cardiac K⁺ channels **(E)** may also contribute to the cardiotoxic effects of LAs by lengthening the cardiac action potential, predisposing the heart to ventricular arrhythmias. LAs have a depressant effect on the Ca²⁺ slow channels **(B)**, attenuating the influx of calcium, which is a vital link to the cardiac excitation-contraction coupling process. LAs may also depress myocardial contraction by interfering with Ca²⁺ release from the sarcoplasmic reticulum **(C)**. Furthermore, LAs bind and inhibit beta-adrenoreceptors **(L)** and adenyl cyclase **(H)**, inhibiting cyclic AMP formation, which may impair resuscitative efforts after cardiotoxicity. Finally, an LA-induced interference with mitochondrial energy metabolism can contribute to the electrical and mechanical depression of the myocardium **(D, F, G, K)**. However, these additional mechanisms of cardiotoxicity may require LA concentrations that are greater than the concentrations that would have produced cardiac standstill from block of cardiac Na⁺ and Ca²⁺ channels. Each of the essential components of mitochondrial metabolism required for oxidative phosphorylation and synthesis of adenosine triphosphate is impaired by lipophilic LAs. These include transport of fatty acids into the mitochondrial matrix, generation of the chemiosmotic gradient, electron transport, and ATP synthesis.
(Adapted from Groban L, Dolinski SY. Differences in cardiac toxicity among ropivacaine, levobupivacaine, bupivacaine, and lidocaine. *Tech Reg Anesth Pain Manag* 2001;5:48–55, with permission.)

result from CNS excitation. At higher plasma concentrations of LA, a dose-dependent prolongation of cardiac conduction is reflected by increases in the PR interval and QRS duration of the electrocardiogram.[59–61] At higher doses still, depression of sinoatrial and atrioventricular nodal activity is manifested by bradycardia and atrioventricular block, potentially leading to asystole.[60] With increased blood concentrations of bupivacaine, the heart becomes increasingly susceptible to prolongation of the QT interval, ventricular tachycardia, torsades, and ventricular fibrillation.[62,63]

Bupivacaine is consistently the most arrhythmogenic LA, regardless of the animal species or experimental protocol. At subconvulsant doses, bupivacaine induced nodal and ventricular arrhythmias, whereas even convulsant lidocaine doses do not induce arrhythmias.[64] Feldman et al. found that at twice the convulsive dose (with no resuscitative attempts), 83% of bupivacaine-treated dogs died as compared to 17% of ropivacaine-treated dogs.[65,66] However, with early

resuscitation, mortality decreased from 83% to 33% in the bupivacaine-treated group and from 17% to 0% in the ropivacaine-treated group. Kotelko et al.[67] reported that in conscious sheep, convulsant bupivacaine doses produced severe arrhythmias whereas convulsant doses of lidocaine produced only transient ST-segment depression or sinus tachycardia.

Ropivacaine is apparently less arrhythmogenic than bupivacaine. In a crossover experimental design, Knudsen et al.[68] found that ropivacaine caused a smaller increase in QRS duration compared to bupivacaine in human volunteers. Since QRS duration have been positively correlated with cardiotoxicity of LAs,[53] these findings provide valuable comparison of the cardiotoxicity of ropivacaine and bupivacaine in humans. A study by Reiz et al.[54] in pigs comparing bupivacaine, ropivacaine, and lidocaine supports this finding. The endpoint being QRS prolongation, the electrophysiologic toxicity ratio was 15:6.7:1 for bupivacaine:ropivacaine:lidocaine.[54]

Levobupivacaine has an intermediate arrhythmogenic risk between ropivacaine and bupivacaine.[69] In nonanesthetized rats, levobupivacaine prolonged the QRS more than ropivacaine. Ventricular tachycardia occurred in seven of eight rats treated with levobupivacaine compared with only one of eight rats treated with ropivacaine.[69] Similarly, in anesthetized rats, the cumulative dose and plasma concentrations of LA at the onset of the first arrhythmia were greater for ropivacaine as compared to levobupivacaine, and both were significantly greater than racemic bupivacaine.[69]

Arrhythmogenicity of a given LA may be different from its LA potency. For peripheral nerve blocks and epidural anesthesia, bupivacaine is about four times more potent than lidocaine (potency ratio of 1:4).[70,71] However, in anesthetized pigs, intracoronary injection of LA produced comparable prolongation of the QRS interval with bupivacaine and lidocaine at a dose ratio of 1:16.[72] Moreover, seven of 15 animals given 4 mg of intracoronary bupivacaine died of ventricular fibrillation, whereas lidocaine-induced ventricular fibrillation occurred at 64 mg. Therefore, it can be concluded that while bupivacaine is four times more potent than lidocaine as an LA, it is 16 times more arrhythmogenic.

Administering LA directly in the coronary artery controls for indirect CNS effects, and such studies indicate that severe bupivacaine-induced ventricular arrhythmias result largely from direct cardiac action, and not CNS activation.[73] Chang et al.[73] studied nonanesthetized sheep receiving intracoronary bupivacaine, levobupivacaine, or ropivacaine. All the three drugs prolonged the QRS duration, but bupivacaine was more potent and produced greater prolongation than ropivacaine. In conscious sheep, IV levobupivacaine produced fewer arrhythmias than bupivacaine.[74,75] Bupivacaine doses of 125 to 200 mg produced fatal ventricular fibrillation in some sheep, whereas, similar life-threatening arrhythmias were not found with levobupivacaine doses <225 mg.

Decreased Myocardial Contractility

Dose-dependent reduction in contractility occurs with systemic LA intoxication and unquestionably contributes to LA-induced cardiovascular instability. The rank order for LA potency as negative inotropes is the same as that for their potency at nerve conduction blockade. More potent LAs (e.g., bupivacaine) tend to reduce cardiac contractility at lower doses and concentrations than the less potent LA agents (e.g., lidocaine).[67,72] However, comparisons of contractile depression among ropivacaine, levobupivacaine, bupivacaine, and lidocaine are not entirely straightforward. Subconvulsant doses of levobupivacaine and bupivacaine given to nonanesthetized sheep produced comparable contractile depression.[75] In sheep, intracoronary ropivacaine produced smaller reductions in myocardial contractility and stroke volume than equivalent doses of bupivacaine or levobupivacaine.[73] Likewise, there was no difference between levobupivacaine and bupivacaine. During incremental LA intoxication in anesthetized dogs, ropivacaine produced less left-ventricular depression than levobupivacaine or racemic bupivacaine (Table 7-2). Similarly, myocardial contractility in nonanesthetized sheep was most severely depressed by bupivacaine, followed by levobupivacaine, and ropivacaine (in decreasing order).[73]

Response to Resuscitation as a Measure of Comparative Cardiac Toxicity

Ease of resuscitation in animal models is a well-defined and clinically relevant endpoint for comparing the intrinsic cardiac toxicity of LAs. Notably, clinical resuscitation from LAST has been changed by the introduction of intravenous lipid emulsion (ILE). Therefore, treatment of LAST *per se* is covered in the next section while the focus of this section is the comparative efficacies of various nonlipid treatments and the relative cardiac toxicity of different LAs.

TABLE 7-2 Concentrations of LAs Inhibiting Myocardial Function

LA	LVEDP (EC$_{50}$ FOR 125% OF BASELINE) (μg/mL)	DP/DTMAX (EC$_{50}$ FOR 65% OF BASELINE) (μg/mL)	%EF (EC$_{50}$ FOR 65% OF BASELINE) (μg/mL)	%FS (EC$_{50}$ FOR 65% OF BASELINE) (μg/mL)	CO (EC$_{50}$ FOR 75% OF BASELINE) (μg/mL)
BUP	2.2 (1.2–4.4)	2.3 (1.7–3.0)	3.2 (2.2–4.7)	2.1 (1.5–3.1)	3.6 (2.1–6.0)
LBUP	1.6 (0.9–3.1)	2.4 (1.9–3.1)	3.1 (1.4–2.9)	1.3 (0.9–1.8)	3.3 (2.0–5.5)
ROP	4.0 (2.1–7.5)[a]	4.0 (3.1–5.2)[b]	4.2 (3.0–6.0)	3.0 (2.1–4.2)[a]	5.0 (3.1–8.3)
LID	6.8 (3.0–15.4)[c]	8.0 (5.7–11.0)[d]	6.3 (4.0–9.9)[c]	5.5 (3.5–8.7)[d]	15.8 (8.3–30.2)[d]

Note: Data represented are EC estimates and 95% confidence intervals.
[a]ROP > LBUP; $p < .05$.
[b]ROP > BUP, LBUP; $p < .05$.
[c]LID > BUP, LBUP; $p < .01$.
[d]LID > BUP, LBUP, ROP; $p < .01$.
EC$_{50}$, effective concentration for 50% of population; BUP, bupivacaine; LBUP, levobupivacaine; ROP, ropivacaine; LID, lidocaine; base, baseline.
Reprinted from Groban L, Dolinski SY. Differences in cardiac toxicity among ropivacaine, levobupivacaine, bupivacaine, and lidocaine. *Tech Reg Anesth Pain Manag* 2001;5:48–55, with permission.

Two studies of anesthetized animals receiving LA infusions suggest that the systemic toxicity of levobupivacaine is intermediate between that of ropivacaine and bupivacaine.[69,76] In anesthetized dogs, an IV overdose of bupivacaine, levobupivacaine, ropivacaine, and lidocaine led to mortality in 50%, 30%, 10%, and 0% of the animals, respectively, after 20 minutes of cardiac massage and administration of vasoactive drugs. Epinephrine-induced arrhythmias occurred more frequently in bupivacaine- (44%) and levobupivacaine- (20%) intoxicated animals than dogs given lidocaine or ropivacaine. Also, significantly less epinephrine was required to treat ropivacaine intoxication than either bupivacaine or levobupivacaine intoxication. These findings confirm the clinical observation that bupivacaine systemic toxicity leads to worse outcomes in terms of cardiac arrest refractory to resuscitation.[3]

Allergic Reactions to LAs

True anaphylaxis appears more likely with ester LAs that are metabolized directly to PABA, such as procaine and benzocaine. Anaphylaxis to amide anesthetics is said to be much less common than to esters although there is limited evidence for this long-standing and widespread belief.[77] Immediate hypersensitivity reactions, albeit rare, do occur in response to amides. Nevertheless, one thing is very clear: True *allergic* reactions to LAs are rare.[78,79] Baluga et al. reviewed the case histories of 5,018 Uruguayan patients receiving LAs during dentistry. They found 25 adverse reactions. Twenty-two were psychogenic or vasovagal episodes or were due to a lapse in technique. One of the patients presented with seeming allergic symptoms (pruritis along the face in the area innervated by the inferior dental nerve) that were related to LA technique complications. The remaining two cases underwent skin and provocative testing with the LA and had allergy ruled out.[80] In another study, 157 asthmatic children (who were allergic to at least one known allergen) and 72 nonasthmatic children underwent skin prick, intradermal, and incremental challenge tests with lidocaine. Although 80% of the children had received LAs in the past, none had an immediate or delayed allergy to lidocaine.[81] In a study of 100 patients referred to an allergist for suspected LA allergic reactions (including 12 who had experienced signs and symptoms of apparent anaphylactoid reactions), not one of these patients had a positive result to intradermal testing.[78] In another study of 236 patients referred for testing after a presumed LA hypersensitivity reaction, only one patient demonstrated any reaction to an LA and that was only local erythema at the site of injection.[82] Thus, none of the patients in these latter two studies had an IgG- or IgE-related cause for their LA reaction. In other words, none of the patients actually had an LA allergy. The preceding discussion should NOT be interpreted as saying that LA allergy never occurs. Crossreactivity is possible. A woman who had experienced anaphylactic reactions to lidocaine and erythema in response to EMLA cream was referred for testing. Positive skin prick tests with full-strength drugs were positive for lidocaine, bupivacaine, and mepivacaine, but negative for ropivacaine. Intradermal testing with 1:100 ropivacaine was positive. All testing with procaine was negative, and this agent was safely used during surgery. A subcutaneous challenge with 0.1 mL of 0.2% ropivacaine resulted in laryngospasm requiring epinephrine.[83] Some patients may react to preservatives such as methylparaben that are often included with LAs. Accidental IV injections of LAs are sometimes misdiagnosed as allergic reactions.

▶ RISK FACTORS

Both physical and pathophysiologic characteristics influence an individual's susceptibility to LAST. LAST increases at the extremes of age, due to decreased clearance, reduced protein binding in infants, and potentially increased absorption. Cardiac disease, particularly ischemia, conduction defects, and low output states appear to lower the threshold for LAST, making these patients more susceptible to LA overdose. Similarly, individuals with altered hepatic function exhibit reduced LA metabolism and are thus susceptible to systemic reactions. Presumably, a reduced clearance rate, reduced protein binding and the resulting increased concentration of free LA contribute to the increased risk of LA toxicity of pregnancy. The pregnant patient also has engorged epidural veins that predispose her to an unintentional systemic administration of LA.

Acid-base status has been well studied. LAST develops more rapidly and with graver consequences in the face of hypoxemia or acidosis. Conversely, alkalemia and respiratory alkalosis have been identified as being protective.[84] While it might seem that the epileptic patient is at higher risk for developing CNS signs of LAST at lower LA plasma concentrations, this has not been confirmed experimentally. In kindled epileptic rats, repeated, subconvulsive electrical stimulation applied to the amygdala did not increase susceptibility to the proconvulsant action of lidocaine.[85] In addition to patient factors and comorbidities, the site of injection of LA, speed of absorption, lipid solubility, and potency of the agent are all risk factors in determining the potential for developing LAST. Notably, LAST generally appears to occur despite the clinician having adhered to suggested clinical doses and methods of administration.[86]

▶ DIAGNOSTIC EVALUATION

The CNS and CVS are the major clinical targets of LAST. CNS is traditionally viewed as more sensitive than the CVS. That is, in experimental animals, CNS intoxication usually manifests before signs of CV toxicity and the relative doses required to produce convulsions with all LAs are usually greater than those causing cardiovascular instability. This is true in experimental models of LAST whether the animal is awake or anesthetized, and regardless of the acid-base status (Box 7-2).

BOX 7-2 Clinical Caveat

Most LAs do not produce CVS toxicity until blood concentrations are at least threefold higher than those that produce convulsions. This may not be the case with racemic bupivacaine and etidocaine, where simultaneous CNS and CVS toxicity have been reported.

The presentation of LA CNS toxicity has been previously described. When LAST occurs secondary to direct intravascular injection (particularly with injection directly into the vertebral or carotid arteries, respectively), premonitory symptoms may be bypassed as the clinical picture rapidly progresses to seizure, leading to CVS excitation followed by collapse.[87] In the latter case, the CVS system response is characterized by hypertension, tachycardia, and ventricular dysrhythmias followed by cardiac depression including bradycardia, decreased contractility and ultimately hypotension, and asystole.[87] This classical progression, however, is only observed in 60% of cases of LAST, which potentially confounds the diagnostic process in some cases.[26] This highlights the requirement for the clinician to maintain vigilance each and every time an LA injection is performed, regardless of the experience of the practitioner and the underlying physiologic state of the patient. In a large review of LAST cases, two-thirds of the patients were female and 15% were <16 years old, while 30% were >60 years old. More than 90% of cases involved either bupivacaine, levobupivacaine, or ropivacaine.[26] Less than 20% of LAST cases involved continuous infusions, and 50% of those were in a pediatric population.[25] Fully one-third of cases involved individuals with underlying cardiac, neurologic, or metabolic disease, further emphasizing the patient group for whom increased vigilance is essential.[25] Observation of the patient and monitoring of vital signs, while maintaining verbal communication and visual observation of patients receiving large doses of LA, is paramount to identifying LAST early enough to minimize the sequelae.

Although CNS side effects from acute overdose, cumulative overdose, or accidental IV injection are undesirable, observable toxic effects are important for providing guidelines for clinical practice. In the past, the primary objective for laboratory studies of acute toxicity was to determine the median lethal dose, LD_{50}, for the classification and standardization of drugs. However, due to extraneous factors that affect the precision of LD_{50}, the ratio of the LA dosage required for irreversible cardiovascular collapse (CC) and the dosage that produces CNS toxicity (convulsions), the CC/CNS ratio, has proven more useful than LD_{50} to compare CV toxicity among LAs. Although, in theory, a high CC/CNS ratio denotes a good safety margin, it is also important that there be a wide margin between clinical dose and convulsant dose. In general, a smaller ratio exists among the longer-acting agents as compared to the short-acting agent, lidocaine. CC/CNS ratio tends to be bupivacaine < levobupivacaine < ropivacaine[88] (Box 7-2).

PREVENTION

In order to minimize the risk of LAST, it remains essential that clinicians use the customary precautions: standard monitoring of the patient, aspiration before injection of LAs, fractionation of the injected dose, test dosing, and the use of the lowest practical concentration of LA to effect conduction blockade. While there is some controversy regarding the risk benefit of using a pharmacologic marker such as low concentration of epinephrine in the LA preparation (e.g., 5 µg/mL or less), the current American Society of Regional Anesthesia and Pain Medicine (ASRA) guidelines recommend using this strategy. Moreover, when large volumes and high concentrations of a long-acting LA are planned for a peripheral nerve block, an agent that provides the least potential for cardiotoxicity in the event of an unrecognized, accidental intravascular injection may be preferred.

Ultrasound guidance in regional anesthesia may have theoretical safety advantages for preventing LAST versus alternative methods of nerve identification for PNB performance including a potential reduction in LA dose/volume for any given block. But, so far, the data are contradictory.[89,90]

TREATMENT

Treatment of LA-induced toxicity has changed dramatically since the last edition of this text, and it is still evolving. Notably, the ASRA published guidelines for managing LA systemic toxicity in the Spring of 2010, and these are presented in Figure 7-3.[87] Nevertheless, several fundamental principles have remained unchanged. Early recognition and intervention are key to a successful recovery, particularly since a potential antidote is now available. The majority of cases occur in a classic sequence of rapid onset of altered mental status or seizures within seconds or minutes of the LA injection and followed in a small fraction of patients by cardiovascular instability, which most often presents as progressive bradycardia and hypotension. However, a substantial percent of patients have an atypical presentation such as rapid progression to CC with no discernable neurologic prodrome, or a delayed onset of more than 5 minutes after the injection.[26] The physician who is aware of the possibility of an atypical toxic syndrome is more likely to entertain the diagnosis and save the patient's life.

The most important component of treatment after making the diagnosis is attention to airway management. It is critical to avoid hypoxemia or respiratory acidosis, which both unquestionably exacerbate the underlying LA toxicity and make resuscitation much more difficult. Credit for developing this approach goes to Dr. Daniel C. Moore[91] who recognized nearly five decades ago the primacy of airway management in treating LA overdose. Mask ventilation with 100% oxygen to assure adequate pulmonary ventilation will suffice in most cases, as intubation is generally not required unless the patient has a full stomach or exhibits cardiovascular instability. The next priority is seizure suppression. This is particularly important since generalized convulsions will produce metabolic acidosis and worsen the underlying toxicity. Benzodiazepines are the preferred antiseizure treatment. Propofol is not an optimal choice since it is a cardiodepressant, shares specific mitochondrial targets of toxicity and could therefore exacerbate LA cardiac depression. Moreover, the lipid content of propofol is not sufficient to have a beneficial partitioning effect.

It is important to consider the infusion of ILE early in the toxic sequence. It is a potential antidote to LA toxicity that was first identified in animal models where it was found to rapidly reverse bupivacaine-induced CC in both rats[92] and dogs[93] (see Fig. 7-4). The leap to clinical practice was made by Rosenblatt et al.[94] who published the first case report of successful reversal of LA toxicity, using ILE in a middle-aged man in full cardiac arrest after a mepivacaine-bupivacaine plexus block. Many published cases have followed,

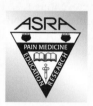

AMERICAN SOCIETY OF
REGIONAL ANESTHESIA AND PAIN MEDICINE

Checklist for Treatment
of Local Anesthetic Systemic Toxicity

The Pharmacologic Treatment of Local Anesthetic Systemic Toxicity (LAST) is Different from Other Cardiac Arrest Scenarios

❑ **Get Help**

❑ **Initial Focus**

  ❑ **Airway management:** ventilate with 100% oxygen

  ❑ **Seizure suppression:** benzodiazepines are preferred; **AVOID propofol** in patients having signs of cardiovascular instability

  ❑ **Alert** the nearest facility having **cardiopulmonary bypass** capability

❑ **Management of Cardiac Arrhythmias**

  ❑ **Basic and Advanced Cardiac Life Support (ACLS)** will require adjustment of medications and perhaps prolonged effort

  ❑ **AVOID vasopressin, calcium channel blockers, beta blockers, or local anesthetic**

  ❑ **REDUCE epinephrine dose to <1 mcg/kg**

❑ **Lipid Emulsion (20%) Therapy** (values in parenthesis are for 70kg patient)

  ❑ **Bolus 1.5 mL/kg** (lean body mass) intravenously over 1 minute (~100mL)

  ❑ **Continuous infusion 0.25 mL/kg/min** (~18 mL/min; adjust by roller clamp)

  ❑ Repeat bolus once or twice for persistent cardiovascular collapse

  ❑ Double the infusion rate to 0.5 mL/kg/min if blood pressure remains low

  ❑ **Continue infusion** for at least10 minutes after attaining circulatory stability

  ❑ Recommended upper limit: Approximately 10 mL/kg lipid emulsion over the first 30 minutes

❑ **Post LAST events at** www.lipidrescue.org and report use of lipid to www.lipidregistry.org

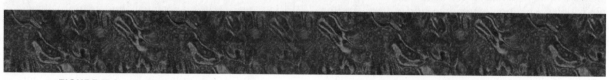

FIGURE 7-3. ASRA guidelines for the treatment of severe LAST. (Reproduced with permission from the American Society of Regional Anesthesia and Pain Medicine.)

indicating efficacy in treating both cardiac and neurologic[95] signs and symptoms of LA overdose, including bupivacaine, mepivacaine, ropivacaine, prilocaine, levobupivacaine, and lidocaine among others.[96,97] Patients that appeared to resist conventional resuscitation measures were often rescued within seconds or minutes of ILE. The Association of Anaesthetists of Great Britain and Ireland and the ASRA have published practice guidelines for treating LA toxicity that include ILE as a key component.[26] Typical dosing recommendations are to administer an initial bolus of 1.5 mL/kg lean body mass over 2 minutes followed by a continuous infusion at roughly 0.25 mL/kg/min. The bolus can be repeated for persistent pulselessness and the infusion rate increased for recurring hypotension. Recently, the American Heart Association has also recommended ILE in this setting, and a systematic analysis of peer-reviewed and non–peer-reviewed cases by Jamaty et al.[98] concluded that, "Current evidence suggests that ILE should be administered as soon as a diagnosis of LA toxicity is established...."

It is important to recognize that the use of ILE is not without limitations or controversy. It is unreasonable to expect that ILE will recover the patient in every case. Patient comorbidities and a variety of treatment factors such as the dose and delivery of LA and the rapidity and appropriateness of the intervention will dictate the success of any resuscitation. Because ILE cannot be expected to work in every instance, it is important to make plans for cardiopulmonary bypass when treating LA toxicity, particularly when cardiovascular instability is apparent. This path is likely to take time; therefore early consideration of this possibility is important so that cardiopulmonary bypass can be instituted as a last resort. Theoretical concerns about possible pulmonary complications related to rapid lipid infusion have so far not been borne out in clinical experience. However, it is important to limit overall volumes of administration to avoid massive volume or lipid overload. Currently, the upper limit for the initial infusion is roughly 12 mL/kg of lean body mass over

the first 30 minutes, though the typical dose, bolus and infusion combined, is usually 4 mL/kg.

ILE will render many standard laboratory measurements invalid for some period of time because of the transient, severe hyperlipemia.[99] Moreover, at least one patient was noted to have developed hyperamylasemia after ILE. While this was self-limited and asymptomatic, the potential for inducing pancreatitis should warrant measuring serum amylase in patients who develop gastrointestinal symptoms after receiving ILE. This same patient developed recurrence of severe cardiac toxicity roughly 40 minutes after an initially successful resuscitation with ILE, indicating that patients should be carefully monitored for several hours following ILE and that treating physicians should be prepared to reinstitute ILE and other supportive measures if signs of toxicity recur. We all learn from such examples and we encourage physicians to report such cases to the educational Web site www.lipidrescue.org and its sister site www.lipidregistry.org, which serves as a repository of clinical experience with ILE.

Perhaps the main clinical question regarding ILE is "When to use it?" The approach to this issue is continuing to evolve. Initially, it was reasonable to wait until all other methods of resuscitation had failed before instituting this largely untested technique. However, with growing understanding of its efficacy, and risk-benefit profile, one can argue against waiting until the patient has proven resistant to all other measures. Several case reports suggest that early use can prevent progression of toxicity and thereby facilitate resuscitation.[100] Since ILE has a favorable safety profile and can be viewed mechanistically as reversing underlying toxicity, logic favors earlier use.

Another major question involves the relationship of ILE, a novel methodology, with more traditional resuscitation medications. Studies using similar rodent models of bupivacaine overdose by Weinberg et al.[101] and Di Gregorio et al.[102] indicate that in these experimental conditions ILE is superior to epinephrine and vasopressin alone or in combination. Measures of cardiac output and tissue perfusion were much better in the group treated with ILE than in any pressor regimen. Moreover, studies by Hiller et al.[103] showed that adding epinephrine to ILE at or above a threshold of 10 μg/kg impaired the efficacy of ILE in reversing bupivacaine-induced CC. Metabolic parameters were severely affected by epinephrine which appeared to promote early recovery of systolic pressure but resulted in severely depressed cardiovascular status by 15 minutes. These findings are in contrast to those of Mayr et al.[104] who showed in a pig model of bupivacaine overdose that high-dose vasopressors were superior to ILE and that of Hicks et al.[105] which found ILE no better than saline controls in another porcine model of bupivacaine overdose. However, the study by Mayr et al. introduced prolonged asphyxia prior to resuscitation and that of Hicks et al. used a very high-dose combined vasopressor (epinephrine and vasopressin) treatment for 10 minutes before animals were randomized to a treatment group. In both instances, a potent confounder that is known either to exacerbate LAST (asphyxia) or to impair ILE (vasopressor therapy) was introduced to the experimental design, making it difficult to compare efficacy of ILE with other treatments. More study of resuscitation from LAST will help identify and optimize treatment of this life-threatening condition. Agreement on

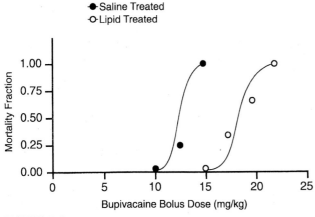

FIGURE 7-4. Mortality after a bolus intravenous dose of bupivacaine, comparing resuscitation with either saline or lipid infusion. Each point represents the mortality fraction in a group of six animals after the corresponding bolus dose of bupivacaine (given over 10 seconds). LD_{50} values are 12.5 mg/kg for saline resuscitation and 18.5 mg/kg for lipid resuscitation. (Reproduced from Knudsen K, Beckman Suurküla M, Blomberg S, et al. Central nervous and cardiovascular effects of i.v. infusions of ropivacaine, bupivacaine and placebo in volunteers. *Br J Anaesth* 1997;78(5):507–514, with permission.)

suitable models and experimental designs is desirable as it should aid in comparing results from various studies and laboratories. The current ASRA guidelines recommend using epinephrine only in small doses (boluses <0.5–1.0 µg/kg) and that vasopressin not be used.

Management of LAST is still evolving. It is expected that with standard precautions, early detection and prompt intervention, the likelihood of severe LA toxicity can be minimized and the probability of good outcome improved substantially. Our goal as a specialty in this regard should be to stamp out fatalities related to LA toxicity. Physician education and increased awareness of LAST are the first steps to this goal.

▶ SUMMARY

LAs are critically important tools for the physician. However, like all tools, even with proper use they can present the clinician with an unexpected danger. Anticipating and preparing for such events will do much to minimize the corresponding morbidity and mortality. Much is known about the interaction of LAs with the Na_v channel, the molecular target for inhibiting propagation of nerve action potentials and the physiologic substrate of nerve block. On the other hand, we still have much to learn about the diverse mechanisms underlying the acute and chronic forms of LA-induced cardiac and neuronal toxicity. Interaction with a variety of ionotropic, metabotropic, and energy transduction systems are all likely to contribute. Moreover, it is important that research continues in this area since identifying safer practice and more effective measures to prevent and treat this complication of regional anesthesia depends on improving our understanding of these phenomena. Most important, such studies are in keeping with our profession's leading role in improving patient safety. We hope that we can eventually eliminate LAST as a major complication of regional anesthesia.

References

1. Strichartz GR. *Local Anesthetics: Handbook of Experimental Pharmacology.* Heidelberg, Germany: Springer-Verlag, 1987.
2. de Jong RH. *Local Anesthetics.* St. Louis, MO: Mosby-Year Book, Inc., 1994.
3. Albright GA. Cardiac arrest following regional anesthesia with etidocaine or bupivacaine. *Anesthesiology* 1979;51:285–287.
4. Sage DJ, Feldman HS, Arthur GR, et al. The cardiovascular effects of convulsant doses of lidocaine and bupivacaine in the conscious dog. *Reg Anesth* 1985;10:175–183.
5. Edde RR, Deutsch S. Cardiac arrest after interscalene brachial-plexus block. *Anesth Analg* 1977;56:446–447.
6. Aberg G. Toxicological and local anaesthetic effects of optically active isomers of two local anaesthetic compounds. *Acta Pharmacol Toxicol* (Copenh) 1972;31:273–286.
7. Aberg G, Dhuner KG, Sydnes G. Studies on the duration of local anaesthesia: structure/activity relationships in a series of homologous local anaesthetics. *Acta Pharmacol Toxicol* 1977;41:432–443.
8. Akerman B, Hellberg IB, Trossvik C. Primary evaluation of the local anaesthetic properties of the amino amide agent ropivacaine (LEA 103). *Acta Anaesthesiol Scand* 1988;32:571–578.
9. Lee LA, Posner KL, Domino KB, et al. Injuries associated with regional anesthesia in the 1980s and 1990s: a closed claims analysis. *Anesthesiology* 2004;101:143–152.
10. Mulroy MF, Norris MC, Liu SS. Safety steps for epidural injection of local anesthetics: review of the literature and recommendations. *Anesth Analg* 1997;85:1346–1356.
11. Auroy Y, Narchi P, Messiah A, et al. Serious complications related to regional anesthesia: results of a prospective surgery in France. *Anesthesiology* 1997;87:479–486.
12. Brown DL, Ransom DM, Hall JA, et al. Regional anesthesia and local anesthetic-induced systemic toxicity: seizure frequency and accompanying cardiovascular changes. *Anesth Analg* 1995;81:321–328.
13. Wang SY, Nau C, Wang GK. Residues in Na(+) channel D3-S6 segment modulate both batrachotoxin and local anesthetic affinities. *Biophys J* 2000;79:1379–1387.
14. Wang SY, Barile M, Wang GK. Disparate role of Na(+) channel D2-S6 residues in batrachotoxin and local anesthetic action. *Mol Pharmacol* 2001;59:1100–1107.
15. Butterworth IV JF, Strichartz GR. Molecular mechanisms of local anesthesia: a review. *Anesthesiology* 1990;72:711–734.
16. Hille B. *Ionic Channels of Excitable Membranes.* 3rd ed. Sunderland, MA: Sinauer Associates, Inc., 2001.
17. Hanck DA, Makielski JC, Sheets MF. Kinetic effects of quaternary lidocaine block of cardiac sodium channels: a gating current study. *J Gen Physiol* 1994;103:19–43.
18. Sugimoto M, Uchida I, Fukami S, et al. The alpha and gamma subunit-dependent effects of local anesthetics on recombinant GABA (A) receptors. *Eur J Pharmacol* 2000;401:329–337.
19. Tetzlaff J. *Clinical Pharmacology of Local Anesthetics.* Woburn, MA: Butterworth-Heinemann, 2000.
20. Covino BG, Vasallo HG. *Local Anesthetics.* New York, NY: Grune & Stratton, 1976.
21. Scott DB, Jebson PJ, Braid DP, et al. Factors affecting plasma levels of lignocaine and prilocaine. *Br J Anaesth* 1972;44:1040–1049.
22. Fragneto RY, Bader AM, Rosinia F, et al. Measurements of protein binding of lidocaine throughout pregnancy. *Anesth Analg* 1994;79:295–297.
23. Strichartz GR, Sanchez V, Arthur GR, et al. Fundamental properties of local anesthetics. II. Measured octanol:butter partition coefficients and pKa values of clinically used drugs. *Anesth Analg* 1990;71:158–170.
24. Groban L, Dolinski SY. Differences in cardiac toxicity among ropivacaine, levobupivacaine, bupivacaine, and lidocaine. *Tech Reg Anesth Pain Manag* 2001;5:48–55.
25. Ash-Bernal R, Wise R, Wright SM. Acquired methemoglobinemia: a retrospective series of 138 cases at 2 teaching hospitals. *Medicine* 2004;83:265–273.
26. Di Gregorio G, Neal J, Rosenquist R, et al. Clinical presentation of local anesthetic toxicity. *Reg Anesth Pain Med* 2010;35:181–187.
27. Satas S, Johannessen S, Hoem NO, et al. Lidocaine pharmacokinetics and toxicity in newborn pigs. *Anesth Analg* 1997;85:306–312.
28. Mather LE. Disposition of mepivacaine and bupivacaine enantiomers in sheep. *Br J Anaesth* 1991;67:239–246, 1991.
29. Denson DD, Behbehani MM, Gregg RV. Enantiomer-specific effects of an intravenously administered arrhythmogenic dose of bupivacaine on neurons of the nucleus tractus solitarus and the cardiovascular system in the anesthetized rat. *Reg Anesth* 1992;17:311–316.
30. Watanabe Y, Dohi S, Iida H, et al. The effects of bupivacaine and ropivacaine on baroreflex sensitivity with or without respiratory acidosis and alkalosis in rats. *Anesth Analg* 1997;84:398–404.
31. Rutten AJ, Nancarrow C, Mather LE, et al. Hemodynamic and central nervous system effects of intravenous bolus doses of lidocaine, bupivacaine, and ropivacaine in sheep. *Anesth Analg* 1989;69:291–299.
32. Scott DB, Lee A, Fagan D, et al. Acute toxicity of ropivacaine compared with that of bupivacaine. *Anesth Analg* 1989;69:563–569.
33. Knudsen K, Beckman Suurkula M, et al. Central nervous and cardiovascular effects of i.v. infusions of ropivacaine, bupivacaine and placebo in volunteers. *Br J Anaesth* 1997;78:507–514.

34. Yi JW, Lee BJ, Kim DO, et al. Effects of bupivacaine and ropivacaine on field potential in rat hippocampal slices. *Br J Anaesth* 2009;102:673–679.

35. Ohmura S, Kawada M, Ohta T, et al. Systemic toxicity and resuscitation in bupivacaine-, levobupivacaine-, or ropivacaine-infused rats. *Anesth Analg* 2001;93:743–748.

36. Huang YF, Pryor ME, Mather LE, et al. Cardiovascular and central nervous system effects of intravenous levobupivacaine and bupivacaine in sheep. *Anesth Analg* 1998;86:797–804.

37. Chang DH, Ladd LA, Wilson KA, et al. Tolerability of large-dose intravenous levobupivacaine in sheep. *Anesth Analg* 2000;91:671–679.

38. Stewart J, Kellett N, Castro D. The central nervous system and cardiovascular effects of levobupivacaine and ropivacaine in healthy volunteers. *Anesth Analg* 2003;97:412–416.

39. Ladd LA, Chang DHT, Wilson KA, et al. Effects of CNS site-directed carotid arterial infusions of bupivacaine, levobupivacaine, and ropivacaine in sheep. *Anesthesiology* 2002;97(2):418–428.

40. Butterworth JF. Models and mechanisms of local anesthetic cardiac toxicity: a review. *Reg Anesth Pain Med* 2010;35(2):167–176.

41. Ahern CA, Eastwood AL, Dougherty DA, et al. New insights into the therapeutic inhibition of voltage-gated sodium channels. *Channels (Austin)* 2008;2(1):1–3.

42. Fozzard HA, Lee PJ, Lipkind GM. Mechanism of local anesthetic drug action on voltage-gated sodium channels. *Curr Pharm Des* 2005;11(21):2671–2686.

43. Courtney KR, Kendig JJ. Bupivacaine is an effective potassium channel blocker in heart. *Biochim Biophys Acta* 1988;939(1):163–166.

44. Mio Y, Fukuda N, Kusakari Y, et al. Comparative effects of bupivacaine and ropivacaine on intracellular calcium transients and tension in ferret ventricular muscle. *Anesthesiology* 2004;101(4):888–894.

45. Rossner KL, Freese KJ. Bupivacaine inhibition of L-type calcium current in ventricular cardiomyocytes of hamster. *Anesthesiology* 1997;87(4):926–934.

46. Coyle DE, Sperelakis N. Bupivacaine and lidocaine blockade of calcium-mediated slow action potentials in guinea pig ventricular muscle. *J Pharmacol Exp Ther* 1987;242(3):1001–1005.

47. McCaslin PP, Butterworth J. Bupivacaine suppresses [Ca(2+)](i) oscillations in neonatal rat cardiomyocytes with increased extracellular K+ and is reversed with increased extracellular Mg(2+). *Anesth Analg* 2000;91(1):82–88.

48. Heavner JE. Cardiac toxicity of local anesthetics in the intact isolated heart model: a review. *Reg Anesth Pain Med* 2002;27(6):545–555.

49. Zhang S, Yao S, Li Q. Effects of ropivacaine and bupivacaine on rabbit myocardial energetic metabolism and mitochondria oxidation. *J Huazhong Univ Sci Technolog Med Sci* 2003;23(2):178–179, 183.

50. Chernoff DM. Kinetic analysis of phasic inhibition of neuronal sodium currents by lidocaine and bupivacaine. *Biophys J* 1990;58(1):53–68.

51. Nau C, Vogel W, Hempelmann G, et al. Stereoselectivity of bupivacaine in local anesthetic-sensitive ion channels of peripheral nerve. *Anesthesiology* 1999;91(3):786–795.

52. Valenzuela C, Delpon E, Tamkun MM, et al. Stereoselective block of a human cardiac potassium channel (Kv1.5) by bupivacaine enantiomers. *Biophys J* 1995;69(2):418–427.

53. Reiz S, Nath S. Cardiotoxicity of local anaesthetic agents. *Br J Anaesth* 1986;58(7):736–746.

54. Reiz S, Haggmark S, Johansson G, et al. Cardiotoxicity of ropivacaine—a new amide local anaesthetic agent. *Acta Anaesthesiol Scand* 1989;33(2):93–98.

55. Pitkanen M, Feldman HS, Arthur GR, et al. Chronotropic and inotropic effects of ropivacaine, bupivacaine, and lidocaine in the spontaneously beating and electrically paced isolated, perfused rabbit heart. *Reg Anesth* 1992;17(4):183–192.

56. Butterworth J, James RL, Grimes J. Structure-affinity relationships and stereospecificity of several homologous series of local anesthetics for the beta2-adrenergic receptor. *Anesth Analg* 1997;85(2):336–342.

57. Butterworth JF, Brownlow RC, Leith JP, et al. Bupivacaine inhibits cyclic-3'',5''-adenosine monophosphate production. A possible contributing factor to cardiovascular toxicity. *Anesthesiology* 1993;79(1):88–95.

58. Moller R, Covino BG. Cardiac electrophysiologic properties of bupivacaine and lidocaine compared with those of ropivacaine, a new amide local anesthetic. *Anesthesiology* 1990;72(2):322–329.

59. Timour Q, Freysz M, Lang J, et al. Electrophysiological study in the dog of the risk of cardiac toxicity of bupivacaine. *Arch Int Pharmacodyn Ther* 1987;287(1):65–77.

60. Gomez De Segura IA, Vazquez Moreno-Planas I, Benito J, et al. Electrophysiologic cardiac effects of the new local anesthetic IQB-9302 and of bupivacaine in the anesthetised dog. *Acta Anaesthesiol Scand* 2002;46(6):666–673.

61. Scott DB, Lee A, Fagan D, et al. Acute toxicity of ropivacaine compared with that of bupivacaine. *Anesth Analg* 1989;69(5):563–569.

62. Lefrant JY, de La Coussaye JE, Ripart J, et al. The comparative electrophysiologic and hemodynamic effects of a large dose of ropivacaine and bupivacaine in anesthetized and ventilated piglets. *Anesth Analg* 2001;93(6):1598–1605, table of contents.

63. de La Coussaye JE, Brugada J, Allessie MA. Electrophysiologic and arrhythmogenic effects of bupivacaine. A study with high-resolution ventricular epicardial mapping in rabbit hearts. *Anesthesiology* 1992;77(1):132–141.

64. de Jong RH, Ronfeld RA, DeRosa RA. Cardiovascular effects of convulsant and supraconvulsant doses of amide local anesthetics. *Anesth Analg* 1982;61(1):3–9.

65. Feldman HS, Arthur GR, Pitkanen M, et al. Treatment of acute systemic toxicity after the rapid intravenous injection of ropivacaine and bupivacaine in the conscious dog. *Anesth Analg* 1991;73(4):373–384.

66. Feldman HS, Arthur GR, Covino BG. Comparative systemic toxicity of convulsant and supraconvulsant doses of intravenous ropivacaine, bupivacaine, and lidocaine in the conscious dog. *Anesth Analg* 1989;69(6):794–801.

67. Kotelko DM, Shnider SM, Dailey PA, et al. Bupivacaine-induced cardiac arrhythmias in sheep. *Anesthesiology* 1984;60(1):10–18.

68. Knudsen K, Beckman Suurkula M, Blomberg S, et al. Central nervous and cardiovascular effects of i.v. infusions of ropivacaine, bupivacaine and placebo in volunteers. *Br J Anaesth* 1997;78(5):507–514.

69. Ohmura S, Kawada M, Ohta T, et al. Systemic toxicity and resuscitation in bupivacaine-, levobupivacaine-, or ropivacaine-infused rats. *Anesth Analg* 2001;93(3):743–748.

70. Morgan M, Russell WJ. An investigation in man into the relative potency of lignocaine, bupivacaine and etidocaine. *Br J Anaesth* 1975;47(5):586–591.

71. Hassan HG, Renck H, Akerman B, et al. On the relative potency of amino-amide local anaesthetics in vivo. *Acta Anaesthesiol Scand* 1994;38(5):505–509.

72. Nath S, Haggmark S, Johansson G, et al. Differential depressant and electrophysiologic cardiotoxicity of local anesthetics: an experimental study with special reference to lidocaine and bupivacaine. *Anesth Analg* 1986;65(12):1263–1270.

73. Chang DH, Ladd LA, Copeland S, et al. Direct cardiac effects of intracoronary bupivacaine, levobupivacaine and ropivacaine in the sheep. *Br J Pharmacol* 2001;132(3):649–658.

74. Chang DH, Ladd LA, Wilson KA, et al. Tolerability of large-dose intravenous levobupivacaine in sheep. *Anesth Analg* 2000;91(3):671–679.

75. Huang YF, Pryor ME, Mather LE, et al. Cardiovascular and central nervous system effects of intravenous levobupivacaine and bupivacaine in sheep. *Anesth Analg* 1998;86(4):797–804.

76. Groban L, Deal DD, Vernon JC, et al. Cardiac resuscitation after incremental overdosage with lidocaine, bupivacaine, levobupivacaine, and ropivacaine in anesthetized dogs. *Anesth Analg* 2001;92(1):37–43.

77. Levy JH. *Anaphylactic Reactions in Anesthesia and Intensive Care*. Boston, MA: Butterworth Publishers, 1992.

78. deShazo RD, Nelson HS. An approach to the patient with a history of local anesthetic hypersensitivity: experience in 90 patients. *J Allergy Clin Immunol* 1979;63:387–394.

79. Gall H, Kaufmann R, Kalveram CM. Adverse reactions to local anesthetics: analysis of 197 cases. *J Allergy Clin Immunol* 1996;97:933–937.

80. Baluga JC, Casamayou R, Carozzi E, et al. Allergy to local anaesthetics in dentistry. Myth or reality? *Allergol Immunopathol (Madr)* 2002;30:14–19.

81. Çetinkaya F. Sensitivity to local anaesthetics among asthmatic children. *Int J Paediatr Dent* 2001;11:405–408.

82. Berkun Y, Ben-Zvi A, Levy Y, et al. Evaluation of adverse reactions to local anesthetics: experience with 236 patients. *Ann Allergy Asthma Immunol* 2003;91:342–345.

83. Morais-Almeida M, Gaspar A, Marinho S, et al. Allergy to local anesthetics of the amide group with tolerance to procaine. *Allergy* 2003;58:827–828.

84. Fujita H, Maru E, Shimada M, et al. A decrease in seizure susceptibility to lidocaine in kindled epileptic rats. *Anesth Analg* 2000;90:1129–1134.

85. Momota Y, Artru A, Powers K, et al. Concentrations of lidocaine and monoethylglycine xylidide in brain, cerebrospinal fluid, and plasma during lidocaine-induced epileptiform electroencephalogram activity in rabbits: the effects of epinephrine and hypocapnia. *Anesth Analg* 2000;91:362–368.

86. Hsu C, Lin T, Yeh C, et al. Convulsions during superior laryngeal nerve block—a case report. *Acta Anaesthesiol Sin* 2000;38:93–96.

87. Neal J, Bernards C, Butterworth J, et al. ASRA practice advisory on local anesthetic systemic toxicity. *Reg Anesth Pain Med* 2010;35:152–161.

88. Groban L. Central nervous system and cardiac effects from long-acting amide local anesthetic toxicity in the intact animal model. *Reg Anesth Pain Med* 2003;28:3–11.

89. Orebaugh S, Williams B, Vallejo M, et al. Adverse outcomes associated with stimulator-based peripheral nerve blocks with versus without ultrasound visualization. *Reg Anesth Pain Med* 2009;34:251–255.

90. Barrington MJ, Watts SA, Gledhill SA, et al. Preliminary results of the Australasian Regional Anaesthesia Collaboration: a prospective audit of more than 7000 peripheral nerve and plexus blocks for neurologic and other complications. *Reg Anesth Pain Med* 2009;34:534–541.

91. Moore DC, Bridenbaugh LD. Oxygen: the antidote for systemic toxic reactions from local anesthetic drugs. *JAMA* 1960;174:102–107.

92. Weinberg GL, VadeBoncouer T, Ramaraju GA, et al. Pretreatment or resuscitation with a lipid infusion shifts the dose-response to bupivacaine-induced asystole in rats. *Anesthesiology* 1998;88:1071–1075.

93. Weinberg G, Ripper R, Feinstein DL, et al. Lipid emulsion infusion rescues dogs from bupivacaine-induced cardiac toxicity. *Reg Anesth Pain Med* 2003;28:198–202.

94. Rosenblatt MA, Abel M, Fischer GW, et al. Successful use of a 20% lipid emulsion to resuscitate a patient after a presumed bupivacaine-related cardiac arrest. *Anesthesiology* 2006;105:217–218.

95. Spence AG. Lipid reversal of central nervous system symptoms of bupivacaine toxicity. *Anesthesiology* 2007;107:516–517.

96. Bern S, Akpa BS, Kuo I, et al. Lipid resuscitation: a life-saving antidote for local anesthetic toxicity. *Curr Pharm Biotechnol* 2011;12:313–319.

97. Rothschild L, Bern S, Oswald S, et al. Intravenous lipid emulsion in clinical toxicology. *Scand J Trauma Resusc Emerg Med* 2010;18:51.

98. Jamaty C, Bailey B, Larocque A, et al. Lipid emulsions in the treatment of acute poisoning: a systematic review of human and animal studies. *Clin Toxicol (Phila)* 2010;48:1–27.

99. Marwick PC, Levin AI, Coetzee AR. Recurrence of cardiotoxicity after lipid rescue from bupivacaine-induced cardiac arrest. *Anesth Analg* 2009;108:1344–1346.

100. McCutchen T, Gerancher JC. Early intralipid therapy may have prevented bupivacaine-associated cardiac arrest. *Reg Anesth Pain Med* 2008;33:178–180.

101. Weinberg GL, Di Gregorio G, Ripper R, et al. Resuscitation with lipid versus epinephrine in a rat model of bupivacaine overdose. *Anesthesiology* 2008;108:907–913.

102. Di Gregorio G, Schwartz D, Ripper R, et al. Lipid emulsion is superior to vasopressin in a rodent model of resuscitation from toxin-induced cardiac arrest. *Crit Care Med* 2009;37:993–999.

103. Hiller DB, Gregorio GD, Ripper R, et al. Epinephrine impairs lipid resuscitation from bupivacaine overdose: a threshold effect. *Anesthesiology* 2009;111:498–505.

104. Mayr VD, Mitterschiffthaler L, Neurauter A, et al. A comparison of the combination of epinephrine and vasopressin with lipid emulsion in a porcine model of asphyxial cardiac arrest after intravenous injection of bupivacaine. *Anesth Analg* 2008;106:1566–1571.

105. Hicks SD, Salcido DD, Logue ES, et al. Lipid emulsion combined with epinephrine and vasopressin does not improve survival in a swine model of bupivacaine-induced cardiac arrest. *Anesthesiology* 2009;111:138–146.

8

Adjuvant and Preservative Toxicity

John C. Rowlingson and Joseph M. Neal

Anesthesiologists have always been concerned about the neurotoxicity of common anesthetic agents, such as local anesthetics and opioids that are deposited around the neuraxis or peripheral nerves. However, the potential adverse effects of the preservatives used during drug formulation or of adjuvants used to potentiate the clinical effects of the primary drug are less well recognized. In an age of expanding understanding about and the discovery of the neuropharmacology of pain impulse transmission and nociceptive processing, awareness of the potential for toxicity from contemporary drug preparations is vital to minimize harm and maximize benefit to patients. This chapter reviews the potential for neurotoxicity related to preservatives and adjuvants.

▶ DEFINITION

The term toxicity, as it is considered in regional anesthesia and pain medicine, refers generally to the effects of substances that are injurious to tissues and/or the body. In considering this definition further, we need to distinguish between toxicity at the tissue level, that is, in the nervous system as with the contemporary concept of neurotoxicity and at systemic sites (Box 8-1). Yaksh[1] highlights concerns about the former by pointing out that the use of untested drugs and drug combinations is rampant in regional anesthesia and pain medicine, and thus our concern is genuine and deserved. Toxicity at the

TABLE 8-1 Local Anesthetics and Their Additives

LOCAL ANESTHETIC	METHYLPARABEN	EDTA	BISULFITE
Bupivacaine	X		X
2-Chloroprocaine	X	X	
Etidocaine			X
Lidocaine	X		X
Mepivacaine	X		
Prilocaine			X
Procaine			X

Note: Levobupivacaine and ropivacaine contain no additives. EDTA, ethylenediaminetetraacetic acid.
Table modified from Weinberg GL. Treatment of local anesthetic systemic toxicity (LAST). *Reg Anesth Pain Med* 2010;35:188–193, with permission.

tissue level is clearly distinct from systemic toxicity. An example of the latter is opioid-induced neurotoxicity, as presented by Sweeney and Bruera.[2] They declare this to be a "recently recognized syndrome of neuropsychiatric consequences of opioid administration." The syndrome includes cognitive impairment, severe sedation, hallucinations, delirium, myoclonus, seizures, hyperalgesia, and allodynia. The syndrome seems to be particularly related to the use of high doses of opioids for prolonged periods of time. Another common example of systemic toxicity would be local anesthetic systemic toxicity (LAST) (Chapter 7).[3–6] This chapter focuses on tissue neurotoxicity as it relates to the neuraxis or peripheral nerves.

▶ SCOPE

Reality dictates that pharmacy, prescription order, and health care provider errors will occur in the provision of *clinical* care, yielding unexpected dosing or effects from drugs placed in the perispinal or peripheral nerve spaces. When this occurs, focal neurotoxicity might be manifested, as might drug withdrawal, overdose, or systemic toxicity. Given the extensive literature addressing the rediscovery of possible local anesthetic toxicity at the tissue level presenting as transient neurologic symptoms (TNSs) (Chapter 13), it is also evident that drugs of long-standing, traditional benefit might also come under new scrutiny.[7,8] As Reichert and Butterworth[9] noted, "clinicians must recognize that even local anesthetics labeled as 'preservative-free' contain 'inactive ingredients'." To be complete, research into single-agent neurotoxicity must isolate the causative agent, separating it from pH, osmolarity, the chemical vehicle of the injected drug, consequences of the use of needles and catheters to place the drugs, and the patient's preexisting physiologic condition.[10] The quest for better adjuvant substances combined with primary drugs to enhance their clinical actions by facilitating additive effects or prolonging the primary drug's action is in part spurred by the desire to reduce total local anesthetic dose, but also raises the potential of toxicity from the adjuvants themselves (Table 8-1).

Indeed, clinicians have been raising more concern about the potential toxicity of everyday drugs in recent years. In a perceptive comment, Sawynok[11] noted that "the demonstration of neurotoxic effects following local administration [of amitriptyline] is an important reminder of the need for careful assessment of novel routes of drug administration." Lavand'homme's[12] editorial from 2006, commenting on the lack of medical science following classic, fundamental steps in the study of intrathecal (IT) midazolam, truly reveals "lessons" that are worth noting. She acknowledges the clinical demand for new agents and their application to, meritoriously, lessen pain. However, "our decision to use spinal analgesics should result from a balance between the risks… and the benefits…. Risks should be our first concern because every spinal drug is potentially neurotoxic and able to produce a local lesion leading to a functional deficit, either temporary or permanent." She outlines the recommended pathway for drug development in this statement—"Ideally, before widespread use, a spinal drug should undergo specific and complete histologic, physiologic, and behavioral testing in at least two different species (a small-animal model and a large-animal model) followed by safety trials in humans."

This growing awareness about a rush of research, embodied only in small-scale studies or case reports, that advocates the premature clinical application of drugs before a strict scientific protocol of development was documented, has necessarily resulted in major anesthesiology journals adopting a more rigorous policy for accepting manuscripts that promote the off-label use of old and new investigational drugs.[13,14] Because all drugs are, indeed, potentially neurotoxic, a journal could give implicit approval by publishing a study that advocates the off-label use of a drug. The new policies contain specific criteria for authors about the submission of manuscripts addressing the off-label use of drugs. Essentially, the editorial boards can ask for more documentation (than even the author's institutional review board required), request more information about relevant animal and human neurotoxicity studies, clarify that the study was done under a Federal Drug Administration-approved investigational new drug status, or acknowledge that the proposed clinical application already represents routine clinical practice. This policy action is appropriate as "… the journals … ultimately bear the ethical and professional burden of promulgating only the best science."[13]

Medical science has validated models to study toxicity. Westin et al.[15] updated the use of the popular implanted lumbar IT catheter technique in 2010. Their report was of a preclinical model for "evaluating dose-dependent efficacy, spinal cord toxicity, and long-term function after IT morphine in the neonatal rat." The emphasis on the preclinical period appropriately reorders the steps taken in getting a drug ready for market and a manuscript into publication quality form. The model is flexible enough such that other drugs can be tested, a wide range of postnatal ages studied, and different animal species utilized.

► PRESERVATIVES AND ADJUVANTS OF HISTORICAL REPUTATION

Parabens

These compounds are added to local anesthetic preparations to provide an antibacterial effect, as in multidose vials. The methyl moieties are more common than the ethyl or propyl varieties. The common concentration is 1 mg/mL. Reichert and Butterworth note that these compounds decrease the microbe load but do not necessarily eliminate it.[9] They state that there is no "convincing evidence" in the literature of a neurotoxic effect of these compounds. This is not a universal belief, as reported by Hetherington and Dooley.[16] There have been reported systemic toxic effects manifested by the metabolism of parabens to paraaminobenzoic acid, which can trigger an allergic reaction in sensitive individuals.[10] This reality is reenforced in a recent case report by Farber et al.,[17] in which they discuss the anesthetic management of a patient with an allergy to propylene glycols and parabens. Their introduction clearly states, "multiple pharmaceutical products contain excipients, or additive chemicals, to improve stability, bioavailability, antimicrobial activity, or palatability. Two of the most common excipients are propylene glycol and parabens." Thus, the potential for a cross-reactivity reaction exists; a neurotoxic event is unlikely. Hodgson et al.[7] concluded that "parabens are safe when administered spinally in the small doses associated with preservative use."

Metabisulfite

Metabisulfite is added to epinephrine-containing local anesthetic solutions as an antioxidant. The intended effect is to increase the stability of the mixture and enhance shelf life.[10] Interestingly, these compounds are also included in many emergency drug preparations such as epinephrine, procainamide, phenylephrine, dopamine, dobutamine, and dexamethasone.[9] It is noted that there is a lack of sensitive and specific challenge tests, and thus the compound does infrequently provoke a hypersensitive reaction, which is characterized clinically by urticaria, flushing, pruritus, and (potentially) airway obstruction.[9]

As to neurotoxicity findings, studies are both mildly positive and negative. Concerns were raised about sodium bisulfite in the 1980s when 2-chloroprocaine, given unintentionally in the IT space, resulted in neural deficits.[7] The explanation put forward was that the bisulfite in a low-pH (pH <4) environment was converted to sulfurous ions that could cross the dura, resulting in injurious concentrations of sulfuric acid in the cerebrospinal fluid (CSF).[7,10] If the pH was >4, inactive sulfonates were formed. The issue of metabisulfite neurotoxicity has returned to the spotlight, as emphasized by Drasner.[18] His editorial in 2005 preceded four articles about "new" trials of 2-chloroprocaine as a spinal anesthetic. His main point was that more careful research *must* precede the broad clinical application of this drug preparation as a replacement for lidocaine, with which there is a high incidence of TNSs. Taniguchi et al.[19] raised an interesting point in their rat model research that compared 2-chloroprocaine with and without bisulfite for creating neurotoxicity. They concluded that clinical deficits previously associated with unintentional IT injection of 2-chloroprocaine may actually have been from the local anesthetic itself, and thus an absolute answer to the toxicity of metabisulfite remains elusive (and may indicate how difficult it is to accurately identify the precise injurious etiology, given the interplay of pharmacodynamics and pharmacokinetics of drugs placed in the body). To be most accurate, it is necessary to note that the doses of 2-chloroprocaine that caused neurotoxicity in Taniguchi et al.'s study would be equivalent to using 1 g of the drug in humans. Furthermore, as they note in their discussion, their findings of the toxicity of 2-chloroprocaine with and without bisulfite are similar to those with lidocaine, using the same experimental paradigm. That the concurrent use of bisulfite seemed to induce a *neuroprotective* effect casts metabisulfite in an entirely different light and certainly begs for further study.

Ethylenediaminetetraacetic Acid and Calcium Chloride

After metabisulfite had been labeled as the offending agent in 2-chloroprocaine neurotoxicity, ethylenediaminetetraacetic acid (EDTA) was substituted as the antioxidant in commercial epidural solutions of 2-chloroprocaine.[10] Thus, the spinal nerves could be at potential risk if unintended doses of EDTA reached the subarachnoid space. Reichert and Butterworth[9] noted that there are papers documenting a dose- and a duration-dependent motor and histopathologic abnormality in animals subjected to IT EDTA (with the effect absent if calcium chloride is administered). This seems to be of only slight import now, in that EDTA is not a common additive. A systemic effect of epidural 2-chloroprocaine containing EDTA was manifested as back muscle spasm, which presented as the epidural block was resolving. It was thought at the time to be caused by the placement of some local anesthetic in the perispinal muscles with the effect that the EDTA chelated calcium, producing the spasm.[20] Hung et al.[21] noted that elevated extracellular calcium ion levels result in diminished nerve excitability. Using a sciatic nerve block model in rats, they showed that the addition of calcium chloride to lidocaine and bupivacaine did, indeed, produce prolonged neural blockade. However, there were histopathologic changes associated with high concentrations of $CaCl_2$ so the authors predicted little clinical enthusiasm for such combinations in the future.

Phenylephrine

This is an additive to local anesthetics used for the purpose of decreasing the systemic blood levels of the associated local anesthetic and prolonging the duration of action of the local anesthetic.[7] In addition to the use of vasoconstrictors such as phenylephrine and epinephrine, other factors that might influence the amount of local anesthetic absorbed include the specific local anesthetic agent used, its volume and concentration, and the anatomic location of its placement.[22] To minimize the chance of a *systemic* toxic reaction, the use of vasoconstrictive agents should be carefully considered in patients with unstable angina, poorly controlled hypertension, arrhythmias, uteroplacental insufficiency, monoamine oxidase (MAO) inhibitor, or tricyclic antidepressant use, as well as in patients having intravenous regional anesthesia. The concern is not gradual systemic uptake of vasoconstrictors but immediate cardiovascular effects consequent to an unintended intravenous bolus injection.

Sakura et al.[23] have reported that TNS symptoms were more frequent after tetracaine spinal anesthesia when phenylephrine was also used, but it was not clear that the symptoms were correlated with definite neurotoxicity. This conclusion was influenced by the possibility that the phenylephrine reduced the spinal cord blood flow, as had been demonstrated in animals (Chapter 12). Hodgson et al.[7] cited a lack of firm data demonstrating direct neurotoxic effects from phenylephrine, as did Haider[22] in his 2004 review. Both authors noted the lack of information about the possible interaction of the drugs lowering the spinal or peripheral nerve blood flow with areas of preexisting "injury" in the targeted nerve(s), leaving open the possibility of synergistic effects causing harm.

Dextrose

Dextrose is commonly used in spinal anesthesia preparations to adjust baricity, which provides some degree of directional control of the local anesthetic and thus the extent and pattern of the subsequent spinal block.[9,10] Although there is some concern about the potential injury from the osmolarity,[7] "Animal and human studies have largely exonerated glucose as a major contribution to neural injury." Kalichman et al.'s[24] study in diabetic rats maintains a concern that defects in glucose metabolism in the host may be a cofactor in neural injury with local anesthetics. Despite these concerns, dextrose has been used in millions of spinal anesthetics in diabetics without obvious harm.

pH Adjusters: Bicarbonate, Carbon Dioxide, HCl, NaOH

The acidic pH of commercial local anesthetics is intentional, as this maintains the stability of the solution. When clinically applied, the low-pH solution does not contain a high content of unionized local anesthetic molecules, the form of the drug that is required for penetrating the surrounding tissues and membranes prior to reaching the site of action, the sodium channel.[6] There is no evidence that pH adjustment with HCl or NaOH, bicarbonate, or carbon dioxide adds to the toxicity of local anesthetic preparations.[7] Although the addition of bicarbonate to commercially available local anesthetic solutions

(and especially lidocaine) was touted as decreasing the block onset time, most studies have revealed this reality is more of statistical fascination than clinical benefit.[25]

Epinephrine

Epinephrine is added to local anesthetics for the purpose of extending block duration, limiting systemic uptake, supplementing analgesic effects, and acting as an indicator of intravascular injection. Historically, concerns have been expressed over adverse effects, including hemodynamic alterations, direct neurotoxicity, enhanced toxicity in diabetic patients, and/or vasoconstriction-induced ischemic complications (Box 8-2).[7,10,22,26]

Direct Neurotoxicity of Epinephrine

Spinal cord injury does not occur following subarachnoid application of epinephrine. Single injection of up to 500 μg of epinephrine failed to cause histopathologic changes in rabbit and rat models, even if delivered in a repeated fashion.[27,28] However, when combined with lidocaine 5% or tetracaine 1% to 2%, epinephrine worsens spinal cord histopathology (see Fig. 11-1).[27,28] This most likely reflects decreased clearance of the local anesthetic rather than direct epinephrine-related neurotoxicity. Epinephrine applied directly to peripheral nerves does not result in tissue damage, provided the blood-nerve barrier remains intact.[29,30]

Epinephrine-induced Ischemia

The vasoconstrictive properties of epinephrine have led to concern that its use could provoke ischemia in the spinal cord. A wealth of clinical experience plus indirect evidence based

---

BOX 8-2 Side Effects of Adjuvant Epinephrine

Hemodynamic effects

- Related to: dose, added local anesthetic, injection site.
- High doses, as from unintentional intravascular injection, result in transient tachycardia, hypertension, and increased cardiac output.
- Low doses, as from epidural uptake, result in decreased systemic vascular resistance and consequent increased cardiac output.

Neurotoxicity

- Epinephrine does not directly cause neurotoxicity, but animal studies show that adjuvant epinephrine may worsen local anesthetic-induced neuraxial or peripheral nerve injury.

Epinephrine-induced ischemia

- Animal studies and clinical surveillance studies strongly suggest that epinephrine does not adversely affect spinal cord blood flow.
- Animal studies show that local anesthetics and epinephrine significantly reduce peripheral nerve blood flow, whereas patient experience suggests that this effect is clinically insignificant.

on human survey studies strongly suggests that epinephrine is not responsible for neuraxial injury in humans (Chapter 12). Indeed, over the past 50 years, published data totaling nearly 27,000 patients document a remarkably low incidence of spinal cord injury subsequent to spinal, epidural, or combined spinal-epidural anesthetic techniques.[31–36] Of those patients who did sustain injury, the vast majority did not receive adjuvant epinephrine, which further suggests that epinephrine is not causally linked to spinal cord injury in the general patient population. Whether patients with compromised blood supply, as from diabetes or atherosclerosis, are at increased risk for injury in the setting of altered spinal cord blood flow autoregulation, trauma, or local anesthetic-induced injury is unknown.[37] Because such patients are often preferentially administered regional anesthesia, vast clinical experience suggests that this risk, if it exists, is exceedingly low.

Peripheral Nerve Ischemia

There is also legitimate concern that perineural epinephrine would decrease the peripheral nerve blood flow, but the clinical significance is unknown. Clinical experience suggests that the risk of neural toxicity is exceedingly low in healthy patients, whereas theoretically increased in patients at risk for compromised peripheral nerve blood flow, as from diabetes or chemotherapy. Studies suggest that epinephrine alone is not toxic to peripheral nerves in diabetic or nondiabetic rats.[30] Furthermore, epinephrine added to lidocaine did not cause more damage in otherwise intact diabetic rat nerves than did lidocaine alone.[30] The ischemic risk of locally applied local anesthetics with epinephrine is very low, even in so-called end-organ circulations. Despite the traditional belief that epinephrine-containing local anesthetic digital blocks could result in ischemia, a comprehensive review of reported cases found no solid evidence that this is the case.[38] Limited indirect clinical evidence notes that epinephrine may worsen outcome if a peripheral nerve has been compromised by mechanical trauma. In Selander et al.'s[29] report of peripheral nerve injury in patients who had also experienced a paresthesia during axillary block, all had received epinephrine. However, most studies of injury following peripheral nerve blocks have not confirmed this association.[39]

Thus, few specific factors increase the risk of epinephrine-associated injury. Adjuvant epinephrine in concentrations >5 μg/mL is unnecessary for clinical anesthesia applications and may theoretically increase ischemic risk. There are no human experimental studies to quantify the risk of adjuvant epinephrine in populations prone to compromised blood flow, such as diabetics, patients with atherosclerosis, or patients with chemotherapy-induced neuropathy. However, on a theoretical basis alone, it is reasonable to weigh the relative risk of adjuvant epinephrine in these patients.[26]

▶ MODERN AGENTS WITH NEUROTOXICITY CONCERNS

Local Anesthetic Systemic Toxicity and Myotoxicity

The potential for local anesthetics and/or their adjuvants to cause neuraxial ischemia or peripheral nerve injury is discussed in detail in Chapters 11 and 12, and in Chapter 14,

respectively. One of the most monumental advances in our specialty has been the management of LAST[3–6] (Chapter 7). Given the prevalence of regional anesthesia and analgesia in current anesthesiology training and everyday practice, having such a simple and effective form of treatment for a dreaded complication is a major factor in the contemporary use of these incredibly valuable clinical techniques, which unmistakably enhance patient outcome and satisfaction.

One clinical circumstance of *tissue* toxicity related to the use of local anesthetics focuses on the myotoxicity of bupivacaine (Chapter 15).

Opioids, Buprenorphine

The application of neuraxial opioids has become commonplace since the sentinel reports of spinal and epidural use in 1979. The rationale was that *smaller doses* of these drugs *placed closer* in the body *to the target site of action* in the spinal cord would provide more intense analgesia (than systemic dosing) and a lower incidence of side effects because of the lower (than systemic) doses.[39–41] That toxicity could be manifested was highlighted early on by DuPen et al.[39] They were using an indwelling epidural-opioid delivery system with a preparation of morphine that contained phenol and formaldehyde. Although pain relief did result, so eventually did neuropathic pain and epidural adhesions. These complications were reversed by the use of preservative-free morphine. Sjoberg et al.[40] reported on the chronic IT administration of morphine with bisulfite and bupivacaine in cancer patients with pain, associated with improved pain relief and functional status of the patients. No definitive postmortem pathologic changes of the spinal cord that were not related to the primary disease were reported. This clinical result is consistent with the general conclusion reached by Hodgson et al.[7] upon a review of the literature of opioid neurotoxicity: "Laboratory studies and extensive clinical experience with morphine, fentanyl, and sufentanil can reasonably assure the safety of limited intrathecal doses of these drugs." That said, a subsequent report by Kakinohana et al.[42] generated reason for concern about a combination of factors involving neuraxial opioids that may result in injury. In a rat model, noninjurious spinal cord ischemia was created. In the presence of IT morphine, CSF glutamate increased, which activated *N*-methyl-D-aspartate (NMDA) receptors and resulted in the degeneration of α-motor neurons (a manifestation of neurotoxicity). Rathmell et al.[43] seemed to have established the safety of IT hydromorphone in a 2005 review. This is important, as this drug is becoming a common component of acute and chronic epidural infusions.

Probably the most frequent manifestation of chronic IT opioid use/toxicity is the formation of catheter-tip granulomas. Allen et al. investigated morphine, hydromorphone, D/L-methadone, L-methadone, D-methadone, and fentanyl, among other substances in dogs, which had had IT catheters implanted.[44] They reported that "opiates at equianalgesic doses present different risks for granuloma formation." Importantly, methadone use resulted in obvious tissue necrosis as well, so the critical demand that research continues to define safe practice is evident.

In a clinical study, Candido et al.[45] furthered our options by reporting on the addition of buprenorphine, an opioid agonist-antagonist, to the analgesic injectate in patients receiving an infragluteal sciatic nerve block. Although all patients receiving either perineural or intramuscular buprenorphine had less postoperative pain, it was clear that the block duration was increased only when the drug was mixed with the bupivacaine. There are no references relevant to toxicity studies in their bibliography, but the technique has been published previously.

Limited data and the infrequent application of opioids used for blocking peripheral nerves make it impossible to realistically comment on this potential toxicity.[25,46] The *systemic* consequences of IT opioid use continue to be documented. In 2003, Rathmell et al.[41] reported a dose-ranging study for IT morphine in patients after total hip and total knee arthroplasty. They found that an IT dose of 0.2 mg morphine combined with patient-controlled analgesia morphine is effective for most patients with these surgical procedures, although post-total knee replacement pain was more difficult to treat. Common opioid side effects (including pruritus, nausea, and vomiting, and oxygen desaturation events) did occur.

In the epidural application of opioids, a new product that slowly released morphine (for up to 48 hours) from a novel liposomal element represented a clinical advance. This mode of drug delivery is to be used for long-acting and controlled-release drug administration. Although not commenting on this specific liposomal vehicle, Rosenberg[47] has some cautionary comments about the neuronal tissue toxicity of some of the lipids previously used in creative liposomal formulations. Rose et al.[48] have also expressed concern regarding the relative lack of neurotoxicity and systemic toxicity data on extended-duration analgesic preparations intended for perineural or neuraxial administration.

Benzyl Alcohol and Polyethylene Glycol

In pain medicine practice, it has been routine that epidural steroid injections are provided as therapy for patients with radicular back pain. Traditionally, preparations of corticosteroids have been chemically engineered to behave as depotsteroids to provide benefit over an extended period of time. The preservatives benzyl alcohol and polyethylene glycol (PEG) have been part of the drugs commonly used (triamcinolone and methylprednisolone). Animal investigations and millions of therapeutic injections in humans have failed to suggest that PEG is toxic at concentrations <3%.[49] The most feared concern was that arachnoiditis would result if such epidural injectates were unexpectedly deposited in the CSF. Although there is little evidence as to the harm of benzyl alcohol, Hodgson et al.[7] offer the caution that *all* alcohols are neurotoxic at certain concentrations. This concern is also repeated by Hetherington and Dooley.[16]

Benzon et al.[50] assessed the particle size of different steroids used in clinical practice in 2007, as a surrogate to explaining the systemic/neurotoxicity of the preparations. Using a confocal microscope, the particulate content of methylprednisolone acetate, triamcinolone acetonide, dexamethasone sodium phosphate, betamethasone sodium phosphate/betamethasone acetate, betamethasone repository (compounded), and betamethasone sodium phosphate was tabulated. The dexamethasone and betamethasone were absent of particles as they are pure liquids. "The proportion of larger particles was significantly greater in the methylprednisolone

and compounded betamethasone preparations compared to the commercial betamethasone." No direct correlation with neurotoxicity was drawn by the authors. There is a proposed relationship between particle size and vascular injury to the spinal cord in the clinical application of these preparations in transforaminal injection techniques (Chapter 28).

In a recent report in the regional anesthesia realm, Parrington et al.[51] reported their findings that the addition of dexamethasone to mepivacaine prolonged the duration of analgesia after supraclavicular blocks. The complication rate did not differ in their study of only 45 adult patients, but it is hard to draw specific conclusions about the neurotoxicity of this combination from such a small study. Williams et al.[26,52] advise caution in considering such use of a steroid preparation in diabetic patients, given the lack of specific studies addressing the safety of the practice and knowing that hyperglycemia can result when steroids are given to diabetics.

Clonidine and Dexmedetomidine

Clonidine is an α-2-adrenergic receptor agonist that binds to such receptors in the substantia gelatinosa and the intermediolateral cell column. The neurophysiologic consequence is to inhibit the release of substance P and the firing of wide dynamic range neurons in the spinal cord dorsal horn.[53] Eisenach et al.[54] demonstrated no toxicity with IT doses of clonidine up to 300 μg, and clinical analgesic effects demonstrated as a decrease in the secondary hyperalgesia of wounds by interaction with DL-alpha-amino-3-hydroxyl-5-methyl-4-isoxazole proprionic acid (AMPA) (excitatory) and gamma-aminobutyric-acid (GABA) (inhibitory) receptors. Yaksh[1] also confirmed a lack of neurotoxic effects (manifested as no change in CSF or histopathology findings) in rats that had been implanted with IT catheters and received 28 days of continuous infusion of clonidine. Hodgson et al.[7] found no evidence of harm from clonidine as reported in their 1999 summary article. A recent review of the clinical analgesic effects of clonidine being added to spinal local anesthetics for surgery was provided by Elia et al.[55] They examined 22 randomized trials including 1,445 patients receiving clonidine mixed with bupivacaine, mepivacaine, prilocaine, or tetracaine. They reported a longer duration of block, less intraoperative pain, and more episodes of hypotension when clonidine was used with the spinal anesthetic. They noted that the optimal dose of added clonidine is still not known and do not comment on there being any evidence of tissue toxicity. Fairbanks et al.[56] amplified the options for choosing an α-2 agonist additive in reporting on the solo or combination use of clonidine and dexmedetomidine in a rat model. The use of both agents produced evidence of synergistic, and not competitive, analgesia, suggesting that the two drugs result in analgesia by two distinct mechanisms of action. There was no report of obvious neurotoxicity.

Peripherally, clonidine appears to act more as a local anesthetic than as a vasoconstrictor. The addition of clonidine has more effect on the duration than the onset of local anesthetic blockade. Systemic side effects such as hypotension, sedation, and dry mouth can occur as with IT dosing.[10] A recent meta-analysis of 20 randomized trials (1,054 patients) of clonidine added to lidocaine for peripheral, single-injection nerve or plexus blocks by Popping et al.[57] highlights the current clinical status of this drug application. With reported doses between 30 and 300 μg, it is evident that clonidine prolongs the duration of sensory and motor block, but also increases the likelihood of hypotension and orthostatic hypotension, fainting, and sedation. The authors noted a lack of evidence of dose responsiveness for beneficial or harmful effects.

It was to be expected that studies about the combination of dexmedetomidine with local anesthetics for peripheral nerve blocks would soon appear. Brummett et al.[58] studied the use of "high-dose" (meaning not clinically relevant in humans) dexmedetomidine added to bupivacaine in a rat sciatic nerve block model. Dexmedetomidine significantly increased the duration of the sensory and motor block, but only when combined with bupivacaine, and did so with no evidence of axonal or myelin injury. These results were duplicated with ropivacaine as the local anesthetic agent in a subsequent study.[59]

Nonsteroidal Anti-inflammatory Agents

Trauma to the body results in the release of inflammatory mediators that activate nociceptors. Prostaglandins from the breakdown of arachidonic acid are part of this cascade.[53] Blockade of prostaglandins should have a potent analgesic effect, and the use of nonsteroidal anti-inflammatory agents is universal and prevalent. Furthermore, Zhu et al.[60] demonstrated that cyclooxygenase-1 in the spinal cord has an important capability to modulate nociceptive input, such as that associated with postoperative pain. Korkmaz et al.[61] utilized the chronic intrathecally implanted rat to study the neurotoxic effects of ketorolac given over 20 days and failed to report any significant evidence of toxicity. Eisenach et al.[62] provided the logical next step in reporting the same (negative) findings in a phase I assessment of IT ketorolac in humans. This same lead investigator broadened the technique in a recent, three-part study of IT ketorolac in humans.[63] The symptoms of five patients already receiving IT morphine were not helped or harmed by the addition of 0.5 to 2 mg of IT ketorolac. Twelve similar patients did not manifest a change in their pain intensity with IT saline compared to 2 mg IT ketorolac. Lastly, 30 patients undergoing vaginal hysterectomy were not distinguished by the receipt of IT saline or 2 mg IT ketorolac when measuring the time to their first request for morphine postoperatively.

Neostigmine

This acetylcholine esterase inhibitor prevents the breakdown of acetylcholine in the spinal cord, which has effects at the muscarinic receptors in the substantia gelatinosa, and results in analgesia.[53] Studies cited in Thannikary and Enneking's[53] review from 2004 failed to demonstrate neurotoxicity with IT administration over 14 days. This theme is repeated in Hodgson et al.'s[7] review from 5 years earlier. Kaya et al.[64] have demonstrated that IT neostigmine has analgesic characteristics, but that nausea is a limiting factor clinically (as can be sedation), even with epidural administration. Joseph and McDonald[25] reported that neostigmine added to peripheral nerve block mixtures offered no beneficial effects to block onset, but only a possible benefit as to block duration, yet consistent, ongoing concerns about common adverse and systemic side effects.

Ketamine

Ketamine is a phencyclidine-related analgesic that binds to gated calcium channels of the NMDA receptor, producing a noncompetitive blockade. It also binds at opioid and monoaminergic receptors and voltage-sensitive calcium channels, and thus its effects and side effects are widespread and variable.[53] Preservative-free solutions of ketamine have proven to be safe for IT injection in a variety of animal models,[7,53] but Errando et al.[65] have shown pathologic findings after repeated dosing with IT injections of commercially available ketamine that contains benzethonium chloride. This concern is only enhanced by the recent study of Braun et al.[66] They specifically investigated the adverse effects of benzethonium, the most widely used preservative in ketamine, in hematopoietic, neuronal, and glial cells. There was definite evidence of additive toxicity for ketamine, benzemethonium, and the combination of the two substances. Severe toxic damage to the spinal cord of rabbits from clinically relevant concentrations and doses of preservative-free S(+) ketamine has also been documented in a study by Vranken et al.[67] A strong word of caution to clinicians about the real, adverse, and potential hazards of "ordinary anesthetic and sedative-hypnotic" drugs, especially on the developing nervous system, is aptly voiced by Drasner[68] in an editorial that precedes an animal study by Walker et al.[69] addressing the detrimental consequences of IT ketamine in neonatal rats. The conjoint concerns relate to apoptosis and neural degenerative changes induced by the drug.

Midazolam

In the modern era, few drugs other than local anesthetics have provoked as much commentary about toxicity as has midazolam.[12,70,71] This is a water-soluble benzodiazepine, and thus it could have therapeutic potential with perineural application. In Hodgson et al.'s[7] review of the neurotoxicity of IT drugs, they concluded that animal data were conflicting (as of their 1999 article), and although there were a few, small studies in humans, the data were genuinely insufficient to draw conclusions about the neural safety of the drug. The issue of neurotoxicity remained largely unsolved until Johansen et al.[72] published a sufficiently sized animal toxicity study that showed a lack of classic neurotoxic effects with the drug given intrathecally. Thus, some of the angst about the conflicting studies in animals was alleviated. This study also set the scene for further discussions about the evidence of toxicity with IT midazolam in humans. Tucker et al.[73] followed up 1,100 patients who had had IT midazolam. They reported no evident neurotoxicity. Yaksh and Allen[71] reviewed this issue and reported in an erudite fashion the entire process by which questions about the neurotoxicity of midazolam were raised and how they should be addressed to arrive at a firm and scientific solution. The theme of more careful, scientific investigation being needed was expressed by Lavand'homme[12] in an editorial that preceded the clinical report of Boussofara et al.[74] about the addition of IT midazolam to a bupivacaine-clonidine mixture in 110 patients having elective lower extremity surgery. Only an increase in the duration of the motor block was a discriminating result. No neurotoxicity or data relevant to lingering clinical consequences were reported.

Amitriptyline

This classic tricyclic antidepressant has raised interest because of the local anesthetic properties attributed to its sodium channel blockade capabilities and that of voltage-gated potassium and calcium channels.[75] Although it was touted as having potential as a long-acting local anesthetic, the dose-related neurotoxic effects manifested with topical application in a rat sciatic nerve model as reported by Estebe and Myers[75] will likely discourage enthusiasm for the IT use of this drug. Sawynok[11] identified "a significant error in the calculation of the total dose [of amitriptyline] administered" in this study in a subsequent letter to the editor. Nonetheless, the opportunity to broadcast caution about the casual use of an obviously neurotoxic drug, albeit dose related, was gained. Fukushima et al.[76] investigated the potential clinical value of low doses of amitriptyline in a dog model of IT administration, but identified worrisome "intense meningeal adhesive arachnoiditis," making it unlikely that this drug will be a spinal adjuvant. Yaksh et al.[77] assessed the toxicity profiles of a number of NMDA antagonists given intrathecally, including amitriptyline, in a canine model. It was evident that IT infusions of amitriptyline, ketamine, MK801, and memantine all contributed to pathological lesions of the neural structures.

Magnesium

This ion is a noncompetitive antagonist at NMDA receptors, which are intimately involved in the CNS processing of nociceptive input. Animal studies of reasonable quality have demonstrated the tissue safety of IT applications of magnesium, referenced by Buvanendran et al.[78] in 2002 in a randomized controlled trial of 52 patients who requested labor analgesia. As in animal studies, fentanyl analgesia was prolonged and no apparent signs or symptoms of neurotoxicity were manifested with the addition of magnesium to the IT injectate. There is little subsequent data upon which to alter this impression of the apparently benign effects of IT magnesium sulfate. As a matter of fact, in an induced spinal cord ischemia model, Jellish et al.[79] showed that concurrent administration of magnesium sulfate in a rabbit model significantly diminished spinal cord motor neuron loss and delayed neuronal degeneration, suggesting perhaps a protective benefit of the drug.

Miscellaneous Agents

Hyaluronidase was used to facilitate the spread of local anesthetics in the past. Because this is now used only in ophthalmologic regional anesthesia, it is not reviewed here.[47] Verapamil and other calcium channel blockers inhibit calcium entry into cells, thereby manifesting the ability to block nociceptive processing in the nervous system. There are too few data to comment on the neurotoxicity of these agents, just as there are for the weak opioid agonist tramadol.[53] Chiari and Eisenach,[80] in addressing the issue of the safety of spinally administered drugs (including somatostatin and calcitonin), stated that as of 1998 there were not enough data to qualify the safety of these agents. Eisenach et al.[81] have also specifically addressed the potential application of IT adenosine. This drug produces receptor-specific analgesia,

especially so at the high density of adenosine receptors in the dorsal horn. Phase I studies failed to identify toxicity with this drug.

The growing application of numerous IT agents in the practice of chronic pain medicine was highlighted by Dougherty and Staats[82] in their 1999 review of this topic. One traditional drug, baclofen (used to treat spasticity), seems to be safe for IT administration given years of such use.[7] Murphy et al.[83] have recently reported the occurrence of a catheter-tip granuloma in a patient receiving only IT baclofen. As might be expected, a clinical investigation was initiated because this previously well-controlled patient developed a significant increase in her spasticity symptoms despite marked increases in her baclofen dosing via an IT pump. Another recent addition to the armamentarium of pain management physicians is ziconotide.[84] This is a conopeptide that is used intrathecally in selected patients with chronic pain. Although its effectiveness was reviewed extensively by a study group, no specific issues about associated neurotoxicity were raised. In a view to the future, Kissin[85] elaborated on the use of vanilloid agonists as adjuvants for peripheral nerve blocks in a rat sciatic nerve block model. It is exciting that initial results failed to demonstrate high levels of toxicity, so such agents may find a clinical application in regional anesthesia and analgesia.

▶ PATHOPHYSIOLOGY

The exact mechanism of injury of adjuvant chemicals, substances, and preservative drugs is not always obvious. If we learn from the local anesthetic experience, even revered drugs of everyday use can provoke toxicity for poorly defined reasons when our ability to survey for such events becomes sophisticated enough. Obviously, a drug can have direct toxic effects on tissue, as might an acid spill on the skin. This is not the general finding with the agents discussed in this chapter. Toxicity is more likely a result of a combination of factors involving some characteristics of the primary drug, which interplay with the physical conditions present such as low pH and osmolarity, and the host's particular preexisting pathologic conditions.

▶ RISK FACTORS

The caution voiced by Yaksh[1] about the multiplicity of untested drugs and drug combinations, all of various concentrations, that are being utilized to obtain analgesia is worth repeating. That medical science got off the usual course of orderly experimental progress and scientific rigor in the evolution of analgesic agents, adjuncts, and preservatives is evident, as highlighted in the intellectual editorials by Drasner,[18] Yaksh and Allen,[71] Chiari and Eisenach,[80] and Lavand'homme.[12] Thus, the necessary preliminary step of tissue testing for safety with a potential analgesic or adjuvant drug must include tests in a variety of animal species before human studies are initiated. We must more fully understand the toxicity of drugs so that the mistakes of the past are not repeated. It is evident that the editorial boards of our journals will hold investigators to this crucial element of scientific method.[13,14]

DIAGNOSIS, TREATMENT, AND PREVENTION

The diagnosis, treatment, and prevention of neuraxial and peripheral nerve injury are discussed in detail in Chapters 10, 11, 12, and 14.

SUMMARY

The pharmacology and physiology of the neurologic response continues to be investigated, and our knowledge expands day by day. When we understand the chemistry and processes involved, drugs tailored to affect specific components of that response system can be created to the benefit of patients. The process by which the neurotoxicity and systemic toxicity of drugs is determined must not be compromised in the rush to clinical application, lest patients be unexpectedly placed in harm's way. There is little direct evidence that most of the classic adjuvants and preservatives have neurotoxic effects. Newer agents must be rigorously tested so that an appropriate balance between risk and benefit is achieved. We are witnessing the creation of reliable models for the scientific study of these matters. There are even signs that protective strategies will be forthcoming. Overall, the sophistication of our approach to neurotoxicity is progressing.

References

1. Yaksh T. Preclinical models for analgesic drug study. In: Godberg AM, Zutphen LFM, eds. *Alternate Methods in Toxicology and the Life Sciences.* New York, NY: Mary Ann Liebert., Inc, 1995: 629–636.
2. Sweeney C, Bruera E. Opioids. In: Melzack R, Wall PD, eds. *Handbook of Pain Medicine.* Philadelphia, PA: Churchill Livingstone, 2003:377–396.
3. Drasner K. Local anesthetic systemic toxicity. A historical perspective. *Reg Anesth Pain Med* 2010;35:162–166.
4. Di Gregorio G, Neal JM, Rosenquist RW, et al. Clinical presentation of local anesthetic systemic toxicity. A review of published cases, 1979 to 2009. *Reg Anesth Pain Med* 2010;35:181–187.
5. Weinberg GL. Treatment of local anesthetic systemic toxicity (LAST). *Reg Anesth Pain Med* 2010;35:188–193.
6. Morau D, Ahern S. Management of local anesthetic toxicity. *Int Anesthesiol Clin* 2010;48:117–140.
7. Hodgson PS, Neal JM, Pollock JE, et al. The neurotoxicity of drugs given intrathecally (spinal). *Anesth Analg* 1999;88:797–809.
8. Rowlingson JC. To avoid "transient neurologic symptoms": the search continues (editorial). *Reg Anesth Pain Med* 2000;25:215–217.
9. Reichert M, Butterworth J. Local anesthetic additives to increase stability and prevent organism growth. *Tech Reg Anesth Pain Mang* 2004;8:106–109.
10. Rowlingson JC. Toxicity of local anesthetic additives. *Reg Anesth* 1993;18:453–460.
11. Sawynok J. Amitriptyline neurotoxicity. *Anesthesiology* 2005;102: 240–241.
12. Lavand'homme P. Lessons from spinal midazolam: when misuse of messages from preclinical models exposes patients to unnecessary risks. *Reg Anesth Pain Med* 2006;31:489–491.
13. Neal JM, Rathmell JP, Rowlingson JC. Publishing studies that involve "off-label" use of drugs. Formalizing *Regional Anesthesia and Pain Medicine's* policy. *Reg Anesth Pain Med* 2009;34:391–392.
14. Anesthesiology information for authors. *Anesthesia and Analgesia* guide for authors. *Anesth Analg* 2009;109:217–231.
15. Westin BD, Walker SM, Deumens R, et al. Validation of a preclinical spinal safety model. Effects of intrathecal morphine in the neonatal rat. *Anesthesiology* 2010;113:183–199.
16. Hetherington NJ, Dooley MJ. Potential for patient harm from intrathecal administration of preserved solutions. *Med J Aust* 2000;173:141–143.
17. Farber MK, Angelo TE, Castells M, et al. Anesthetic management of a patient with an allergy to propylene glycol and parabens. *Anesth Analg* 2010;110:839–842.
18. Drasner K. Chloroprocaine spinal anesthesia: back to the future? (editorial). *Anesth Analg* 2005;100:549–552.
19. Taniguchi M, Bollen AW, Drasner K. Sodium bisulfite: scapegoat for chloroprocaine neurotoxicity? *Anesthesiology* 2004;100:85–91.
20. Stevens RA, Urmey WF, Urquhart BL, et al. Back pain after epidural anesthesia with chloroprocaine. *Anesthesiology* 1993;78:492–497.
21. Hung YC, Suzuki S, Chen CC, et al. Calcium chloride prolongs the effects of lidocaine and bupivacaine in rat sciatic nerve. *Reg Anesth Pain Med* 2009;34:333–339.
22. Haider N. Additives used to limit systemic absorption. *Tech Reg Anesth Pain Mang* 2004;8:119–122.
23. Sakura S, Sumi M, Sakaguchi Y, et al. The addition of phenylephrine contributes to the development of transient neurologic symptoms after spinal anesthesia with 0.5% tetracaine. *Anesthesiology* 1997;87:771–778.
24. Kalichman MW, Calcutt NA. Local anesthetic-induced conduction block and nerve fiber injury in streptozotocin-diabetic rats. *Anesthesiology* 1992;77:941–947.
25. Joseph RS, McDonald SB. Facilitating the onset of regional anesthetic blocks. *Tech Reg Anesth Pain Mang* 2004;8:110–113.
26. Williams BA, Murinson BB, Grable BR, et al. Future considerations for pharmacologic adjuvants in single-injection peripheral nerve blocks for patients with diabetes mellitus. *Reg Anesth Pain Med* 2009;34:445–457.
27. Oka S, Matsumoto M, Ohtake K, et al. The addition of epinephrine to tetracaine injected intrathecally sustains an increase in glutamate concentrations in the cerebrospinal fluid and worsens neuronal injury. *Anesth Analg* 2001;93:1050–1057.
28. Hashimoto K, Hampl KF, Nakamura Y, et al. Epinephrine increases the neurotoxic potential of intrathecally administered lidocaine in the rat. *Anesthesiology* 2001;94:876–881.
29. Selander D, Edshage S, Wolff T. Paresthesiae or no paresthesiae? Nerve lesions after axillary blocks. *Acta Anaesthesiol Scand* 1979;23:27–33.
30. Kroin JS, Buvanendran A, Williams DK, et al. Local anesthetic sciatic nerve block and nerve fiber damage in diabetic rats. *Reg Anesth Pain Med* 2010;35:343–350.
31. Dripps RD, Vandam LD. Long term follow-up of patients who received 10,098 spinal anesthetics: failure to discover major neurological sequelae. *JAMA* 1954;156:1486–1491.
32. Horlocker TT, McGregor DG, Matsushige DK, et al. Neurologic complications of 603 consecutive continuous spinal anesthetics using macrocatheter and microcatheter techniques. *Anesth Analg* 1997;84:1063–1070.
33. Horlocker TT, McGregor DG, Matsushige DK, et al. A retrospective review of 4767 consecutive spinal anesthetics: central nervous system complications. *Anesth Analg* 1997;84:578–584.
34. Moore DC, Bridenbaugh LD. Spinal (subarachnoid) block: a review of 11,574 cases. *JAMA* 1966;195:907–912.
35. Vandam LD, Dripps RD. Long-term follow-up of patients who received 10,098 spinal anesthetics. IV. Neurological disease incident to traumatic lumbar puncture during spinal anesthesia. *JAMA* 1960;172:1483–1487.
36. Hebl JR, Kopp SL, Schroeder DR, et al. Neurologic complications after neuraxial anesthesia or analgesia in patients with preexisting peripheral sensorimotor neuropathy or diabetic polyneuropathy. *Anesth Analg* 2006;103:1294–1299.
37. Denkler K. A comprehensive review of epinephrine in the finger: to do or not to do. *Plast Reconstr Surg* 2001;108:114–124.

38. Neal JM. Effects of epinephrine in local anesthetics on the central and peripheral nervous systems: neurotoxicity and neural blood flow. *Reg Anesth Pain Med* 2003;28:124–134.

39. DuPen SL, Ramsey D, Chin S. Chronic epidural morphine and preservative-induced injury. *Anesthesiology* 1987;67:987–988.

40. Sjoberg M, Karlsson PA, Nordborg C, et al. Neuropathologic findings after long-term intrathecal infusion of morphine and bupivacaine for pain treatment in cancer patients. *Anesthesiology* 1992;76:173–186.

41. Rathmell JP, Pino CA, Taylor R, et al. Intrathecal morphine for postoperative analgesia: a randomized, controlled, dose-ranging study after hip and knee arthroplasty. *Anesth Analg* 2003;97:1452–1457.

42. Kakinohana M, Kakinohana O, Jun JH, et al. The activation of spinal N-methyl-D-aspartate receptors may contribute to degeneration of spinal motor neurons induced by neuraxial morphine after a noninjurious interval of spinal cord ischemia. *Anesth Analg* 2005;100:327–334.

43. Rathmell JP, Lair TR, Nauman B. The role of intrathecal drugs in the treatment of acute pain. *Anesth Analg* 2005;101(5 suppl): S30–S43.

44. Allen JW, Horais KA, Tozier NA, et al. Opiate pharmacology of intrathecal granulomas. *Anesthesiology* 2006;105:590–598.

45. Candido KD, Hennes J, Gonzales S, et al. Buprenorphine enhances and prolongs the postoperative analgesic effect of bupivacaine in patients receiving infragluteal sciatic nerve block. *Anesthesiology* 2010;113:1419–1426.

46. Weller R, Butterworth J. Opioids as local anesthetic adjuvants for peripheral nerve block. *Tech Reg Anesth Pain Mang* 2004;8: 123–128.

47. Rosenberg PH. Additives to increase tissue spread of local anesthetics. *Tech Reg Anesth Pain Mang* 2004;8:114–118.

48. Rose JS, Neal JM, Kopacz DJ. Extended-duration analgesia: update on microspheres and liposomes. *Reg Anesth Pain Med* 2005;30:275–285.

49. McQuillan PM, Kafiludali R, Hahn M. Interventional techniques. In: Raj PP, ed. *Pain Medicine: A Comprehensive Review*. 2nd ed. St. Louis, MO: Mosby, 2003:286–287.

50. Benzon HT, Chew TL, McCarthy RJ, et al. Comparison of the particle sizes of different steroids and the effect of dilution. A review of the relative neurotoxicities of the steroids. *Anesthesiology* 2007;106:331–338.

51. Parrington SJ, O'Donnell D, Chan VWS, et al. Dexamethasone added to mepivacaine prolongs the duration of analgesia after supraclavicular brachial plexus block. *Reg Anesth Pain Med* 2010;35:422–426.

52. Williams BA. Toward a potential paradigm shift for the clinical care of diabetic patients requiring perineural analgesia; strategies for using the diabetic rodent model. *Reg Anesth Pain Med* 2010;35:229–232.

53. Thannikary LJ, Enneking FK. Non-opioid additives to local anesthetics. *Tech Reg Anesth Pain Mang* 2004;8:129–140.

54. Eisenach JC, De Kock M, Klimscha W. Alpha 2-adrenergic agonists for regional anesthesia: a clinical review of clonidine (1984–1995). *Anesthesiology* 1996;85:655–674.

55. Elia N, Culebras X, Mazza C, et al. Clonidine as an adjuvant to intrathecal local anesthetics for surgery: systemic review of randomized trials. *Reg Anesth Pain Med* 2008;33:159–167.

56. Fairbanks CA, Kitto KF, Nguyen O, et al. Clonidine and dexmedetomidine produce antinociceptive synergy in mouse spinal cord. *Anesthesiology* 2009;110:638–647.

57. Popping DM, Elia N, Marret E, et al. Clonidine as an adjuvant to local anesthetics for peripheral nerve and plexus blocks. *Anesthesiology* 2009;111:406–415.

58. Brummett CM, Norat MA, Palmisano JM, et al. Perineural administration of dexmedetomidine in combination with bupivacaine enhances sensory and motor blockade in sciatic nerve block without inducing neurotoxicity in rat. *Anesthesiology* 2008;109:502–511.

59. Brummett CM, Padda AK, Amodeo FS, et al. Perineural dexmedetomidine added to ropivacaine causes a dose-dependent increase in the duration of thermal antinociception in sciatic nerve block in rat. *Anesthesiology* 2009;111:1111–1119.

60. Zhu X, Conklin D, Eisenach JC. Cyclooxygenase-1 in the spinal cord plays an important role in postoperative pain. *Pain* 2003;104:15–23.

61. Korkmaz HA, Maltepe F, Erbayraktar S, et al. Antinociceptive and neurotoxicologic screening of chronic intrathecal administration of ketorolac tromethamine in the rat. *Anesth Analg* 2004;98: 148–152.

62. Eisenach JC, Curry R, Hood DD, et al. Phase I safety assessment of intrathecal ketorolac. *Pain* 2002;99:599–604.

63. Eisenach JC, Curry R, Rauck R, et al. Role of spinal cyclooxygenase in human postoperative and chronic pain. *Anesthesiology* 2010;112:1225–1233.

64. Kaya FN, Sahin S, Owen MD, et al. Epidural neostigmine produces analgesia but also sedation in women after cesarean delivery. *Anesthesiology* 2004;100:381–385.

65. Errando CL, Sifre C, Moliner S, et al. Subarachnoid ketamine in swine, pathological findings after repeated doses: acute toxicity study. *Reg Anesth Pain Med* 1999;24:146–152.

66. Braun S, Werdehausen R, Gaza N, et al. Benzethonium increases the cytotoxicity of S(+)-ketamine in lymphoma, neuronal and glial cells. *Anesth Analg* 2010;111:1389–1393.

67. Vranken JH, Troost D, de Haan P, et al. Severe toxic damage to the rabbit spinal cord after intrathecal administration of preservative-free S(+)-ketamine. *Anesthesiology* 2006;105:813–818.

68. Drasner K. Anesthetic effects on the developing nervous system. If you aren't concerned, you haven't been paying attention. *Anesthesiology* 2010;113:10–12.

69. Walker SM, Westin D, Deumens R, et al. Effects of intrathecal ketamine in the neonatal rat. Evaluation of apoptosis and long-term functional outcome. *Anesthesiology* 2010;113:147–159.

70. Cousins MJ, Miller RD. Intrathecal midazolam: an ethical editorial dilemma (editorial). *Anesth Analg* 2004;98:1507–1508.

71. Yaksh TL, Allen JW. Preclinical insights into the implementation of intrathecal midazolam: a cautionary tale (editorial). *Anesth Analg* 2004;98:1509–1511.

72. Johansen MJ, Gradert TL, Satterfield WC, et al. Safety of continuous intrathecal midazolam infusion in the sheep model. *Anesth Analg* 2004;98:1528–1535.

73. Tucker AP, Lai C, Nadeson R, et al. Intrathecal midazolam I: a cohort study investigating safety. *Anesth Analg* 2004;98:1512–1520.

74. Boussofara M, Carles M, Raucoules-Aime M, et al. Effects of intrathecal midazolam on postoperative analgesia when added to a bupivacaine-clonidine mixture. *Reg Anesth Pain Med* 2006;31: 501–505.

75. Estebe JP, Myers RR. Amitriptyline neurotoxicity: dose-related pathology after topical application to rat sciatic nerve. *Anesthesiology* 2004;100:1519–1525.

76. Fukushima FB, Barros GAM, Marques MEA, et al. The neuraxial effects of intraspinal amitriptyline at low concentrations. *Anesth Analg* 2009;109:965–971.

77. Yaksh TL, Tozier N, Horais KA, et al. Toxicology profile of N-methyl-D-aspartate antagonists delivered by intrathecal infusion in the canine model. *Anesthesiology* 2008;108:938–949.

78. Buvanendran A, McCarthy RJ, Kroin JS, et al. Intrathecal magnesium prolongs fentanyl analgesia: a prospective, randomized, controlled trial. *Anesth Analg* 2002;95:661–666.

79. Jellish WS, Zhang X, Langen KE, et al. Intrathecal magnesium sulfate administration at the time of experimental ischemia improves neurological functioning by reducing acute and delayed loss of motor neurons in the spinal cord. *Anesthesiology* 2008;108:78–86.

80. Chiari A, Eisenach JC. Spinal anesthesia: mechanisms, agents, methods, and safety. *Reg Anesth Pain Med* 1998;23:357–362, 384–387.

81. Eisenach JC, Hood DD, Curry R. Phase I safety assessment of intrathecal injection of an American formulation of adenosine in humans. *Anesthesiology* 2002;96:24–28.

82. Dougherty PM, Staats PS. Intrathecal drug therapy for chronic pain: from basic science to clinical practice. *Anesthesiology* 1999;91:1891–1918.

83. Murphy PM, Skouvaklis DE, Amadeo RJJ, et al. Intrathecal catheter granuloma associated with isolated baclofen infusion. *Anesth Analg* 2006;102:848–852.

84. Wallace MS, Rauck R, Fisher R, et al. Intrathecal ziconotide for severe chronic pain: safety and tolerability results of an open-label, long-term trial. *Anesth Analg* 2008;106:628–637.

85. Kissin I. Vanilloid-induced conduction analgesia: selective, dose-dependent, long-lasting, with a low level of potential neurotoxicity. *Anesth Analg* 2008;107:271–281.

COMPLICATIONS SPECIFIC TO NEURAXIS BLOCK

9

Meningeal Puncture Headache

Brian E. Harrington

Postural headache following interventions that disrupt meningeal integrity is most commonly and, in the International Classification of Headache Disorders, officially labeled "postdural puncture headache" (PDPH).[1] However, this terminology has been criticized as confusing[2] and probably inaccurate,[3] as explained further below. The anatomically supported and less ambiguous "meningeal puncture headache" (MPH) has been proposed as an alternate term[4,5] and will be used throughout this chapter. It is also important to acknowledge that references to "dural puncture" throughout the medical literature (including this chapter) actually describe puncture of the dura and arachnoid mater, and are more correctly termed "meningeal puncture."

Regardless of terminology, practitioners of anesthesia are universally aware of MPH. Yet, our understanding of this serious complication remains surprisingly incomplete. This chapter summarizes the current state of knowledge regarding this familiar iatrogenic problem as well as the closely related topics of unintentional dural puncture (UDP) and the epidural blood patch (EBP).

► HISTORY AND CURRENT RELEVANCE

As one of the earliest recognized complications of regional anesthesia, MPH has a long and colorful history.[6] Dr. August Bier noted this adverse effect in the first patient to undergo successful spinal anesthesia on August 16, 1898. Bier[7] observed: "Two hours after the operation his back and left leg became painful and the patient vomited and complained of severe headache. The pain and vomiting soon ceased, but *headache was still present the next day*" (italics added). The following week, Bier and his assistant, Dr. August Hildebrandt, performed experiments with cocainization of the spinal cord on themselves. In a description of MPH scarcely improved upon in an intervening century, Bier[7] later reported firsthand his experience in the days to follow: "I had a feeling of very strong pressure on my skull and became rather dizzy when I stood up rapidly from my chair. All these symptoms vanished at once when I lay down flat, but returned when I stood up … I was forced to take to bed and remained there for nine days, because all the manifestations recurred as soon as I got up …. The symptoms finally resolved nine days after the lumbar puncture." In medical history, few complications have come to be considered as closely linked to a specific technique as MPH with spinal anesthesia.

Employing the methods of the early 20th century, spinal anesthesia was frequently followed by severe and prolonged headache, casting a long shadow over the development and acceptance of this modality. Investigations into the cause of these troubling symptoms eventually led to the conclusion that they were due to persistent cerebrospinal fluid (CSF) loss through the rent created in the meninges. The most notable successful efforts to minimize the loss of CSF were through the use of smaller gauge and "noncutting" needles (as convincingly demonstrated in the 1950s by Vandam and Dripps[8] and Hart and Whitacre,[9] respectively). Despite these significant advances in prevention, MPH remained a frustratingly common occurrence.

The extensive search for effective treatments for MPH dates to Bier's time. Yet efforts through the first half of the 20th century, while often intensive and creative, were questionably worthwhile. In a monograph intended to be a comprehensive review of MPH from the 1890s through 1960, Dr. Wallace Tourette et al.[10] cite dozens of separate and far-ranging treatment recommendations, including such interventions as intravenous ethanol, x-rays to the skull, sympathetic blocks, and manipulation of the spine. Unfortunately, prior to the introduction of the EBP, there were no treatment measures that could be described as significant improvements over the simple passage of time. In his 1955 textbook, *Complications of Regional Anesthesia*, Dr. Daniel C. Moore[11] describes in detail a full 3-day treatment protocol for MPH. He concludes by noting that 3 days is the usual duration of untreated mild-to-moderate headaches, but that "nevertheless, the patient feels an attempt to help his problem is being made."

The EBP, a startlingly unique medical procedure, proved to be the major breakthrough in the treatment of MPH. The concept of using autologous blood to "patch" a hole in the meninges was introduced in late 1960 by Dr. James Gormley,[12] a general surgeon. Yet, Gormley's brief report went largely unnoticed for nearly a decade because, to the practitioners of the day, an iatrogenic epidural hematoma raised serious concerns of scarring, infection, and nerve damage. The procedure was only later popularized in anesthesiology circles, and performed as a true epidural injection, largely through the work of Drs. Anthony DiGiovanni and Burdett Dunbar.[13] The EBP procedure was further refined through the 1970s as the volume of blood commonly utilized increased to 20 mL.[14] Today, the EBP is nearly universally employed as the cornerstone of treatment for severe MPH.[15]

MPH remains a prominent clinical concern to the present day. Largely due to modifications in practice that followed the identification of risk factors, rates of MPH following spinal anesthesia have steadily declined—from an incidence exceeding 50% in Bier's time to around 10% in the 1950s,[8] until currently a rate of 1% or less can be reasonably expected. However, as perhaps the highest risk group, an unfortunate 1.7% of obstetric patients continue to experience MPH after spinal anesthesia using 27-gauge Whitacre needles.[16] Intending to avoid meningeal puncture, epidural techniques are an attractive alternative to spinal anesthesia. Yet occasional UDP, either with the needle or the catheter, is unavoidable (and may be unrecognized at the time in over 25% of patients who eventually develop MPH[17]). In nonobstetric situations (e.g., interlaminar epidural steroid injections), the rate of UDP should be <0.5%. However, UDP is of greatest concern in the obstetric anesthesia setting, where the incidence of this adverse event is around 1.5%.[16] Over half of all patients who experience UDP with epidural needles will eventually develop headache symptoms, with many studies in obstetric populations reporting MPH rates of 75% or greater. In addition to anesthesia interventions, MPH remains a too-common iatrogenic complication following myelography and diagnostic/therapeutic lumbar puncture (LP). In these situations, rates of MPH around 10% are still commonly cited as practitioners often continue to use Quincke needles, and large-gauge needles are considered necessary due to the viscosity of contrast material and to facilitate the timely collection of CSF. Consequently, there is evidence to suggest that the majority of instances of MPH now have a non–anesthesia-related origin.[18]

The practical significance of MPH is illustrated in being noted in the American Society of Anesthesiologists Closed Claims Project database as one of the most frequent claims for malpractice involving obstetric anesthesia,[19] regional anesthesia,[20] and chronic pain management.[21] Justifiably, headache is the most commonly disclosed risk when obtaining consent for spinal and epidural anesthesia.[22] The potentially serious nature of this complication necessitates inclusion in informed consent involving any procedure that may result in MPH. As part of this discussion, patients should also be apprised of the normal delayed onset of symptoms and given clear instructions for the timely provision of advice or management should they experience adverse effects.

▶ PATHOPHYSIOLOGY

It has long been accepted that MPH results from a disruption of normal CSF homeostasis. However, despite a great deal of research and observational data, the pathophysiology of MPH remains incompletely understood.[23]

CSF is produced primarily in the choroid plexus at a rate of approximately 0.35 mL/min and reabsorbed through the arachnoid villa. The total CSF volume in adults is maintained around 150 mL, of which approximately half is extracranial, and gives rise to normal lumbar opening pressures of 5 to 15 cm H_2O in the horizontal position (40–50 cm H_2O in the upright position). It has been shown experimentally that the loss of approximately 10% of total CSF volume predictably results in the development of typical MPH symptoms, which resolve promptly with the reconstitution of this deficit.[24] It is agreed that MPH is due to the loss of CSF through a persistent leak in the meninges. In this regard, it has been postulated that the cellular arachnoid mater (containing frequent tight junctions and occluding junctions) is perhaps more important than the more permeable and acellular dura mater in the genesis of symptoms.[3] Thus, preference for the term "meningeal puncture headache" over "postdural puncture headache". The apparent role of the arachnoid mater in this disorder further calls into question the significance of many published studies that involve isolated dura mater *in vitro*.

The actual means by which CSF hypotension generates headache is controversial and currently ascribed to a bimodal mechanism involving both loss of intracranial support and cerebral vasodilation (predominantly venous). Diminished buoyant support is thought to allow the brain to sag in the upright position, resulting in traction and pressure on pain-sensitive structures within the cranium (dura, cranial nerves, bridging veins, and venous sinuses) (Fig. 9-1). Passive and adenosine-mediated vasodilation may occur secondary to diminished intracranial CSF (in accordance with the Monro-Kellie hypothesis, which states that intracranial volume must remain constant) and reflexively secondary to traction on intracranial vessels.

Multiple neural pathways are involved in generating the symptoms of MPH. These include the ophthalmic branch of the trigeminal nerve (CN V_1) in frontal head pain, cranial nerves IX and X in occipital pain, and cervical nerves C1-3 in neck and shoulder pain.[25] Nausea is attributed to vagal stimulation (CN X). Auditory and vestibular symptoms are secondary to the direct communication between the CSF and the perilymph via the cochlear aqueduct, which results in decreased perilymphatic pressures in the inner ear and an imbalance between the endolymph and perilymph.[26] Significant visual disturbances may represent a transient palsy of the nerves supplying the extraocular muscles of the eye (CN III, IV, and VI). Here, the lateral rectus muscle is most

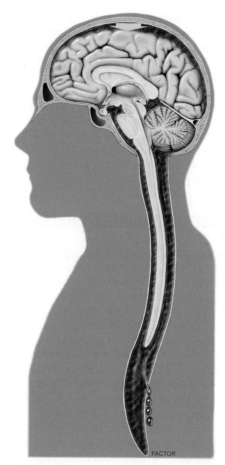

FIGURE 9-1. Schematic drawing illustrating diminished buoyant support of intracranial structures in the upright position (*arrow*) secondary to persistent extracranial CSF loss. (Image by David Factor [Mayo Clinic, Rochester, MN], with his permission.)

often involved, which is attributed to the long, vulnerable intracranial course of the abducens nerve (CN VI).[27] Other, much less frequent cranial nerve palsies of the trigeminal (CN V), facial (CN VII), and auditory (CN VIII) nerves have also been reported.[28]

▶ CLINICAL PRESENTATION AND CHARACTERISTICS

Although many clinical variations have been described, most cases of MPH are characterized by their typical onset, presentation, and associated symptoms.

Onset

Onset of symptoms is generally delayed, with headache usually beginning 12 to 48 hours and rarely more than 5 days following meningeal puncture. In their landmark observational study, Vandam and Dripps[8] reported onset of headache symptoms within 3 days of spinal anesthesia in 84.8% of patients for whom such data were available. More recently, Lybecker et al.[29] performed a detailed analysis of 75 consecutive patients with MPH following spinal anesthesia (primarily using 25-gauge cutting-point needles). While none of their patients noted the onset of symptoms during the first hour following meningeal puncture, 65% experienced symptoms within 24 hours and 92% within 48 hours. An onset of symptoms within 1 hour of neuraxial procedures is suspicious for pneumocephalus, especially in the setting of an epidural loss-of-resistance technique using air.[30] Occasional reports of unusually delayed onset of MPH highlight the importance of seeking a history of central neuraxial instrumentation whenever positional headaches are evaluated.[31]

Presentation

The cardinal feature of MPH is its postural nature, with headache symptoms worsening in the upright position and relieved, or at least improved, with recumbency. The International Classification of Headache Disorders further describes this positional quality as worsening within 15 minutes of sitting or standing and improving within 15 minutes after lying.[1] Headache is always bilateral, with a distribution that is frontal (25%), occipital (27%), or both (45%).[29] Headaches are typically described as "dull/aching," "throbbing," or "pressure-type."

The severity of headache symptoms, a feature with important ramifications for treatment, varies considerably among patients. Although there is no widely accepted severity scale, one practical approach is to have patients simply rate their headache intensity using a 10-point analog scale, with 1 to 3 classified as "mild,", 4 to 6 "moderate," and 7 to 10 "severe." Lybecker et al.[29] further categorized patients according to restriction in physical activity, degree of confinement to bed, and presence of associated symptoms (Box 9-1). A prospective analysis of MPH after spinal anesthesia using Lybecker's classification system demonstrated that 11% were mild, 23% moderate, and 67% severe.

Associated Symptoms

If headaches are severe, they are more likely to be accompanied by a variety of other symptoms. Pain and stiffness in the neck and shoulders is common and seen in nearly half of all patients experiencing MPH.[32] With questioning, nausea may be reported by a majority of patients and can lead to vomiting.[29]

Uncommonly, patients may experience auditory or visual symptoms,[26] and the risk for either appears to be directly related to needle size.[27,33] In Vandam and Dripps'[8] large study of MPH, each was seen to a clinically apparent degree in 0.4% of patients. Auditory symptoms include hearing loss, tinnitus, and even hyperacusis and can be unilateral. It is interesting to note that subclinical hearing loss, especially in the lower frequencies, has been found to be common following spinal anesthesia, even in the absence of MPH.[33] Closely associated with auditory function, vestibular disturbances (dizziness or vertigo) may also occur. Visual problems include blurred vision, difficulties with accommodation, mild photophobia, and diplopia. In contrast to headache complaints, which are consistently bilateral, nearly 80% of episodes of diplopia secondary to meningeal puncture involve unilateral cranial nerve palsies.[27]

▶ RISK FACTORS

Risk factors for MPH can be broadly categorized into patient characteristics and procedural details.

Patient Characteristics

The patient characteristic having the greatest impact on risk of MPH is age. Uncommonly reported in children <10 years of age, MPH has a peak incidence in the teens and early 20s.[34]

BOX 9-1 Classification of Severity of MPH

Severity of MPH

Mild	Postural headache slightly restricting daily activities Patient is not bedridden at any time during the day No associated symptoms
Moderate	Postural headache that significantly restricts daily activities Patient is bedridden part of the day Associated symptoms may or may not be present
Severe	Postural headache severe enough to stay in bed all day Associated symptoms always present

Associated Symptoms of MPH

Vestibular	Nausea, vomiting, dizziness
Cochlear	Hearing loss, hyperacusis, tinnitus
Ocular	Photophobia, teichopsia, diplopia, difficulty with accommodation
Musculoskeletal	Neck stiffness, scapular pain

Adapted from Lybecker H, Djernes M, Schmidt JF. Postdural puncture headache (PDPH): onset, duration, severity, and associated symptoms. An analysis of 75 consecutive patients with PDPH. *Acta Anaesthesiol Scand* 1995;39:606–12, with permission.

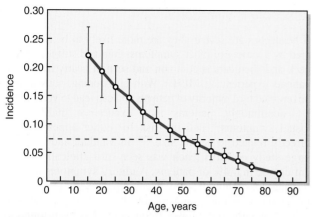

FIGURE 9-2. Logistic regression of the incidence of MPH as a function of age: Pa = [1 + exp (0.633 + 0.039 × age)]⁻¹. Age-specific incidence means and 95% confidence limits are shown as *vertical lines*. The overall incidence of MPH for this study, which used cutting needles only, was 7.3% (*dashed horizontal line*). (Redrawn and used from Lybecker H, Moller JT, May O, et al. Incidence and prediction of postdural puncture headache: a prospective study of 1021 spinal anesthesias. *Anesth Analg* 1990;70:389–394, with permission.)

The incidence then declines over time, becoming much less frequent in patients over 50 years of age (Fig. 9-2). Females have long been recognized as being at increased risk for MPH, and a systematic review of published studies found the odds of developing MPH were significantly lower for male than age-matched nonpregnant female subjects (odds ratio = 0.55; 95% confidence interval, 0.44–0.67).[35] The etiology behind this gender difference is not clear. Body mass index (BMI) appears to be a mixed risk factor. Morbid obesity presents obvious technical difficulties for central neuraxial procedures, increasing the likelihood of multiple needle passes and UDP.[36] Yet, low BMI has been reported as an independent risk factor for MPH[37] and high BMI (i.e., obesity) may actually decrease the risk, possibly due to a beneficial effect of increased intra-abdominal pressure.[38]

Pregnancy has traditionally been regarded as a risk factor for MPH,[8] but this consideration largely reflects a young female cohort as well as the high incidence of UDP in the gravid population. Although controversial, pushing during the second stage of labor, thought to promote the loss of CSF through a hole in the meninges, has been reported to influence the risk of MPH following UDP. Angle et al.[39] noted that the cumulative duration of bearing down correlated with the risk of developing MPH in patients who had experienced UDP. They also found that patients who avoided pushing altogether (proceeded to cesarean delivery prior to reaching second-stage labor) had a much lower incidence of MPH (10%) than those who pushed (74%).

MPHs appear to have an interesting association with other headaches. Patients who report having had a headache within the week prior to LP have been observed to have a higher incidence of MPH.[37] Upon further analysis, only those with chronic bilateral tension-type headaches were found to be at increased risk.[40] A history of unilateral headache[40] or migraine[41] has not been linked to an increased risk of MPH. Menstrual cycle, a factor in migraine headaches, did not influence the rate of MPH in one small pilot study.[42] Patients with a history of previous

MPH, particularly women, appear to have an increased risk for new MPH after spinal anesthesia.[43] With epidural procedures, patients with a history of UDP have been shown to be at slightly increased risk for another UDP (and subsequent MPH).[44]

Procedural Details

Needle size and tip design are the most important procedural factors related to MPH[45] (Fig. 9-3). Needle size is directly related to the risk of MPH. Meningeal puncture with larger needles is associated with a higher incidence of MPH,[8] more severe headache and associated symptoms,[45] a longer duration of symptoms,[46] and a greater need for definitive treatment measures.[47] Needle tip design is also a major influence, with "noncutting" needles clearly associated with a reduced incidence of MPH when compared with "cutting" (usually Quincke) needles of the same gauge. In general, noncutting needles have an opening set back from a tapered ("pencil-point") tip and include the Whitacre, Sprotte, European, Pencan, and Gertie Marx needles. Adding to this somewhat confusing terminology, noncutting needles are sometimes still incorrectly referred to as "atraumatic" needles, this despite being shown with electron microscopy to produce a more traumatic rent in the dura than cutting needles (perhaps resulting in a better inflammatory healing response).[48] The influence of needle size on the risk of MPH appears to be greatest for cutting needles (e.g., the reduction seen in the incidence of MPH between 22- and 26-gauge sizes is greater for cutting than noncutting needles). Insertion of cutting needles with the bevel parallel to the long axis of the spine significantly reduces the incidence of MPH.[49] This observation was for many years attributed to a spreading rather than the cutting of longitudinal-oriented dural fibers. However, scanning electron microscopy reveals the dura to be made of many layers of concentrically directed fibers,[50] and the importance of needle bevel insertion is now thought to be due

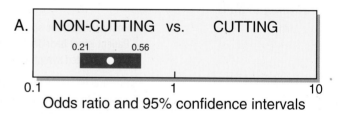

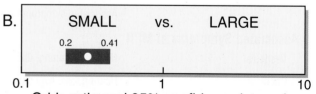

FIGURE 9-3. Pooled odds ratios and 95% confidence intervals (from meta-analysis of nonheterogeneous studies) for risk of MPH based on (A) needle type and (B) needle size. (Redrawn and used from Halpern S, Preston R. Postdural puncture headache and spinal needle design. Metaanalysis. *Anesthesiology* 1994;81:1376–1383, with permission.)

to longitudinal tension on the meninges, particularly in the upright position, and its influence on CSF leakage through holes having differing orientations.

Not surprisingly, a larger number of meningeal punctures have been shown to increase the rate of MPH.[51] The degree of experience/comfort/skill of the operator is clearly associated with the incidence of UDP during epidural procedures, with higher UDP rates consistently reported when procedures are performed by residents.[52,53] The risk of UDP also appears to be higher for procedures done at night, strongly suggesting a significant contribution of operator fatigue.[54]

A number of procedural details do not appear to influence the rate of development of MPH, including patient position at the time of meningeal puncture, "bloody tap" during spinal anesthesia, addition of opiates to spinal block, and volume of CSF removed (for diagnostic purposes).[6]

▶ PREVENTION

Although prophylaxis is most simply thought of as preventing any symptoms of MPH, in the clinical context this issue is deceptively complex. It is important to appreciate that significant "prevention" may encompass a number of other endpoints, such as a reduced incidence of severe MPH, a shorter duration of symptoms, or decreased need for EBP. Unfortunately, despite the clear relevance of this issue, the overall quality of evidence for preventive measures is generally weak.[55–57]

General Measures

As with all regional techniques, appropriate patient selection is crucial in minimizing complications. In this regard, anesthesiologists should take pause when caring for patients having known risk factors for MPH. As age is a major risk factor, spinal anesthesia is perhaps best avoided in patients under 40 years of age unless the benefits are sufficiently compelling (such as in the obstetric population). Practitioners (and patients alike) may also wish to avoid central neuraxial techniques in those with a previous history of UDP or MPH (particularly females). Other patient-related factors (e.g., obesity) should be considered on a case-by-case basis, weighing the risks of MPH with the benefits of regional anesthesia.

Neuraxial procedures should be performed with needles having the smallest gauge possible. However, extremely small spinal needles are more difficult to place, have a slow return of CSF, may be associated with multiple punctures of the meninges, and can result in a higher rate of unsuccessful block. The ideal choice for spinal anesthesia is generally a 24- to 27-gauge noncutting needle. Epidural options are limited, especially with catheter techniques, but the risk of MPH following UDP can probably also be reduced by always using the smallest feasible epidural needles.

While only recently utilized for neuraxial techniques, the use of ultrasound for regional anesthesia holds some promise in reducing the risk of MPH. Ultrasound can decrease the number of needle passes required for regional procedures and has been shown to accurately predict the depth of the epidural space.[58] Further study is ongoing to define this potential for ultrasound to reduce the incidence of UDP and MPH.

Pharmacologic measures, notably caffeine, continue to be widely used in hopes of decreasing the incidence of MPH following meningeal puncture.[15] In support of this practice, one small study ($n = 60$) found that intravenous caffeine (500 mg caffeine sodium benzoate within 90 minutes after spinal anesthesia) significantly reduced the incidence of moderate-to-severe headache.[59] However, generalizing these results to other clinical settings is difficult as this investigation involved the use of 22-gauge Quincke needles in a relatively young patient population. In another study, oral caffeine (75 or 125 mg) administered every 6 hours during the first 3 days following spinal anesthesia failed to influence the rate of MPH.[60] A critical review of the available evidence fails to support the use of caffeine in the prevention of MPH.[61] More recently, a small pilot study raised the possibility of using the long-acting 5-HT receptor agonist frovatriptan (2.5 mg/d orally for 5 days) in the prevention of MPH.[62] Currently, however, there is no proven pharmacologic prophylaxis for MPH.

A recent survey of United States (US) anesthesiologists reported that bed rest and aggressive oral and intravenous hydration continue to be employed by a sizable majority as prophylactic measures against MPH.[15] However, a systematic review of the literature regarding bed rest versus early mobilization after dural puncture failed to show any evidence of benefit from bed rest and suggested that the risk of MPH may actually be decreased by early mobilization.[63] It is notable that the practice of US anesthesiologists regarding bed rest is in direct contrast to that seen in United Kingdom (UK) maternity units, where 75% encourage mobilization as early as possible following UDP as prophylaxis against MPH.[64] Likewise, a randomized prospective trial of increased oral hydration following LP failed to decrease the incidence or duration of MPH.[63] In summary, at this time there is no evidence to support the common recommendations of bed rest or aggressive hydration in the prevention of MPH.

Spinal Technique

Attention to needle tip design is an important technical means of reducing the risk of MPH with spinal anesthesia. If available, noncutting needles should be employed. If cutting-tip needles are used, the bevel should be directed parallel to the long axis of the spine.

Replacing the stylet after CSF collection but prior to needle withdrawal is an effective means of lowering the incidence of MPH after LP. This recommendation is based on a prospective, randomized study of 600 patients using 21-gauge Sprotte needles. In this setting, replacing the stylet reduced the incidence of MPH from 16.3% to 5.0% ($p < 0.005$).[65] This safe and simple maneuver is theorized to decrease the possibility of a wicking strand of arachnoid mater from extending across the dura (Fig. 9-4).

Continuous spinal anesthesia (CSA) has been reported by some to be associated with surprisingly low incidences of MPH compared with single-dose spinal techniques using similar gauge needles.[66] This observation has been attributed to the reaction to the catheter, which may promote better sealing of a breach in the meninges.

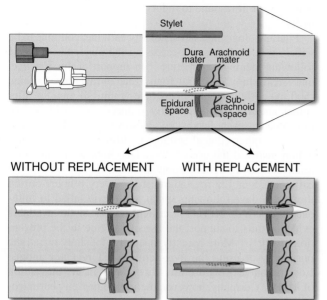

FIGURE 9-4. Schematic drawing of the proposed mechanism of decreased incidence of MPH seen with stylet replacement. **Upper:** Flow of CSF from the subarachnoid space may draw strands of arachnoid mater into the needle. **Lower left:** Removal of the needle without stylet replacement results in threading of arachnoid across the dura, promoting prolonged CSF leak. **Lower right:** Replacing the stylet fully prior to needle removal either pushes out or cuts the arachnoid mater, reducing the risk of CSF loss into the epidural space. (Used from Strupp M, Brandt T, Muller A. Incidence of post-lumbar puncture syndrome reduced by reinserting the stylet: a randomized prospective study of 600 patients. *J Neurol* 1998;245:589–592, with permission.)

CSA with small-gauge needles and catheters ("microcatheters") is an appealing option when titration of the spinal drug is desirable and duration of surgery is uncertain, but microcatheters have usually been unavailable in the US, where the risk of MPH with CSA remains a concern when using approximately 20-gauge "macrocatheters." For this reason, although the technique may have clinical advantages, deliberate CSA has been investigated almost exclusively in low-risk populations.

Epidural Technique

The issue of air versus liquid for identification of the epidural space with the loss-of-resistance technique has long been a source of controversy. Each method has acknowledged advantages and disadvantages but neither has been shown convincingly to result in a lower risk of UDP.[67] In this case, operator preference and experience would be expected to strongly influence performance, and the overriding significance of this factor is illustrated in fewer instances of UDP noted when the medium is chosen at the anesthesiologist's discretion.[68]

Bevel orientation for epidural needle insertion remains a matter of debate. Norris et al.[69] found that the incidence of moderate-to-severe MPH after UDP was only 24% when the needle bevel was oriented parallel to the long axis of the spine (compared to 70% with perpendicular insertion).

This resulted in fewer therapeutic EBPs administered to patients in the parallel group ($p < 0.05$). However, this technique necessitates a controversial 90-degree rotation of the needle for catheter placement.[70] It appears that a number of concerns regarding parallel needle bevel insertion (lateral needle deviation, difficulties with catheter insertion, and dural trauma with needle rotation) are of greater concern to practitioners. Most respondents (71.3%) to a survey of US anesthesiologists preferred to insert epidural needles with the bevel perpendicular to the long axis of the spine (consistent with the intended direction of catheter travel).[15]

Combined spinal-epidural (CSE) techniques have been reported to be associated with a low incidence of MPH. While providing the advantages of a spinal anesthetic, CSE appears to have no increased incidence of MPH or the need for EBP when compared to plain epidural analgesia.[71] This observation may be due to several factors, including the ability to successfully use extremely small (e.g., 27-gauge) noncutting spinal needles, and tamponade provided by epidural infusions.

Measures to Reduce the Risk of MPH after UDP

The risk-to-benefit ratio of prophylaxis should be most favorable in situations having the greatest likelihood of developing severe MPH. Therefore, most efforts to reduce the risk of MPH after UDP have been in the obstetric patient population. Several prophylactic measures, discussed below, are worthy of consideration and have been utilized alone or in combination.[72] However, since not all patients who experience UDP will develop MPH, and only a portion of those who do will require definitive treatment (i.e., an EBP), a cautious approach in this regard is still generally warranted.

Stylet Replacement

Although there have not been any studies to support the use of this technique in the setting of UDP, replacing the stylet is a simple and effective means of lowering the incidence of MPH after LP.[65] Given the innocuous nature of this maneuver, if no other prophylactic measures are taken, there appears to be little reason not to replace the stylet prior to epidural needle removal in the event of UDP.

Subarachnoid Saline

Limited evidence indicates that the subarachnoid injection of sterile preservative-free saline following UDP may be associated with a significant reduction in the incidence of MPH and the need for EBP. In one small study ($n = 43$), immediate injection of 10 mL saline through the epidural needle substantially reduced the incidence of MPH (32%, compared with 62% in a matched control group) and resulted in a significant reduction in the need for EBP ($p = 0.004$).[73] The injection of saline and the reinjection of CSF have been speculated as important in the prevention of MPH by maintaining CSF volume.[72] However, given the relatively rapid rate of CSF regeneration, it may be that the benefit of fluid injection following UDP is actually in preventing a wicking strand of arachnoid (as proposed for stylet replacement). Further investigation into this issue is needed.

Intrathecal Catheters

Immediately placing an intrathecal catheter (ITC) after UDP has the advantages of being able to rapidly provide spinal analgesia as well as eliminate the possibility of another UDP under challenging clinical circumstances. However, the potential benefits of ITC use must be weighed against the readily appreciated risks involved (accidental use, misuse, and infection). Although evidence is extremely limited, ITC use has also been proposed to reduce the risk of MPH after UDP.[56] Ayad et al.[74] placed and maintained an ITC for 24 hours following UDP. In their obstetric population, catheter placement resulted in an MPH rate of only 6.2%, with an expected incidence of >50% in this setting. A similar reduction in the development of MPH with 24-hour ITC maintenance after UDP has been noted in orthopedic patients.[75] This impressive reduction in the incidence of MPH has generally not been reported from studies where catheters have been left in place for <24 hours. It has been proposed that the mechanism of benefit from ITC maintenance may be due to reaction to the catheter, with inflammation or edema preventing further CSF loss after removal. There are also preliminary data to suggest that the incidence of MPH may be further reduced by the injection of preservative-free saline through an ITC immediately prior to removal.[73] With some accepted and other possible benefits, rates of ITC use following UDP have clearly increased during the past decade. Recent surveys of US, UK, and Australian practice have noted rates of routine intrathecal catheterization following UDP in obstetric patients of 18%, 28%, and 35%, respectively.[15,64,76]

Although ITC use has increased, reattempting an epidural at an adjacent interspace remains the preferred action following UDP.[15] Provided an epidural catheter can be successfully placed, several epidural approaches have been used in the hope of reducing the incidence and severity of MPH:

Epidural Saline

Efforts have included both bolus (usually around 50 mL as a single or repeated injection) and continuous infusion techniques (commonly 600–1,000 mL over 24 hours). As these measures are resource intensive and may only serve to delay the inevitable onset of symptoms, they have generally not been continued beyond 36 hours. In one large analysis (n = 241), Stride and Cooper[77] reported a reduction in the incidence of MPH from 86% in a conservatively treated control group to 70% with epidural saline infusion. Trivedi et al.[78] noted a similar reduction in MPH (from 87% to 67%) in 30 patients who received a single prophylactic "saline patch" (40–60 mL) following completion of an obstetric procedure. Other studies of epidural saline have noted this modest decrease in the incidence of MPH. Stride and Cooper[77] also reported a lower incidence of severe headache (from 64% to 47%), but this effect has been inconsistently seen by other investigators, and there is no convincing evidence that epidural saline reduces the eventual need for EBP.

Epidural Opiates

Epidural opiates (especially morphine), while long utilized for the treatment of MPH, have been thought unlikely to influence the natural history of the disorder. However, recently revisiting the issue of opiates as prophylaxis after UDP, Al-metwalli[79] found that two epidural injections of morphine (3 mg in 10 mL), compared with epidural injections of an equal volume of saline, resulted in fewer episodes of MPH (p = 0.014) and decreased the need for EBP (p = 0.022). Due to the small number of patients involved (n = 25), further prospective investigation is warranted.

Prophylactic Epidural Blood Patch

The impressive efficacy of the EBP when used as treatment for MPH has fueled interest in the technique for prophylaxis. Research into the efficacy of the EBP for prophylaxis has yielded mixed results, and closer scrutiny indicates that optimism should be guarded. The strongest investigation to date has been by Scavone et al.,[80] who performed a prospective, randomized, double-blind study in 64 parturients comparing the prophylactic epidural blood patch (PEBP) to a sham EBP. In this study, an identical 56% of patients in each group went on to develop MPH. Although there was a trend toward fewer therapeutic EBPs recommended and performed in the prophylactic group, the difference was not statistically significant (p = 0.08). The primary benefit of the PEBP was a shorter total duration of symptoms (from a median of ~5 days to 2 days) and, consequently, a reduction in the overall pain burden (Fig. 9-5).

A recent systematic review of the evidence concluded that the relative risk for MPH after PEBP was 0.48 (95% confidence interval: 0.23–0.99) in five nonrandomized controlled trials (total n = 436) and 0.32 (95% confidence interval: 0.10–1.03) in four randomized controlled trials (total n = 173, with 64 of these patients from the Scavone study mentioned above).[57] With such inconclusive support, the PEBP is not currently recommended as a routine measure based upon available evidence.[56,81] Due to concerns of

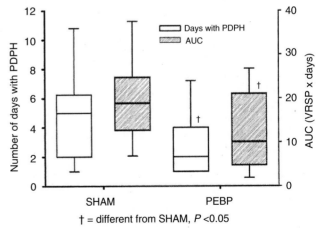

† = different from SHAM, P <0.05

FIGURE 9-5. Plot of the duration of MPH (PDPH) (*open boxes*, with scale on left) and the pain intensity duration (*shaded boxes*, with scale on right) for sham injection and PEBP. Area under the curve (AUC) consists of the verbal rating score for pain (VRSP) multiplied by the number of days with MPH. Boxes are the interquartile range, solid lines within the boxes represent the median value, and whiskers are the 10th and 90th percentiles. (Used from Scavone BM, Wong CA, Sullivan JT, et al. Efficacy of a prophylactic epidural blood patch in preventing post dural puncture headache in parturients after inadvertent dural puncture. *Anesthesiology* 2004;101:1422–1427, with permission.)

exposing patients to a potentially unnecessary and marginally beneficial procedure, prophylactic application of the EBP has declined substantially in recent years.[15,64] If used for prophylaxis, the EBP should be performed only after any spinal or epidural local anesthetic has worn off, as premature administration has been associated with excessive cephalad displacement of local anesthetic.[82] Residual epidural local anesthetic may also inhibit coagulation of blood, further decreasing the efficacy of the EBP.[83]

Pharmacologic Measures

As mentioned above, there is no convincing evidence that systemic pharmacologic measures are beneficial in the prevention of MPH. However, based on a number of theoretical mechanisms, adrenocorticotrophic hormone (ACTH) and its analogues have long been used in the treatment of MPH.[84] Hakim recently reported randomizing 90 parturients experiencing UDP to receive either 1 mg cosyntropin or saline intravenously 30 minutes after delivery.[85] The incidence of MPH and EBP was 33% and 11% in the cosyntropin group versus 69% and 30% in the saline group. No serious reactions were associated with cosyntropin use. These limited data are encouraging but will need to be supported through further study.

Limiting/Avoiding Pushing

In the event of UDP, limiting the duration of the second stage of labor (usually to 30–60 minutes) and avoiding pushing may reduce the risk of MPH. While these measures are not uncommonly recommended in UK maternity units,[64] such management is rare in US practice.[15]

▶ DIAGNOSTIC EVALUATION

MPH remains a diagnosis of exclusion. Although headache following meningeal puncture will naturally be suspected to be MPH, it remains critical to rule out other etiologies (Box 9-2). Fortunately, a careful history with a brief consideration of other possible diagnoses is usually all that is necessary to differentiate MPH from other causes of headache. While numerous clinical variations have been reported, most cases of MPH will have: (a) a history of known or possible meningeal puncture, (b) delayed onset of symptoms (but within 48 hours), and (c) bilateral postural headache (possibly accompanied by associated symptoms if moderate or severe). Importantly, most nonmeningeal puncture headaches will not have a strong positional nature. Laboratory studies are usually not necessary for the diagnosis of MPH and, if obtained, are generally unremarkable (most commonly, MRI may show meningeal enhancement and LP may reveal low opening pressures and increased CSF protein).

Physical exam plays a limited role in the diagnosis of MPH. Vital signs (normal blood pressure and absence of fever) and a basic neurologic exam (gross motor and sensory function plus ocular and facial movements) should be documented. Firm bilateral jugular venous pressure, applied briefly (10–15 seconds), tends to worsen headaches secondary to intracranial hypotension.[24] Conversely, the "sitting epigastric pressure test" may result in transient relief of MPH symptoms.[86] For this test, the patient is placed in a sitting position until headache symptoms become manifest. Firm, continuous abdominal pressure is applied with one

---

BOX 9-2 Differential Diagnosis of MPH

Benign Etiologies

Non-specific headache
Exacerbation of chronic headache (e.g. tension-type headache)
Hypertensive headache
Pneumocephalus
Sinusitis
Drug side-effect
Spontaneous intracranial hypotension
Other

Serious Etiologies

Meningitis
Subdural hematoma
Subarachnoid hemorrhage
Preeclampsia/eclampsia
Intracranial venous thrombosis
Other

---

hand, while the other hand is secure against the patient's back. In cases of MPH, some improvement is usually noted within 15 to 30 seconds with prompt return of symptoms upon the release of abdominal pressure.

It must be appreciated that benign headaches are frequently encountered in the perioperative setting, even in the absence of meningeal puncture, but have generally been noted to be less severe than MPH (proposed etiologies include dehydration, hypoglycemia, anxiety, and caffeine withdrawal). With spinal anesthesia, the specific local anesthetic used, as well as the addition of dextrose or epinephrine, may influence the occurrence of nonspecific headache but do not affect the rate of true MPH.[87] The majority of headaches following meningeal puncture will be benign nonspecific headaches. In a careful analysis of headache following spinal anesthesia using strict criteria for MPH, Santanen et al.[88] found an incidence of nonmeningeal puncture headache of 18.5%, with an incidence of true MPH of only 1.5%. Headaches and neck/shoulder pain are also common in the postpartum period.[32] In one study, 39% of postpartum patients were noted to be symptomatic, but the etiology in over 75% of these was determined to be primary headache (migraine, tension-type, cervicogenic, and cluster).[53] In this analysis, while 89% of patients received neuraxial anesthesia, only 4.7% of postpartum headaches were MPH.

Benign headaches can often be differentiated from MPH by characteristic features. Exacerbation of chronic headache (e.g., tension-type, cluster, or migraine) is usually notable for a history of similar headaches. In the study cited immediately above, a previous headache history was a significant risk factor for postpartum headache (adjusted odds ratio = 2.25, if >12 episodes per year).[53] Significant hypertension may cause headaches and should be detected through routine vital sign assessment. Stella et al.[89] studied severe and unrelenting postpartum headaches with onset >24 hours from the time of delivery and found that 39% were tension-type headaches, 24% were due to preeclampsia/eclampsia, and only 16% were MPH (despite neuraxial anesthesia in 88% of patients). Based on this observation, they developed a treatment algorithm for severe postpartum headache that recommends treatment of tension/migraine headache prior to consideration of MPH (Fig. 9-6). Pneumocephalus can produce a positional headache that can be difficult to distinguish from MPH and does not respond to EBP, but is readily diagnosed with computerized tomography.[90] Sinusitis may be associated with purulent nasal discharge and tenderness over the affected sinus and is often improved with assuming an upright position. It should be kept in mind that headache is also a side effect of some commonly utilized pharmacologic agents, such as ondansetron.[91] Although certainly unusual, classic MPH symptoms may even conceivably represent a coincidental case of spontaneous intracranial hypotension (SIH). A number of other benign etiologies are possible.

Serious causes of headache will be rare but must be excluded. It is important to remember that lateralizing neurologic signs (with the exception of cranial nerve palsies), fever/chills, seizures, or changes in mental status are not consistent with a diagnosis of MPH. Meningitis tends to be associated with fever, leukocytosis, changes in mental status, and meningeal signs (such as nuchal rigidity).[92] Subdural hematoma (SDH) is a recognized complication of dural puncture and is believed under these circumstances to be due to intracranial hypotension resulting in excessive traction on cerebral vessels, leading to their disruption. Practitioners must maintain a high index of suspicion for SDH, which is often preceded by typical MPH symptoms but progresses to lose its postural component and may evolve to include disturbances in mentation and focal neurologic signs. It has been proposed that early definitive treatment of severe MPH may serve to prevent SDH.[93] Subarachnoid hemorrhage, most commonly due to rupture of a cerebral aneurysm or arteriovenous malformation, is usually associated with the sudden onset of excruciating headache followed by a decreased level of consciousness or coma.[94] Preeclampsia/eclampsia often presents with headache and may only become evident in the postpartum period.[95] Intracranial venous thrombosis (ICVT) is most often seen in the postpartum obstetric population, where headache symptoms are easily confused with MPH but may progress to seizures,

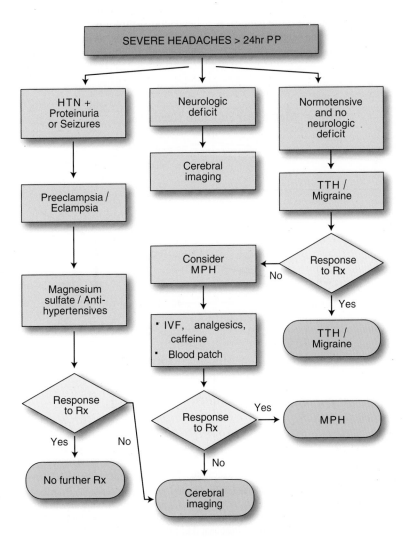

FIGURE 9-6. Suggested treatment algorithm for the management of severe postpartum headache present >24 hours after delivery. (PP, postpartum; HTN, hypertension; MPH, meningeal puncture headache; TTH, tension-type headache; IVF, intravenous fluid.). (Redrawn after Stella CL, Jodicke CD, How HY, et al. Postpartum headache: is your work-up complete? *Am J Obstet Gynecol* 2007;196:318.e1–318.e7, with permission.)

focal neurologic signs, and coma.[96] Predisposing factors for ICVT include hypercoagulability, dehydration, and inflammatory and infectious diseases. Reports of other intracranial pathology (intracranial tumor, intracerebral hemorrhage, etc.) misdiagnosed as MPH are extremely uncommon and will be detected with a thorough neurologic evaluation.[97]

Diagnosis of MPH can be particularly challenging in patients who have undergone LP as part of a diagnostic workup for headache. In these situations, a change in the quality of headache, most commonly a new postural nature, points toward MPH. Occasionally, if the benign diagnostic possibilities cannot be narrowed down with certainty, a favorable response to EBP can provide definitive evidence for a diagnosis of MPH.

▶ TREATMENT

Once a diagnosis of MPH has been made, patients should be provided a straightforward explanation of the presumed etiology (Fig. 9-1), anticipated natural course (factoring in the time from meningeal puncture), and a realistic assessment of treatment options (with consideration of needle gauge). A treatment algorithm, based primarily on the severity of symptoms, can serve as a useful guide for management (Fig. 9-7).

Time

Because MPH is a complication that tends to resolve spontaneously, the simple passage of time plays an important role in the appropriate management of this disorder. Prior to the introduction of the EBP as definitive therapy, the natural history of MPH was documented by Vandam and Dripps[8] as they followed 1,011 episodes of MPH after spinal anesthesia using cutting needles of various sizes. While their analysis is flawed by a lack of information regarding duration in 9% of patients, if one considers their observed data, spontaneous resolution of MPH was seen in 59% of cases within 4 days and 80% within 1 week. More recently, Lybecker et al.[29] closely followed 75 episodes of MPH and, while providing an EBP to 40% of their patients (generally to those having the most severe symptoms), observed in the untreated patients a median duration of symptoms of 5 days with a range of 1 to 12 days. van Kooten et al.,[98] in a small but prospective, randomized, blinded study of patients with moderate or severe MPH (most following lumbar puncture with 20 gauge cutting needles), noted 18 of 21 patients (86%) in the control treatment group (24-hour bed rest, at least 2 L of fluids by mouth daily, and prn analgesics) still having headache symptoms at 7 days, with over half of these still rating symptoms as moderate or severe (Fig. 9-8). These data serve to illustrate the unpredictable and occasionally

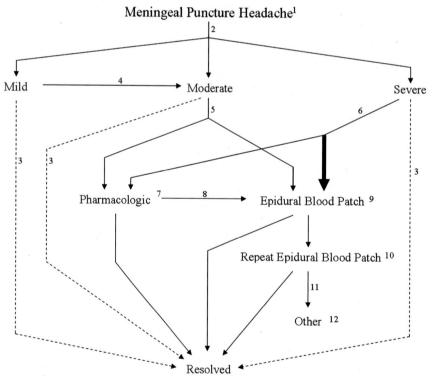

FIGURE 9-7. Treatment algorithm for established MPH. See text for further details. (1) Patient education, reassurance, and supportive measures. (2) Triage by severity of symptoms. (3) Resolution over time without further treatment. (4) Worsening symptoms or failure to improve substantially within 5 days. (5) Choice of EBP or less effective pharmacologic measures based on patient preference. (6) Definitive treatment (EBP) is recommended (*bold arrow*). (7) Caffeine or other agents. (8) Failure, worsening of symptoms, or recurrence. (9) Patch materials other than blood remain preliminary. (10) Generally performed no sooner than 24 hours after a first EBP. (11) Serious reconsideration of diagnosis. (12) Radiologic guidance is recommended if another EBP is performed.

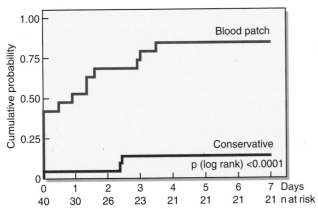

FIGURE 9-8. Cumulative probability of recovery from moderate or severe MPH. Full recovery was noted in 3.5 days, and unchanged by 7 days, in 16 of 19 patients (84%) in the blood patch group and 3 of 21 patients (14%) in the control treatment ("conservative") group. (Redrawn after van Kooten F, Oedit R, Bakker SLM, et al. Epidural blood patch in post dural puncture headache: a randomized, observer-blind, controlled clinical trial. *J Neurol Neurosurg Psychiatry* 2008;79:553–558, with permission.)

prolonged duration of untreated MPH. Indeed, Vandam and Dripps[8] reported 4% of patients still experiencing symptoms 7 to 12 months after spinal anesthesia. Given this reality, it is not surprising that there are a number of case reports of successful treatment of MPH months and even years after known or occult meningeal puncture.

Largely due to the self-limited nature of MPH, the optimal time course of treatment has not been well-defined. Clinically, the practical issue is how long definitive therapy (i.e., the EBP) can appropriately be delayed. Most practitioners currently advocate a trial, most commonly 24 to 48 hours, of conservative management.[15] However, the rationale behind this approach is questionable, given the often severely disabling nature of symptoms, particularly in the postpartum period when newborn care may be significantly impaired.

Supportive Measures

Reassurance and measures directed toward minimizing symptoms, while not expected to alter the natural course of the disorder, are advised for all patients. By definition, the majority of patients with moderate-to-severe MPH will naturally seek a recumbent position for symptomatic relief. Despite a lack of supportive evidence, aggressive hydration continues to be the most frequently recommended practice utilized in the treatment of MPH.[15] Although aggressive hydration does not appear to influence the duration of symptoms,[63] patients should and often must be encouraged to avoid dehydration.

Analgesics (acetaminophen, nonsteroidal anti-inflammatory agents [NSAIDS], opiates, etc.) may be administered by a number of different routes and are commonly used, yet the relief obtained is often unimpressive, especially with severe headaches. Antiemetics and stool softeners should be prescribed when indicated. Abdominal binders have been advocated but are uncomfortable and seldom used in modern practice. Alternative measures that have been suggested in the management of MPH include acupuncture[99] and bilateral greater occipital nerve block.[100]

Pharmacologic Therapies

A number of pharmacologic agents have been advocated as treatments for MPH.[101] While appealing, these options have generally been poorly studied and are of questionable value due to the small numbers of patients treated, methodologic flaws in published reports, and the self-limited nature of the disorder.

Methylxanthines are used for their cerebral vasoconstrictive effect and include aminophylline, theophylline, and (the most familiar) caffeine. Experimentally, caffeine has been used intravenously (usually 500 mg caffeine sodium benzoate, which contains 250 mg caffeine) and orally (e.g., 300 mg). Published studies of caffeine for MPH consistently demonstrate improvement at 1 to 4 hours in over 70% of patients treated.[101] However, a single oral dose of 300 mg caffeine for treatment of MPH is statistically no better than placebo at 24 hours.[102] With a terminal half life of generally <6 hours, repeated doses of caffeine would seem necessary for the treatment of MPH, yet few studies have evaluated more than two doses for efficacy or safety (of particular concern in the nursing parturient). Furthermore, there is no convincing evidence that any pharmacologic agents reduce the eventual need for EBP. Overall, the use of caffeine for MPH does not appear to be supported by the available literature.[61] Nevertheless, surveys indicate that it continues to be widely used in the treatment of MPH.[15,64] Clinically, encouraging unmonitored caffeine intake is of extremely uncertain value, especially considering the general lack of awareness of caffeine content in readily available beverages and medications. The temporary benefit often observed with caffeine would indicate that, if used, it is perhaps most appropriate for the treatment of MPH of moderate (and possibly mild or severe) intensity while awaiting spontaneous resolution of the condition. While the familiarity of caffeine for nonmedical purposes would argue for its general safety, practitioners should note that its use is contraindicated in patients with seizure disorders, pregnancy-induced hypertension, or a history of supraventricular tachyarrhythmias.

In addition to the methylxanthines, experiences with other pharmacologic approaches to MPH continue to be reported. Some recent examples: sumatriptan, a serotonin type-1d receptor agonist that causes cerebral vasoconstriction, is commonly used for migraine headache and has been used to treat MPH. Corticosteroidogenics (ACTH and its synthetic analogs [i.e., cosyntropin/tetracosactin]) have long been proposed as treatments for MPH. Although the mechanism of action remains speculative, ACTH is known to have multiple physiologic effects that could theoretically improve symptoms of MPH.[84] However, neither sumatriptan[103] nor a synthetic ACTH analog[104] was found to be effective in small randomized, prospective studies for treatment of severe MPH. Hydrocortisone (100 mg IV every 8 hours for 6 doses) has been reported to be effective in the treatment of severe MPH following spinal anesthesia using a 25-gauge Quincke needle.[105] A small, uncontrolled pilot study of methylergonovine (0.25 mg orally three times daily for 24–48 hours) indicated that this vasoconstrictive agent may hasten the resolution of MPH.[106] A case report of gabapentin (400 mg orally every 8 hours for 3 days) suggested that this agent may also be useful in the setting of severe MPH.[107] Reports of the successful use of these and other pharmacologic agents are intriguing, but their proper place in the management of MPH awaits further study. However, given the initial optimism but eventually disproven role for so many pharmacologic agents through the years, practitioners are advised to have guarded expectations in this regard, especially when dealing with severe MPH.

Epidural Therapies

While not a contraindication to epidural treatments, a history of significant technical difficulties with attempted neuraxial techniques should naturally encourage a trial of less invasive measures. However, the appeal of epidural approaches is evident if access to the epidural space is deemed reasonable or if the patient already has a correctly placed catheter *in situ*.

Epidural Saline

Epidural saline, as bolus and infusion, has a long history of use for treatment of MPH. Bolus injections of epidural saline (usually 20–30 mL, repeated as necessary if a catheter is present) have been reported to produce prompt and virtually universal relief of MPH, yet the practice is plagued by an extremely high rate of headache recurrence. The transient nature of this effect is not surprising as increases in epidural pressure following bolus administration of saline have been demonstrated to return to baseline within 10 minutes.[108] Favorable results achieved with this approach have been speculated to represent the mechanical reapproximation of a dural flap (the "tin-lid" phenomenon).[6] However, bolus administration of saline for treatment of MPH has been convincingly shown to be inferior to the EBP, especially when headaches are secondary to large-bore needle punctures.[109] Overall, epidural saline appears to be of limited value for established MPH.[56] Nevertheless, the successful use of epidural saline, administered as bolus and/or infusion, continues to be reported occasionally under exceptional circumstances.[110]

Epidural Blood Patch

During the past several decades, the EBP has emerged as the "gold standard" for treatment of MPH.[6] A Cochrane review (a systematic assessment of the evidence) regarding the EBP recently concluded that the procedure now has proven benefit over more conservative treatment.[81] The mechanism of action of the EBP, while not entirely elucidated, appears to be related to the ability to stop further CSF loss by the formation of clot over the defect in the meninges as well as a tamponade effect with cephalad displacement of CSF (the "epidural pressure patch").[111] The appropriate role of the EBP in individual situations will depend on multiple factors including the duration and severity of headache and associated symptoms, type and gauge of original needle used, and patient wishes. The EBP should be encouraged in patients experiencing UDP with an epidural needle and those whose symptoms are categorized as severe (i.e., pain score >6 on a 1–10 scale). Informed consent for the EBP should include a discussion with the patient regarding the common as well as serious risks involved, true success rate, and anticipated side effects. Finally, patients should be provided clear instructions for the provision of timely medical attention should they experience a recurrence of symptoms.

A number of controversies surround the EBP, reflecting the scarcity of adequately powered, randomized trials. The procedure itself has been well described and consists of the sterile injection of fresh autologous blood near the previous dural puncture (Box 9-3). An MRI study of the EBP in five young patients (ages 31–44) using 20 mL blood noted a spread of 4.6 ± 0.9 intervertebral spaces (mean ± SD), averaging 3.5 levels above and 1 level below the site of injection.[111] This and other observations of a preferential cephalad spread of blood in the lumbar epidural space has led to the common recommendation to perform the EBP "at or below" the meningeal puncture level. However, the influence on efficacy of the level of blood placement and use of an epidural catheter (often situated considerably cephalad to a meningeal puncture) for EBP have never been clinically evaluated.

The optimal timing of the EBP is a matter of debate. After diagnosis, most practitioners prefer to delay performing the EBP, possibly to further confirm the diagnosis as well as to allow an opportunity for spontaneous resolution. A 1996 survey of UK neurologic departments found that only 8% would consider the EBP before 72 hours had passed following

---

BOX 9-3 The EBP Procedure

- Obtain written informed consent.
- Establish intravenous access. An 18-gauge or larger saline lock is sufficient.
- Position the patient for epidural needle placement (mindful that a lateral decubitus position may be more comfortable for the patient).
- Using standard sterile technique, place an epidural needle into the epidural space at or below the level of previous meningeal puncture.
- Collect 20 mL fresh autologous venous blood using strict sterile technique (this is usually readily accomplished using the previously placed saline lock).
- Without delay, steadily inject blood through the epidural needle until the patient reports fullness or discomfort in the back, buttocks, or neck.
- Maintain the patient in a recumbent position for a period of time (1-2 hours may result in more complete resolution of symptoms). Intravenous infusion of 1 liter crystalloid during this interval is often helpful.
- Instructions for discharge:
  - Over-the-counter analgesics as needed (patient preference).
  - Avoid lifting, straining, or air travel for 24 hours.
  - Contact anesthesia for inadequate relief or recurrence of symptoms.

LP.[112] A recent survey of UK maternity units reported that 71% would perform the EBP only "after the failure of conservative measures."[64] Likewise, the majority of respondents to recent surveys of practice in the US and Nordic countries usually waited at least 24 hours from the onset of symptoms before performing the EBP.[15,113] Several studies have suggested that the EBP procedure may become more effective with the passage of time.[114,115] Safa-Tisseront et al.[115] found a delay of <4 days from meningeal puncture before performing an EBP to be an independent risk factor for failure of the procedure. Yet, these authors were careful to state that failure of the EBP may be primarily related to the severity of the CSF leak (with larger, harder-to-treat situations demanding earlier attention) and that their study should not be grounds for delaying the EBP. Sandesc et al.[116] performed a prospective, randomized, double-blind study of the EBP versus conservative management (IV/PO fluids up to 3 L/d, NSAIDS, and caffeine sodium benzoate 500 mg IV every 6 hours) in 32 patients with severe MPH symptoms (mean pain intensity = 8.1). At the time treatment was initiated, none of these patients had experienced symptoms for longer than 24 hours. While all patients in the EBP group had satisfactory resolution of symptoms at 24-hour follow-up, the control group was essentially unchanged (mean pain intensity = 7.8). Notably, 14 of 16 patients in the conservatively treated group then elected for EBP treatment. These investigators concluded that there was no reason to delay the EBP for more than 24 hours after making a diagnosis of severe MPH. This recommendation is further supported by a prospective analysis of 79 patients with MPH that determined early EBP in those with moderate-to-severe symptoms minimized overall patient suffering.[117]

The ideal volume of blood for EBP is unclear. Conceptually, the volume of blood used should be sufficient to form an organized clot over the meningeal defect as well as to produce some degree of epidural tamponade.[111] When performing the EBP, anesthesiologists commonly inject as much blood as was drawn (usually around 20 mL), stopping when the patient complains of discomfort or fullness in the back, buttocks, or neck. There appear to be geographic preferences regarding blood volume. The largest analysis of the EBP to date ($n = 504$) utilized a blood volume of 23 ± 5 mL (mean ± SD).[115] Importantly, this French study found no significant difference in blood volumes between successful and failed EBP. Notably, they reported "discomfort" in 78% of injections with 19 ± 5 mL and "pain" in 54% with 21 ± 5 mL, with the only independent risk factor for pain during EBP being age <35 years. A recent survey of US anesthesiologists reported general unanimity for a smaller blood volume, with two-thirds (66.8%) most commonly using between 16 and 20 mL.[15] As previously mentioned, there may be some experimental support for using a blood volume of 15 to 20 mL, as early studies of CSF drainage in volunteers reported consistently producing positional headache symptoms with loss of 10% of total CSF volume (~15 mL).[24] Furthermore, the reduction in CSF pressures produced by this degree of fluid loss would be expected to reduce or eliminate transmeningeal driving pressure, resulting at that point in a relative CSF volume homeostasis (in the supine position). Formal studies designed to determine an ideal volume of blood for EBP in the treatment of MPH have generally failed to achieve better results with volumes

>10 mL, and there are little data to encourage the use of volumes >20 mL.[118] It is notable that although the value of the EBP in the treatment of SIH is uncertain,[56] much larger blood volumes (up to 100 mL) are commonly recommended for this indication.[119] However, recent case reports highlight some potential complications, such as severe radiculopathy, from large-volume EBP,[120,121] and practitioners are therefore generally encouraged to use the smallest effective volume.

To allow for clot organization and regeneration of CSF (~0.35 mL/min), it is common practice to have patients remain recumbent for a period of time following the EBP. While the optimal duration of bed rest immediately following an EBP remains unknown, one small study suggested that maintaining the decubitus position for at least 1 and preferably 2 hours may result in a more complete resolution of symptoms.[122] Patients are usually advised to avoid lifting, Valsalva maneuvers (e.g., straining with bowel movement), and air travel for 24 to 48 hours after EBP to minimize the risk of patch disruption.

Contraindications to the EBP are similar to those of any epidural needle placement: coagulopathy, systemic sepsis, fever, infection at the site, and patient refusal. Theoretical concerns have been expressed regarding the possibility of neoplastic seeding of the central nervous system in patients with cancer.[123] Although not free from concern and controversy, the EBP has been safely provided to patients with HIV infection[124] and acute varicella.[125] Modifications of usual EBP technique have been suggested to accommodate the special needs of Jehovah's Witnesses.[126] The EBP may also be indicated and performed, with decreased volumes of blood, in the pediatric population (0.2–0.3 mL/kg has been associated with successful EBP in adolescents)[127] and at extralumbar sites (e.g., cervical).[128]

Minor side effects are common following the EBP. Patients should be warned to expect aching in the back, buttocks, or legs (seen in ~25% of patients).[114] While usually short-lived, backache was noted to be persistent in 16% of patients following EBP and lasted 3 to 100 days (with a mean duration in this subgroup of 27.7 days).[129] Despite these lingering symptoms, patient satisfaction with the EBP is high. Other frequent but benign aftereffects of the EBP include transient neckache,[129] bradycardia,[130] and modest temperature elevation.[129]

Largely through extensive clinical experience, the EBP has been sufficiently proven to be safe. Risks are essentially the same as with other epidural procedures (infection, bleeding, nerve damage, and UDP). Uncommonly, the temporary back and lower extremity radicular pain mentioned above has been reported to be severe. With proper technique, infectious complications are vanishingly rare. Although still controversial, a previous EBP does not appear to significantly influence the success of future epidural interventions.[131] Serious complications secondary to the EBP do occur but have usually consisted of isolated case reports and have often been associated with significant deviations from standard practice.[6]

Other Epidural Therapies

For various reasons, a number of alternatives to blood have been promoted as patch materials. The most commonly proposed materials (dextran-40, hydroxyethylstarch, gelatin, and fibrin glue) have been adapted for a perceived ability to provide prolonged epidural tamponade and/or result in sealing of a meningeal rent. In a rat model, experimental support for a "blood-like" effect was best shown for fibrin glue.[108] Yet, clinical use of these alternatives is limited to case reports and small series, and their use is uncommon in the US.[15] While not necessarily without merit, these options remain poorly defined and are not without potential for serious risk (e.g., allergic reactions to dextran), and reports of their use should still be considered preliminary.

► PERSISTENT OR RECURRENT MPH

Early reports of the EBP frequently cited success rates between 90% and 100%, but often did not include a strict definition of "success," had little or no follow-up, and failed to consider the influence of such confounding factors as needle size and tip design, severity of symptoms, or natural history of MPH. The true efficacy of the EBP procedure is now known to be significantly lower than once thought. Persistent or recurrent headaches following the EBP, while not necessarily requiring consultation, warrant follow-up and thoughtful reevaluation.

The EBP is associated with nearly immediate symptomatic relief in >90% of cases, but appropriate follow-up reveals a number of patients experiencing incomplete relief, failure, and recurrence. In an uncontrolled, prospective, observational study of 504 consecutive patients treated with EBP following meningeal puncture with needles of various sizes, Safa-Tisseront et al.[115] reported some relief of symptoms in 93%. Yet, upon closer analysis, complete relief of symptoms was seen in only 75% of patients, with 18% experiencing incomplete relief. They also found that the EBP was more likely to fail if the original meningeal puncture was made with needles larger than 20 gauge (Fig. 9-9). For needles larger than 20 gauge, the unqualified success rate of the EBP was only 62%, with 17% of patients reporting

incomplete relief of symptoms and 21% experiencing failure. Not surprisingly, the majority of these large needles were Tuohy epidural needles.

Expectations of success with the EBP must be further tempered in obstetric patients (all young and female) following UDP with epidural needles. Under these circumstances, Williams et al.[132] noted complete relief of symptoms with EBP in only 34% of patients, partial relief in 54%, and no relief in 7% (results unknown in 5%). If performed, a second EBP resulted in complete relief in 50%, partial relief in 36%, and no relief in 14%. In a similar patient population, Banks et al.,[114] despite initially observing complete or partial relief with EBP in 95% of patients, reported the return of moderate-to-severe symptoms in 31%, with a mean time to development of recurrent headache of 31.8 hours (range 12–96 hours). The rates of repeat EBP for the Williams and Banks studies were 27% and 19%, respectively. These studies clearly demonstrate the reduced efficacy of the EBP following meningeal punctures made with large needles, which not uncommonly make it necessary to consider repeating the procedure. Overall, success rates of a second EBP appear to be approximately equal to that of a first. The ideal timing and blood volume for repeat EBP is even more uncertain than for a primary procedure. A majority of US anesthesiologists would wait at least 24 hours after recurrence of MPH before performing a second EBP.[15] If more than one EBP is performed within a short period of time, practitioners should remain cognizant of the cumulative amount of blood used, as excessive volumes under these circumstances have been implicated in adverse outcomes.[120,121]

Insufficient evidence exists to guide management following a second failed EBP. Given the frequency of MPH and significant failure rate of the EBP, instances of sequential EBP failure are not unheard of, especially following large-gauge meningeal punctures. In an analysis of outcomes following UDP with 18-gauge Tuohy needles in an obstetric unit, Sadashivaiah[133] reported three of 48 patients (6.25%) requiring a third EBP to relieve the headache. Obviously, each failure of the EBP necessitates an even more critical reconsideration of the diagnosis. While experiences with managing repeated EBP failure have been published,[134] such sporadic case reports are insufficient to guide others. However, one frequently cited and logical recommendation regarding repeat EBP, and particularly a third EBP, is to use some form of radiologic guidance to ensure accurate epidural blood placement. Other measures under these difficult circumstances may include any of the aforementioned "treatments," with open surgical repair usually constituting a last resort.

► WHEN TO SEEK FURTHER CONSULTATION

Since MPH tends to improve even without specific treatment and the EBP has a relatively high rate of success, many practitioners reasonably seek neurologic consultation in situations where symptoms have failed to resolve after an arbitrary duration (e.g., 7–10 days) or number of EBPs (usually two or three).

Consultation is always indicated in situations where serious non-MPH is suspected or cannot reasonably be ruled out. As previously mentioned, lateralizing neurologic

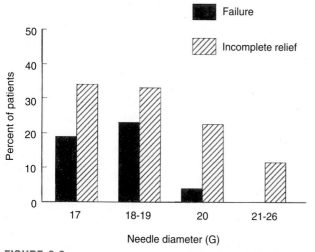

FIGURE 9-9. Percentages of patients with incomplete relief of symptoms (including failures) and failure of the EBP versus the gauge of the needle performing meningeal puncture. (Reprinted from Safa-Tisseront V, Thormann F, Malassiné P, et al. Effectiveness of epidural blood patch in the management of post-dural puncture headache. *Anesthesiology* 2001;95: 334–9, with permission.)

signs, fever/chills, seizures, or change in mental status are not consistent with a diagnosis of MPH or benign headache. Consultation is also appropriate for any headaches with atypical features. Proceeding with treatment measures directed toward MPH under uncertain circumstances may hinder a correct diagnosis, cause critical delays in proper treatment, and can prove harmful. The EBP, for example, has occasionally been reported to produce detrimental increases in intracranial pressure.

Because MPH can be anticipated to resolve spontaneously, headaches that worsen over time and no longer have a positional nature should be strongly suspected to be secondary to SDH (especially if there are focal neurologic signs or decreases in mental status). Under these circumstances, a neurologic consultation should be obtained and diagnostic radiologic studies performed.

Although headache and most associated symptoms, including auditory symptoms,[33] resolve quickly following EBP, cranial nerve palsies generally resolve slowly (within 6 months) and may appropriately prompt a neurology consult for ongoing management and reassurance.[27] Although there are no accepted treatments for cranial nerve palsy associated with MPH, it seems reasonable to treat these conditions similar to idiopathic facial nerve (CN VII) palsy ("Bell's palsy"). There is some evidence, for example, to suggest that corticosteroids administered early (within 72 hours of onset) may hasten the resolution of symptoms from Bell's palsy,[135] and similar treatment has been suggested for cranial nerve palsy following meningeal puncture.[28]

▶ SUMMARY

Over a century after being first described, MPH remains a significant clinical concern for a number of medical specialties. As with any complication, prevention is preferable to treatment. Identification and consideration of the risk factors for MPH has resulted in an impressive reduction in the incidence of this iatrogenic problem.

Unintentional meningeal puncture with epidural needles continues to be a major concern and challenge. The consequent MPH symptoms tend to be more severe, of longer duration, and more difficult to treat than those seen with smaller gauge needles. It should be noted that there is no evidence to support the two most commonly practiced prophylactic measures in this setting—aggressive hydration and encouraging bed rest. Several other prophylactic interventions after UDP appear promising, but each seems likely to be of limited value. Heterogeneity between studies and apparent publication bias toward small nonrandomized controlled trials with positive results limits the value of the available evidence.[57] Large, multicenter randomized comparative studies are needed to determine the optimal management following UDP.

Many episodes of MPH, especially those of mild-to-moderate severity, will resolve in time without specific treatment. Despite being commonly advised, hydration, bed rest, and caffeine are all of questionable value in the treatment of established MPH. Although alternatives have been proposed, the EBP remains the definitive and sole proven treatment for MPH and should be encouraged and performed early (within 24 hours of diagnosis) if symptoms are severe.

Unfortunately, the published literature concerning MPH has generally been of poor quality.[56,81,136] Many questions remain regarding the optimal means of preventing and treating this troublesome complication. Even much of what is "known" to this point has not been confirmed in follow-up studies. It is anticipated that these issues will be resolved in the future through well-designed clinical investigations.

References

1. International Headache Society. International classification of headache disorders. 2nd ed. *Cephalalgia* 2004;24(suppl 1):79.
2. Colclough GW. "Postdural" is an ambiguity. *Reg Anesth Pain Med* 2005;30:317–318.
3. Bernards CM. Sophistry in medicine: lessons from the epidural space. *Reg Anesth Pain Med* 2005;30:56–66.
4. Harrington BE. Reply to Dr. Colclough. *Reg Anesth Pain Med* 2005;30:318.
5. Neal JM, Bernards C. Reply to Dr. Colclough. *Reg Anesth Pain Med* 2005;30:318.
6. Harrington BE. Postdural puncture headache and the development of the epidural blood patch. *Reg Anesth Pain Med* 2004;29:136–163.
7. Bier A. Versuche ueber cocainsirung des rueckenmarkes. *Deutsche Zeitschrift Chirurgie* 1899;51:361–368.
8. Vandam LD, Dripps RD. Long-tern follow-up of patients who received 10,098 spinal anesthetics. Syndrome of decreased intracranial pressure (headache and ocular and auditory difficulties). *JAMA* 1956;161:586–591.
9. Hart JR, Whitacre RJ. Pencil-point needle in prevention of postspinal headache. *JAMA* 1951;147:657–658.
10. Tourtellotte WW, Haerer AF, Heller GL, et al. *Post-Lumbar Puncture Headaches.* Springfield, IL:Charles C. Thomas, 1964.
11. Moore DC. Headache. *Complications of Regional Anesthesia.* Springfield, IL: Charles C. Thomas, 1955:177–196.
12. Gormley JB. Treatment of postspinal headache. *Anesthesiology* 1960;21:565–566.
13. DiGiovanni AJ, Dunbar BS. Epidural injections of autologous blood for postlumbar-puncture headache. *Anesth Analg* 1970;49:268–271.
14. Crawford JS. Experiences with epidural blood patch. *Anaesthesia* 1980;35:513–515.
15. Harrington BE, Schmitt AM. Meningeal (postdural) puncture headache, unintentional dural puncture, and the epidural blood patch. A national survey of United States practice. *Reg Anesth Pain Med* 2009;34:430–437.
16. Choi PT, Galinski SE, Takeuchi L, et al. PDPH is a common complication of neuraxial blockade in parturients: a meta-analysis of obstetrical studies. *Can J Anesth* 2003;50:460–469.
17. Paech M, Banks S, Gurrin L. An audit of accidental dural puncture during epidural insertion of a Tuohy needle in obstetric patients. *Int J Obstet Anesth* 2001;10:162–167.
18. Vercauteren MP, Hoffmann VH, Mertens E, et al. Seven-year review of requests for epidural blood patches for headache after dural puncture: referral patterns and the effectiveness of blood patches. *Eur J Anaesthesiol* 1999;16:298–303.
19. Davies JM, Posner KL, Lee LA, et al. Liability associated with obstetric anesthesia. A closed claims analysis. *Anesthesiology* 2009;110:131–139.
20. Lee LA, Posner KL, Domino KB, et al. Injuries associated with regional anesthesia in the 1980s and 1990s: a closed claims analysis. *Anesthesiology* 2004;101:143–152.
21. Fitzgibbon DR, Posner KL, Domino KB, et al. Chronic pain management: American Society of Anesthesiologists Closed Claims Project. *Anesthesiology* 2004;100:98–105.
22. Brull R, McCartney CJL, Chan VWS, et al. Disclosure of risks associated with regional anesthesia: a survey of academic regional anesthesiologists. *Reg Anesth Pain Med* 2007;32:7–11.

23. Levine DN, Rapalino O. The pathophysiology of lumbar puncture headache. *J Neurol Sci* 2001;192:1–8.

24. Kunkle EC, Ray BS, Wolff HG. Experimental studies on headache. Analysis of the headache associated with changes in intracranial pressure. *Arch Neurol Psychiatry* 1943;49:323–358.

25. Larrier D, Lee A. Anatomy of headache and facial pain. *Otolaryngol Clin North Am* 2003;36:1041–1053.

26. Day CJE, Shutt LE. Auditory, ocular, and facial complications of central neural block. A review of possible mechanisms. *Reg Anesth* 1996;21:197–201.

27. Nishio I, Williams BA, Williams JP. Diplopia. A complication of dural puncture. *Anesthesiology* 2004;100:158–164.

28. Fang JY, Lin JW, Li Q, et al. Trigeminal nerve and facial nerve palsy after combined spinal-epidural anesthesia for cesarean section. *J Clin Anesth* 2010;22:56–58.

29. Lybecker H, Djernes M, Schmidt JF. Postdural puncture headache (PDPH): onset, duration, severity, and associated symptoms. An analysis of 75 consecutive patients with PDPH. *Acta Anaesthesiol Scand* 1995;39:605–612.

30. Aida S, Taga K, Yamakura T, et al. Headache after attempted epidural block: the role of intrathecal air. *Anesthesiology* 1998;88:76–81.

31. Reamy BV. Post-epidural headache: how late can it occur? *J Am Board Fam Med* 2009;22:202–205.

32. Chan TM, Ahmed E, Yentis SM, et al. Postpartum headaches: summary report of the National Obstetric Anaesthetic Database (NOAD) 1999. *Int J Obstet Anesth* 2003;12:107–112.

33. Sprung J, Bourke BA, Contreras MG, et al. Perioperative hearing impairment. *Anesthesiology* 2003;98:241–257.

34. Lybecker H, Moller JT, May O, et al. Incidence and prediction of postdural puncture headache: a prospective study of 1021 spinal anesthesias. *Anesth Analg* 1990;70:389–394.

35. Wu CL, Rowlingson AJ, Cohen SR, et al. Gender and post-dural puncture headache. *Anesthesiology* 2006;105:613–618.

36. Vallejo MC. Anesthetic management of the morbidly obese parturient. *Curr Opin Anaesthesiol* 2007;20:175–180.

37. Kuntz KM, Kokmen E, Stevens JC, et al. Post-lumbar puncture headaches: experience in 501 consecutive procedures. *Neurology* 1992;42:1884–1887.

38. Faure E, Moreno R, Thisted R. Incidence of postdural puncture headache in morbidly obese parturients. *Reg Anesth* 1994;19:361–363.

39. Angle P, Thompson D, Halpern S, et al. Second stage pushing correlates with headache after unintentional dural puncture in parturients. *Can J Anaesth* 1999;46:861–866.

40. Hannerz J. Postlumbar puncture headache and its relation to chronic tension-type headache. *Headache* 1997;37:659–662.

41. Bader AM. The high risk obstetric patient: neurologic and neuromuscular disease in the obstetric patient. *Anesthesiol Clin North Am* 1998;16:459–476.

42. Echevarria M, Caba F, Rodriguez R. The influence of the menstrual cycle in postdural puncture headache. *Reg Anesth Pain Med* 1998;23:485–490.

43. Amorim JA, Valenca MM. Postdural puncture headache is a risk factor for new postdural puncture headache. *Cephalalgia* 2007;28:5–8.

44. Blanche R, Eisenach JC, Tuttle R, et al. Previous wet tap does not reduce success rate of labor epidural analgesia. *Anesth Analg* 1994;79:291–294.

45. Halpern S, Preston R. Postdural puncture headache and spinal needle design. Metaanalysis. *Anesthesiology* 1994;81:1376–1383.

46. Kovanen J, Sulkava R. Duration of postural headache after lumbar puncture: effect of needle size. *Headache* 1986;26:224–226.

47. Lambert DH, Hurley RJ, Hertwig L, et al. Role of needle gauge and tip configuration in the production of lumbar puncture headache. *Reg Anesth* 1997;22:66–72.

48. Reina MA, de Leon-Casasola OA, Lopez A, et al. An *in vitro* study of dural lesions produced by 25-gauge Quincke and Whitacre needles evaluated by scanning electron microscopy. *Reg Anesth Pain Med* 2000;25:393–402.

49. Richman J, Joe E, Cohen S, et al. Bevel direction and postdural puncture headache. A meta-analysis. *Neurologist* 2006;12:224–228.

50. Reina MA, Dittmann M, Garcia AL, et al. New perspectives in the microscopic structure of human dura mater in the dorsolumbar region. *Reg Anesth* 1997;22:161–166.

51. Seeberger MD, Kaufmann M, Staender S, et al. Repeated dural punctures increase the incidence of postdural puncture headache. *Anesth Analg* 1996;82:302–305.

52. Singh S, Chaudry SY, Phelps AL, et al. A 5-year audit of accidental dural punctures, postdural puncture headaches, and failed regional anesthetics at a tertiary-care medical center. *ScientificWorldJournal* 2009;9:715–722.

53. Goldszmidt E, Kern R, Chaput A, et al. The incidence and etiology of postpartum headaches: a prospective cohort study. *Can J Anesth* 2005;52:971–977.

54. Aya AGM, Manguin R, Robert C, et al. Increased risk of unintentional dural puncture in night-time obstetric epidural anaesthesia. *Can J Anesth* 1999;46:665–669.

55. Paech MJ, Whybrow T. The prevention and treatment of post dural puncture headache. *ASEAN J Anaesthesiol* 2007;8:86–95.

56. Warwick WI, Neal JM. Beyond spinal headache: prophylaxis and treatment of low-pressure headache syndromes. *Reg Anesth Pain Med* 2007;32:455–461.

57. Apfel CC, Saxena OS, Cakmakkaya OS, et al. Prevention of postdural puncture headache after accidental dural puncture: a quantitative systematic review. *Br J Anaesth* 2010;105:255–263.

58. Perlas A. Evidence for the use of ultrasound in neuraxial blocks. *Reg Anesth Pain Med* 2010;35 (suppl 1):S43–S46.

59. Yucel A, Ozyalcin S, Talu GK, et al. Intravenous administration of caffeine sodium benzoate for postdural puncture headache. *Reg Anesth Pain Med* 1999;24:51–54.

60. Esmaoglu A, Akpinar H, Ugur F. Oral multidose caffeine-paracetamol combination is not effective for the prophylaxis of postdural puncture headache. *J Clin Anesth* 2005;17:58–61.

61. Halker RB, Demaerschalk BM, Wellik KE, et al. Caffeine for the prevention and treatment of postdural puncture headache: debunking the myth. *Neurologist* 2007;13:323–327.

62. Bussone G, Tullo V, d'Onofrio F, et al. Frovatriptan for the prevention of postdural puncture headache. *Cephalalgia* 2007;27:809–813.

63. Sudlow C, Warlow C. Posture and fluids for preventing postdural puncture headache. *Cochrane Database Syst Rev* 2002;(2):CD001790.

64. Baraz R, Collis R. The management of accidental dural puncture during labor epidural analgesia: a survey of UK practice. *Anaesthesia* 2005;60:673–679.

65. Strupp M, Brandt T, Muller A. Incidence of post-lumbar puncture syndrome reduced by reinserting the stylet: a randomized prospective study of 600 patients. *J Neurol* 1998;245:589–592.

66. Moore JM. Continuous spinal anesthesia. *Am J Ther* 2009;16:289–294.

67. Schier R, Guerra D, Aguilar J, et al. Epidural space identification: a meta-analysis of complications after air versus liquid as the medium for loss of resistance. *Anesth Analg* 2009;109:2012–2021.

68. Segal S, Arendt KW. A retrospective effectiveness study of loss of resistance to air or saline for identification of the epidural space. *Anesth Analg* 2010;110:558–563.

69. Norris MC, Leighton BL, DeSimone CA. Needle bevel direction and headache after inadvertent dural puncture. *Anesthesiology* 1989;70:729–731.

70. Duffy B. Don't turn the needle! *Anaesth Intensive Care* 1993;21:328–330.

71. Simmons SW, Cyna AM, Dennis AT, et al. Combined spinal-epidural versus epidural analgesia in labour. *Cochrane Database Syst Rev* 2009;(1):CD003401.

72. Kuczkowski KM, Benumof JL. Decrease in the incidence of postdural puncture headache: maintaining CSF volume. *Acta Anaesthesiol Scand* 2003;47:98–100.

73. Charsley MM, Abram SE. The injection of intrathecal normal saline reduces the severity of postdural puncture headache. *Reg Anesth Pain Med* 2001;26:301–305.

74. Ayad S, Bemian Y, Narouze S, et al. Subarachnoid catheter placement after wet tap for analgesia in labor: influence on the risk of headache in obstetric patients. *Reg Anesth Pain Med* 2003;28:512–515.

75. Turkoz A, Kocum A, Eker HE, et al. Intrathecal catheterization after unintentional dural puncture during orthopedic surgery. *J Anesth* 2010;24(1):43–48.

76. Newman M, Cyna A. Immediate management of inadvertent dural puncture during insertion of a labour epidural: a survey of Australian obstetric anaesthetists. *Anaesth Intensive Care* 2008;36:96–101.

77. Stride PC, Cooper GM. Dural taps revisited: a 20-year survey from Birmingham maternity hospital. *Anaesthesia* 1993;48:247–255.

78. Trivedi NS, Eddi D, Shevde K. Headache prevention following accidental dural puncture in obstetric patients. *J Clin Anesth* 1993;5:42–45.

79. Al-metwalli RR. Epidural morphine injections for prevention of post dural puncture headache. *Anaesthesia* 2008;63:847–850.

80. Scavone BM, Wong CA, Sullivan JT, et al. Efficacy of a prophylactic epidural blood patch in preventing post dural puncture headache in parturients after inadvertent dural puncture. *Anesthesiology* 2004;101:1422–1427.

81. Boonmak P, Boonmak S. Epidural blood patching for preventing and treating post-dural puncture headache. *Cochrane Database Syst Rev* 2010;(1):CD001791.

82. Leivers D. Total spinal anesthesia following early prophylactic epidural blood patch. *Anesthesiology* 1990;73:1287–1289.

83. Tobias MD, Pilla MA, Rogers C, et al. Lidocaine inhibits blood coagulation: implications for epidural blood patch. *Anesth Analg* 1996;82:766–769.

84. Carter BL, Pasupuleti R. Use of intravenous cosyntropin in the treatment of postdural puncture headache. *Anesthesiology* 2000;92:272–274.

85. Hakim SM. Cosyntropin for prophylaxis against postdural puncture headache after accidental dural puncture. *Anesthesiology* 2010;113:413–420.

86. Gutsche BB. Lumbar epidural analgesia in obstetrics: taps and patches. In: Reynolds F, ed. *Epidural and Spinal Blockade in Obstetrics*. London, UK: Balliere Tindall, 1990:75–106.

87. Naulty JS, Hertwig L, Hunt CO, et al. Influence of local anesthetic solution on postdural puncture headache. *Anesthesiology* 1990;72:450–454.

88. Santanen U, Rautoma P, Luurila H, et al. Comparison of 27-gauge (0.41-mm) Whitacre and Quincke spinal needles with respect to post-dural puncture headache and non-dural puncture headache. *Acta Anaesthesiol Scand* 2004;48:474–479.

89. Stella CL, Jodicke CD, How HY, et al. Postpartum headache: is your work-up complete? *Am J Obstet Gynecol* 2007;196:318.e1–318.e7.

90. Somri M, Teszler CB, Vaida SJ, et al. Postdural puncture headache: an imaging-guided management protocol. *Anesth Analg* 2003;96:1809–1812.

91. Sharma R, Panda A. Ondansetron-induced headache in a parturient mimicking postdural puncture headache. *Can J Anesth* 2010;57:187–188.

92. van de Beek D, Drake JM, Tunkel AR. Nosocomial bacterial meningitis. *N Engl J Med* 2010;362:146–154.

93. Machurot PY, Vergnion M, Fraipont V, et al. Intracranial subdural hematoma following spinal anesthesia: case report and review of the literature. *Acta Anaesthesiol Belg* 2010;61:63–66.

94. Bleeker CP, Hendriks IM, Booij LHDJ. Postpartum post-dural puncture headache: is your differential diagnosis complete? *Br J Anaesth* 2004;93:461–464.

95. Matthys LA, Coppage KH, Lambers DS, et al. Delayed postpartum preeclampsia: an experience of 151 cases. *Am J Obstet Gynecol* 2004;190:1464–1466.

96. Lockhart EM, Baysinger CL. Intracranial venous thrombosis in the parturient. *Anesthesiology* 2007;107:652–658.

97. Vanden Eede H, Hoffmann VLH, Vercauteren MP. Post-delivery postural headache: not always a classical post-dural puncture headache. *Acta Anaesthesiol Scand* 2007;51:763–765.

98. van Kooten F, Oedit R, Bakker SLM, et al. Epidural blood patch in post dural puncture headache: a randomized, observer-blind, controlled clinical trial. *J Neurol Neurosurg Psychiatry* 2008;79:553–558.

99. Sharma A, Cheam E. Acupuncture in the management of postpartum headache following neuraxial analgesia. *Int J Obstet Anesth* 2009;18:417–419.

100. Takmaz SA, Kantekin CU, Kaymak C, et al. Treatment of postdural puncture headache with bilateral greater occipital nerve block. *Headache* 2010;50:869–872.

101. Choi A, Laurito CE, Cummingham FE. Pharmacologic management of postdural puncture headache. *Ann Pharmacother* 1996;30:831–839.

102. Camann WR, Murray RS, Mushlin PS, et al. Effects of oral caffeine on postdural puncture headache. A double-blind, placebo-controlled trial. *Anesth Analg* 1990;70:181–184.

103. Connelly NR, Parker RK, Rahimi A, et al. Sumatriptan in patients with postdural puncture headache. *Headache* 2000;40:316–319.

104. Rucklidge MWM, Yentis SM, Paech MJ, et al. Synacthen depot for the treatment of postdural puncture headache. *Anaesthesia* 2004;59:138–141.

105. Ashraf N, Sadeghi A, Azarbakht Z, et al. Hydrocortisone in post-dural puncture headache. *Middle East J Anesthesiol* 2007;19:415–422.

106. Hakim S, Khan RM, Maroof M, et al. Methylergonovine maleate (methergine) relieves postdural puncture headache in obstetric patients. *Acta Obstet Gynecol Scand* 2005;84:100.

107. Lin YT, Sheen MJ, Huang ST, et al. Gabapentin relieves postdural puncture headache—a report of two cases. *Acta Anaesthesiol Taiwan* 2007;45:47–50.

108. Kroin JS, Nagalla SKS, Buvanendran A, et al. The mechanisms of intracranial pressure modulation by epidural blood and other injectates in a postdural puncture rat model. *Anesth Analg* 2002;95:423–429.

109. Bart AJ, Wheeler AS. Comparison of epidural saline placement and epidural blood placement in the treatment of post-lumbar-puncture headache. *Anesthesiology* 1978;48:221–223.

110. Liu SK, Chen KB, Wu RSC, et al. Management of postdural puncture headache by epidural saline delivered with a patient-controlled pump—a case report. *Acta Anaesthesiol Taiwan* 2006;44:227–230.

111. Vakharia SB, Thomas PS, Rosenbaum AE, et al. Magnetic resonance imaging of cerebrospinal fluid leak and tamponade effect of blood patch in postdural puncture headache. *Anesth Analg* 1997;84:585–590.

112. Serpell MG, Haldane GJ, Jamieson DR, et al. Prevention of headache after lumbar puncture: questionnaire survey of neurologists and neurosurgeons in United Kingdom. *Br Med J* 1998;316:1709–1710.

113. Darvish B, Gupta A, Alahuhta S, et al. Management of accidental dural puncture and post-dural puncture headache after labour: a Nordic survey. *Acta Anaesthesiol Scand* 2011;55:46–53.

114. Banks S, Paech M, Gurrin L. An audit of epidural blood patch after accidental dural puncture with a Tuohy needle in obstetric patients. *Int J Obstet Anesth* 2001;10:172–176.

115. Safa-Tisseront V, Thormann F, Malassine P, et al. Effectiveness of epidural blood patch in the management of post-dural puncture headache. *Anesthesiology* 2001;95:334–339.

116. Sandesc D, Lupei MI, Sirbu C, et al. Conventional treatment or epidural blood patch for the treatment of different etiologies of post dural puncture headache. *Acta Anaesthesiol Belg* 2005;56:265–269.

117. Vilming ST, Kloster R, Sandvik L. When should an epidural blood patch be performed in postlumbar puncture headache? A theoretical approach based on a cohort of 79 patients. *Cephalalgia* 2005;25:523–527.

118. Chen LK, Huang CH, Jean WH, et al. Effective epidural blood patch volumes for postdural puncture headache in Taiwanese women. *J Formos Med Assoc* 2007;106:134–140.

119. Schievink WI. Spontaneous spinal cerebrospinal fluid leaks and intracranial hypotension. *JAMA* 2006;295:2286–2296.

120. Riley CA, Spiegel JE. Compliations following large-volume epidural blood patches for postdural puncture headaches. Lumbar subdural hematoma and arachnoiditis: initial cause or final effect? *J Clin Anesth* 2009;21:355–359.

121. Desai MJ, Dave AP, Martin MB. Delayed radicular pain following two large volume epidural blood patches for post-lumbar puncture headache: a case report. *Pain Physician* 2010;13:257–262.

122. Martin R, Jourdain S, Clairoux M, et al. Duration of decubitus position after epidural blood patch. *Can J Anaesth* 1994;41:23–25.

123. Bucklin BA, Tinker JH, Smith CV. Clinical dilemma: a patient with postdural puncture headache and acute leukemia. *Anesth Analg* 1999;88:166–167.

124. Tom DJ, Gulevich SJ, Shapiro HM, et al. Epidural blood patch in the HIV-positive patient. *Anesthesiology* 1992;76:943–947.

125. Martin DP, Bergman BD, Berger IH. Epidural blood patch and acute varicella. *Anesth Analg* 2004;99:1760–1762.

126. Jagannathan N, Tetzlaff JE. Epidural blood patch in a Jehovah's Witness patient with post-dural puncture cephalgia. *Can J Anaesth* 2005;52:113.

127. Janssens E, Aerssens P, Alliet P, et al. Post-dural puncture headaches in children: a literature review. *Eur J Pediatr* 2003;162:117–121.

128. Waldman SD, Feldstein GS, Allen ML. Cervical epidural blood patch: a safe effective treatment for cervical post-dural puncture headache. *Anesthesiol Rev* 1987;14:23–24.

129. Abouleish E, de La Vega S, Blendinger I, et al. Long-term follow-up of epidural blood patch. *Anesth Analg* 1975;54:459–463.

130. Andrews PJD, Ackerman WE, Juneja M, et al. Transient bradycardia associated with extradural blood patch after inadvertent dural puncture in parturients. *Br J Anaesth* 1992;69:401–403.

131. Hebl JR, Horlocker TT, Chantigian RC, et al. Epidural anesthesia and analgesia are not impaired after dural puncture with or without epidural blood patch. *Anesth Analg* 1999;89:390–394.

132. Williams EJ, Beaulieu P, Fawcett WJ, et al. Efficacy of epidural blood patch in the obstetric population. *Int J Obstet Anesth* 1999;8:105–109.

133. Sadashivaiah J. 18-G Tuohy needle can reduce the incidence of severe post dural puncture headache. *Anaesthesia* 2009;64:1379–1380.

134. Ho KY, Gan TJ. Management of persistent post-dural puncture headache after repeated epidural blood patch. *Acta Anaesthesiol Scand* 2007;51:633–636.

135. Sullivan FM, Swan IRC, Donnan PT, et al. Early treatment with prednisone or acyclovir in Bell's palsy. *N Engl J Med* 2007;357:1598–1607.

136. Choi PTL, Galinski SE, Lucas S, et al. Examining the evidence in anesthesia literature: a survey and evaluation of obstetrical post-dural puncture headache reports. *Can J Anaesth* 2002;49:49–56.

Neuraxis Mechanical Injury

Joseph M. Neal

Mechanical injury to the neuraxis as a consequence of regional anesthesia techniques may occur directly or indirectly. Direct spinal cord injury results from mechanical damage secondary to needle or catheter placement. Indirect spinal cord injury may result from a variety of conditions that lead to spinal cord ischemia, such as space-occupying lesions in the form of spinal hematoma, epidural abscess, or spinal stenosis. Once mechanical damage occurs, previously innocuous agents such as local anesthetics or additives may worsen the damage, particularly if the blood/spinal cord barrier becomes compromised. Many of these processes are presented in detail in chapters on bleeding complications (Chapter 4), infectious complications (Chapter 5), local anesthetic neurotoxicity (Chapter 11), and ischemic complications (Chapter 12). The intent of this chapter is to focus on isolated mechanical injury and the pathophysiology of mass lesions within the neuraxis.

DEFINITION

This chapter defines mechanical neuraxis injury as fulfilling one of two criteria. The first, direct mechanical injury, encompasses those circumstances in which a needle or catheter directly damages the spinal vasculature, the spinal cord, or a spinal nerve. The second way in which mechanical damage is defined is indirect mechanical injury. In these circumstances, a mass lesion competes for area within the spinal canal, epidural space, or subarachnoid space and exerts sufficient pressure on blood inflow and/or outflow to cause spinal cord ischemia. Examples of such space-occupying lesions include hematoma, abscess, epidural fat, and spinal stenosis from bony overgrowth or soft tissue hyperplasia[1] (Box 10-1).

SCOPE

Neuraxis injury consequent to mechanical trauma is a decidedly rare event, and therefore reliable incidence data do not exist. Awareness of these complications comes from isolated case reports and large surveys of regional anesthesia complications. In the American Society of Anesthesiologists (ASA) Closed Claims Study,[2] approximately half of major nerve damage claims were the direct result of neuraxis injury from hematoma, abscess, direct trauma, or vascular insults. Only 12 of 84 (12%) neuraxial injuries were associated with anterior spinal artery syndrome (ASAS) or spinal cord infarct; while 25% of permanent spinal cord injuries during chronic pain management procedures were associated with direct needle trauma.[2] A recognized limitation of the Closed Claims Study is that denominators are unknown, and therefore precise incidences cannot be determined. This methodology may also suffer reporting bias consequent to

BOX 10-1 Causes of Mechanical Injury to the Spinal Cord

Direct needle or catheter injury

    Spinal cord injury
    Spinal nerve injury
    Spinal vasculature injury
    Anterior spinal artery syndrome

Indirect spinal cord injury

    Intradural mass lesions
    Extradural mass lesions
    Epidural hematoma or abscess
    Epidural lipomatosis or tumor
    Spinal stenosis
    Positioning-associated injury

its medicolegal source. French regional anesthesia surveillance data[3,4] do not specifically report direct spinal cord or nerve root mechanical injury, but the 95% confidence interval for neurologic injury after 40,640 spinal anesthetics was 3.5 to 8.3 per 10,000 and 0.4 to 3.6 per 10,000 after 30,413 epidural anesthetics.[4] ASAS is particularly rare. Only 1 of 57 cases of acute spinal cord ischemia syndrome that presented over a 12-year period to a single referral institution was associated with neuraxial anesthesia.[5] In the 2006 to 2007 National Audit Project of the Royal College of Anaesthetists (RCA), spinal cord ischemia occurred in 4 of an estimated 700,000 neuraxial procedures, but it was difficult to determine in these frail, elderly patients whether the etiology was directly attributable to their epidural anesthetic or other factors.[6] Although the exact incidence is difficult to determine, it is clear that once neuraxial injury occurs it is often permanent. For instance, 100% of spinal cord infarct claims, 88% of epidural hematoma claims, and 80% of ASAS claims in the ASA Closed Claims database were associated with permanent injury.[2] In the 1997 French surveillance study, 15% of all neurologic injuries remained after 3 months[4]; while the RCA study reported 30% of nerve injuries after neuraxial block remaining after 6 months, and permanence after all ischemic cord injuries.[6]

In contrast to data on direct spinal cord injury, information regarding spinal cord ischemia as a consequence of mass lesions is more readily available. Analysis of 1990 to 1999 Swedish data for hematoma after neuraxial block reveals an incidence of 1.9 hematomas per 100,000 patients. Furthermore, the incidence varied widely between patient groups—from 1:200,000 for young obstetrical patients to 1:3,600 for elderly females undergoing knee replacement.[7] The high rates in the knee replacement group may reflect an increased rate of hematoma consequent to the increased use of powerful perioperative thromboprophylaxis drugs and increased propensity for neuraxial compression because of underlying spinal stenosis, both of which are not typical comorbidities in young parturients. Epidural abscess occurs in 1:1,930 to 5,000 catheters. The higher incidence is associated with immunocompromised patients with longer duration of catheterization and/or anticoagulation.[8]

▶ PATHOPHYSIOLOGY

Direct Mechanical Injury

In case of direct spinal cord injury, the mechanism of injury is seldom known with certainty. Similarly, with the exception of a small number of animal studies, the explanations offered to explain vascular injury (that needles directly injure feeding vasculature or that vascular irritation from needles or injected substances leads to vasospasm) are speculative.[9]

Spinal Cord Injury

The spinal cord or spinal nerves can be traumatized directly by needle or catheter placement. How this complication can occur and yet at the time be unrecognized by the anesthesiologist or the patient is of particular interest.

That needle- or catheter-induced spinal cord trauma is not reported more frequently is remarkable considering vertebral column surface anatomy and the anatomy of the neuraxis itself. Direct trauma to the spinal cord can occur by several mechanisms. First is misidentification of vertebral interspace level during the performance of spinal anesthesia.[7] Traditional teaching states that the caudad terminus of the spinal cord is the L1-2 interspace. However, the pediatric spinal cord typically ends several interspaces caudad to this and the adult spinal cord terminates as low as L4-5 in a small percentage of individuals.[10] Moreover, anesthesiologists commonly misidentify the lumbar interspace by plus or minus one interspace.[7,11] Particularly in patients in whom surface landmark identification is problematic, the spinal cord may actually reside directly beneath the selected interspace, even when using a low lumbar approach. Two anatomic peculiarities further complicate this situation. First, the ligamentum flavum may incompletely fuse at its most posterior point,[12,13] thus failing to provide a sufficient firmness from which to appreciate the loss of resistance and thereby risking unintended meningeal puncture. Second, as one moves cephalad along the vertebral column the distance between the ligamentum flavum and the dura progressively narrows, from 4 to 5 mm in the lumbar area to 1 to 2 mm in the cervical and high thoracic levels.[14] Indeed, it is rather surprising that needles or catheters do not contact the spinal cord more frequently than they apparently do. Alternatively, inconsequential spinal cord contact may occur but be unrecognized.

A common misconception is that needle or catheter contact with the spinal cord is always heralded by a painful paresthesia-like sensation.[15] Like the brain the spinal cord is devoid of sensory innervation. Case reports document neuroimaging evidence of spinal cord penetration that occurred without recognition by unanesthetized patients undergoing spinal or epidural anesthesia.[16–18] In some cases, patients become aware of the presence of a foreign object near the spinal cord when sensory fibers within the meninges[19] are stimulated.[20,21] Why patients inconsistently recognize[20] or fail to recognize[16–18] the presence of a needle or catheter touching or penetrating the spinal cord is incompletely understood, although the presence of local anesthetic in the epidural space can significantly lessen the awareness of meningeal puncture.[22] Furthermore, medullary penetration does not necessarily result in permanent injury. For example, a patient who sustained unintentional intramedullary spinal catheter placement noted pain upon awakening from general anesthesia, but ultimately suffered no permanent neurologic injury.[23] Conversely, an elderly man who suffered permanent injury after placement of a thoracic epidural under general anesthesia was initially unaware of sensory and motor deficits probably because of the infusion of local anesthetic through an unrecognized intramedullary catheter.[24]

Paresthesia elicited during spinal and epidural needle placement is relatively common (6.3% in a retrospective series of 4,767 spinal anesthetics).[25] A needle-induced paresthesia during subarachnoid block has been shown in 87% of occurrences to herald presumably the correct needle placement (as evidenced by the return of cerebrospinal fluid [CSF]).[26] Although a paresthesia during block placement has been associated with an increased risk of a persistent paresthesia,[25] this relationship is inconsistent.[2–4] Moreover, the incidence of paresthesia is vastly greater than the incidence of neuraxial injury. In summary, case reports note that spinal cord penetration with or without injection of local anesthetic may not always be apparent to a patient or anesthesiologist and may not always be associated with neurologic deficit.

Injection of local anesthetic, opioid, or additives into the spinal cord may present a different scenario, in terms of both recognition and injury. Case reports of spinal cord injury associated with injection of anesthetic solution[21] suggest that patients are more likely to recognize this event, presumably because volume-induced deformation of the spinal cord results in massive neural discharge as compared to the relatively atraumatic passage of a needle. Permanent neurologic damage may follow intramedullary injection, as a consequence of physical deformity and/or local anesthetic neurotoxicity.[24] For example, the intramedullary injection of local anesthetic during intended interscalene brachial plexus block performed on anesthetized patients has resulted in central syrinx formation and permanent paralysis.[27] In awake patients, the sequence of painful injection of neuraxial local anesthetic followed by magnetic resonance imaging (MRI) documentation of an intramedullary lesion and permanent neural deficit has been described in several case series and individual case reports.[21,28]

Spinal Nerve Injury

The spinal nerves represent the joined anterior and posterior nerve roots as they pass through the intervertebral foramen. Temporary and permanent injury to the spinal nerves, presumably from direct needle trauma, has been reported in the French surveillance, the ASA Closed Claims, and other large-scale studies.[2–4,6,7] During standard interlaminar approaches, needles and catheters are directed toward the central cord and thus spinal nerve injury is unlikely. However, transforaminal techniques, perivertebral approaches (such as posterior lumbar plexus or paravertebral blocks), or needles that are unintentionally off target could encounter a spinal nerve either within the foramen or as the nerve exits toward the periphery (Fig. 10-1). Stenosis of the intervertebral foramina might further increase the likelihood of nerve root trauma, because a relatively tethered nerve would be less likely to slip away from an approaching needle.

Vascular Injury

Spinal cord blood supply consists of a variable and incomplete network of arteries and arterioles that branches from larger segmental arteries (Fig. 10-2). The spinal cord is primarily served by three to four major spinal medullary arteries, which

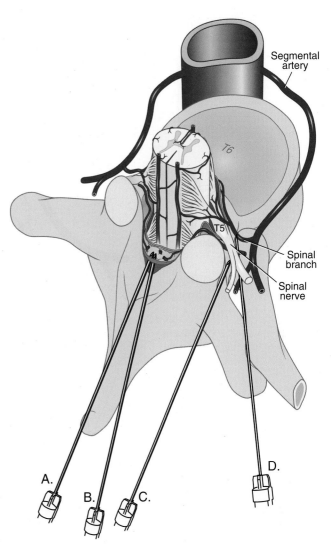

FIGURE 10-1. **Potential sites of needle injury to the neuraxis.** Midline **(A)** or paramedian interlaminar approaches **(B)** are unlikely to be associated with needle contact with a spinal nerve. Intentionally, lateral approaches **(C)**, such as would be used for celiac plexus block or paravertebral block, or transforaminal injections **(D)** potentially allow needle contact with spinal nerves or spinal arteries.

are extensions of spinal radicular arteries and supply oxygen and nutrients to three major territories: the cervical cord, the upper and midthoracic cord, and the lower thoracic/lumbosacral cord[29] (see Fig. 12–2). The cervical cord arterial supply is typically derived from the vertebral or costocervical arteries, whereas the upper and midthoracic arterial supply comes from a cervicothoracic or a high thoracic segment from the aorta. A single major artery (the radicularis magna or artery of Adamkiewicz) typically supplies the lower thoracic/lumbosacral cord. The cervical and lower thoracic/lumbosacral spinal cord segments are functionally larger than the midthoracic segment, reflecting their innervation of the extremities. Major spinal cord feeder arteries tend to be unilateral (most often left-sided), and, in the case of the radicularis magna, most commonly originate between the T9 and L1 levels[30,31] (Chapter 12). The anterior spinal artery and paired posterior spinal arteries are ultimately supplied by this network of segmental reinforcing arteries. Because of their vulnerability as they course laterally along the vertebral bodies and through the intervertebral foramina, it is the segmental arteries and

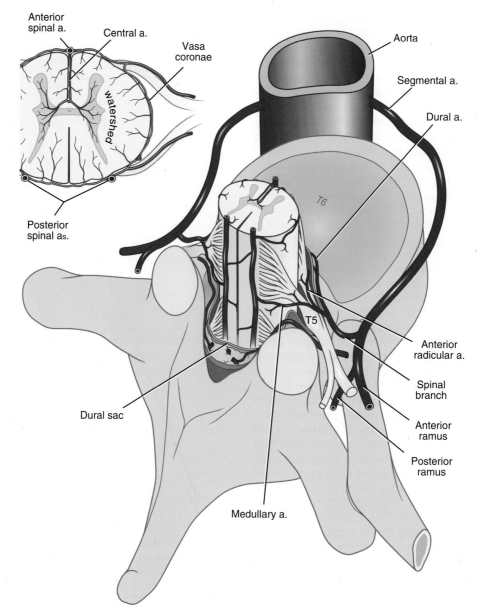

FIGURE 10-2. **Arterial vascular supply to the spinal cord.** Segmental vessels branch from the vertebral or costocervical arteries, or from the aorta. Most spinal segmental arteries become a single anterior or posterior radicular artery that supplies the spinal nerve roots. Radicular arteries that continue on to the spinal cord are termed medullary arteries, which anastomose across spinal segment levels to become the anterior spinal artery and the paired posterior spinal arteries.

their immediate branches that are most at risk for mechanical injury.

The radicularis magna represents the most commonly implicated artery for direct needle injury. Judging by anatomy, direct injury to this artery should be very rare during spinal or epidural anesthesia because the midline or interlaminar approaches are distant from the intervertebral foramina (through which the major feeder arteries pass). However, anesthetic or pain management techniques that use a more lateral approach to their target (celiac plexus, paravertebral, or transforaminal blocks) may contact a major segmental artery. Needle trauma could damage the artery, or more likely mechanical irritation or injection of substances such as alcohol or phenol could cause vasospasm[32] and compromise spinal circulation (Fig. 10-3). Indeed, several case reports of neurologic symptoms after celiac plexus block

have postulated chemically induced vasospasm as the mechanism of injury.[33,34]

Mechanical damage to an individual spinal segmental artery as it courses through an intervertebral foramen is unlikely to precipitate spinal cord ischemia. This pathophysiologic assumption recognizes that the majority of spinal segmental arteries terminate as radicular arteries and that most of the few radicular arteries that continue to the spinal cord as medullary arteries will make only minor contributions to the anterior or posterior spinal arteries. A nonrobust collateral arterial circulation also exists between adjacent spinal cord segments. In contradistinction to true mechanical injury, injection of particulate material into a spinal segmental artery as it enters the intervertebral foramen has been proposed to explain spinal cord or brain stem infarction, or cortical blindness after transforaminal injection of particulate

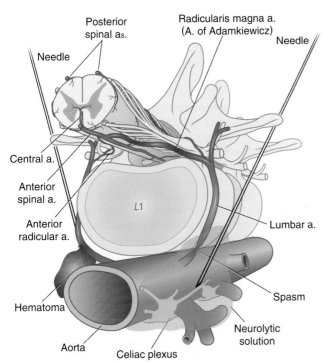

FIGURE 10-3. Needles may directly injure segmental arteries during celiac plexus block or other paravertebral approaches. The left-hand needle illustrates direct vascular trauma with hematoma formation. The right-hand needle precipitated vasospasm as a result of mechanical irritation or chemical irritation from phenol or alcohol. These mechanisms of injury are speculative and have not been proven in humans.

steroid preparations.[35] In these cases, it is speculated that steroidal particulate matter blocks circulation to watershed areas of the spinal cord[36,37] (Chapter 28).

Anterior Spinal Artery Syndrome

ASAS describes the sudden painless onset of lower extremity weakness and variable sensory deficit, with relative preservation of proprioception. This entity has been postulated as a cause of paralysis after neuraxial regional anesthetic techniques, yet critical review of pathophysiology and case reports gives reason to question these assumptions. ASAS likely occurs as a result of a vascular accident affecting the anterior spinal artery, which supplies the cauda equina and the anterior two-thirds of the spinal cord, or a primary spinal medullary artery that feeds the anterior spinal artery. Mechanical injury to a major feeder artery (e.g., the radicularis magna) is improbable during neuraxial techniques because the needle path should be well clear of the artery's course within the intervertebral foramina. Further, direct needle injury to the anterior spinal artery can only occur if the needle penetrates the spinal cord, which would likely be seen on subsequent neuroimaging (Fig. 10-1).

Another proposed mechanism for ASAS is intraoperative hypotension, which assumes that decreased blood pressure results in spinal cord ischemia. In normal patients, this explanation is unlikely because: (i) spinal cord blood flow is autoregulated within mean arterial blood pressures (MAPs) of 50–65 to 120 mm Hg,[38,39] (ii) spinal cord metabolic need is reduced by the presence of volatile and local anesthetics,[40,41] and (iii) patients with little to no blood pressure for brief periods

of time (cardiac arrest survivors) or with longer periods of reduced MAP (normothermic cardiopulmonary bypass or induced hypotension techniques) very rarely suffer spinal cord infarction. The precise lower limits of autoregulation in humans have been questioned.[42] A more detailed discussion of this topic can be found in Chapter 12. Vasoconstrictors such as epinephrine are unlikely to cause ASAS, as they do not adversely affect blood flow to otherwise normal spinal cords.[43] The most likely etiology of ASAS during the perioperative period is atherosclerosis with or without embolization of plaque material to the spinal circulation.[44] Importantly, the exact mechanism of ASAS is poorly understood and may well involve a combination of spinal vasculature atherosclerosis and postlesion hypoperfusion, neither of which are predictable or under the anesthesiologist's direct control.

Indirect Spinal Cord Injury

Mass lesions within the neuraxis can either directly compress the spinal cord (Fig. 10-4) or cause increases in epidural or subarachnoid space pressures as compensatory CSF volume displacement reaches its limit. Blood flow to the spinal cord becomes compromised as extrinsic pressure exceeds arterial inflow, venous outflow, and/or capillary perfusion pressure. The result is spinal cord ischemia, which if uncorrected within minutes to hours may cause spinal cord infarction.

Intradural Mass Lesions

Most spinal cord tumors of sufficient size to affect neuraxial pressure-volume dynamics are typically accompanied by obvious neurologic deficit. A more insidious intrathecal mass lesion complicates long-term continuous intrathecal opioid infusion. Case reports describe intrathecal granulomas that form around implanted subarachnoid catheters used to deliver central nervous system (CNS) opioids, including tramadol.[45–47] These granulomas apparently form as a function of opioid dose and infusion duration and are unaffected by the presence or absence of additives such as clonidine. The patient and treating physician are unaware of the presence of the granuloma until rapidly escalating dosing requirements are needed to achieve the same level of analgesia. The granuloma may cause neurologic symptoms such as radicular pain and/or motor weakness, which can present suddenly.

Extradural Mass Lesions
Epidural Hematoma and Epidural Abscess

Blood or infection within the epidural space can exert a mass effect that impedes arterial blood ingress and/or venous blood egress, which results in spinal cord ischemia and eventual infarction. Details of these two major complications can be found in Chapters 4 and 5.

Epidural Lipomatosis and Epidural Tumor Metastasis

Rarely, individuals may have excess epidural fat stores—an unpredictable condition known as epidural lipomatosis, which has been associated with neurologic symptoms during otherwise routine epidural anesthesia. Isolated case reports describe patients whose neuraxial block fails to resolve. Subsequent neuroimaging and/or decompressive laminectomy reveal large deposits of epidural fat.[48] The proposed pathophysiology involves sustained epidural space pressures from the combination of local anesthetic and fat stores competing

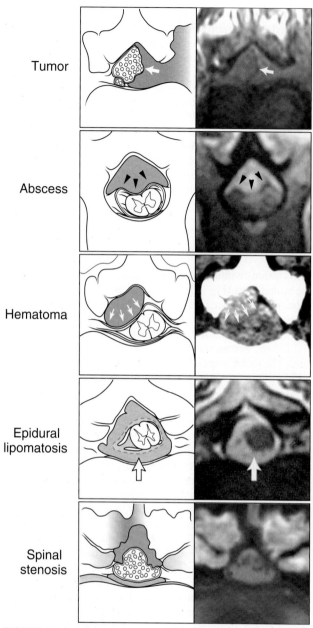

Tumor

Abscess

Hematoma

Epidural
lipomatosis

Spinal
stenosis

FIGURE 10-4. **Various extradural lesions can exert a mass effect on the neuraxis.** *Arrows* represent compression of the spinal cord or cauda equina. In the top frame, perispinal metastasis extends into the epidural space. In the second and third frames, an epidural abscess and epidural hematoma compress and displace the spinal cord. The fourth frame illustrates spinal cord impingement by massive epidural lipomatosis. The final frame shows reduced cross-sectional area of the central canal secondary to hypertrophy of the ligamentum flavum and surrounding bony elements.

for limited volume within the epidural space. Alternatively, the fat can directly compress the spinal cord. If abnormal pressures are sustained, spinal cord blood flow is compromised (Fig. 10-4). These clinical observations are consistent with experimental evidence that disease within the epidural space alters its pressure/volume relationships.[49]

A similar mechanism is proposed for those patients who have suffered neurologic deficits associated with epidural anesthesia, and in whom the diagnosis of previously unrecognized epidural tumor is made[50] (Fig. 10-4). Patients with multiple myeloma, lung, prostate, and breast cancer

are particularly predisposed to epidural metastasis.[51] Other mass lesions—such as lumbar ependymoma,[52] diabetic scleredema,[53] or synovial cysts[54,55]—have also been associated with paraplegia after neuraxial anesthesia.[1]

Spinal Stenosis

Spinal stenosis is a nonspecific term that refers to decreased cross-sectional area of the central spinal canal. Several anatomic abnormalities contribute to spinal stenosis, most of which are associated with degenerative spine disease or aging. Bony hypertrophic changes, such as spurs or facet enlargement, may diminish central canal cross-sectional area. The ligamentum flavum can also thicken and reduce the space within the canal (Fig. 10-4). Bony hypertrophy around the intervertebral foramen not only diminishes central canal volume but disrupts the natural spillover pathway that allows excess volumes of epidural local anesthetic solutions to egress into the perispinal periphery, thereby preventing abnormal pressure buildup. The true clinical significance of spinal stenosis as a cause of neuraxial anesthesia-related neural injury is unknown. This is in part due to the lack of clearly defined degrees of spinal stenosis reported in the anesthesiology literature. In a large series of neural deficits following spinal and epidural anesthesia, spinal pathology was linked to 6 of 33 cases of spinal hematoma.[7] A 15-year retrospective study from the Mayo Clinic noted that the presence of preexisting spinal pathology (especially compressive radiculopathy or multiple neurologic diagnoses) led to a 1.1% (95% CI 0.5%, 2.0%) incidence of neurologic complications after neuraxial blockade, which is slightly higher than expected for patients without these pathologies.[56] Importantly, these findings only identify an association between patients with postoperative paralysis who also were discovered to have spinal stenosis. A cause-and-effect relationship has not been proven. Indeed, there are also reports of patients with previously unrecognized spinal stenosis who sustained neuraxial injury after general anesthesia.[57] Pathophysiologically, the presence of spinal stenosis may reduce the volume of blood, pus, or local anesthetic that can accumulate around the neuraxis before pressure/volume relationships are adversely affected. One can reasonably speculate that such competition for central canal space might explain in part why epidural hematoma is seen more commonly in elderly patients.[7]

Exaggerated patient positioning has also been postulated to contribute to spinal cord ischemia by a mechanism similar to spinal stenosis. In these cases, spinal deformity from the lithotomy,[54] lateral,[44,58] or hyperlordotic[59] positions is postulated to have altered epidural/subarachnoid pressure/volume characteristics, the integrity of spinal vessels, and/or the egress of epidural fluids.

▶ RISK FACTORS

Although most mechanical neuraxis injury is unpredictable, there are certain risk factors that may be avoidable. Special care should be taken when ascertaining vertebral interspace levels by surface landmarks, particularly in obese patients. Ultrasound prescanning has been shown to more accurately identify spinal interspaces than physical examination.[60] Patients receiving long-term intrathecal opioid therapy are at risk for intrathecal granuloma. Over 90% of cancer patients with back pain have vertebral metastasis.[51] Although back pain in cancer patients is only rarely indicative of epidural metastasis, this condition should be considered prior to epidural placement.[61] The most controversial risk factor is whether or not spinal, epidural, or other perineuraxial blocks should be placed in patients who are anesthetized or heavily sedated[15] (Box 10-2). The American Society of Regional Anesthesia and Pain Medicine (ASRA) has taken the position that neuraxial blockade should not routinely be performed in anesthetized or heavily sedated adult patients.[9]

► DIAGNOSIS AND TREATMENT

The clinical presentation of motor block out of proportion to that expected from the regional anesthetic technique, prolonged motor block, or recrudescence of a motor or sensory block that had shown previous signs of resolution should always prompt the practitioner to suspect neuraxis injury. As with all unexpected neurological deficits associated with neuraxial anesthesia, rapid diagnosis and treatment is paramount. Patterns of onset and presentation may facilitate differential diagnosis. Rapid painless onset of lower extremity sensory deficit in an elderly patient is most consistent with vascular injury or ASAS. Conversely, a more progressive onset of neurologic symptoms, particularly if associated with back pain or fever, is more consistent with epidural hematoma or abscess. Ultimately, definitive diagnosis must be made with neuroimaging, (preferably) MRI,

BOX 10-2 Clinical Controversy

The advisability of performing neuraxial regional anesthesia or peripheral nerve blocks near the neuraxis in adult patients receiving general anesthesia or heavy sedation is controversial. The argument to perform these blocks in awake or lightly sedated patients is based on the assumption that unintentional needle placement and/or local anesthetic injection near or within the spinal cord or spinal nerves is heralded by warning signs such as paresthesia, pain upon injection, or atypical discomfort. Case reports describe devastating medullary injury suffered by anesthetized patients who received neuraxial blocks or perineuraxial peripheral nerve blocks. Conversely, many of the reported cases of spinal cord injury from needle and/or injection trauma occurred in awake patients, some of whom were unaware of any untoward symptoms during block placement. Furthermore, the spinal cord itself is devoid of sensory innervation and injection or needle contact with the meninges inconsistently elicits a warning sensation. In summary, performing neuraxial techniques in awake patients cannot consistently prevent spinal cord injury. Arguably, awake patients at least have a chance of reporting symptoms that could potentially warn the anesthesiologist of undesirable needle-to-neuraxis proximity. The American Society of Regional Anesthesia and Pain Medicine's (ASRA) Practice Advisory on Neurologic Complications takes the position that adult neuraxial blocks should not *routinely* be performed in anesthetized or deeply sedated patients.[12,19]

or computerized tomography (CT).[62] Importantly, imaging findings consistent with fluid should not be misconstrued as residual products of epidural infusion.[63] In the case of needle trauma or vascular infarct, early MRI may be nondiagnostic, but repeat imaging several days later may demonstrate signs of infarction, edema, or intracord hemorrhage (Table 10-1).

Although there are no beneficial treatments for completed vascular lesions, those that are suspected and in progress may empirically respond to induced hypertension, high-dose steroids, and/or reduced CSF volume. These therapies are unproven and inadequately studied, although some animal studies and case reports tout their benefit. When neuroimaging reveals a mass lesion (whether containing blood, pus, or another form of intraspinal mass), immediate neurosurgical consultation is critical because surgical decompression within 8 hours of symptom onset affords the best chance of full or partial recovery.[64]

► PREVENTION

A sobering reality of mechanical neuraxis injury is that it is largely unpredictable and not always preventable. Avoidance of or carefully timed neuraxial intervention in anticoagulated or soon-to-be anticoagulated patients is key to preventing intraspinal hematoma. Accurate determination of spinal interspace level, careful needle advancement, meticulous technique, and possibly avoiding placement of neuraxial and peripheral nerve blocks near the spinal cord in anesthetized adult patients (Box 10-2) might diminish the likelihood of these otherwise rare complications. A high index of suspicion may help to identify patients at risk for epidural tumor metastasis.[61] In those patients with known spinal stenosis, the location and severity of the disease may lead the anesthesiologist to alter their approach to the spine or consider other anesthetic or analgesic options, such as substituting a low-volume subarachnoid technique for a high-volume epidural technique or avoiding neuraxial anesthesia. Unfortunately, the incomplete state of the literature obviates a firm, evidence-based recommendation (Box 10-3).

Yet even with excellent technique by experienced anesthesiologists, spinal injury can occur. Most worrisome are those extremely rare conditions that may make an individual prone to injury—for instance, abnormal caudad termination of the spinal cord, tethered spinal cord, unstable plaque formation in a major spinal cord feeding vessel, epidural lipomatosis, or critically reduced cross-sectional central canal area from spinal stenosis. The vast majority of these conditions are unknown to the patient and the anesthesiologist.

► SUMMARY

Mechanical neuraxis injuries associated with regional anesthesia and pain management are exceedingly rare. Although an awake patient may not always interpret warning signs of direct spinal cord needle or catheter trauma, this author believes that awake patients have at least some chance of reporting unusual sensations during needle placement or injection of anesthetic solutions. With the exception of transforaminal techniques and some perivertebral pain blocks, direct injury to spinal cord vasculature is anatomically unlikely. ASAS associated with neuraxial block is often

TABLE 10-1 Differential Diagnosis of Mechanical Neuraxis Injury

	NEEDLE-INDUCED MYELOPATHY	NEEDLE-INDUCED VASCULAR INJURY	ANTERIOR SPINAL ARTERY SYNDROME (ASAS)	EPIDURAL HEMATOMA	EPIDURAL ABSCESS	EPIDURAL LIPOMATOSIS OR TUMOR
Risk factors	Nonspecific; misidentification of vertebral level	Paravertebral approaches	Atherosclerosis, prolonged severe hypotension	Anticoagulation	Infection	Metastatic carcinomas
Patient age	Nonspecific	Nonspecific	Elderly	Elderly at greater risk	Nonspecific	Nonspecific
Onset	Sudden to hours	Sudden to hours	Sudden to hours	Sudden to 1 to 3 d	1 to 3 d	Sudden to hours
Motor signs	Weakness to flaccid	Weakness to flaccid	Weakness to flaccid	Increasing motor block	Increasing motor block	Weakness to flaccid
Sensory signs	Variable	Variable	Variable to preserved	Increasing sensory block	Increasing sensory block	Variable
Generalized symptoms	None	None	None	Variable back pain, bowel/bladder dysfunction	Fever, malaise, back pain	Exacerbation of previous back pain
Imaging	MRI may initially be normal	MRI may initially be normal	Spinal cord infarction; may initially be normal	Extradural compression	Extradural compression	Extradural compression

BOX 10-3 Prevention of Mechanical Spinal Cord Injury

The following may reduce the risk of mechanical spinal cord injury:

- Avoidance of neuraxial techniques in patients with compromised coagulation.
- Meticulous technique, including strict asepsis, careful identification of spinal vertebral level, and controlled needle and catheter advancement.
- Placement of blocks in awake or minimally sedated patients. This may allow the adult patient to report warning symptoms that would otherwise be masked by general anesthesia or heavy sedation.
- Consideration of risk-to-benefit before placing neuraxial blocks in patients with known epidural tumor mass.
- Realization that radiographic guidance may aid precise needle placement in some blocks but does not always prevent injury.
- Realization that mechanical spinal cord injury is possible despite exacting technique and vigilance. Many conditions that theoretically predispose a patient to neuraxis injury are unknown to the patient or to the anesthesiologist.

unjustifiably linked to intraoperative hypotension or the use of vasoconstrictors. Subarachnoid or epidural mass lesions can impair spinal cord blood flow and result in ischemia or infarction. In these cases, rapid diagnosis and treatment are paramount to meaningful recovery of neurologic function.

References

1. Neal JM. Anatomy and pathophysiology of spinal cord injuries associated with regional anesthesia and pain medicine. *Reg Anesth Pain Med* 2008;33:423–434.
2. Lee LA, Posner KL, Domino KB, et al. Injuries associated with regional anesthesia in the 1980s and 1990s. *Anesthesiology* 2004;101:143–152.
3. Auroy Y, Benhamou D, Bargues L, et al. Major complications of regional anesthesia in France. The SOS regional anesthesia hotline service. *Anesthesiology* 2002;97:1274–1280.
4. Auroy Y, Narchi P, Messiah A, et al. Serious complications related to regional anesthesia. Results of a prospective survey in France. *Anesthesiology* 1997;87:479–486.
5. Nedeltchev K, Loher TJ, Stepper F, et al. Long-term outcome of acute spinal cord ischemia syndrome. *Stroke* 2004;35:560–565.
6. Cook TM, Counsell D, Wildsmith JAW. Major complications of central neuraxial block: report of the Third National Audit Project of the Royal College of Anaesthetists. *Br J Anaesth* 2009;102:179–190.
7. Moen V, Dahlgren N, Irestedt L. Severe neurological complications after central neuraxial blockades in Sweden 1990–1999. *Anesthesiology* 2004;101:950–959.
8. Wang LP, Hauerberg J, Schmidt JR. Incidence of spinal epidural abscess after epidural analgesia. *Anesthesiology* 1999;91:1928–1936.
9. Neal JM, Bernards CM, Hadzic A, et al. ASRA Practice Advisory on neurologic complications in regional anesthesia and pain medicine. *Reg Anesth Pain Med* 2008;33:404–422.
10. Kim J, Bahk J, Sung J. Influence of age and sex on the position of the conus medullaris and Tuffier's line in adults. *Anesthesiology* 2003;99:1359–1363.
11. Render CA. The reproducibility of the iliac crest as a marker of lumbar spine level. *Anaesthesia* 1996;51:1070–1071.
12. Lirk P, Kolbitsch C, Putz G, et al. Cervical and high thoracic ligamentum flavum frequently fails to fuse in the midline. *Anesthesiology* 2003;99:1387–1390.
13. Lirk P, Moriggl B, Colvin J, et al. The incidence of ligamentum flavum midline gaps. *Anesth Analg* 2004;98:1178–1180.
14. Hogan QH. Epidural anatomy examined by cryomicrotome section. Influence of age, vertebral level, and disease. *Reg Anesth* 1996;21:395–406.
15. Bernards CM, Hadzic A, Suresh S, et al. Regional anesthesia in anesthetized or heavily sedated patients. *Reg Anesth Pain Med* 2008;33:449–460.
16. Jacob AK, Borowiec JC, Long TR, et al. Transient profound neurologic deficit associated with thoracic epidural analgesia in an elderly patient. *Anesthesiology* 2004;101:1470–1471.
17. Tripathi M, Nath SS, Gupta RK. Paraplegia after intracord injection during attempted epidural steroid injection in an awake patient. *Anesth Analg* 2005;101:1209–1211.
18. Tsui BCH, Armstrong K. Can direct spinal cord injury occur without paresthesia? A report of delayed spinal cord injury after epidural placement in an awake patient. *Anesth Analg* 2005;101:1212–1214.
19. Kumar R, Berger RJ, Dunsker SB, et al. Innervation of the spinal dura: myth or reality? *Spine* 1996;21:18–26.
20. Absalom AR, Martinelli G, Scott NB. Spinal cord injury caused by direct damage by local anaesthetic infiltration needle. *Br J Anaesth* 2001;87:512–515.
21. Hamandi K, Mottershead J, Lewis T, et al. Irreversible damage to the spinal cord following spinal anaesthesia. *Neurology* 2002;59:624–626.
22. van den Berg AA, Sadek M, Swanson S. Epidural injection of lidocaine reduces the response to dural puncture accompanying spinal needle insertion when performing combined spinal-epidural anesthesia. *Anesth Analg* 2005;101:882–885.
23. Huntoon MA, Hurdle M-FB, Marsh RW, et al. Intrinsic spinal cord catheter placement: implications of new intractable pain in a patient with a spinal cord injury. *Anesth Analg* 2004;99:1763–1765.
24. Kao M-C, Tsai S-K, Tsou M-Y, et al. Paraplegia after delayed detection of inadvertent spinal cord injury during thoracic epidural catheterization in an anesthetized elderly patient. *Anesth Analg* 2004;99:580–583.
25. Horlocker TT, McGregor DG, Matsushige DK, et al. A retrospective review of 4767 consecutive spinal anesthetics: central nervous system complications. *Anesth Analg* 1997;84:578–584.
26. Pong RP, Gmelch BS, Bernards CM. Does a paresthesia during spinal needle insertion indicate intrathecal needle placement? *Reg Anesth Pain Med* 2009;34(1):29–32.
27. Benumof JL. Permanent loss of cervical spinal cord function associated with interscalene block performed under general anesthesia. *Anesthesiology* 2000;93:1541–1544.
28. Reynolds F. Damage to the conus medullaris following spinal anaesthesia. *Anaesthesia* 2001;56:238–247.
29. Hoy K, Hansen ES, He S-Z, et al. Regional blood flow, plasma volume, and vascular permeability in the spinal cord, the dural sac, and lumbar nerve roots. *Spine* 1994;19:2804–2811.
30. Morishita K, Murakamik G, Fujisawa Y, et al. Anatomical study of blood supply to the spinal cord. *Ann Thor Surg* 2003;76:1967–1971.
31. Sliwa JA, Maclean IC. Ischemic myelopathy: a review of spinal vasculature and related clinical syndromes. *Arch Phys Med Rehabil* 1992;73:365–371.
32. Brown DL, Rorie DK. Altered reactivity of isolated segmental lumbar arteries of dogs following exposure to ethanol and phenol. *Pain* 1994;56:139–143.
33. Lo JN, Buckley JJ. Spinal cord ischemia: a complication of celiac plexus block. *Reg Anesth* 1982;7:66–68.
34. Wong GY, Brown DL. Transient paraplegia following alcohol celiac plexus block. *Reg Anesth* 1995;20:352–355.

35. Rathmell JP, April C, Bogduk N. Cervical transforaminal injection of steroids. *Anesthesiology* 2004;100:1595–1600.

36. Benzon HT, Chew TL, McCarthy R, et al. Comparison of the particle sizes of the different steroids and the effect of dilution: a review of the relative neurotoxicities of the steroids. *Anesthesiology* 2007;106:331–338.

37. Rathmell JP, Benzon HT. Transforaminal injection of steriods: should we continue? *Reg Anesth Pain Med* 2004;29:397–399.

38. Kobrine AI, Doyle TF, Martins AN, et al. Autoregulation of spinal cord blood flow. *Clin Neurosurg* 1975;22:573–581.

39. Hickey R, Albin MS, Bunegin L, et al. Autoregulation of spinal cord blood flow: is the cord a microcosm of the brain? *Stroke* 1986;17:1183–1189.

40. Cole DJ, Lin DM, Drummond JC, et al. Spinal tetracaine decreases central nervous system metabolism during somatosensory stimulation in the rat. *Can J Anaesth* 1990;37:231–237.

41. Kuroda Y, Sakabe T, Nakakimura K, et al. Epidural bupivacaine suppresses local glucose utilization in the spinal cord and brain of rats. *Anesthesiology* 1990;73:944–950.

42. Drummond JC. The lower limit of autoregulation: time to revise our thinking? *Anesthesiology* 1997;86:1431–1433.

43. Neal JM. Effects of epinephrine in local anesthetics on the central and peripheral nervous systems: neurotoxicity and neural blood flow. *Reg Anesth Pain Med* 2003;28:124–134.

44. Bhuiyan MS, Mallick A, Parsloe M. Post-thoracotomy paraplegia coincident with epidural anaesthesia. *Anaesthesia* 1998;53:583–586.

45. Peng P, Massicotte EM. Spinal cord compression from intrathecal catheter-tip inflammatory mass: case report and a review of etiology. *Reg Anesth Pain Med* 2004;29:237–242.

46. Shields DC, Palma C, Khoo LT, et al. Extramedullary intrathecal catheter granuloma adherent to the conus medullaris presenting as cauda equia syndrome. *Anesthesiology* 2005;102:1059–1061.

47. Toombs JD, Follett KA, Rosenquist R, et al. Intrathecal catheter tip inflammatory mass: a failure of clonidine to protect. *Anesthesiology* 2005;102:687–690.

48. Guegan Y, Fardoun R, Launois B, et al. Spinal cord compression by extradural fat after prolonged corticosteroid therapy. *J Neurosurg* 1982;56:267–269.

49. Rocco AG, Philip JH, Boas RA, et al. Epidural space as a Starling resistor and elevation of inflow resistance in a diseased epidural space. *Reg Anesth* 1997;22:167–177.

50. Graham GP, Dent CM, Matthews P. Paraplegia following spinal anaesthesia in a patient with prostatic metastasis. *Br J Urol* 1992;70:445–452.

51. Loblaw DA, Laperriere NJ. Emergency treatment of malignant extradural spinal cord compression: an evidence-based guideline. *J Clin Oncol* 1998;16:1613–1624.

52. Jaeger M, Rickels E, Schmidth A, et al. Lumbar ependymoma presenting with paraplegia following attempted spinal anaesthesia. *Br J Anaesth* 2002;88:438–440.

53. Eastwood DW. Anterior spinal artery syndrome after epidural anesthesia in a pregnant diabetic patient with scleroderma. *Anesth Analg* 1991;73:90–91.

54. Wills JH, Wiesel S, Abram SE. Synovial cysts and the lithotomy position causing cauda equina syndrome. *Reg Anesth Pain Med* 2004;29:234–236.

55. de Seze M-P, Sztark F, Janvier G, et al. Severe and long-lasting complications of the nerve root and spinal cord after central neuraxial blockade. *Anesth Analg* 2007;104:975–979.

56. Hebl JR, Horlocker TT, Kopp SL, et al. Neuraxial blockade in patients with preexisting spinal stenosis, lumbar disc disease, or prior spinal surgery: efficacy and neurological complications. *Anesth Analg* 2010;111:1511–1519.

57. Lewandrowski K-U, McLain RF, Lieberman I, et al. Cord and cauda equina injury complicating elective orthopedic surgery. *Spine* 2006;31:1056–1059.

58. Hong DK, Lawrence HM. Anterior spinal artery syndrome following total hip arthroplasty under epidural anaesthesia. *Anaesth Intens Care* 2001;29:62–66.

59. Beloeil H, Albaladejo P, Hoen S, et al. Bilateral lower limb hypoesthesia after radical prostatectomy in the hyperlordotic position under general anesthesia. *Can J Anaesth* 2003;50:653–656.

60. Perlas A. Evidence for the use of ultrasound in neuraxial blocks. *Reg Anesth Pain Med* 2010;35:S43–S46.

61. Rathmell JP, Roland T, DuPen SL. Management of pain associated with metastatic epidural spinal cord compression: use of imaging studies in planning epidural therapy. *Reg Anesth Pain Med* 25:113–118.

62. Sorenson EJ. Neurological injuries associated with regional anesthesia. *Reg Anesth Pain Med* 2008;33:442–448.

63. Davidson EM, Sklar E, Bhatia R, et al. Magnetic resonance imaging findings after uneventful continuous infusion neuraxial analgesia: a prospective study to determine whether epidural infusion produces pathologic magnetic resonance imaging findings. *Anesth Analg* 2010;110:233–237.

64. Horlocker TT, Wedel DJ, Rowlingson JC, et al. Regional anesthesia in the patient receiving antithrombotic or thrombolytic therapy: American Society of Regional Anesthesia and Pain Medicine Evidence-Based Guidelines (Third Edition). *Reg Anesth Pain Med* 2010;35:64–101.

11

Local Anesthetic Neurotoxicity and Cauda Equina Syndrome

Kenneth Drasner

Local anesthetics can manifest two forms of toxicity: systemic toxicity, in which translocation of local anesthetics via the vascular system to the central nervous system and/or cardiac system results in various physiologic perturbations, and neurotoxicity, in which contact with the local anesthetic results in direct toxicity specific to the affected neural tissue. This chapter examines neurotoxicity, particularly as it is manifested within the central nervous system (spinal cord and spinal nerve roots), often presenting as cauda equina syndrome. Neurotoxicity of peripheral nerves is discussed in Chapter 14.

▶ DEFINITION

Recent clinical experience and experimental data define a rather narrow therapeutic index for local anesthetics with respect to their potential for neurotoxic injury.[1] The actual risk varies based on the definition used or the threshold for detection. For example, persistent or clinically significant functional impairment remains a rare occurrence when local anesthetics are properly employed for spinal and epidural anesthesia. In contrast, minor or subtle deficits are not infrequent, and although such effects reflect alterations in neurologic function and/or architecture they are generally transient or fully reversible. Strictly speaking, anesthetic action could be considered a form of neurotoxicity. However, in common usage, neurotoxicity refers to those neurologic effects that do not derive from the reversible binding and blockade of the sodium channel, but rather extend beyond these effects. Despite such simplicity, causation is often difficult to establish, because it is frequently difficult to distinguish anesthetic neurotoxicity from other potential etiologies. In addition, adverse effects of the local anesthetics may be indirect, being mediated through mechanisms such as disturbance in nerve blood flow.[2,3] To further complicate matters, other factors or adjuvants that are coadministered may potentiate toxicity. For example, there is experimental data to suggest that epinephrine can enhance the neurotoxicity of spinally administered lidocaine[4] (Fig. 11-1), an effect presumably due to greater exposure to local anesthetic resulting from delayed clearance.

Abundant experimental animal data support the concept that all currently used local anesthetics are capable of inducing disturbances in function and/or morphology at very low concentrations, at times below those commonly used for clinical anesthesia.[5,6] Such information is critical for determining mechanisms of injury, and for developing clinical strategies for minimizing or eliminating the risk of toxicity. However, extrapolation to clinical practice is challenging,

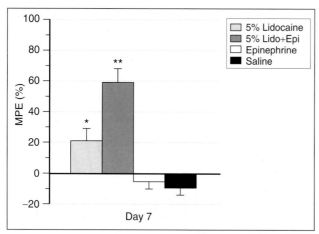

FIGURE 11-1. Sensory function 7 days after intrathecal administration of 5% lidocaine, 5% lidocaine with epinephrine (0.2 mg/mL; Lido Epi), epinephrine (0.2 mg/mL), or saline. Sensory function assessed by tail flick and expressed as percentage maximum possible effect (MPE): [(tail-flick latency − baseline)/(cutoff − baseline)] Å ~ 100. Data represent mean ± SD. *$p < .05$ versus epinephrine or saline. **$p < .05$ versus all other groups. (Adapted from Hashimoto K, Hampl KF, Nakamura Y, et al. Epinephrine increases the neurotoxic potential of intrathecally administered lidocaine in the rat. *Anesthesiology* 2001;94:876–881, with permission.)

and the clinical significance of data obtained primarily from animals can be easily overstated. Thus, if one were to consider minor or transient effects and the possibility of subclinical injury as defined by experimental laboratory studies, anesthetic neurotoxicity might be a relatively common occurrence. However, this chapter is narrowly restricted to the rare significant clinical deficits for which there is clear evidence supporting local anesthetic neurotoxicity as the mechanism of injury. As such, it does not consider transient neurologic symptoms (TNS) because of the uncertain relationship of TNS to neural injury (Chapter 13). Although the primary emphasis is overt clinical injury, experimental work is reviewed as necessary to provide an appreciation of mechanisms of injury and the factors that may promote or attenuate damage.

▶ SCOPE

Since the introduction of local anesthetics into clinical practice, sporadic reports of neurologic injury associated with spinal and epidural anesthesia have periodically raised concern that local anesthetics are potentially neurotoxic. These concerns first coalesced with a report in 1937 by Ferguson and Watkins of 14 cases of cauda equina syndrome associated with the use of "heavy" Durocaine, an anesthetic formulation containing 10% procaine, 15% ethanol, glycerin, and gum acacia or gliadin.[7] Although experimental studies in cats demonstrated that 10% procaine alone could induce similar injury, the nature of the vehicle components distracted focus from the local anesthetic.

Concern for anesthetic neurotoxicity was again heightened in the early 1980s by reports of injury associated with apparent unintentional intrathecal injection of doses of 2-chloroprocaine (Nesacaine-CE) intended for the epidural space.[8] However, similar to the injuries associated with

Durocaine, questions concerning the toxicity of one of the components of the Nesacaine-CE solution (the antioxidant sodium bisulfite) created uncertainty regarding the actual toxicity of the local anesthetic.[9] Although the experimental data were somewhat conflicted,[10] most concluded that 2-chloroprocaine was not neurotoxic (or at least no more so than other local anesthetics).

Although the issue of 2-chloroprocaine neurotoxicity was never actually settled, concern for local anesthetic neurotoxicity again subsided, only to reemerge a decade later with reports of injuries associated with continuous spinal anesthesia (CSA).[11] The initial report contained four cases: three involved the administration of 5% lidocaine with 7.5% dextrose that was administered through a small-bore (28-gauge) microcatheter specifically marketed for CSA. The other case occurred with 0.5% tetracaine with 5% glucose administered though a standard epidural catheter intentionally positioned within the subarachnoid space for CSA.[11] Despite differences in technique, all four cases shared certain elements critical to the development of neurotoxicity: administration of anesthetic produced a restricted sacral block; repetitive doses of local anesthetic were required to achieve adequate surgical anesthesia; and a cumulative dose exceeding that normally used with a single-injection spinal technique. It was suggested that the combination of maldistribution and the high dose of anesthetic led to neurotoxic anesthetic concentrations in a restricted area of the subarachnoid space, a mechanism that gained support from subsequent *in vitro* and *in vivo* experimental studies[12,13] (Box 11-1). Within a year, eight additional cases were reported,[14] all consistent with this etiology.

The occurrence of these cases led the Food and Drug Administration (FDA) to withdraw approval for microcatheters (defined as 27-gauge and smaller) and to issue a bulletin to all health care providers to alert them to "a serious hazard associated with CSA."[14] However, this action did

---

BOX 11-1 Continuous Spinal Anesthesia: Guidelines for Anesthetic Administration

- Insert catheter just far enough to confirm and maintain placement.
- Use the lowest effective anesthetic concentration.
- Place a limit on the amount of local anesthetic to be used.
- Administer a subarachnoid test dose and assess the extent of block.
- If maldistribution is suspected, use maneuvers to increase the spread of local anesthetic (e.g., change the patient's position, alter the lumbosacral curvature, switch to a solution with a different baricity).
- If well-distributed sensory anesthesia is not achieved before the dose limit is reached, abandon the technique.

Adapted from Rigler ML, Drasner K, Krejcie TC, et al. Cauda equina syndrome after continuous spinal anesthesia. *Anesth Analg* 1991;72: 275–281, with permission.)

not eliminate risk, as practitioners remained at liberty to use large-bore (epidural) catheters for CSA, a practice that remains particularly common following unintentional dural puncture during attempted epidural placement. Moreover, small-bore catheters may be reintroduced into clinical practice in the near future.[15] Avoidance of injury therefore requires an understanding of the factors that contribute to neurotoxicity and appropriate clinical management (Box 11-1).

The factors that can lead to neurotoxic injury with CSA are not unique to this technique, but are also present with single-injection spinal anesthesia. Specifically, maldistribution can and does occur with single-injection spinals. In fact, maldistribution is likely the most common cause of a "failed spinal." In this case, as with CSA, repeat injection following such failure may confer risk because the second injection may produce a similar restricted distribution (albeit less than with a catheter in fixed position). Here again, the combination of maldistribution and the relatively high anesthetic dose has the potential to achieve neurotoxic concentrations of anesthetic within the subarachnoid space. A 1991 review of the closed claims database, and subsequent case reports, provide compelling support for this mechanism of injury.[16]

There is a third mechanism by which relatively high doses of anesthetic may be administered intrathecally during routine anesthetic practice. While attempting an epidural anesthetic, a practitioner may fail to appreciate that the needle or catheter has been unintentionally positioned in the subarachnoid space and administer an "epidural dose" that far exceeds that appropriate for spinal block. Although the excessive spread of spinal anesthesia and the hemodynamic and respiratory consequences have often been the focus of attention, these complications can be readily managed without long-term sequelae. In contrast, the effects of local tissue toxicity are likely to be permanent. As previously noted, concern for neurotoxicity under these clinical circumstances initially surfaced in the early 1980s with reports of injuries associated with 2-chloroprocaine.[8] Beginning in 1992, similar cases have been reported with lidocaine,[17] an anesthetic once considered the "gold standard" for safety.

The reports of injury with CSA, repetitive injection after a failed spinal, and intrathecal injection of an "epidural dose" of anesthetic served to establish the significant risk of toxicity with doses of intrathecal anesthetic exceeding those commonly used for single-injection spinal anesthesia. Far more surprising, and of greater concern, two subsequent reports raised suspicion that injury can occur with lidocaine administered within the dose range generally recommended for single-injection spinal anesthesia. One described a case in which cauda equina syndrome followed otherwise uncomplicated administration of 100 mg of hyperbaric lidocaine with epinephrine.[18] The second report contained data from a prospective study of regional anesthesia in France.[19] In this database, which contained roughly 10,000 single-injection lidocaine spinals, there were eight persistent deficits that could not be explained on any basis other than neurotoxicity. All of these injuries occurred with doses at the high end of the normal dosage range (≥ 75 mg), and the two that were permanent followed injection of the highest recommended dose (100 mg). The lack of an alternative etiology and this clustering of injury at the high end of the dose range made toxicity the most likely etiology.[20]

Recent reports of injury associated with lidocaine, combined with supportive experimental data, have generated interest in alternative local anesthetics for spinal anesthesia. This interest has been reinforced by the common occurrence of TNS associated with this agent (Chapter 13). Despite a rather blemished record, considerable attention is now focused on 2-chloroprocaine, and based on early systemic volunteer studies,[21–23] small clinical reports,[24] and fairly extensive off-label use, it would appear to hold promise, although additional clinical data are required to establish safety.[25] Clinical use of 2-chloroprocaine has rested on the assumption that the neurotoxicity associated with the Nesacaine-CE formulation was due to the presence of bisulfite (at a low pH) rather than to the anesthetic *per se*.[9] However, as mentioned previously, this etiology was never clearly established, and recent experimental data suggest that bisulfite might actually be neuroprotective[26] (Chapter 8). Ironically, these data also suggest that the toxicity of 2-chloroprocaine is roughly equivalent to lidocaine on a milligram-for-milligram basis, a fact that could be used to support the use of spinal 2-chloroprocaine and to provide guidance regarding an acceptable dose range for this agent. (It should be recalled that previously reported injuries associated with 2-chloroprocaine likely involved administration of high doses intended for the epidural space.)

PATHOPHYSIOLOGY

Despite a century of clinical concern, the pathophysiology of anesthetic neurotoxicity is still poorly understood. The issue rests not in the lack of an effect that might underlie the toxicity of these compounds but with which of the many identified injurious effects of the local anesthetics play a role in clinical toxicity. Specifically, studies using cell culture[6,27,28] or isolated segments of frog,[5] crayfish,[29] rabbit,[30] or rat[31] axon demonstrate myriad detrimental effects with "clinical" concentrations of local anesthetics, including conduction failure, membrane damage, enzyme inhibition, loss of membrane potential, enzyme leakage, cytoskeleton disruption, accumulation of intracellular calcium, disruption of axonal transport, growth cone collapse, neurite degeneration, and cell death. As anticipated, blockade or attenuation of some of these effects may reduce or prevent toxicity. For example, preventing the anesthetic-induced rise in intracellular calcium by preloading cultured dorsal root ganglion (DRG) neurons with the Ca buffer BAPTA can inhibit anesthetic-induced cell death.[6] However, the manner in which the diverse deleterious factors interact and (specifically) in which effects are "upstream" has yet to be defined, though membrane disruption (perhaps via a detergent effect) is likely to be an early event.[32] Further complicating the matter, the concentration having a specific effect in an isolated segment of axon or in cell culture must be interpreted with caution, as the relevant concentrations achieved at the neuronal or cellular level *in vivo* are largely speculative.

Although the underlying mechanisms of toxicity have yet to be clearly defined, *in vivo* studies demonstrate the potential clinical relevance of anesthetic toxicity. To this end, spinal administration of clinical concentrations of anesthetic in an intact animal can induce functional loss corresponding to clinical injury and histologic damage consistent with

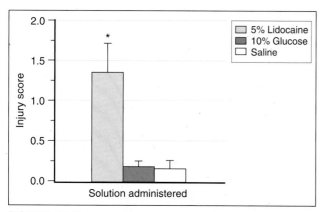

FIGURE 11-2. Nerve injury score for sections obtained 7 days after an intrathecal infusion of 5% lidocaine, 10% glucose, or normal saline. Data reflect the mean ± SEM. (Adapted from Hashimoto K, Sakura S, Bollen AW, et al. Comparative toxicity of glucose and lidocaine administered intrathecally in the rat. *Reg Anesth Pain Med* 1998;23:444–450, with permission.)

impairment.[4,33,34] Substantial evidence suggests that these effects are due to the anesthetic *per se*, rather than to the presence of glucose or to high osmolarity (e.g., hyperbaric 5% lidocaine has an osmolarity of roughly 857 mOsm). Specifically, dose-dependent loss of sensory function produced by intrathecal lidocaine is unaffected by the presence of 7.5% glucose, and in contrast to 5% lidocaine, administration of 10% glucose does not induce functional impairment or morphologic damage[34] (Fig. 11-2). Moreover, when applied directly to an axon *in vitro*, 7.5% glucose does not affect the compound action potential or potentiate conduction failure induced by lidocaine.[5]

Although neurotoxicity results from a direct effect of the local anesthetic, it is not the result of blockade of the voltage-gated sodium channel or inhibition of axonal transmission—as demonstrated in experiments using tetrodotoxin (TTX), a paralytic poison first isolated from puffer fish.[35] Similar to the local anesthetics, TTX blocks axonal conduction by binding to the sodium channel. However, TTX is extremely potent and highly selective—contrasting sharply with traditional local anesthetics, which are weakly bound and have diverse biologic effects at concentrations required for channel blockade. Intrathecal administration of TTX produces spinal anesthesia of extremely long duration. Nonetheless, functional recovery is complete and without evidence of histologic damage, even at a dose 10 times that required for spinal block. In contrast, equivalent doses of any of the traditional local anesthetics will consistently produce extensive functional impairment and widespread histologic damage. Thus, anesthetic effect and toxicity are not mediated by the same mechanism.

▶ RISK FACTORS

The clinical experience and experimental studies of the last two decades have clarified the role of a number of factors in anesthetic toxicity, which in turn form the basis for recommended modifications in practice. These factors relate to technique, anesthetic agent, and components or characteristics of the anesthetic solution.

Dose, Concentration, and Anesthetic Distribution

The most important factor affecting anesthetic neurotoxicity is the concentration of anesthetic that bathes the nerves in the subarachnoid space, where they are particularly vulnerable due to their high surface-to-volume ratio and the fact that they lack the protective sheath of peripheral nerves (Fig. 11-3). This concentration will in turn be determined by three factors: the concentration of anesthetic in the spinal anesthetic solution, the dose administered, and the distribution of anesthetic within the subarachnoid space. With respect to these factors, it should be appreciated that limiting dose will be a more effective strategy than reducing anesthetic concentration. Barring extreme maldistribution, it is the dose rather than the concentration that is the primary determinant of subarachnoid anesthetic concentration.

Restricted anesthetic distribution may be unintentional (e.g., failed spinal) or deliberate (e.g., saddle block). Unintentional distribution, known as maldistribution, is more likely with solutions at the extreme of hyperbaricity, with more caudal interspaces selected for spinal anesthesia, and with slow injection rates. The effect of a slow injection rate accounts for the greater likelihood of maldistribution with small-bore catheters used for spinal anesthesia, in that the high resistance to injection encountered with small-bore catheters limits the achievable flow rate. When a restricted distribution is deliberately sought, the dose should be adjusted accordingly because less drug is required for the desired effect and the risk of toxicity increases inversely with the subarachnoid spread of anesthetic.

Anesthetic Agent

The clinical reports of deficits associated with the use of lidocaine for spinal anesthesia suggest a higher incidence, or greater risk, of injury than the use of bupivacaine or tetracaine. This impression is supported by the data from the aforementioned prospective study of regional anesthesia from France.[19] Nine of the twelve nontraumatic deficits were associated with the use of lidocaine despite greater use of bupivacaine in the investigators' clinical practice. This clinical impression finds support by both *in vitro* and *in vivo* experimental studies in which lidocaine induces greater conduction failure in isolated nerves,[5] and more profound sensory dysfunction and histologic damage in the intact animal when compared with bupivacaine or tetracaine.[33] In contrast, there is evidence to suggest that the toxicity of lidocaine is roughly equivalent to that of prilocaine or 2-chloroprocaine.[25,36] With respect to 2-chloroprocaine, lidocaine actually appears to have a slightly more favorable therapeutic index; as most assessments find lidocaine to have greater potency, less drug would be required to achieve the desired anesthetic effect.

Vasoconstrictors

Vasoconstrictors are commonly added to spinal anesthetic solutions to increase the intensity and prolong the duration of anesthesia. However, vasoconstrictors might contribute to toxicity by promoting ischemia, decreasing anesthetic uptake, or directly affecting neural elements. Recent laboratory data indicate that epinephrine potentiates injury induced

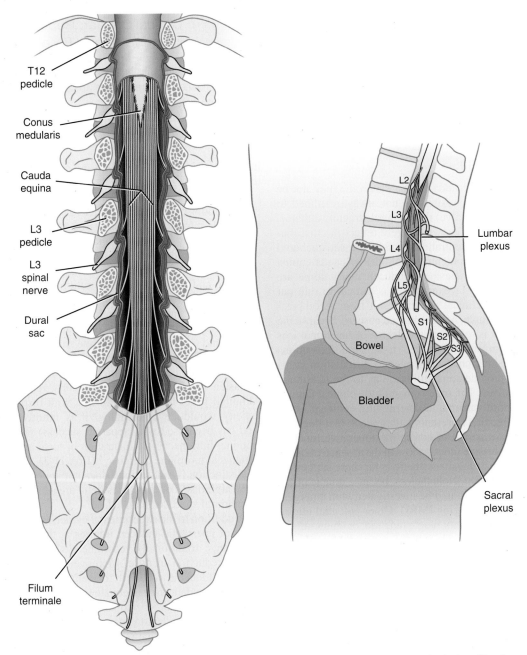

FIGURE 11-3. The cauda equina. Note the relatively long course that spinal nerve roots travel prior to exiting the intervertebral foramina, thereby increasing exposure to possible neurotoxic substances. Injury to the cauda equina may result in lower extremity weakness, bowel or bladder dysfunction, and/or perineal sensory loss.

by intrathecal lidocaine[4] (Fig. 11-1). Importantly, spinal administration of epinephrine in the absence of local anesthetic induces neither persistent functional impairment nor histologic damage.

▶ DIAGNOSTIC EVALUATION

Clinical Characteristics

With respect to spinal and epidural anesthesia, the characteristic clinical manifestations of anesthetic neurotoxicity generally reflect the distinctive arrangement of the rostral cord, lumbosacral nerve roots, and the subarachnoid space. In the fetus, the spinal cord extends the entire length of the canal. However, the caudal termination comes to lie at the level of the third lumbar vertebra at birth and most commonly lies at the lower border of the first lumbar vertebra by adulthood. Consequently, spinal needles are not routinely introduced above L2 in the adult, and the highest concentrations of anesthetic are thus achieved in the region rostral to the conus. The same holds true for unintentional intrathecal injections of anesthetic intended for the epidural space, in that most high-dose epidurals are performed in this region.

Below the termination of the cord, the nerve roots of the lower segments run parallel, forming the cauda equina (named for its resemblance to a horse's tail) (Fig. 11-3). These roots must travel a significant distance to reach the corresponding neural foramina, and this greater distance provides greater opportunity for anesthetic exposure and toxicity. As they travel together, they are subject to collective damage—resulting in the characteristic multiple-root involvement of cauda equina syndrome, clinically manifested by varying degrees of bowel and bladder dysfunction, perineal sensory loss, and lower extremity motor weakness.

Differential Diagnosis

Although diagnosis of cauda equina syndrome may not be a diagnostic challenge, toxicity is not always confined to (and might not even involve) these neural structures, that is, the clinical manifestations will largely reflect the distribution of anesthetic concentrations within the subarachnoid space. There are other potential etiologies of cauda equina syndrome, and unlike anesthetic-induced injury some are potentially treatable. For example, it is critical to rule out the possibility that clinical deficits result from a compressive lesion, for example, hematoma and abscess, because the extent of recovery is related to the degree of functional loss and the time from onset of deficits to surgical decompression. The clinical circumstances, such as coagulation status or sepsis, may provide some guidance as to the likelihood of these alternatives. The time course of the clinical deficits may be even more valuable in determining etiology. Local anesthetic neurotoxicity presents with a block that does not resolve, whereas a period of normal postoperative function followed by progressive function loss in the absence of ongoing administration of local anesthetic is far more suggestive of a compressive lesion. Nonetheless, because time is of the essence any suspicion should be investigated with emergent magnetic resonance imaging (MRI). Other potential etiologies (such as trauma, immunologic reaction, or unintentional administration of neurotoxic substances) may be evaluated in a less urgent fashion.

▶ PREVENTION

Because there is no effective treatment for deficits induced by local anesthetics, preventive measures are paramount. Fortunately, although the pathophysiology remains somewhat ill defined, the factors contributing to clinical injury have become quite evident over the last two decades (Box 11-1). First and foremost, injury is dose dependent, and clinical strategies have been advocated to minimize if not eliminate the possibility that an excessively high dose of anesthetic will reach the subarachnoid space. Thus, guidelines for CSA include placing a limit on the amount of anesthetic used to establish surgical anesthesia.[11] If this limit is reached prior to achieving adequate anesthesia, the technique is abandoned, most often in favor of a general anesthetic.

With repetitive injection after a failed spinal, the clinical circumstances are a bit more complex, as technical failures do occur, that is, failure to inject the anesthetic in the subarachnoid space. Consequently, guidelines have been proposed for the management of repetitive spinal injection after a failed spinal, which include an assessment of the likelihood of technical error and adjustment of dosage for the second

> **BOX 11-2** Clinical Caveat: Repetitive Injection After a Failed Spinal
>
> Limit the combined anesthetic dosage to the maximum amount one would consider reasonable to administer as a single intrathecal injection.

injection.[16] However, a simpler (and even safer) approach is to adopt a strategy similar to that used for CSA. Namely, to merely limit the combined anesthetic dosage to the maximum amount one would consider reasonable to administer as a single intrathecal injection (Box 11-2).

The injuries associated with unintentional intrathecal injection of epidural doses of 2-chloroprocaine and lidocaine have served to highlight the critical importance of the test dose and fractional administration of anesthetic during epidural anesthesia. If, however, high doses of local anesthetic are unintentionally administered through a misplaced catheter, repetitive withdrawal of small volumes (5–10 mL) of CSF and replacement with saline should be considered—again regardless of the anesthetic used. This maneuver was initially promoted by Lemmon and Paschal as a method to hasten block recovery in their early reports of CSA.[37] Although proof of clinical efficacy with respect to neurotoxicity would be challenging, it is intuitively attractive (and has been used with apparent success) following unintentional intrathecal administration of local anesthetic[38] and intrathecal morphine overdose[39] (Box 11-3). Of note, a critical distinction is that toxicity does not appear to be an issue when high doses of local anesthetic are administered within the epidural space as intended.

In addition to the experimental evidence, the likely occurrence of anesthetic-induced injuries at the high end of the dose range traditionally recommended for lidocaine warrants a reduction in dose. Moreover, 100 mg exceeds the dose of lidocaine required for reliable spinal anesthesia. Although the data are inadequate to make firm recommendations, it is the author's personal practice not to exceed 60 mg. It would seem prudent to apply the same 60 mg dose limitation if 2-chloroprocaine is to be used for spinal anesthesia, although this recommendation is based on limited animal data assuming equivalent toxicity on a milligram-for-milligram basis, reinforcing the need for additional clinical data to confirm its perceived safety.

Toxicity is to some extent concentration dependent. However, as previously discussed, the actual concentration

> **BOX 11-3** Clinical Caveat: Unintentional Intrathecal Injection of an Epidural Dose of Anesthetic
>
> If high doses of local anesthetic are unintentionally administered intrathecally, repetitive withdrawal of small volumes (5–10 mL) of CSF and replacement with saline should be considered, regardless of the local anesthetic used.

achieved in the subarachnoid space will be far more dependent on the dose administered rather than the injectate concentration because of its dilution by cerebrospinal fluid. Nonetheless, the lowest effective anesthetic concentration should be selected for spinal anesthesia, as there remains some advantage to lowering concentration with respect to toxicity and there is no clinical disadvantage; for example, 5% lidocaine offers no benefit over 2% lidocaine with respect to clinical efficacy.

Experimental data suggest that epinephrine potentiates sensory impairment and histologic damage induced by intrathecal lidocaine.[4] Combined with the clinical report of a deficit following intrathecal injection of 100 mg lidocaine with epinephrine,[18] these data argue against using a vasoconstrictor with lidocaine for spinal anesthesia. Although some have questioned the clinical relevance of these findings and the significance of this single case report, the principal rationale for continued use of spinal lidocaine is the lack of an alternative short-acting anesthetic with well-documented safety and efficacy. There is, however, an acceptable alternative to the longer-acting lidocaine with epinephrine. Bupivacaine will produce comparable anesthesia, and it has a better therapeutic index, even ignoring the issue of vasoconstrictors (or TNS). In addition, in cases in which potentiation of spinal lidocaine is sought, fentanyl might be used without increasing the risk of toxicity, although it will not be as effective in prolonging the anesthetic effect. Consequently, it is difficult to imagine a rational argument for the continued use of epinephrine with intrathecal lidocaine. A somewhat similar case can be made for avoidance of epinephrine with spinal 2-chloroprocaine. In addition, coadministration of epinephrine with 2-chloroprocaine was associated with the occurrence of flu-like symptoms in a limited volunteer study.[23] These symptoms have been postulated to derive from trace quantities of bisulfite in the epinephrine solution having liberated sulfur dioxide at low pH of the commercial 2-chloroprocaine. Although this theory remains to be established (as does the reproducibility of these symptoms), the occurrence of the symptoms in this small volunteer study reinforces the recommendation to avoid vasoconstrictors if using 2-chloroprocaine for spinal anesthesia.

▶ TREATMENT

Unfortunately, there is no effective treatment for neurotoxic injury to the spinal cord or nerve roots induced by local anesthetics. Although some have advocated regimens of high-dose steroids (similar to those employed for traumatic spinal cord injury), these agents have no proven benefit.

Efforts at rehabilitation rest on the nature and the extent of the deficits. In most cases of cauda equina syndrome resulting from anesthetic neurotoxicity, motor function is minimally impaired, and bowel and (particularly) bladder dysfunction predominate. These may require considerable supportive care to avoid secondary complications.

▶ SUMMARY

Neurotoxic damage to the spinal cord and nerve roots remains a concern in contemporary anesthetic practice. Although the actual incidence varies considerably in relation to how one chooses to define toxicity, clinically significant injury rarely occurs. Nonetheless, the potential severity of these injuries requires the practitioner to understand and appreciate the factors that may contribute to anesthetic toxicity in order to eliminate, or at least minimize, the possibility of their occurrence.

References

1. Drasner K. Local anesthetic neurotoxicity: clinical injury and strategies that may minimize risk. *Reg Anesth Pain Med* 2002;27:576–580.
2. Kalichman MW, Lalonde AW. Experimental nerve ischemia and injury produced by cocaine and procaine. *Brain Res* 1991;565:34–41.
3. Kozody R, Ong B, Palahniak RJ, et al. Subarachnoid bupivacaine decreases spinal cord blood flow in dogs. *Can Anaesth Soc J* 1985;32:216–222.
4. Hashimoto K, Hampl KF, Nakamura Y, et al. Epinephrine increases the neurotoxic potential of intrathecally administered lidocaine in the rat. *Anesthesiology* 2001;94:876–881.
5. Lambert LA, Lambert DH, Strichartz GR. Irreversible conduction block in isolated nerve by high concentrations of local anesthetics. *Anesthesiology* 1994;80:1082–1093.
6. Gold MS, Reichling DB, Hample KF, et al. Lidocaine toxicity in primary afferent neurons from the rat. *J Pharmacol Exp Ther* 1998;285:413–421.
7. Ferguson F, Watkins K. Paralysis of the bladder and associated neurologic sequelae of spinal anaesthesia (cauda equina syndrome). *Br J Surg* 1937;25:735–752.
8. Ravindran RS, Bond VK, Tasch MD, et al. Prolonged neural blockade following regional analgesia with 2-chloroprocaine. *Anesth Analg* 1980;59:447–451.
9. Gissen A, Datta S, Lambert D. The chloroprocaine controversy. II. Is chloroprocaine neurotoxic? *Reg Anesth* 1984;9:135–144.
10. Kalichman MW, Powell MW, Reisner LS, et al. The role of 2-chloroprocaine and sodium bisulfite in rat sciatic nerve edema. *J Neuropathol Exp Neurol* 1986;45:566–575.
11. Rigler ML, Drasner K, Krejcie TC, et al. Cauda equina syndrome after continuous spinal anesthesia. *Anesth Analg* 1991;72:275–281.
12. Rigler ML, Drasner K. Distribution of catheter-injected local anesthetic in a model of the subarachnoid space. *Anesthesiology* 1991;75:684–692.
13. Drasner K. Models for local anesthetic toxicity from continuous spinal anesthesia. *Reg Anesth* 1993;18:434–438.
14. FDA Safety Alert. Cauda equina syndrome associated with the use of small-bore catheters in continuous spinal anesthesia. May 29, 1992.
15. Arkoosh VA, Palmer CM, Yun EM, et al. A randomized, double-masked, multicenter comparison of the safety of continuous intrathecal labor analgesia using a 28-gauge catheter versus continuous epidural labor analgesia. *Anesthesiology* 2009;108:286–298.
16. Drasner K, Rigler M. Repeat injection after a "failed spinal": at times, a potentially unsafe practice. *Anesthesiology* 1991;75:713–714.
17. Drasner K, Rigler ML, Sessler DI, et al. Cauda equina syndrome following intended epidural anesthesia. *Anesthesiology* 1992;77:582–585.
18. Gerancher J. Cauda equina syndrome following a single spinal administration of 5% hyperbaric lidocaine through a 25-gauge Whitacre needle. *Anesthesiology* 1997;87:687–689.
19. Auroy Y, Messiah A, Litt L, et al. Serious complications related to regional anesthesia: results of a prospective survey in France. *Anesthesiology* 1997;87:479–486.
20. Drasner K. Lidocaine spinal anesthesia: a vanishing therapeutic index? *Anesthesiology* 1997;87:469–472.
21. Kopacz DJ. Spinal 2-chloroprocaine: minimum effective dose. *Reg Anesth Pain Med* 2005;30:36–42.

22. Kouri ME, Kopacz DJ. Spinal 2-chloroprocaine: a comparison with lidocaine in volunteers. *Anesth Analg* 2004;98:75–80.

23. Smith KN, Kopacz DJ, McDonald SB. Spinal 2-chloroprocaine: a dose-ranging study and the effect of added epinephrine. *Anesth Analg* 2004;98:81–88.

24. Casati A, et al. Intrathecal 2-chloroprocaine for lower limb outpatient surgery: a prospective, randomized, double-blind, clinical evaluation. *Anesth Analg* 2006;103:234–238.

25. Drasner K. Chloroprocaine spinal anesthesia: back to the future? *Anesth Analg* 2005;100:549–552.

26. Taniguchi M, Bollen AW, Drasner K. Sodium bisulfite: scapegoat for chloroprocaine neurotoxicity? *Anesthesiology* 2004;100: 85–91.

27. Radwan IA, Saito S, Goto F. Growth cone collapsing effect of lidocaine on DRG neurons is partially reversed by several neurotrophic factors. *Anesthesiology* 2002;97:630–635.

28. Johnson ME, Saenz JA, Da Silva AD, et al. Effect of local anesthetic on neuronal cytoplasmic calcium and plasma membrane lysis (necrosis) in a cell culture model. *Anesthesiology* 2002;97:1466–1476.

29. Kanai Y, Katsuki H, Takasaki M. Graded, irreversible changes in crayfish giant axon as manifestations of lidocaine neurotoxicity in vitro. *Anesth Analg* 1998;86:569–573.

30. Byers MR, Fink BR, Kennedy RD, et al. Effects of lidocaine on axonal morphology, microtubules, and rapid transport in rabbit vagus nerve in vitro. *J Neurobiol* 1973;4:125–143.

31. Kanai Y, Katsuki H, Takasaki M. Lidocaine disrupts axonal membrane of rat sciatic nerve in vitro. *Anesth Analg* 2000;91:944–948.

32. Kitagawa N, Oda M, Totoki T. Possible mechanism of irreversible nerve injury caused by local anesthetics: detergent properties of local anesthetics and membrane disruption. *Anesthesiology* 2004;100:962–967.

33. Drasner K, Sakura S, Chan VW, et al. Persistent sacral sensory deficit induced by intrathecal local anesthetic infusion in the rat. *Anesthesiology* 1994;80:847–852.

34. Hashimoto K, Sakura S, Bollen AW, et al. Comparative toxicity of glucose and lidocaine administered intrathecally in the rat. *Reg Anesth Pain Med* 1998;23:444–450.

35. Sakura S, Bollen AW, Ciriales R, et al. Local anesthetic neurotoxicity does not result from blockade of voltage-gated sodium channels. *Anesth Analg* 1995;81:338–346.

36. Kishimoto T, Bollen AW, Drasner K. Comparative spinal neurotoxicity of prilocaine and lidocaine. *Anesthesiology* 2002;97: 1250–1253.

37. Lemmon W, Paschal G. Continuous-serial, fractional, controllable intermittent-spinal anesthesia, with observations on 1000 cases. *Surg Gynecol Obstet* 1942;74:948–956.

38. Tsui BC, et al. Reversal of an unintentional spinal anesthetic by cerebrospinal lavage. *Anesth Analg* 2004;98:434–436.

39. Kaiser K, Bainton C. Treatment of intrathecal morphine overdose by aspiration of cerebrospinal fluid. *Anesth Analg* 1987;66: 475–477.

12

Neuraxis Ischemic Injury

Christopher M. Bernards and Joseph M. Neal

Ischemic spinal cord injury is an extremely rare perioperative complication that is feared by patient and practitioner alike because of its devastating nature. Unfortunately, the low incidence of this complication makes it difficult to study prospectively. Consequently, we lack experimental data that clearly identify the demographic and/or technical risk factors that predispose to ischemic spinal cord injury. In the absence of such data, this chapter describes the normal anatomy and physiology of spinal cord blood flow (SCBF) in the hope of providing anesthesiologists with the necessary background to identify those rare situations in which patients may be at risk for ischemic complications during regional anesthesia.

▶ DEFINITION

Broadly speaking, the spinal cord is at risk of ischemic injury under any circumstances in which the supply of oxygen or nutrients is insufficient to meet metabolic demands. Thus, severe hypoxia, anemia, or hypoglycemia can cause spinal cord "ischemia" even if SCBF is normal or elevated. However, ischemia is probably more likely to occur because of reduced SCBF, such as that which may result from extrinsic compression of vessels supplying the spinal cord (e.g., epidural hematoma), elevated spinal cerebrospinal fluid (CSF) pressure (e.g., intrathecal injection of a large fluid volume), spontaneous thrombosis of spinal blood vessels, iatrogenic occlusion of vessels supplying the spinal cord (e.g., aortic surgery), and severe prolonged hypotension, among others.[1] Most worrisome are situations in which multiple risk factors exist concurrently (e.g., when anemia, hypotension, epidural local anesthetic injection, and aortic occlusion occur simultaneously in a patient with occlusive vascular disease undergoing resection of an abdominal aortic aneurysm).

▶ SCOPE

Ischemic injury to the neuraxis can occur spontaneously[2,3] during surgery under general anesthesia[4] and following neuraxial blocks.[5] The incidence of ischemic injury to the spinal cord following spinal or epidural anesthesia is not precisely known, but it is rare. For example, Auroy et al.[6] noted no ischemic complications following 41,079 spinal anesthetics and 35,293 epidural anesthetics voluntarily reported to the French SOS Regional Anesthesia Service over 10 months in 1998 and 1999. Nedeltchev et al.[2] reviewed 57 cases of anterior spinal artery syndrome presenting to their institution (University Hospital of Bern, Switzerland) between 1990 and 2002 and reported 1 case associated with epidural anesthesia. These investigators made it clear that epidural anesthesia was not a proven cause but was chosen as the etiologic factor because no other clear etiology existed.

▶ SPINAL CORD VASCULAR ANATOMY, PHYSIOLOGY, AND PHARMACOLOGY

Vascular Anatomy

Arterial System

The arterial supply to the spinal cord is both complex and variable (Fig. 12-1). Much of the variability relates to differences among individuals in terms of the exact sites of origin of vessels that perfuse the spinal cord.

In general, two posterior spinal arteries and a single anterior spinal artery supply the spinal cord. The posterior vessels originate from either the vertebral arteries or the posterior inferior cerebellar arteries. The anterior spinal artery originates from paired branches of the vertebral arteries that meet in the midline near where the vertebral arteries merge to form the basilar artery. The single anterior spinal artery supplies the anterior two-thirds of the spinal cord and the cauda equina. The posterior arteries supply the posterior third of the spinal cord but do not generally contribute to the cauda equina nerve roots. The fact that the single anterior spinal artery supplies two-thirds of the spinal cord likely accounts for the fact that the anterior spinal artery syndrome is far more common than the posterior spinal artery syndrome.

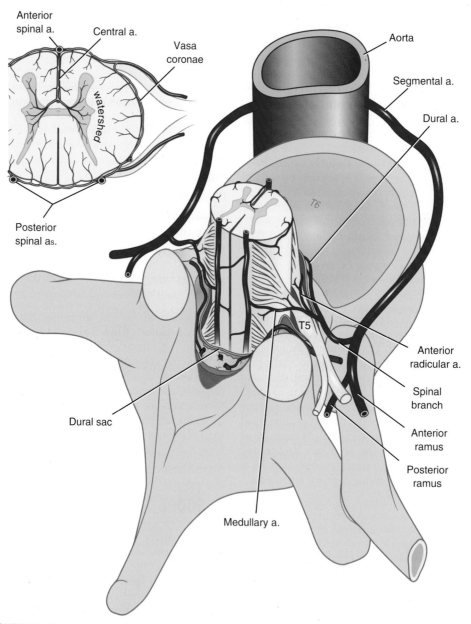

FIGURE 12-1. Arterial supply to the spinal cord, transverse view. (Modified from Sliwa JA, Maclean IC. Ischemic myelopathy: a review of spinal vasculature and related clinical syndromes. *Arch Phys Med Rehabil* 1992;73:365–372, with permission. Ref. 7.)

The anterior and posterior arteries connect via branches that encircle the spinal cord (vasa coronae), thereby providing a limited capacity for communication between the anterior and posterior circulations (Fig. 12-1). The limited capacity for communication between the anterior and posterior spinal circulations is demonstrated by the fact that ischemic syndromes in the anterior and posterior circulations are recognized as distinct clinical entities. The anterior, posterior, and vasa coronae arteries give rise to penetrating arterioles that supply the deeper layers of the spinal cord. There are no anastomoses between the penetrating arterioles, and thus the center of the cord represents a watershed area.

Blood flow through both the anterior and the posterior spinal arteries is augmented by segmental contributions from a variable number of "reinforcing" arteries (Fig. 12-2). The classification system used to describe these vessels varies throughout the literature, giving rise to some confusion about the underlying anatomy. For the purposes of this text, vessels arising from the aorta or its main branches and reaching the intervertebral foramen are termed segmental arteries. Those extending from the intervertebral foramen across the epidural space and along the nerve roots are termed spinal radicular arteries. The terminal portions of radicular arteries that reach the spinal cord are termed spinal medullary arteries.

In the early embryo, there are bilateral segmental arteries associated with each spinal segment (62 total), but many of these degenerate during embryogenesis. The remaining segmental arteries vary greatly in number, size, and location among individuals. Those segmental arteries that persist take their origin from the closest artery adjacent to the spinal column (i.e., vertebral, costocervical trunk, thyrocervical trunk, intercostal branches of the aorta, lumbar arteries, iliolumbar arteries, and lateral sacral arteries).

The segmental arteries enter the spinal canal via the intervertebral foramina, at which point they become radicular branches. The radicular arteries divide into anterior and posterior branches that accompany the corresponding nerve roots (Fig. 12-1). Most of these radicular branches do not reach the spinal cord but terminate on the spinal nerve roots. The terminal branches of the few radicular arteries that do reach the spinal cord are termed spinal medullary arteries. Tureen[9] reported that on average there are only 24 medullary arteries that reach the spinal cord, and most of these anastomose with the posterior spinal arteries. In fact, Mettler[10] reported that the anterior spinal artery receives contributions from only between 4 and 10 medullary vessels.

The most important segmental artery is the arteria radicularis magna (artery of Adamkiewicz), which is responsible for the blood supply to 25% to 50% of the anterior spinal cord. The origin and course of the arteria radicularis magna is both variable and clinically important. Biglioli et al.[11] have reported that the artery originates on the left 71% of the time and between L_1 and L_3 65% of the time. They also noted origins as high as T_9 and as low as L_5. In fact, origins as high as T_5 have been reported. The arteria radicularis magna's origin is clinically important because interruption of flow through this critical vessel (e.g., during aortic cross-clamping) puts the spinal cord at risk of ischemia.

In general, spinal cord segments cephalad of T_2 and caudad of T_8 are relatively highly vascularized, whereas the intermediate thoracic cord is less vascularized. Thus, some have suggested that the midthoracic cord is at greater risk of hypoperfusion. However, it is important to note that the midthoracic cord contains less gray matter and fewer neurons than the cervical and lumbar enlargements and therefore requires less blood flow. Thus, it is not clear that the midthoracic cord is physiologically at greater risk of reduced blood flow than are the more highly perfused regions.

Venous System

As in other organs, the venous drainage from the spinal cord is highly variable. In general, blood drains from the center of the cord centrifugally into an anterior central vein, a posterior central vein, and variously positioned peripheral veins lying on the surface of the cord. These venous channels drain into anterior and posterior radicular veins that follow the spinal nerve away from the spinal cord. Although radicular veins are more uniformly distributed than radicular arteries, they

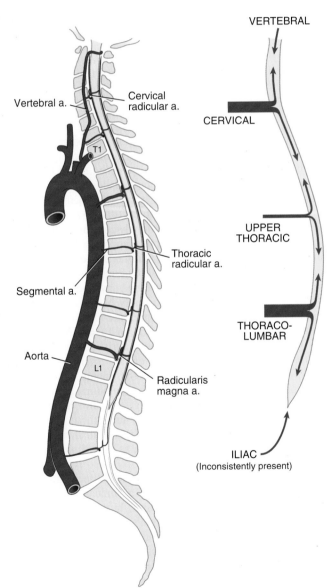

FIGURE 12-2. Arterial supply to the spinal cord, longitudinal view. (Modified from Neal JM. Neurologic complications. In: Rathmell JP, Neal JM, Viscomi CM, eds. *Regional Anesthesia: The Requisites in Anesthesiology.* Philadelphia, PA: Elsevier-Mosby, 2004:157–163, with permission. Ref. 8.)

are not present at each spinal segment and their diameter is highly variable. If both anterior and posterior radicular veins are present at a given spinal cord segment, they unite to form a single radicular vein, which courses adjacent to the spinal nerve.

After traversing the dura mater, the radicular veins join the vertebral venous plexus (Batson's plexus). This plexus lies primarily in the anterior lateral epidural space[12] and runs the entire length of the spinal column. It also drains the vertebral bodies and the paraspinous muscles. In addition, the vertebral venous plexus has connections to systemic veins from the pelvis to the base of the brain.

Vascular Physiology

Technical barriers make studies of SCBF difficult in humans. However, animal models suggest that control of SCBF is qualitatively similar to the control of cerebral blood flow (CBF). For example, like the cerebral vasculature, blood flow in the spinal vasculature is autoregulated. That is, within defined limits of spinal cord perfusion pressure (SCPP) SCBF remains constant (Box 12-1). Using rhesus monkeys, Kobrine et al.[13] demonstrated that SCBF was maintained constant between a mean arterial pressure (MAP) of 50 and 135 mm Hg. Above and below these limits, the flow was pressure passive. Similarly, Hickey et al.[14] used a rat model to demonstrate that autoregulatory thresholds for the brain and spinal cord were identical (roughly 60–120 mm Hg). Further, they demonstrated that global CBF and global SCBF were identical (~60 mL/100 g/min) (Fig. 12-3).

Autoregulation has not been as well studied in humans, but both Abe et al.[15] and Tsuji et al.[16] measured human SCBF during PGE_1-induced hypotension in humans undergoing spinal surgery. Both studies found that SCBF was maintained constant when MAP was decreased to 60 mm Hg. However, what is largely unknown is what constitutes the ischemic threshold in most humans. Using an electroencephalogram model in humans undergoing carotid endarterectomy, Sharbrough et al.[17] saw no reduction in neurophysiologic function until CBF was reduced by 50% in these patients. In recent years, Drummond[18] and others have questioned whether the commonly published 50 mm Hg lower limit of cerebral autoregulation (LLA) is in fact too low for a subset of humans, particularly those with underlying hypertension. This potentially meritorious theory admittedly has limited corroborating human outcome data, but has led some practitioners to rethink the lower limits of autoregulation in their patients. Thus, Drummond[18] suggested in

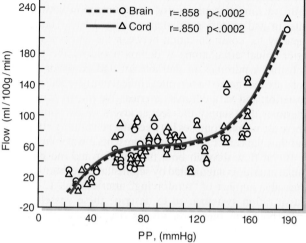

FIGURE 12-3. Simultaneous blood flow to the brain and spinal cord as a function of perfusion pressure (PP = MAP − ICP) in rats. For both brain and spinal cord, flow is essentially constant between a perfusion pressure of 60 and 120 mm Hg. (Redrawn from Hickey R, Albin MS, Bunegin L, et al. Autoregulation of spinal cord blood flow: is the cord a microcosm of the brain? *Stroke* 1986;17:1183–1189, with permission.)

a 1997 letter-to-the-editor that the LLA for normotensive, unanesthetized adults may be closer to 65 mm Hg, while the point at which CBF reserve is exceeded might be 40% below baseline MAP. Because volatile and local anesthetics may themselves reduce the LLA because of their vasodilation and metabolic uncoupling effects (discussed below), it is possible that what we have previously considered the LLA in awake patients may more closely approximate the LLA in the anesthetized state. Further study is needed to improve our understanding of these critical relationships.

Importantly, SCPP is determined by the difference between the inflow pressure (normally MAP) and outflow resistance (the higher of venous pressure [VP] or cerebrospinal fluid pressure [CSFP]). That is, SCPP = MAP − CSFP (or VP). Thus, the spinal cord is put at risk of ischemia by systemic hypotension, occlusion of any arterial vessel(s) contributing to SCBF (e.g., aortic cross-clamp, atherosclerotic disease, traumatic vascular injury, epidural hematoma, and so on), increases in CSFP (e.g., epidural hematoma, epidural injection), occlusion of venous outflow (e.g., epidural hematoma, epidural injection), mechanical ventilation during certain pathologic states such as acute lung injury,[19] and so on.

The impact of CSFP on SCBF deserves special attention because it has been shown to play a clinically significant role in SCPP during low-flow states. In particular, animal studies demonstrate that CSF drainage (i.e., reducing CSFP) significantly increases SCBF and reduces the risk of spinal cord ischemia during aortic cross-clamp.[20,21] Similar studies in humans suggest the same.[22] More important, epidural local anesthetic injections have been shown to produce a significant volume-related increase in CSFP.[23–25] Although this increase in pressure is clearly well tolerated by most patients, it is reasonable to infer that injections into the epidural space during periods of reduced spinal cord perfusion (i.e., during

BOX 12-1 Determinants of SCBF

SCBF is autoregulated in a way similar to cerebral blood flow. Spinal cord perfusion pressure is determined by:

- Mean arterial pressure
- The greater of venous pressure or cerebrospinal fluid pressure
- Spinal vasculature exhibits CO_2 reactivity
- SCBF exhibits flow-metabolism coupling

aortic cross-clamp) may put patients at increased risk of spinal cord ischemia.

In addition to autoregulation, animal models demonstrate that the spinal vasculature (like the cerebral vasculature) has CO_2 reactivity. Specifically, SCBF increases with increasing P_aCO_2 and decreases with decreasing P_aCO_2.[26,27] Importantly, CO_2 reactivity is preserved following spinal cord transection, indicating that CO_2 reactivity is a local phenomenon and is not mediated by higher centers. Thus, the risk of spinal cord ischemia is increased in the presence of hyperventilation (hypocapnia), especially if there is a simultaneous decrease in SCPP.

Like the brain, the spinal cord displays flow-metabolism coupling. That is, increased or decreased metabolic activity results in a commensurate increase or decrease in SCBF. This was shown in a study by Sakamoto and Monafo,[28] who found that decreasing metabolic activity by local cooling of the spinal cord resulted in a significant decrease in SCBF. Importantly, decreases in blood flow that result from decreased metabolic activity do not put the spinal cord at risk of ischemia because the flow is exactly matched to the metabolic needs of the tissue. It is crucial to keep this fact in mind when interpreting the effects of local anesthetics on SCBF.

Pharmacology

Identifying the effects of spinally administered drugs on SCBF is essential for understanding the ischemia-related risks of neuraxial blocks. In particular, it is necessary to know whether intrathecally administered drugs have direct effects on SCBF. In this respect, the scientific literature is somewhat wanting. The principal difficulty in interpreting the available data is that investigators often failed to control for, or to account for, the effects of changes in MAP, P_aCO_2, temperature, drug-mediated decreases in spinal cord metabolic rate (either the study drug or the concomitant general anesthetic), drug-mediated effects on autoregulation, and so on. In the absence of appropriate controls, it is often difficult to determine whether the observed effect on SCBF is a direct effect of the local anesthetic or the result of effects on MAP, metabolic rate, and so on.

Local Anesthetics

Intrathecal

Studies of the effects of local anesthetics on SCBF have produced all possible results (i.e., increased flow, decreased flow, and no change in flow). The variability of the results may reflect differences in the local anesthetic employed, the animal model studied, the method used to measure blood flow, the concomitant general anesthetic administered, whether MAP was maintained in the autoregulatory range, and so on.[29,30]

Kozody et al.[31] used radioactive microspheres to measure the effect of intrathecal bupivacaine (20 mg) on SCBF in pentobarbitone-anesthetized mechanically ventilated dogs. They found that bupivacaine alone produced an approximately 37% decrease in SCBF and an approximately 30% decrease in MAP.

These data may be interpreted in several ways. For example, the decrease in flow could be explained by a local anesthetic–mediated loss of SCBF autoregulatory mechanisms, which in the face of the decreased MAP (i.e., decreased SCPP) would result in a decrease in SCBF comparable to the MAP decrease. However, there are data suggesting that autoregulatory mechanisms are intact during spinal anesthesia. For example, Dohi et al.[32] found that tetracaine spinal anesthesia alone did not decrease SCBF despite a significant decrease in MAP from 110 to 89 mm Hg. However, when animals were hemorrhaged to a MAP of 66 mm Hg, SCBF decreased significantly. These data are consistent with the hypothesis that autoregulation was intact and that SCBF decreased only when MAP was decreased below the autoregulatory threshold.

An alternative explanation is that local anesthetic–mediated blockade of neuronal activity may have decreased neuronal metabolic rate, resulting in a commensurate decrease in blood flow because of flow-metabolism coupling. Consistent with the latter explanation is a study by Kuroda et al.,[33] who measured the metabolic rate for glucose in the spinal cord of rats before and after epidural bupivacaine block. They reported that epidural bupivacaine block produced an 18% to 29% decrease in glucose metabolism. Similarly, Crosby[34] has shown that intrathecal bupivacaine reduces glucose metabolism by 15% to 21% in superficial regions of the spinal cord. Using a different approach to studying local anesthetic effects on spinal cord metabolic activity, both Cole et al.[35] and Breckwoldt et al.[36] have shown that intrathecal tetracaine markedly increases the spinal cord's ability to tolerate ischemia, presumably because of decreased metabolic rate.

Although they do not offer definitive proof, these studies suggest that the decrease in SCBF observed by Kozody following intrathecal bupivacaine may be the result of a decrease in spinal cord metabolic rate, and not a loss of autoregulatory mechanisms. Studies of tetracaine's effects on SCBF are variable. Using a pentobarbitone-anesthetized mechanically ventilated dog model, Kozody et al.[37] reported that tetracaine (20 mg) produced an approximately 140% increase in SCBF. The mechanism(s) responsible for the increase in blood flow is unclear, but tetracaine-mediated disruption of flow-metabolism coupling is one possibility. Loss of autoregulation is an unlikely explanation because spinal block was not associated with an increase in MAP.

In contrast, using a halothane-anesthetized mechanically ventilated dog model, Dohi et al.[32] found that 5 mg of intrathecal tetracaine had no effect on SCBF. Similarly, Porter et al.[38] used a pentobarbitone-anesthetized cat model to demonstrate that 5 mg intrathecal tetracaine had no effect on SCBF.

It is tempting to ascribe the differences in the effect of intrathecal tetracaine on SCBF solely to differences in the tetracaine doses used in these studies (Kozody et al., 20 mg; Dohi et al. and Porter et al., 5 mg). However, in the absence of a clear study of dose-related effects of intrathecal tetracaine on SCBF, it is difficult to unquestioningly accept this conclusion.

Dohi et al.,[39] using an anesthetized dog model, performed a dose-ranging study of intrathecal lidocaine's effect on SCBF. These investigators found that 10, 20, 30, or 50 mg of plain lidocaine did not have any statistically significant effect on SCBF despite significant decreases in MAP at all doses. Similarly, using a pentobarbitone-anesthetized cat model, Porter et al.[38] found that neither intrathecal lidocaine (15 mg) nor mepivacaine (10 mg) had any effect on SCBF despite a significant decrease in MAP.

Epidural

Studies of the effects of epidural local anesthetics are fewer in number than studies of intrathecal local anesthetics. Mitchell et al.[40] used an opioid-anesthetized dog model to study the effects of 100 mg of lumbar epidural lidocaine (5 mL, 2%) on SCBF. They found that blood flow was reduced in all regions of the spinal cord by 20% to 40% and that the magnitude of the reduction was generally greater the closer the measurement was made to the site of local anesthetic injection. The reduction in SCBF occurred despite the fact that MAP was maintained at baseline by infusion of lactated Ringer's solution. In addition, they used evoked potentials to document that spinal cord neuronal activity was reduced by epidural blockade, a finding that suggests that the reduction in SCBF was in response to a reduction in spinal cord metabolic activity.

Bouaziz et al.[41] used pentobarbitone-anesthetized rabbits to investigate the effects of 20 mg epidural lidocaine (1 mL; 2%) in young and adult animals. They found that lumbar SCBF was not altered in adult animals despite a significant decrease in MAP. Conversely, in young animals, lumbar SCBF decreased significantly and the decrease was correlated with the decrease in MAP. These findings suggest that adult animals maintained normal autoregulation but that autoregulation was impaired in immature animals. Whether there are similar age-related differences in humans is unknown.

Vasoactive Adjuncts: Intrathecal

Phenylephrine and epinephrine are sometimes added to local anesthetics to increase the duration and/or to improve the quality of spinal and epidural blockade. The conventional wisdom has been that these drugs exert their salutary effects on block duration by decreasing local anesthetic clearance by way of alpha$_1$-adrenergic receptor-mediated vasoconstriction. The problem with this simplistic view is that it fails to explain why the dose of phenylephrine required to prolong spinal blockade is approximately 10 to 20 times greater than the dose of epinephrine, even though both drugs are approximately equipotent as alpha$_1$-adrenergic agonists. One reasonable answer to this question is that the block-prolonging effects of epinephrine and phenylephrine are not mediated by vasoconstriction.

Consistent with the idea that spinal cord vasoconstriction is not the mechanism by which epinephrine and phenylephrine prolong spinal anesthesia is the observation by Kozody et al.[42] (using a radioactive microsphere technique) that neither epinephrine (200 µg) nor phenylephrine (5 mg) had any effect on SCBF in pentobarbitone-anesthetized dogs. Dohi et al.[32] also reported that intrathecal epinephrine (100, 300, and 500 µg) had no effect on SCBF in halothane-anesthetized dogs using a hydrogen clearance technique to measure blood flow.

In contrast to the results of Kozody et al., Dohi et al.[39] reported a dose-dependent decrease (25%–45%) in SCBF following intrathecal phenylephrine doses of 2, 3, and 5 mg. A 1-mg phenylephrine dose produced a statistically insignificant decrease in SCBF. Why the effects of phenylephrine reported by Kozody and Dohi are so divergent is unclear. However, it is worth noting that Dohi et al. used the hydrogen clearance technique to measure blood flow and that Kozody used the "gold-standard" microsphere technique. The hydrogen clearance technique requires the insertion of a hydrogen-sensitive electrode into the spinal cord, and electrode insertion itself has been shown to decrease blood flow.[43]

Iida et al.[44] attempted to determine the effects of vasoactive drugs on spinal cord circulation by applying a variety of drugs directly to pial vessels on the surface of the spinal cord and measuring the change in vessel diameter. They found that topical application of epinephrine (5 µg/mL) and phenylephrine (5 µg/mL) produced a modest reduction in the diameter of pial vessels (~8%–11%). These investigators did not measure resultant SCBF, but previous studies have shown that the diameter of superficial pial arterioles does not correlate well with blood flow in the underlying tissue.[45]

Thus, with respect to the direct effect of epinephrine and phenylephrine on SCBF, the available data would suggest that intrathecal epinephrine does not have a significant effect on SCBF.[46] The data are not as clear for the effects of phenylephrine, but the best data (Kozody et al. and Iida et al.) would suggest that phenylephrine probably does not have a significant effect either. This begs the question as to how these drugs prolong and improve local anesthetic block if they do not decrease SCBF. One possibility is that a vascular site other than the spinal cord is the vasoconstrictor effect site. In particular, the dura mater is possibly the site, as it has an abundant vascular supply. In fact, Kozody et al. showed that although intrathecal epinephrine and phenylephrine did not affect SCBF, they did significantly reduce dural blood flow. Another possibility is that the alpha$_2$-adrenergic receptor effects of epinephrine and phenylephrine are responsible for their ability to improve local anesthetic block. That is, these drugs may prolong the block by inhibiting nociceptive transmission just as the alpha$_2$-agonist clonidine does. An attractive aspect of this hypothesis is that it would explain why the required dose of phenylephrine is so much greater than that of epinephrine. Specifically, because phenylephrine is a very weak alpha$_2$ agonist at usual clinical doses, a supraphysiologic dose is necessary to produce a measurable alpha$_2$-mediated block-prolonging effect (Box 12-2).

BOX 12-2 Mechanisms by Which Vasoconstrictors Prolong Neuraxial Local Anesthetic Block

- Epinephrine and probably phenylephrine do not decrease SCBF.
- Epinephrine and phenylephrine significantly decrease dural blood flow, which reduces the clearance of local anesthetics.
- Epinephrine and (to a lesser extent) phenylephrine provide direct analgesia as agonists of alpha$_2$-adrenergic receptors in the spinal cord.

Local Anesthetics Plus Vasoconstrictors

Although studies of the effects of epinephrine and phenylephrine alone on SCBF are informative, the effect of vasoactive drugs when combined with local anesthetics is more relevant clinically.

Intrathecal

Unfortunately, the available data give a mixed picture as to the effect of adding vasoactive agents to local anesthetics for spinal anesthesia. For example, Porter et al. added epinephrine (10 µg/mL) to intrathecal tetracaine (5 mg), lidocaine (15 mg), and mepivacaine (10 mg) and reported that none of these solutions had any effect on SCBF.[31] In contrast, Kristensen et al.[47] reported that bupivacaine (0.025, 0.125, and 0.25 mg) alone decreased SCBF in a dose-dependent manner in a rat model wherein laser Doppler was used to measure the blood flow. The addition of epinephrine to the 0.125- and 0.25-mg bupivacaine doses did not decrease SCBF further. However, when added to the lowest dose of bupivacaine, epinephrine did decrease the blood flow further (from a 10% reduction to a 37% reduction).

These authors did not examine the mechanism responsible for the decrease in SCBF in response to bupivacaine alone, but the most likely explanation is a local anesthetic mediated decrease in spinal cord metabolic activity and a commensurate decrease in the blood flow because of flow-metabolism coupling. Consistent with this hypothesis are the studies discussed previously demonstrating that spinal anesthesia decreases spinal cord metabolic activity. The additional reduction in SCBF observed by Kristensen when adding epinephrine to the lowest dose of bupivacaine may have resulted from an alpha$_2$-mediated further reduction in neuronal metabolic activity. The failure of epinephrine to further reduce SCBF when added to the larger doses of bupivacaine is consistent with the possibility that the larger doses produced a maximal decrease in CMRO$_2$ that could not be further reduced by the addition of epinephrine.

Dohi et al.[39] examined the effect of lidocaine plus phenylephrine on SCBF in a dog model ($n = 5$) of spinal anesthesia. They reported that lidocaine alone had no effect on SCBF but that the addition of phenylephrine (5 mg) caused a decrease. However, this claim is difficult to evaluate because the authors did not report the average change in SCBF, whether the change was statistically significant, or whether MAP decreased simultaneously.

Epidural

Bouaziz et al.[41] examined the effect of adding epinephrine (5 µg/mL) to epidural lidocaine (20 mg) in a rabbit model. The authors reported that lidocaine plus epinephrine had no significant effect on SCBF in adult rabbits. In immature animals, lidocaine alone decreased SCBF in parallel with MAP, but the addition of epinephrine had no additional effect on SCBF.

As the reader can now appreciate, studies of the effects of spinally and epidurally administered drugs on SCBF are not "clean." The available studies are at once contradictory, inadequately controlled, and incomplete. However, the animal data suggest that to the extent that local anesthetics decrease SCBF they do so by decreasing spinal cord metabolic activity and are in fact protective in the setting of experimental spinal cord ischemia. In addition, the addition of vasoactive agents (particularly epinephrine) does not appear to put the spinal cord at added risk of ischemia (Chapter 8).

Importantly, clinical experience also suggests that neuraxial block with or without vasoactive adjuncts is unlikely to have a clinically significant effect on SCBF in the overwhelming majority of patients.[46] Whether there are rare patients or clinical situations in which a local anesthetic or vasoactive adjunct in and of itself puts the spinal cord at significant risk of ischemia is currently unknown, and given the rarity of the phenomenon this may be effectively unknowable.

▶ RISK FACTORS

The most common cause of regional anesthesia-related ischemic injury to the spinal cord is arguably epidural (and occasionally intrathecal) hematoma. The pathophysiology of ischemia in this setting is fairly clear: the pressure exerted by the expanding hematoma impairs the venous outflow and arterial inflow. The presence of the hematoma makes the determination of the source of spinal cord ischemia reasonably clear.

Spinal cord ischemia and infarction have also been associated with transforaminal epidural steroid injections performed for cervical radicular pain.[48-51] The mechanism by which blood flow is impaired in these cases is not clear. One possibility is that the needle disrupts a major feeding artery traversing the intervertebral foramen. Consistent with this mechanism, Huntoon[52] found in an autopsy study of 10 cadavers that 7 of the 95 foramina dissected had a radicular vessel traversing the posterior aspect of the intervertebral foramen that could potentially be injured by transforaminal needle placement. A second possibility is that a particulate steroid suspension (e.g., triamcinolone-hexacetonide) is injected into a radicular artery and carried to the spinal cord, where it occludes the spinal capillaries.[53,54] Consistent with this mechanism, Baker et al.[55] have demonstrated the injection of contrast into a radicular artery and its passage to the spinal cord during a trial injection prior to attempted transforaminal epidural steroid injection. Regardless of which of these potential mechanisms is responsible for the cases of spinal cord injury associated with transforaminal injections, it is clear that the spinal cord is at risk during these procedures and that the necessary techniques to reduce the risk, for example, the use of nonparticulate steroid preparations and real-time test injection of a contrast agent under fluoroscopy, remain to be better defined (Chapter 28).[56]

Cases in which patients develop ischemic spinal cord injury following a transforaminal injection or because of an epidural hematoma following a neuraxial block clearly implicate the regional anesthetic procedure as causative. More vexing are cases in which spinal cord ischemia occurs in the absence of a clear etiology. Unfortunately, in these cases identifying the cause often devolves into "rounding up the usual suspects," and if the patient has had a regional anesthetic it will often head the list of potential causes. Systemic hypotension is probably the most common etiologic mechanism blamed for perioperative spinal cord ischemia. Given that SCBF is pressure dependent, it is not unreasonable to consider hypotension (or more specifically, hypoperfusion) as a possible mechanism. However, the critical question is: What level of hypotension, maintained for what period of time, puts a patient at increased risk of spinal cord ischemia?

Unfortunately, there are no studies that specifically address this issue for SCBF. A large-scale study of blood pressures during noncardiac anesthesia could not link 1-year mortality to a specific minimal blood pressure. At best, this study by Bijker et al.[57] found a trend for increased hazard ratio in elderly patients who sustained a relative 40% decrease in systolic blood pressure or MAP, and found that the risk of death increased as the corresponding time at these pressures increased. It is reasonable to speculate that hypoperfusion of the spinal cord may also follow a similar paradigm wherein lower perfusion pressures are tolerated for a shorter duration of time. However, there are many studies of deliberate hypotension that also provide relevant information. In these studies, hundreds of patients have had their MAP lowered to between 34 and 60 mm Hg for periods ranging from 20 minutes to several hours without causing spinal cord injury.[16,58-70] Patients who survive the more extreme hypotension that accompanies cardiac arrest often develop brain injury, but only rarely do they develop spinal cord injury. Thus, despite frequent claims that intraoperative hypotension is a cause of postoperative spinal cord ischemia, hypotension *per se* does not appear to be a significant cause of this entity. Importantly, clinical experience demonstrates that organs other than the spinal cord (e.g., brain, myocardium) are more susceptible to ischemic injury during systemic hypotension. Thus, spinal cord ischemia in the absence of other end-organ injury is unlikely to have resulted from hypotension alone.

That said, systemic hypotension might conceivably contribute to spinal cord ischemia when other risk factors are simultaneously present. For example, vascular disease (particularly vertebral, carotid, and aortic) can magnify the impact of hypotension because the fall in perfusion pressure is greater within stenotic blood vessels than in normal vessels. Embolic phenomena (from atherosclerosis, air, or fat) or vasoocclusive sludging (from sickle cell disease or other hemoglobinopathies) can also be worsened by hypotension. Anemia and/or hypoxia reduce oxygen delivery that may already be reduced by a hypotension-mediated fall in SCBF. Similarly, hypermetabolic states (e.g., hyperthermia, thyrotoxicosis, and myoclonic seizures) may increase the oxygen demand above that which can be met during hypotension-mediated decreases in SCBF. Elevated spinal CSFP (e.g., following epidural injections) has an exaggerated impact on SCBF when systemic pressure is low (recall that SCPP = MAP – CSFP). Although CSFP elevation after epidural injections is generally transient (~15 minutes maximal effect), this may be sufficient to cause ischemia in a severely compromised patient. Other pressure-related conditions, such as severe spinal stenosis, epidural lipomatosis, or tumor, are discussed in Chapter 10.

Exaggerated patient positioning during surgery with consequent impingement of spinal cord vasculature (both intrinsic and extrinsic) has also been implicated as a cause of spinal cord ischemia. For example, Deinsberger et al.[71] used somatosensory-evoked potentials (SSEPs) to monitor spinal cord integrity while patients were placed in a semi-sitting position with the neck flexed and rotated for posterior fossa surgery. They observed that 14.5% of patients had a significant decrease in SSEPs requiring a change in position. The authors hypothesized that spinal cord ischemia from vascular compression was a potential cause of the decrease in SSEP. Similarly, Bhuiyan et al.[72] reported a case of spinal cord infarction believed to have been caused by positioning in exaggerated lateral flexion during thoracotomy in a patient with stenosed spinal arteries. Finally, postoperative spinal cord injury has also been reported to result from exaggerated spinal flexion in patients with herniated disks that compress the spinal cord.[73]

These position-related injuries demonstrate that spinal cord ischemia does occur during surgery by mechanisms unrelated to anesthesia, and they help to illustrate the types of situations (e.g., thoracic epidural block for thoracotomy or spinal block in patients with herniated disks) in which regional anesthesia procedures may be incorrectly blamed for causing spinal cord ischemia.

▶ DIAGNOSTIC EVALUATION

Diagnosing perioperative spinal cord ischemia in the setting of a regional anesthetic, especially neuraxial block, can be very difficult. The primary difficulty arises from the fact that there is a natural tendency to assume that the early sensory-motor changes that are the pathopneumonic signs/symptoms of spinal cord ischemia are simply the result of the block and that the appropriate first response is to simply wait for the resolution of the block, or in the case of a continuous epidural infusion to decrease the local anesthetic infusion rate. The unfortunate result of this mindset is a delay in definitive diagnosis and appropriate therapy (particularly in the setting of epidural hematoma), with potentially devastating consequences. Clinicians must maintain a high index of suspicion and have a low threshold for ordering appropriate diagnostic studies to rule out correctable causes of spinal cord ischemia (e.g., hematoma).[74]

A second pitfall in the early diagnosis of spinal cord ischemia is that imaging studies may not be sufficiently sensitive for the detection of early spinal cord ischemia. T2-weighted MR images may miss spinal cord ischemia in the first hours after onset, although diffusion-weighted images have detected ischemia as early as 3 hours after symptom onset.[75,76] CT myelography has been insensitive in some cases of acute spinal cord ischemia.[3] Importantly, although CT and MRI techniques may miss early spinal cord ischemia, both techniques are sensitive for the diagnosis of mass lesions (e.g., epidural hematoma) causing spinal cord ischemia.

▶ PREVENTION

Preventing spinal cord ischemia caused by regional anesthesia must focus on the highest-incidence cause: spinal hematoma. In this regard, the single-most important preventive measure is a thorough history and medication review to determine if the patient is at risk of coagulopathy. Readers are referred to the American Society of Regional Anesthesia Consensus Conference on Neuraxial Anesthesia and Anticoagulation[77] (www.asra.com) for a current review and recommendations for performing central neuraxial blocks in patients who are taking, or who have taken, drugs that impair coagulation (e.g., coumadin, platelet inhibitors, NSAIDS, heparins, and so on) (Chapter 4).

The other increasingly clear connection between regional anesthesia and spinal cord injury is the rare interruption of SCBF that can occur during transforaminal injections. Without additional controlled data, it is difficult to make recommendations for preventing this complication except to suggest that there may be a role for contrast injection under fluoroscopy (ideally using a digital subtraction technique) to rule out intravascular injection prior to injecting a particulate-free steroid suspension[54,56,78] (Chapter 28).

Apart from these two areas, it is impossible to make recommendations for preventing regional anesthesia-caused spinal cord ischemia that are supported by data. Some have speculated that spinal stenosis is a risk factor, but currently available data make it difficult to ascertain whether the linkage of severe spinal stenosis with heightened risk of neuraxial injury is association or truly cause-and-effect[79,80] (Chapters 10 and 20).

▶ TREATMENT

Treatment of spinal cord ischemia must obviously focus on treatable causes. Chief among these is the evacuation of epidural or intrathecal hematomas, which must occur "early" to improve the chances of neurologic recovery. For example, Lawton et al.[81] showed in a series of 30 patients with epidural hematomas that both severity of neurologic symptoms and time from symptom onset to surgical evacuation correlated with degree of neurologic recovery. In this study, surgical evacuations performed within 12 hours of symptom onset resulted in significantly greater recovery than those performed later. Others have reported time to decompression should be 8 hours or less.[74,82]

If no correctable causes of ischemia can be identified, appropriate supportive measures should be instituted. As in any neurologic injury, situations that contribute to secondary neurologic injury should be avoided. Chief among these is hypotension (i.e., hypoperfusion). Maintaining "normal" to slightly higher than normal MAPs is important. In addition, CSF drainage (which improves spinal cord perfusion by decreasing CSFP) has been shown to be effective in situations in which spinal cord ischemia developed during recovery from aortic aneurysm repair.[83,84] Other contributors to secondary neurologic injury include hyperglycemia, hyperthermia, hypoxia, and anemia.

Several therapeutic strategies have a credible scientific rationale but lack sufficient supportive clinical evidence in the context of spinal cord ischemia. For example, high-dose methylprednisolone is a controversial therapy shown to have some modest benefit in recovery from traumatic spinal cord injury in some, but not all, human clinical trials. However, its value in the context of spinal cord ischemia is unknown. Similarly, naloxone, magnesium, mannitol, estrogen, dextromethorphan, and cyclosporine-A, among others, have been shown to reduce secondary neurologic injury in some experimental systems, but there are insufficient data in the context of human spinal cord ischemia to permit a recommendation regarding their use.

▶ SUMMARY

With the exception of epidural and intrathecal hematomas, ischemic injury to the spinal cord that is clearly caused by neuraxial block is a very rare event. The majority of case reports of ischemic injury occurring in the setting of neuraxial blocks fail to clearly identify the block as the proximate

BOX 12-3 Clinical Caveat

There is minimal, if any, scientific evidence to link neuraxial ischemic injury to the use of neuraxial regional anesthetic techniques or the concurrent use of local anesthetics and/or vasoactive additives. Known causes of neuraxial ischemia include direct vascular trauma, intravascular injection of toxins or drugs that block blood flow in spinal cord feeding vessels, and vascular compression from space-occupying lesions such as epidural hematoma or abscess. The majority of perioperative spinal cord ischemic injuries are unrelated to anesthetic technique.

cause and too often amount to little more than "guilt by association."

That said, knowledge of spinal vascular anatomy and physiology provides insights into potential mechanisms by which spinal and epidural anesthesia may increase the risk of spinal cord ischemia. "Disruption" of an important radicular artery is an obvious potential mechanism, and it is certainly theoretically possible for an epidural or spinal needle to encounter radicular vessels in the epidural space (Chapter 10). Prolonged systemic hypotension below the patient's autoregulatory/ischemic threshold, especially in a patient with precarious blood flow to the spinal cord, may conceivably produce ischemia. This risk would be increased if P_aCO_2 is low because of hyperventilation or epidural pressures are raised by volume injection. Importantly, the available animal data would suggest that spinal or epidural local anesthetic block would reduce the risk of ischemia in this setting because of decreased metabolic rate and therefore greater vascular reserve. There is no reason to believe that local anesthetics put the spinal cord at risk of ischemia. In fact, local anesthetics may have neuroprotective qualities.

The available data would also seem to suggest that the addition of epinephrine to local anesthetics does not adversely affect SCBF, and the wealth of clinical experience with this adjuvant is consistent with this view. The impact of phenylephrine on SCBF is less clear from animal experiments, but again clinical experience would suggest that phenylephrine *per se* is not a cause of spinal cord ischemia (Box 12-3). Thus, in the absence of direct vascular injury, unintentional intravascular injection of injurious materials (e.g., colloidal drug suspension), or spinal hematoma formation, neuraxial block is unlikely to cause spinal cord ischemia.

References

1. Neal JM. Anatomy and pathophysiology of spinal cord injuries associated with regional anesthesia and pain medicine. *Reg Anesth Pain Med* 2008;33:423–434.
2. Nedeltchev K, Loher TJ, Stepper AF, et al. Long-term outcome of acute spinal cord ischemia syndrome. *Stroke* 2004;35:560–565.
3. Elksnis SM, Hogg JP, Cunningham ME. MR imaging of spontaneous spinal cord infarction. *J Comput Assist Tomogr* 1991;15:228–232.
4. Beloeil H, Albaladejo P, Hoen S, et al. Bilateral lower limb hypoesthesia after radical prostatectomy in the hyperlordotic position under general anesthesia. *Can J Anaesth* 2003;50:653–656.

5. Hong DK, Lawrence HM. Anterior spinal artery syndrome following total hip arthroplasty under epidural anaesthesia. *Anaesth Intensive Care* 2001;29:62–66.

6. Auroy Y, Benhamou D, Bargues L, et al. Major complications of regional anesthesia in France: the SOS Regional Anesthesia Hotline Service. *Anesthesiology* 2002;97:1274–1280.

7. Sliwa JA, Maclean IC. Ischemic myelopathy: a review of spinal vasculature and related clinical syndromes. *Arch Phys Med Rehabil* 1992;73:365–372.

8. Neal JM. Neurologic complications. In: Rathmell JP, Neal JM, Viscomi CM, eds. *Regional Anesthesia: The Requisites in Anesthesiology.* Philadelphia, PA: Elsevier-Mosby, 2004:157–163.

9. Tureen L. Circulation of the spinal cord and the effect of vascular occlusion. *Res Nerv Ment Disc Proc* 1938;18:394–437.

10. Mettler F. *Neuroanatomy.* St. Louis, MO: Mosby, 1948.

11. Biglioli P, Roberto M, Cannata A, et al. Upper and lower spinal cord blood supply: the continuity of the anterior spinal artery and the relevance of the lumbar arteries. *J Thorac Cardiovasc Surg* 2004;127:1188–1192.

12. Hogan QH. Lumbar epidural anatomy: a new look by cryomicrotome section. *Anesthesiology* 1991;75:767–775.

13. Kobrine AI, Doyle TF, Rizzoli HV. Spinal cord blood flow as affected by changes in systemic arterial blood pressure. *J Neurosurg* 1976;44:12–15.

14. Hickey R, Albin MS, Bunegin L, et al. Autoregulation of spinal cord blood flow: is the cord a microcosm of the brain? *Stroke* 1986;17:1183–1189.

15. Abe K, Nishimura M, Kakiuchi M. Spinal cord blood flow during prostaglandin E1 induced hypotension. *Prostaglandins Leukot Essent Fatty Acids* 1994;51:173–176.

16. Tsuji T, Matsuyama Y, Sato K, et al. Evaluation of spinal cord blood flow during prostaglandin E1-induced hypotension with power Doppler ultrasonography. *Spinal Cord* 2001;39:31–36.

17. Sharbrough FW, Messick JM, Sundt TM. Correlation of continuous electroencephalograms with cerebral blood flow measurements during carotid endarterectomy. *Stroke* 1973;4:674–683.

18. Drummond JC. The lower limit of autoregulation: time to revise our thinking? *Anesthesiology* 1997;86:1431–1433.

19. Kreyer S, Putensen C, Berg A, et al. Effects of spontaneous breathing during airway pressure release ventilation on cerebral and spinal cord perfusion in experimental acute lung injury. *J Neurosurg Anesthesiol* 2010;22:323–329.

20. Uceda P, Basu S, Robertazzi RR, et al. Effect of cerebrospinal fluid drainage and/or partial exsanguination on tolerance to prolonged aortic cross-clamping. *J Card Surg* 1994;9:631–637.

21. Bower TC, Murray MJ, Gloviczki P, et al. Effects of thoracic aortic occlusion and cerebrospinal fluid drainage on regional spinal cord blood flow in dogs: correlation with neurologic outcome. *J Vasc Surg* 1989;9:135–144.

22. Cina CS, Abouzahr L, Arena GO, et al. Cerebrospinal fluid drainage to prevent paraplegia during thoracic and thoracoabdominal aortic aneurysm surgery: a systematic review and meta-analysis. *J Vasc Surg* 2004;40:36–44.

23. Kopacz DJ, Carpenter RL, Mulroy MF. The reliability of epidural anesthesia for repeat ESWL: a study of changes in epidural compliance. *Reg Anesth* 1990;15:199–203.

24. Usubiaga JE, Wikinski JA, Usubiaga LE. Epidural pressure and its relation to spread of anesthetic solutions in epidural space. *Anesth Analg* 1967;46:440–446.

25. Usubiaga JE, Usubiaga LE, Brea LM, et al. Effect of saline injections on epidural and subarachnoid space pressures and relation to postspinal anesthesia headache. *Anesth Analg* 1967;46:293–296.

26. Scremin OU, Decima EE. Control of blood flow in the cat spinal cord. *J Neurosurg* 1983;58:742–748.

27. Marsala M, Vanicky I, Yaksh TL. Effect of graded hypothermia (27 degrees to 34 degrees C) on behavioral function, histopathology, and spinal blood flow after spinal ischemia in rat. *Stroke* 1994;25:2038–2046.

28. Sakamoto T, Monafo WW. Regional spinal cord blood flow during local cooling. *Neurosurgery* 1990;26:958–962.

29. Hodgson PS, Neal JM, Pollock JE, et al. The neurotoxicity of drugs given intrathecally (spinal). *Anesth Analg* 1999;88:797–809.

30. Iida H, Iida M. Effects of spinal analgesics on spinal circulation. The safety standpoint. *J Neurosurg Anesthesiol* 2008;20:180–187.

31. Kozody R, Ong B, Palahniuk RJ, et al. Subarachnoid bupivacaine decreases spinal cord blood flow in dogs. *Can Anaesth Soc J* 1985;32:216–222.

32. Dohi S, Takeshima R, Naito H. Spinal cord blood flow during spinal anesthesia in dogs: the effects of tetracaine, epinephrine, acute blood loss, and hypercapnia. *Anesth Analg* 1987;66:599–606.

33. Kuroda Y, Sakabe T, Nakakimura K, et al. Epidural bupivacaine suppresses local glucose utilization in the spinal cord and brain of rats. *Anesthesiology* 1990;73:944–950.

34. Crosby G. Local spinal cord blood flow and glucose utilization during spinal anesthesia with bupivacaine in conscious rats. *Anesthesiology* 1985;63:55–60.

35. Cole DJ, Shapiro HM, Drummond JC, et al. Halothane, fentanyl/nitrous oxide, and spinal lidocaine protect against spinal cord injury in the rat. *Anesthesiology* 1989;70:967–972.

36. Breckwoldt WL, Genco CM, Connolly RJ, et al. Spinal cord protection during aortic occlusion: efficacy of intrathecal tetracaine. *Ann Thorac Surg* 1991;51:959–963.

37. Kozody R, Palahniuk RJ, Cumming MO. Spinal cord blood flow following subarachnoid tetracaine. *Can Anaesth Soc J* 1985;32:23–29.

38. Porter SS, Albin MS, Watson WA, et al. Spinal cord and cerebral blood flow responses to subarachnoid injection of local anesthetics with and without epinephrine. *Acta Anaesthesiol Scand* 1985;29:330–338.

39. Dohi S, Matsumiya N, Takeshima R, et al. The effects of subarachnoid lidocaine and phenylephrine on spinal cord and cerebral blood flow in dogs. *Anesthesiology* 1984;61:238–244.

40. Mitchell P, Goad R, Erwin CW, et al. Effect of epidural lidocaine on spinal cord blood flow. *Anesth Analg* 1989;68:312–317.

41. Bouaziz H, Okubo N, Malinovsky JM, et al. The age-related effects of epidural lidocaine, with and without epinephrine, on spinal cord blood flow in anesthetized rabbits. *Anesth Analg* 1999;88:1302–1307.

42. Kozody R, Palahniuk RJ, Wade JG, et al. The effect of subarachnoid epinephrine and phenylephrine on spinal cord blood flow. *Can Anaesth Soc J* 1984;31:503–508.

43. Verhaegen MJ, Todd MM, Warner DS, et al. The role of electrode size on the incidence of spreading depression and on cortical cerebral blood flow as measured by H2 clearance. *J Cereb Blood Flow Metab* 1992;12:230–237.

44. Iida H, Ohata H, Iida M, et al. Direct effects of alpha1- and alpha2-adrenergic agonists on spinal and cerebral pial vessels in dogs. *Anesthesiology* 1999;91:479–485.

45. Haberl RL, Heizer ML, Ellis EF. Laser-Doppler assessment of brain microcirculation: effect of local alterations. *Am J Physiol* 1989;256:H1255–H1260.

46. Neal JM. Effects of epinephrine in local anesthetics on the central and peripheral nervous systems: neurotoxicity and neural blood flow. *Reg Anesth Pain Med* 2003;28:124–134.

47. Kristensen JD, Karlsten R, Gordh T. Spinal cord blood flow after intrathecal injection of ropivacaine and bupivacaine with or without epinephrine in rats. *Acta Anaesthesiol Scand* 1998;42:685–690.

48. Brouwers PJ, Kottink EJ, Simon MA, et al. A cervical anterior spinal artery syndrome after diagnostic blockade of the right C6-nerve root. *Pain* 2001;91:397–399.

49. Hodges SD, Castleberg RL, Miller T, et al. Cervical epidural steroid injection with intrinsic spinal cord damage. Two case reports. *Spine* 1998;23:2137–2142.

50. Ludwig MA, Burns SP. Spinal cord infarction following cervical transforaminal epidural injection: a case report. *Spine* 2005;30:E266–E268.

51. McMillan MR, Crumpton C. Cortical blindness and neurologic injury complicating cervical transforaminal injection for cervical radiculopathy. *Anesthesiology* 2003;99:509–511.

52. Huntoon MA. Anatomy of the cervical intervertebral foramina: vulnerable arteries and ischemic neurologic injuries after transforaminal epidural injections. *Pain* 2005;117:104–111.

53. Benzon HT, Chew TL, McCarthy R, et al. Comparison of the particle sizes of the different steroids and the effect of dilution: a review of the relative neurotoxicities of the steroids. *Anesthesiology* 2007;106:331–338.

54. Rathmell JP, Benzon HT. Transforaminal injection of steroids: should we continue? (editorial). *Reg Anesth Pain Med* 2004;29:397–399.

55. Baker R, Dreyfuss P, Mercer S, et al. Cervical transforaminal injection of corticosteroids into a radicular artery: a possible mechanism for spinal cord injury. *Pain* 2003;103:211–215.

56. Neal JM, Bernards CM, Hadzic A, et al. ASRA Practice Advisory on neurologic complications in regional anesthesia and pain medicine. *Reg Anesth Pain Med* 2008;33:404–422.

57. Bijker JB, van Klei WA, Vergouwe Y, et al. Intraoperative hypotension and 1-year mortality after noncardiac surgery. *Anesthesiology* 2009;111:1217–1226.

58. Bernard JM, Passuti N, Pinaud M. Long-term hypotensive technique with nicardipine and nitroprusside during isoflurane anesthesia for spinal surgery. *Anesth Analg* 1992;75:179–185.

59. Lam AM, Gelb AW. Cardiovascular effects of isoflurane-induced hypotension for cerebral aneurysm surgery. *Anesth Analg* 1983;62:742–748.

60. Lessard MR, Trepanier CA, Baribault JP, et al. Isoflurane-induced hypotension in orthognathic surgery. *Anesth Analg* 1989;69:379–383.

61. Lessard MR, Trepanier CA, Brochu JG, et al. Effects of isoflurane-induced hypotension on renal function and hemodynamics. *Can J Anaesth* 1990;37:S42.

62. Lustik SJ, Papadakos PJ, Jackman KV, et al. Nicardipine versus nitroprusside for deliberate hypotension during idiopathic scoliosis repair. *J Clin Anesth* 2004;16:25–33.

63. Prys-Roberts C, Lloyd JW, Fisher A, et al. Deliberate profound hypotension induced with halothane: studies of haemodynamics and pulmonary gas exchange. *Br J Anaesth* 1974;46:105–116.

64. Sum DC, Chung PC, Chen WC. Deliberate hypotensive anesthesia with labetalol in reconstructive surgery for scoliosis. *Acta Anaesthesiol Sin* 1996;34:203–207.

65. Thompson GE, Miller RD, Stevens WC, et al. Hypotensive anesthesia for total hip arthroplasty: a study of blood loss and organ function (brain, heart, liver, and kidney). *Anesthesiology* 1978;48:91–96.

66. Toivonen J, Kaukinen S. Clonidine premedication: a useful adjunct in producing deliberate hypotension. *Acta Anaesthesiol Scand* 1990;34:653–657.

67. Toivonen J, Kaukinen S, Oikkonen M, et al. Effects of deliberate hypotension induced by labetalol on renal function. *Eur J Anaesthesiol* 1991;8:13–20.

68. Toivonen J, Kuikka P, Kaukinen S. Effects of deliberate hypotension induced by labetalol with isoflurane on neuropsychological function. *Acta Anaesthesiol Scand* 1993;37:7–11.

69. Toivonen J, Virtanen H, Kaukinen S. Deliberate hypotension induced by labetalol with halothane, enflurane or isoflurane for middle-ear surgery. *Acta Anaesthesiol Scand* 1989;33:283–289.

70. Toivonen J, Virtanen H, Kaukinen S. Labetalol attenuates the negative effects of deliberate hypotension induced by isoflurane. *Acta Anaesthesiol Scand* 1992;36:84–88.

71. Deinsberger W, Christophis P, Jodicke A, et al. Somatosensory evoked potential monitoring during positioning of the patient for posterior fossa surgery in the semisitting position. *Neurosurgery* 1998;43:36–40; discussion 40–42.

72. Bhuiyan MS, Mallick A, Parsloe M. Post-thoracotomy paraplegia coincident with epidural anaesthesia. *Anaesthesia* 1998;53:583–586.

73. Brower RS, Herkowitz HN, Weissman ML. Conus medullaris injury due to herniated disk and intraoperative positioning for arthroscopy. *J Spinal Disord* 1995;8:163–165.

74. Sorenson EJ. Neurological injuries associated with regional anesthesia. *Reg Anesth Pain Med* 2008;33:442–448.

75. Fujikawa A, Tsuchiya K, Takeuchi S, et al. Diffusion-weighted MR imaging in acute spinal cord ischemia. *Eur Radiol* 2004;14:2076–2078.

76. Kuker W, Weller M, Klose U, et al. Diffusion-weighted MRI of spinal cord infarction: high resolution imaging and time course of diffusion abnormality. *J Neurol* 2004;251:818–824.

77. Horlocker TT, Wedel DJ, Rowlingson JC, et al. Regional anesthesia in the patient receiving antithrombotic or thrombolytic therapy: American Society of Regional Anesthesia and Pain Medicine Evidence-Based Guidelines (Third Edition). *Reg Anesth Pain Med* 2010;35:64–101.

78. Rathmell JP, April C, Bogduk N. Cervical transforaminal injection of steroids. *Anesthesiology* 2004;100:1595–1600.

79. Hebl JR, Horlocker TT, Kopp SL, et al. Neuraxial blockade in patients with preexisting spinal stenosis, lumbar disc disease, or prior spinal surgery: efficacy and neurological complications. *Anesth Analg* 2010;111:1511–1519.

80. Moen V, Dahlgren N, Irestedt L. Severe neurological complications after central neuraxial blockades in Sweden 1990–1999. *Anesthesiology* 2004;101:950–959.

81. Lawton MT, Porter RW, Heiserman JE, et al. Surgical management of spinal epidural hematoma: relationship between surgical timing and neurological outcome. *J Neurosurg* 1995;83:1–7.

82. Vandermeulen EP, Van Aken H, Vermylen J. Anticoagulants and spinal-epidural anesthesia. *Anesth Analg* 1994;79:1165–1177.

83. Blacker DJ, Wijdicks EF, Ramakrishna G. Resolution of severe paraplegia due to aortic dissection after CSF drainage. *Neurology* 2003;61:142–143.

84. Tiesenhausen K, Amann W, Koch G, et al. Cerebrospinal fluid drainage to reverse paraplegia after endovascular thoracic aortic aneurysm repair. *J Endovasc Ther* 2000;7:132–135.

13

Transient Neurologic Symptoms

Julia E. Pollock

Since its introduction in 1948, 5% hyperbaric lidocaine has been used for millions of spinal anesthetics. The predictable onset and limited duration of action made lidocaine one of the most popular spinal anesthetics. Concern about the use of spinal lidocaine began in 1991 with published reports of cauda equina syndrome (CES) after continuous spinal anesthesia,[1,2] and this was heightened in 1993 by case reports of four patients undergoing spinal anesthesia who experienced postoperative aching and pain in the buttocks and lower extremities.[3] The constellation of this latter group of symptoms is currently referred to as transient neurologic symptoms (TNS).

▶ DEFINITION AND HISTORY

The first prospective safety study of intrathecal lidocaine was performed by Phillips et al.[4] and published in 1968. This study evaluated 10,440 patients (93% obstetric) undergoing spinal anesthesia with lidocaine. The authors concluded that lidocaine was safe for spinal anesthesia. Analyses of these data reveal that during the study period 284 patients complained of back pain. Of these patients, 91 refused subsequent spinal anesthesia because of postspinal back pain. Subsequently, millions of patients underwent spinal anesthesia with 5% hyperbaric lidocaine, with only rare published reports of complications. Scrutiny of lidocaine began in 1991, with case reports documenting CES after continuous

spinal anesthesia.[1,2] Of the initial case reports of CES following continuous spinal anesthesia, all but one involved the use of lidocaine. It was postulated that the mechanics of spinal microcatheters (which allowed the pooling of local anesthetic at the lumbosacral roots), in combination with an extremely large dose of the local anesthetic, were the cause of CES in these patients. Subsequently, at the direction of the United States (US) Food and Drug Administration (FDA), spinal microcatheters were withdrawn from the US market.

Concern over the use of single-dose 5% hyperbaric lidocaine for spinal anesthesia began in 1993 when Schneider et al.[3] published a report of four patients undergoing spinal anesthesia in the lithotomy position who experienced postoperative aching and pain in the buttocks and lower extremities. Initial reports used the term transient radicular irritation to describe this syndrome. Eventually, the terminology was changed to TNS to better reflect the symptomatology and lack of definitive etiology. All of Schneider's patients recovered completely. Nonetheless, subsequent case reports and editorials questioned the continued use of 5% hyperbaric lidocaine and suggested that a fresh appraisal of its safety by the appropriate regulatory agencies might be in order.[5,6]

The term TNS is used to describe both unilateral and bilateral pain occurring within 24 hours after spinal anesthesia that involves the buttocks and may radiate to the lower extremities. The lower back may or may not be included. The term TNS is itself controversial because it implies a neurologic etiology, which has yet to be proven (Box 13-1).

BOX 13-1 Diagnostic Components of TNS

- Symptoms begin within 24 hours after the resolution of spinal anesthesia.
- Most patients experience aching and/or pain of the unilateral or bilateral buttocks. Fewer patients will experience dysesthesia radiating into the anterior or posterior thighs.
- Back pain may not be present in all patients.
- Symptoms resolve in 6 hours to 4 days.
- There are no neurologic findings upon physical exam or imaging.

▶ SCOPE

After Schneider's initial case report, multiple case reports and a few laboratory and clinical studies evaluated the components of TNS after spinal anesthesia. Prospective randomized controlled studies[7–25] have shown a remarkable variability in the incidence of TNS among patients undergoing spinal anesthesia with lidocaine (Fig. 13-1). Clearly, the incidence of TNS is the highest following lidocaine spinal anesthesia versus other local anesthetics. The association of TNS with lidocaine spinal anesthesia has also been supported by two separate meta-analyses.[26,27] Randomized studies, as well as an epidemiologic study by Freedman et al.,[28] have shown that the incidence of TNS varies with the type of surgery performed (Table 13-1). For example, patients undergoing surgery in the lithotomy position have an incidence of TNS of approximately 30% to 36%,[7,9,12] patients undergoing arthroscopic knee surgery an incidence of 18% to 22%,[8,10,15,16] and patients undergoing surgery in the supine position an incidence of 4% to 8%.[18,19] This observation makes it easier to explain the variation reported in studies evaluating the incidence of TNS.

Because the symptoms of TNS are transitory and result in no abnormalities on physical exam or neurologic testing, many physicians have questioned the clinical importance of the syndrome. One study attempted to quantify the degree of functional impairment found in patients experiencing TNS[24] by randomizing 453 patients to undergo either 1% or 5% hyperbaric 80-mg lidocaine spinal anesthesia for urologic surgery. The patients were assessed for the incidence of TNS and functional impairment. The incidence of TNS was 21% with 1% lidocaine and 18% with 5% lidocaine, and the patients experiencing TNS reported significant impairment of daily functional activities such as walking, sitting, and sleeping.

▶ PATHOPHYSIOLOGY

Possible causes of TNS include specific local anesthetic toxicity,[5,6] needle trauma, neural ischemia secondary to sciatic stretching,[3] patient positioning, pooling of local anesthetics secondary to small-gauge pencil-point needles,[29] muscle spasm, myofascial trigger points,[30] early mobilization, and/or irritation of the dorsal root ganglion.[31] Because few patients receiving intrathecal bupivacaine report TNS, it appears that TNS is not the result of having a subarachnoid block *per se*. Hence, epiphenomena of subarachnoid block (spinal needle placement, bed-to-bed transfer, or surgery) are not the sole causative factors of TNS.[32]

Several authors have assumed that TNS is a symptom of direct neurotoxicity. Local anesthetics clearly exert significant neurotoxicity in laboratory models, and indeed lidocaine, tetracaine, and prilocaine seem to be more neurotoxic in animal models than are bupivacaine and chloroprocaine.[33] Concentrations of lidocaine within its clinically useful range (1%–5%) have been shown to inhibit nerve conduction in isolated frog sciatic nerve models.[34,35] However, one argument against local anesthetic toxicity as the etiology of TNS is that factors reported to increase the incidence of TNS are not the same factors that increase the incidence of CES, which is known to result from local anesthetic toxicity. For example, the incidence of CES is increased by higher doses and concentrations of local anesthetics and

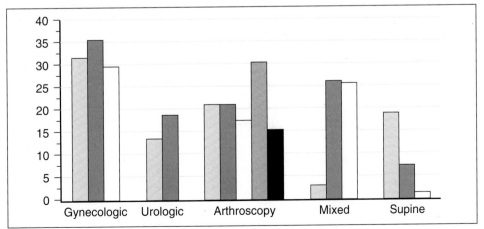

FIGURE 13-1. **Incidence of TNS as a function of surgical position.** All patients received spinal lidocaine. Most gynecologic and urologic patients were in lithotomy position. All arthroscopy patients were knee arthroscopy. Mixed patients refer to studies where surgical position varied. Vertical bars represent individual studies, which are referenced to the following citations: gynecologic,[7,9,12] urologic,[13,24] knee arthroscopy,[8,10,15,16,25] mixed surgery,[11,14,17] and supine.[8,19,20]

TABLE 13-1 Randomized Controlled Studies of TNS

PRIMARY AUTHOR AND YEAR PUBLISHED	SURGERY TYPE AND NUMBER OF SUBJECTS	INCIDENCE OF TNS RELATIVE TO LOCAL ANESTHETIC
Hampl (1995)[7]	Gynecology 44	5% Lidocaine 32% 0.5% Bupivacaine 0%
Pollock (1996)[8]	Knee arthroscopy, inguinal herniorrhaphy 159	5% Lidocaine 16% 2% Lidocaine 16% 0.75% Bupivacaine 0%
Hampl (1996)[9]	Gynecology 50	5% Lidocaine 32% 2% Lidocaine 40%
Liguori (1998)[10]	Knee arthroscopy 60	2% Lidocaine 22% 1.5% Mepivacaine 0%
Martinez-Bourio (1998)[11]	Mixed surgical 200	5% Lidocaine 4% 5% Prilocaine 1%
Salmela (1998)[13]	Mostly urologic 90	2.5% Lidocaine 20% 4% Mepivacaine 37% 5% Bupivacaine 0%
Hampl (1998)[12]	Gynecology 90	2% Lidocaine 30% 2% Prilocaine 3% 0.5% Bupivacaine 0%
Pollock (1999)[15]	Knee arthroscopy 109	2% Lidocaine 16% 1.0% Lidocaine 22% 0.5% Lidocaine 17%
Hiller (1999)[14]	Mixed surgical 60	5% Lidocaine 27% General Anesthesia 3%
Hodgson (2000)[16]	Knee arthroscopy 70	5% Lidocaine 31% 10% Procaine 6%
Keld (2000)[17]	Mixed surgical 70	5% Lidocaine 26% 0.5% Bupivacaine 3%
Ostgaard (2000)[18]	Urologic 100	2% Lidocaine 14% 2% Prilocaine 1%
DeWeert (2000)[19]	Supine mixed surgical 70	2% Lidocaine 3% 2% Prilocaine 0%
Salazar (2001)[20]	Supine orthopedics 80	2% Lidocaine 2.5% 2% Mepivacaine 2.5%
Lindh (2001)[21]	Ambulation after inguinal hernia 107	2% Lidocaine—early 23% 2% Lidocaine—late 23%
Philip (2001)[22]	Postpartum tubal ligation 58	5% Lidocaine 3% 0.75% Bupivacaine 7%
Aouad (2001)[23]	Cesarean delivery 200	5% Lidocaine 0% 0.75% Bupivacaine 0%
Tong (2003)[24]	Urologic 453	5% Lidocaine 18% 1% Lidocaine 21%
Silvanto (2004)[25]	Knee arthroscopy 120	2% Lidocaine—early 7.5% 2% Lidocaine—6 h 28% 2% Lidocaine—late 13%

by the addition of vasoconstrictors, but none of these factors appear to increase the incidence of TNS. One study attempted to determine if TNS was the result of direct neurotoxicity of lidocaine by evaluating volunteers with electromyography, nerve conduction studies, and somatosensory-evoked potentials before and during episodes of TNS. Volunteers in this small study had no abnormalities in electrophysiologic tests even in areas susceptible to the effects of local anesthetic toxicity such as the posterior nerve roots.[36]

The etiology of TNS has been the subject of ongoing laboratory and clinical research. It does appear that TNS is associated predominately with the use of lidocaine spinal anesthesia, that decreasing the concentration from 5% to 0.5% does not decrease the incidence of TNS,[15,24] and that hyperosmolarity,[7] hyperbaricity, or the addition of glucose are not contributing factors. Why surgical position contributes to the development of TNS remains unclear, but potential etiologies include musculoskeletal strain or sciatic nerve stretching.

▶ RISK FACTORS

Clinical studies have attempted to determine which patients may be at risk for the development of TNS. Lidocaine spinal anesthesia and the lithotomy position[24] are important contributing factors. In the epidemiologic study by Freedman et al.,[28] outpatient status was shown to be a significant risk factor for the development of TNS, but subsequent randomized controlled studies[21,25] have not confirmed early ambulation as an additional risk factor. One of these studies[21] randomized inguinal hernia patients to early (immediate) or late (12 hours) ambulation following 100-mg hyperbaric 2% lidocaine spinal anesthesia and found no difference in the incidence of TNS (23%) between the groups. Arthroscopic knee surgery and obesity may also affect the incidence of TNS (Box 13-2).

Despite the concern that pregnant patients may be at increased risk for neurologic deficits or pain after spinal anesthesia, randomized controlled trials have revealed a low incidence of TNS in women undergoing cesarean delivery (0%–8%)[23] or postpartum tubal ligation (3%).[22] The incidence in these patients seems consistent with other studies of nonpregnant patients undergoing surgery in the supine position.

▶ DIAGNOSTIC EVALUATION

Several randomized studies have included descriptions of the characteristics of TNS reported by patients experiencing the syndrome. The majority of patients experience bilateral

symptoms in the anterior or posterior aspects of the thighs, which they describe variously as burning, aching, cramping, or radiating. Approximately half the patients report that the pain radiates into their lower extremities and 50% to 100% report low back pain (Fig. 13-2). When asked to rate their pain on a scale of 1 to 10, the average number is 6.2 (range 1–9).[8,15] The onset is within 12 to 24 hours after surgery and the duration is between 6 hours and 4 days. The onset of this syndrome is markedly different from that of back pain following 2-chloroprocaine epidural anesthesia, which occurs immediately upon the resolution of the epidural block and is confined to the lower back without a radicular component. No patients with TNS have exhibited abnormal neurologic exams or motor weakness. Thus, if a patient presents with an abnormal neurologic exam or motor weakness, other possible etiologies such as an epidural hematoma or nerve root damage must be considered (Box 13-3).

▶ PREVENTION

Because current treatment options for TNS are not always successful, prevention is important. Although total abandonment of spinal lidocaine is probably not warranted, careful patient selection is crucial. Because the primary risk factors for the development of TNS are lidocaine spinal anesthesia in patients undergoing knee arthroscopy or surgery in the lithotomy position,[24] avoidance of lidocaine spinal anesthesia in these patients is justified. Because

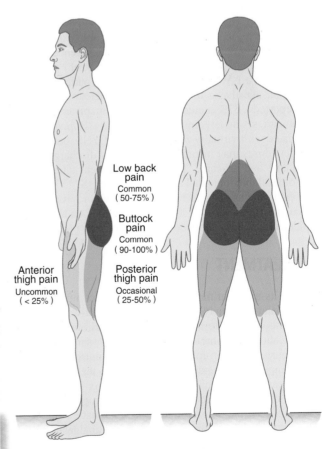

FIGURE 13-2. Distribution and frequency of the symptoms associated with TNS.

Low back pain
Common
(50-75%)

Buttock pain
Common
(90-100%)

Anterior thigh pain
Uncommon
(< 25%)

Posterior thigh pain
Occasional
(25-50%)

BOX 13-2 Primary Risk Factors for TNS

- Lidocaine > other local anesthetics >> bupivacaine.
- Patient position: lithotomy or knee arthroscopy.
- Ambulation and obesity: conflicting data.

BOX 13-3 When to Suspect a More Ominous Diagnosis Than TNS

- Presence of any neurologic sign other than dysesthesia to the legs
- Lower extremity weakness
- Bowel or bladder dysfunction
- Fever

If any of the previous symptoms are present, consider alternative diagnoses such as:

- Epidural hematoma
- Epidural abscess
- Cauda equina syndrome

BOX 13-4 Treatment Options for TNS

- Reassurance as to its transient nature
- Nonsteroidal anti-inflammatory drugs: therapy of choice
- Symptomatic therapy (heat, comfortable positioning)
- Muscle relaxants: if muscle spasm is present
- Opioids: moderately effective adjunct to previous options
- Trigger-point injections: anecdotal reports, but low risk

---

the incidence of TNS after lidocaine spinal anesthesia in patients undergoing inguinal hernia repair is between 4% and 8%,[8] this is perhaps an acceptable risk, as a limited number of other effective short-acting spinal agents are available. Dilution of lidocaine from 5% to 0.5% does not decrease the incidence of TNS.[15,24] The selection of alternative spinal anesthetics for high-risk patients is not an easy one. Procaine, mepivacaine, bupivacaine, prilocaine, and 2-chloroprocaine have all been evaluated, but no ideal alternative exists.

Procaine may have an incidence of TNS that is less than lidocaine but produces less reliable anesthesia and increased nausea and pruritus when combined with fentanyl.[16] Mepivacaine has been used routinely in Europe for spinal anesthesia in a 4% hyperbaric concentration. The true incidence of TNS with mepivacaine is controversial. Liguori et al.[10] reported no TNS with a 1.5% mepivacaine solution in patients receiving spinal anesthesia for arthroscopy, whereas Salmela et al.[13] reported a 37% incidence with a 4% mepivacaine solution in patients undergoing urologic surgery. Bupivacaine is associated with virtually zero incidence of TNS, but even in very low doses may inconsistently prolong discharge times. Prilocaine and articaine, potentially excellent alternatives, are not available for spinal anesthesia in the US.[12,37,38] Recent studies on the use of preservative-free 2-chloroprocaine for spinal anesthesia show encouraging results as an alternative to lidocaine in both volunteers and ambulatory patients.[39–47]

▶ TREATMENT

Despite its transient nature, TNS is very uncomfortable for patients and extremely difficult to treat effectively. Current treatment options remain limited to traditional classes of medications and some interventional therapy and include opioids, nonsteroidal anti-inflammatory drugs, muscle relaxants, and symptomatic therapy. Unfortunately, these treatment reports remain predominantly anecdotal (Box 13-4).

One of the most successful classes of drugs for treating TNS has been the nonsteroidal anti-inflammatory drugs. In general, this class of drugs accomplishes analgesia by the inhibition of prostaglandin synthesis. The propionic acid derivatives are all effective cyclooxygenase inhibitors, although there is considerable variation in their potency.

Patients generally report good pain relief with these drugs. Ibuprofen, naproxen, and ketorolac have all been used successfully. If significant muscle spasm is an accompanying component of TNS, patients may benefit from the addition of muscle relaxants such as cyclobenzaprine. These drugs work at the brain stem as opposed to spinal cord levels, although action on the latter may contribute to overall skeletal muscle relaxant activity. Evidence suggests that the net effect is a reduction of tonic somatic motor activity, influencing both gamma and alpha motor neurons. Symptomatic therapy, including leg elevation on pillows and using heating pads, may provide an additional measure of patient comfort.

In addition to systemic medications, there have been case reports describing the use of trigger-point injections to treat TNS after lidocaine spinal anesthesia.[30] In the first case report to describe this therapy, the patients were treated 2 weeks after their spinal anesthetic. It is very difficult to determine if the symptoms that these patients experienced 2 weeks postoperatively were TNS or more classic muscle spasm that may have been initiated by TNS. Nonetheless, trigger-point injection is a relatively easy therapy to administer and has few risks. It is thus a good option for patients who are so uncomfortable that they return to the hospital or outpatient clinic for treatment.

When a patient complains of symptoms following neuraxial block, other more serious causes of leg and back pain must be eliminated (Box 13-3). Motor weakness is not a symptom of TNS and always suggests other etiologies including spinal hematoma. Once other possible etiologies (hematoma, abscess, and CES) have been eliminated, treatment may begin. Reassure the patient that their symptoms, though uncomfortable, are transient in nature and typically resolve within 1 to 4 days.

▶ SUMMARY

Local anesthetic agents all have the potential to be neurotoxic, particularly in concentrations and doses greater than those used clinically. Despite local anesthetics having the potential for neurotoxicity in the laboratory model, large-scale surveys of the complications of spinal anesthesia attest to the relative safety of intrathecal local anesthetics. Neurotoxicity has not been determined to be the etiology of TNS after single-dose spinal anesthesia. However, because TNS does lead to functional impairment and a confusing differential diagnosis, the use of lidocaine for spinal anesthesia is best avoided in patients considered at high risk for the development of the syndrome, including those undergoing surgery in the lithotomy position or knee arthroscopy.

References

1. Rigler M, Drasner K, Krejcie T, et al. Cauda equina syndrome after continuous spinal anesthesia. *Anesth Analg* 1991;72:275–281.
2. Schell R, Brauer F, Cole D, et al. Persistent sacral root deficits after continuous spinal anesthesia. *Can J Anaesth* 1991;38:908–911.
3. Schneider M, Ettlin T, Kaufmann M, et al. Transient neurologic toxicity after hyperbaric subarachnoid anesthesia with 5% lidocaine. *Anesth Analg* 1993;76:1154–1157.
4. Phillips O, Ebner H, Nelson A, et al. Neurologic complications following spinal anesthesia with lidocaine: a prospective review of 10,440 cases. *Anesthesiology* 1969;30:284–289.
5. deJong R. Last round for a "heavyweight"? *Anesth Analg* 1994;78:3–4.
6. Drasner K. Lidocaine spinal anesthesia: a vanishing therapeutic index? *Anesthesiology* 1997;87:469–471.
7. Hampl KF, Schneider MC, Thorin D, et al. Hyperosmolarity does not contribute to transient radicular irritation after spinal anesthesia with hyperbaric 5% lidocaine. *Reg Anesth* 1995;20:363–368.
8. Pollock JE, Neal JM, Stephenson CA, et al. Prospective study of the incidence of transient radicular irritation in patients undergoing spinal anesthesia. *Anesthesiology* 1996;84:1361–1367.
9. Hampl KF, Schneider MC, Pargger H, et al. A similar incidence of transient neurologic symptoms after spinal anesthesia with 2% and 5% lidocaine. *Anesth Analg* 1996;83:1051–1054.
10. Liguori GA, Zayas VM, Chisholm M. Transient neurologic symptoms after spinal anesthesia with mepivacaine and lidocaine. *Anesthesiology* 1998;88:619–623.
11. Martinez-Bourio R, Arzuaga M, Quintana JM, et al. Incidence of transient neurologic symptoms after hyperbaric subarachnoid anesthesia with 5% lidocaine and 5% prilocaine. *Anesthesiology* 1998;88:624–628.
12. Hampl KF, Heinzmann-Wiedmer S, Luginbuehol I, et al. Transient neurologic symptoms after spinal anesthesia. *Anesthesiology* 1998;88:629–633.
13. Salmela L, Aromma U. Transient radicular irritation after spinal anesthesia induced with hyperbaric solutions of cerebrospinal fluid-diluted lidocaine 50 mg/ml or mepivacaine 40 mg/ml or bupivacaine 5 mg/ml. *Acta Anaesthesiol Scand* 1998;42:765–769.
14. Hiller A, Karjalainen K, Balk M, et al. Transient neurologic symptoms after spinal anaesthesia with hyperbaric 5% lidocaine or general anaesthesia. *Br J Anaesth* 1999;82:575–579.
15. Pollock J, Liu S, Neal J, et al. Dilution of spinal lidocane does not alter the incidence of transient neurologic symptoms. *Anesthesiology* 1999;90:445–449.
16. Hodgson P, Liu S, Batra M, et al. Procaine compared with lidocaine for incidence of transient neurologic symptoms. *Reg Anesth Pain Med* 2000;25:218–222.
17. Keld DB, Hein L, Dalgaard M, et al. The incidence of transient neurologic symptoms after spinal anaesthesia in patients undergoing surgery in the supine position: hyperbaric lidocaine 5% versus hyperbaric bupivacaine 0.5%. *Acta Anaesthesiol Scand* 2000;44:285–290.
18. Ostgaard G, Hallaraker O, Ulveseth OK, et al. A randomised study of lidocaine and priolocaine for spinal anaesthesia. *Acta Anaestheiol Scand* 2000;44:436–440.
19. DeWeert K, Traksel M, Gielen M, et al. The incidence of transient neurologic symptoms after spinal anaesthesia with lidocaine compared to prilocaine. *Anaesthesia* 2000;55:1003–1024.
20. Salazar F, Bogdanovich A, Adalia R, et al. Transient neurologic symptoms after spinal anaesthesia using isobaric 2% mepivacaine and isobaric 2% lidocaine. *Acta Anaesthesiol Scand* 2001;45:240–245.
21. Lindh A, Andersson AS, Westman L. Is transient lumbar pain after spinal anaesthesia with lidocaine influence by early mobilisation? *Acta Anaesthesiol Scand* 2001;45:290–293.
22. Philip J, Sharma S, Gottumukkla V, et al. Transient neurologic symptoms after spinal anesthesia with lidocaine in obstetric patients. *Anesth Analg* 2001;92:405–409.
23. Aouad M, Siddik S, Jalbout M, et al. Does pregnancy protect against intrathecal lidocaine-induced transient neurologic symptoms? *Anesth Analg* 2001;92:401–404.
24. Tong D, Wong J, Chung F, et al. Prospective study on incidence and functional impact of transient neurologic symptoms associated with 1% versus 5% hyperbaric lidocaine in short urologic procedures. *Anesthesiology* 2003;98:485–494.
25. Silvanto M, Tarkkila P, Makela ML, et al. The influence of ambulation time on the incidence of transient neurologic symptoms after lidocaine spinal anesthesia. *Anesth Analg* 2004;98:542–546.
26. Eberhart LH, Morin AM, Kranke P, et al. Transiente neurologishce symptome nach spinalanasthesie. *Der Anaesthesist* 2002;7:539–546.
27. Zaric D, Christiansen C, Pace NL, et al. Transient neurologic symptoms after spinal anesthesia with lidocaine versus other local anaesthetics: a systematic review. *Anesth Analg* 2005;6:1811–1816.
28. Freedman J, Li D, Drasner K, et al. Risk factors for transient neurologic symptoms after spinal anesthesia. *Anesthesiology* 1998;89:633–641.
29. Beardsley D, Holman S, Gantt R, et al. Transient neurologic deficit after spinal anesthesia: Local anesthetic maldistribution with pencil point needles? *Anesth Analg* 1995;81:314–320.
30. Naveira FA, Copeland S, Anderson M, et al. Transient neurologic toxicity after spinal anesthesia, or is it myofascial pain? Two case reports. *Anesthesiology* 1998;88:268–270.
31. Dahlgren N. Transient radicular irritation after spinal anaesthesia-reply 2. *Acta Anaesthesiol Scand* 1996;40:865.
32. Frey K, Holman S, Mikat-Stevens M, et al. The recovery profile of hyperbaric spinal anesthesia with lidocaine, tetracaine and bupivacaine. *Reg Anesth Pain Med* 1998;23:159–163.
33. Ready L, Plumer M, Haschke R. Neurotoxicity of intrathecal local anesthetics in rabbits. *Anesthesiology* 1985;63:364–370.
34. Lambert L, Lambert D, Strichartz G. Irreversible conduction block in isolated nerve by high concentrations of local anesthetics. *Anesthesiology* 1994;80:1082–1093.
35. Bainton C, Strichartz G. Concentration dependence of lidocaine-induced irreversible conduction loss in frog nerve. *Anesthesiology* 1994;81:657–667.
36. Pollock J, Burkhead D, Neal J, et al. Spinal nerve function in five volunteers experiencing transient neurologic symptoms after lidocaine subarachnoid anesthesia. *Anesth Analg* 2000;90:658–665.
37. Kallio H, Snall EVT, Loude T, et al. Hyperbaric articaine for day-case spinal anaesthesia. *Br J Anaesth* 2006;97:704–709.
38. Hendriks MP, de Weert CJM, Snoeck MMJ, et al. Plain articaine or prilocaine for spinal anaesthesia in day- case knee arthroscopy: a double-blind randomized trial. *Br J Anaesth* 2008;102:259–263.
39. Kouri M, Kopacz D. Spinal 2-chloroprocaine: a comparison with lidocaine in volunteers. *Anesth Analg* 2004;98:75–80.
40. Smith K, Kopacz D, McDonald S. Spinal 2-chloroprocaine: a dose-ranging study and the effect of added epinephrine. *Anesth Analg* 2004;98:81–88.
41. Vath J, Kopacz D. Spinal 2-chloroprocaine: the effect of added fentanyl. *Anesth Analg* 2004;98:89–94.
42. Warren D, Kopacz D. Spinal 2-chloroprocaine: the effect of added dextrose. *Anesth Analg* 2004;98:95–101.
43. Casati A, Fanelli G, Danelli G, et al. Spinal anaesthesia with lidocaine or preservative free 2-chloroprocaine for outpatient knee arthroscopy: a prospective, randomized, double blind comparison. *Anesth Analg* 2007;104:959–964.
44. Casati A, Danelli G, Berti M, et al. Intrathecal 2-chloroprocaine for lower limb outpatient surgery: a prospective, randomized, double-blind, clinical evaluation. *Anesth Analg* 2006;103:234–238.
45. Sell A, Tein T, Pitkanen M. Spinal 2-chloroprocaine: effective dose for ambulatory surgery. *Acta Anaesthesiol Scand* 2008;52:695–699.
46. Hejtmanek MR, Pollock JE. Chloroprocaine for spinal anesthesia: a retrospective analysis. *Acta Anaesthesiol Scand* 2011;55:267–272.
47. Forster JG, Kallio H, Rosenberg PH, et al. Chloroprocaine vs. articaine as spinal anaesthetics for day-case knee arthroscopy. *Acta Anaesthesiol Scand* 2011;55:273–281.

COMPLICATIONS SPECIFIC TO PERIPHERAL NERVE BLOCK

14

Peripheral Nerve Injury

James R. Hebl

Peripheral nerve injury has long been recognized as a potential complication of regional anesthesia. Neuhof[1] in 1914 described musculospiral nerve paralysis following brachial plexus anesthesia that could not be attributed to the original injury. Subsequently, Woolley and Vandam[2] reviewed the available literature in 1959 and found several cases of persistent neurologic symptoms following brachial plexus blockade. They reported frequencies of nerve injury ranging from 0.1%[3] to 5.6%[4] and speculated that many of the injuries may be attributed to mechanical trauma or local anesthetic toxicity. Woolley and Vandam[2] recommended that, "an atraumatic technic with the use of small gauge needles

and avoidance of hematoma formation" be the primary goal. Furthermore, they suggested that the patient be "carefully prepared with sedatives so that the experience of nerve injection is not disagreeable nor the recollection too vivid."

Since this time, several basic science and clinical investigations have examined the issue of peripheral nerve injury in an attempt to identify risk factors commonly associated with postoperative neurologic dysfunction. As a result of this work, a multitude of patient, surgical, and anesthetic risk factors have been identified that may contribute to perioperative nerve injury (Box 14-1). This chapter will examine the estimated risk of peripheral nerve injury, review the relevant anatomy

BOX 14-1 Risk Factors Contributing to Perioperative Nerve Injury

Patient Risk Factors

- Male gender
- Tobacco use
- Increasing age
- Preexisting diabetes mellitus
- Extremes of body habitus
- Preexisting neurologic disorders

Surgical Risk Factors

- Surgical trauma or stretch
- Tourniquet ischemia
- Vascular compromise
- Perioperative inflammation
- Hematoma
- Cast compression or irritation
- Postoperative infection or abscess formation
- Patient positioning

Anesthetic Risk Factors

- Needle- or catheter-induced mechanical trauma
- Intrafascicular injection
- Ischemic injury (vasoconstrictors)
- Perineural edema
- Local anesthetic toxicity

BOX 14-2 Variables Contributing to Differences in Rates of Perioperative Nerve Injury

Sample sizes

- Small vs. large studies

Surgical procedures and block techniques

- Multiple surgical procedures vs. single surgical intervention
- Upper extremity block techniques vs. lower extremity block techniques vs. both

Providers performing the blocks

- Experienced vs. novice

Patient status during block placement

- Awake vs. sedated vs. general anesthesia

Exclusion criteria

- Variable (may or may not include patients with preexisting neurologic deficits)

Definition of perioperative nerve injury

- New deficits vs. worsening of preexisting deficits vs. both
- Anesthesia-related injuries vs. surgical related injuries vs. both

Method of postoperative evaluation

- Direct contact by anesthesiologist vs. patient self-reports vs. surgical follow-up vs. voluntary patient or provider surveys

Time of follow-up evaluation

- Variable (48 hours to 6 months)

as it pertains to practicing clinicians, and discuss the relative contribution of several risk factors commonly associated with peripheral nerve injury. Specifically, anesthetic related risk factors will be examined in depth and comment made with regard to preventative measures clinicians may take to potentially avoid catastrophic or devastating long-term sequelae.

▶ DEFINITION

Perioperative nerve injury may be defined as the presence of pain, paresthesias, sensory or motor deficits, or other neurologic abnormalities (e.g., cranial nerve dysfunction) after surgery. The deficit(s) may be newly diagnosed (i.e., no prior history) or a progression of preexisting neurologic findings. A *persistent* neurologic deficit occurring after regional anesthesia refers to a sensory or motor abnormality that lasts beyond the expected duration of an administered local anesthetic. While the majority of perioperative neurologic deficits are transient and self-limited, those remaining unchanged after 12 months are considered *permanent* by many neurologists and neurosurgeons.

▶ SCOPE

Background and Incidence

Several investigators have examined the incidence of perioperative nerve injury with varying results. For example, during the past decade, prospective randomized studies have reported the frequency of perioperative nerve injury after regional anesthesia to range from 0.02%[5] to 11%.[6] Several differences in study methodology likely account for the tremendous variation in reported rates of neurologic complications (Box 14-2).[7]

Welch et al.[8] examined the frequency of perioperative nerve injury in 380,680 surgical cases at a single institution over a 10-year period of time. Overall, they identified a neurologic complication rate of 0.03%. General and epidural anesthesia were more often associated with neurologic injury than spinal anesthesia or peripheral nerve blockade (PNB). Significant associations were also found among patients undergoing neurosurgical interventions, cardiac surgery, general surgery, and orthopedic surgery. In contrast, Jacob et al.[9] recently found that the type of anesthesia (general vs. neuraxial) or PNB was *not* associated with an increased risk of perioperative nerve injury in 12,329 patients undergoing total knee arthroplasty.

Auroy et al.[10] performed one of the first large-scale prospective investigations evaluating the risk of serious complications related to regional anesthesia. In this French survey, a total of 103,730 regional anesthetics, including 71,053 neuraxial anesthetics, 21,278 peripheral nerve blocks (PNB), and 11,229 intravenous regional anesthetics, were performed over a 5-month period of time. Neurologic complications related to regional anesthetic techniques occurred in 34 (0.03%) patients. This represented 26% of all complications related to regional anesthesia. Of the 34 neurologic complications, 24 (70%) occurred during spinal anesthesia, 6 (18%) during epidural anesthesia, and 4 (12%) during PNB. All neurologic complications occurred within 48 hours of surgery and resolved within 3 months in 85% of patients. In all cases of neurologic injury after PNB, needle placement was associated with either a paresthesia during needle insertion or pain on injection. In all cases, the sensory deficit had the same topography as the associated paresthesia during block placement.

In a follow-up investigation, Auroy et al.[5] further examined 158,083 regional anesthetics—including 50,223 PNB —over a 10-month period. The overall incidence of serious complications related to regional anesthesia (all techniques) was found to be approximately 4/10,000 (0.04%) (Table 14-1). Interestingly, when they specifically examined the risk associated with PNB, they found an identical incidence of 4/10,000 (0.04%). However, a significantly higher percentage of complications were noted with the posterior lumbar plexus block, when compared to other peripheral techniques (Table 14-2). Similar to their initial findings, the incidence of cardiac arrest and neurologic complications was found to be significantly higher after spinal anesthesia when compared to other types of regional anesthesia (Table 14-1). Neurologic complications attributed specifically to the regional technique occurred in 26 (0.02%) patients; recovery was complete within 6 months in 16 (62%) of the 26 patients. Of the 12 patients experiencing a neurologic complication after PNB, 7 (58%) persisted for >6 months. Of these, nine had been performed with the use of a peripheral nerve stimulator.

More recently, Barrington et al.[11] performed a prospective audit of more than 7,000 PNB performed in nine Australian hospitals. Ultrasound imaging was used as the primary mode of neural localization in more than 63% of the procedures. Overall, they identified a neurologic injury rate of 0.5%. However, only 10% of these injuries were attributed to PNB, suggesting that the vast majority of perioperative nerve injuries have a nonanesthesia-related etiology. The nerve injury rate attributed to PNB was found to be 0.04%—a rate similar to other large-scale investigations.[5,10] Horlocker et al.[12] have also found that nearly 90% of perioperative nerve injures are secondary to surgical (i.e., nonanesthesia) causes. Of the patients experiencing neurologic deficits secondary to regional anesthesia, the vast majority (66%) had their deficits persist beyond 6 months, with 33% of deficits extending for >1 year.[11] Jacob et al.[9] have suggested that anesthesia-related neurologic deficits (i.e., deficits occurring after PNB) may be less likely to have a complete neurologic recovery when compared to nerve injuries from surgical causes.

Many investigators speculate that the risk of peripheral nerve injury may be higher in patients undergoing continuous perineural catheter placement versus single-injection techniques. The frequency of minor neurologic deficits (e.g., hypoesthesias, dysesthesias, persistent numbness) occurring within the first few days after perineural catheter placement is variable, ranging from 0%[13] to 8%.[14] However, severe neural lesions or long-term (i.e., 3–6 months) neurologic deficits occur at rates comparable to single-injection techniques.[13–18]

Based upon these and other findings, most authors conclude that needle-induced mechanical trauma and local anesthetic neurotoxicity are the primary etiologies of

TABLE 14-1 Serious Complications Related to Regional Anesthesia

TECHNIQUE	CARDIAC ARREST	RESPIRATORY FAILURE	DEATH	SEIZURE	NEUROLOGIC INJURY
Spinal (N = 41,251)	10 (2.4)	2 (0.5)	3 (0.7)	1 (0.2)	14 (3.4)
Epidural (N = 35,379)	0	3 (0.8)	0	3 (0.8)	0
Peripheral blocks (N = 50,223)	1 (0.2)	2 (0.4)	1 (0.2)	6 (1.2)	12 (2.4)
IV regional (N = 4,448)	0	0	0	0	0
Peribulbar blocks (N = 17,071)	0	0	0	0	0
Total regional blocks (N = 158,083)	11 (0.7)	7 (0.4)	4 (0.3)	10 (0.6)	26 (1.6)

Data presented are number and the estimated (n/10,000) where applicable.

Reprinted from Auroy Y, Benhamou D, Bargues L, et al. Major complications of regional anesthesia in France: the SOS Regional Anesthesia Hotline Service. *Anesthesiology* 2002;97:1274–1280, with permission.

TABLE 14-2 Serious Complications Related to PNB

TECHNIQUE	CARDIAC ARREST	RESPIRATORY FAILURE	DEATH	SEIZURE	NEUROLOGIC INJURY
Interscalene block (N = 3,459)	0	0	0	0	1 (2.9)
Supraclavicular block (N = 1,899)	0	0	0	1 (5.3)	0
Axillary block (N = 11,024)	0	0	0	1 (0.9)	2 (1.8)
Mid-humeral block (N = 7,402)	0	0	0	1 (1.4)	1 (1.4)
Posterior lumbar plexus (N = 394)	1 (25.4)	2 (50.8)	1 (25.4)	1 (25.4)	0
Femoral block (N = 10,309)	0	0	0	0	3 (3)
Sciatic nerve block (N = 8,507)	0	0	0	2 (2.4)	2 (2.4)
Popliteal nerve block (N = 952)	0	0	0	0	3 (32)
Total peripheral nerve blocks (N = 50,223)	1 (0.2)	2 (0.4)	1 (0.2)	6 (1.2)	12 (2.4)

Data presented are number and the estimated (n/10,000) where applicable.

Reprinted from Auroy Y, Benhamou D, Bargues L, et al. Major complications of regional anesthesia in France: the SOS Regional Anesthesia Hotline Service. *Anesthesiology* 2002;97:1274–1280, with permission.

neurologic complications attributed to regional anesthesia. Although most of these studies found that the incidence of severe anesthesia-related complications is extremely low, they have also demonstrated that serious complications may occur in the presence of experienced anesthesiologists—and that continued vigilance in patients undergoing regional anesthesia is not only warranted, but critical to minimize perioperative nerve injuries.

Closed Claims Analysis

Cheney et al.[19] examined the American Society of Anesthesiologists Closed Claims database to further delineate the role of nerve damage in malpractice claims filed against anesthesia care providers. Of the 4,183 claims reviewed, 670 (16%) were for anesthesia-related nerve injury. The most frequent sites of injury were the ulnar nerve (28%), the brachial plexus (20%), the lumbosacral nerve roots (16%), and the spinal cord (13%). Additional mononeuropathies comprised the remaining 22% of claims. Overall, regional anesthesia was more frequently associated with nerve damage claims when compared to general anesthesia. The only exception was ulnar nerve injuries, which were predominantly associated with general anesthesia (85%).

Regional anesthetic techniques (axillary, interscalene, and supraclavicular blockade) were attributed specifically to 16% of all brachial plexus injuries, in which 31% experienced a paresthesia either during needle placement or with injection of local anesthetic. In contrast, 30% of ulnar nerve injuries were attributed to regional anesthetic techniques in which a mechanism of injury was explicitly stated. Interestingly, none of these claims involved the elicitation of a paresthesia. In these cases, the onset of symptoms occurred immediately within the postoperative period in 21% of patients and was delayed from 1 to 28 days postoperatively (median 3 days) in 62% of cases.[19] It has been suggested that neurologic deficits that arise within the first 24 hours of surgery most likely represent extra- or intraneural hematoma, intraneural edema, or a lesion involving a sufficient number of nerve fibers to allow immediate diagnosis.[12,20] In contrast, several investigations have reported a delay in neurologic findings, in which symptoms develop several days or even weeks following surgery.[10,12,19–21] The presentation of late disturbances in nerve function may suggest an alternate etiology, such as a tissue reaction, scar formation, or inflammatory process leading to the degeneration of nerve fibers.[20,22] However, it is not possible from the available data to determine whether this reaction may be due to mechanical trauma, local anesthetic neurotoxicity, or a combination of both.

In a more recent review of the American Society of Anesthesiologists Closed Claims database, Lee et al.[23] specifically examined serious injuries associated with regional anesthesia during the period 1980 to 1999. During this time, a total of 1,005 regional anesthesia claims were identified, of which 368 (37%) were obstetric related claims and 637 (63%) nonobstetric claims. All obstetric claims were related to complications associated with neuraxial anesthesia or analgesia. In contrast, 134 of the 637 (21%) nonobstetric claims were related specifically to complications occurring during PNB. An updated review of the Closed Claims database reported that axillary blocks were used in the majority of peripheral nerve block claims (40%), followed by interscalene blocks (23%), intravenous regional anesthesia (19%), supraclavicular blocks (8%), intercostal nerve blocks (2%), cervical plexus blocks (2%), and ankle blockade (2%).[24] Nerve damage was associated with 59% of peripheral nerve block claims and was evenly divided between temporary and permanent injury. The damaging event was related to the block technique in over 50% of cases. Overall, temporary or permanent peripheral nerve injury occurred in 79 (59%) of 134 peripheral nerve claims. Upper extremity techniques were more commonly associated with peripheral nerve claims than lower extremity techniques.[23,24] Additional complications occurring during PNB included death or brain damage (13%), pneumothorax (10%), emotional distress (2%), inflammatory skin reactions (2%), and miscellaneous causes (14%).[23] Peripheral nerve block claims were associated with substandard care in 21% of claims.[24]

▶ PATHOPHYSIOLOGY

Peripheral Nerve Anatomy

The peripheral nervous system (PNS) comprises <0.1% of all nerve tissue. The somatic PNS, when defined anatomically by the presence of Schwann cells, includes the primary nerve roots, dorsal root ganglions, mixed spinal nerves, plexuses, nerve trunks, and the autonomic nervous system. Each peripheral nerve is composed of individual myelinated nerve fibers embedded within an endoneurial connective tissue layer and grouped into discrete bundles termed fascicles. Each fascicle is surrounded by a squamous epithelial sheath called the perineurium that regulates the microenvironment, or homeostatic milieu, of the myelinated nerve fibers. Nerve fascicles are surrounded by a connective tissue environment (i.e., perineural space) and encased by the peripheral nerve's outer epineurial membrane (Fig. 14-1).

The PNS consists of both sensory and motor components. The cell bodies of sensory nerves are located within the dorsal root ganglion, while those for motor nerves are located within the anterior horn of the spinal cord. The normal function of myelinated nerve fibers depends upon the integrity of both the axon and its myelin sheath. Nerve action potentials "jump" from one node of Ranvier to the next—propagating neural signal transmission. This rapid saltatory conduction depends on the insulating properties of the myelin sheath for proper and efficient functioning.

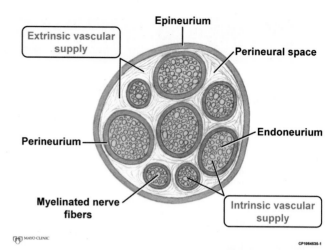

FIGURE 14-1. Cross-sectional peripheral nerve anatomy. Cross-section of a peripheral nerve with its vascular supply. (By permission of Mayo Foundation for Medical Education and Research.)

The functional integrity of a peripheral nerve is highly dependent upon its microcirculation,[25] which consists of an intrinsic supply of exchange vessels within the endoneurium and an extrinsic supply of larger, non-nutritive vessels located within the perineural space[26] (Fig. 14-1). The extrinsic circulation is under adrenergic control and thus highly responsive to epinephrine-containing solutions.

Pathogenesis of Peripheral Nerve Injury

Peripheral nerve injury may occur through a variety of mechanisms, with patient, surgical, and anesthetic risk factors all being major contributors (Box 14-1). However, regardless of the etiology, the pathogenesis of peripheral nerve injury remains fairly constant. Once injury occurs, those components distal to the site of injury will degenerate and be destroyed by phagocytosis. This process—termed secondary or Wallerian degeneration—may require up to 4 weeks for completion. However, morphologic changes will begin to occur within the first 72 hours. During this time period, the nerve may retain a variable degree of functionality while distal axonal segments begin to shrink secondary to fragmentation and fluid loss. As a result, these components assume a more oval or globular appearance, which promotes subsequent phagocytosis. At approximately 1 week postinjury, macrophages have reached the site of injury in greater numbers—clearing nearly all debris within 2 to 4 weeks. Schwann cell division by mitosis occurs simultaneously with this process, increasing the number of cells available to "fill" the area once occupied by the distal axon and myelin sheath.[27]

The reaction proximal to the site of injury is referred to as primary or retrograde degeneration. The time required for this process to occur is somewhat dependent upon sensory and motor segments, as well as the on the relative size and myelination of nerve fibers. Retrograde degeneration proceeds for at least one internodal space—being highly dependent upon the degree of proximal insult. Morphologic changes in the parent cell body vary to some degree with the type of cell and its proximity to the site of injury. The more proximal the site of injury, the more pronounced the changes within the axonal cell body. Histologically, severe injury may be evident by chromatolysis, or the swelling of the cytoplasm with eccentric displacement of the cell's nucleus. If present, this will generally occur within the first 5 to 7 days, with death or evidence of recovery beginning over the next 4 to 6 weeks. With recovery, the edema begins to subside, the nucleus once again migrates to the center of the cell, and Nissl substance begins to reaccumulate.[27]

Axonal regeneration may begin within the first 24 hours after injury. During this process, endoneurial tubes and their associated Schwann cells will reorganize distal to the site of injury at the most proximal point of retrograde degeneration. In this location, the endoneurial tubes are optimally positioned to accept regenerating nerve sprouts from the axonal stump. All nerve sprouts are initially unmyelinated, whether they arise from myelinated or unmyelinated nerve fibers. If the endoneurial tube has been uninterrupted during the injury, axonal sprouts may readily pass along their former courses, innervating endorgans over the course of several weeks to months. However, if the injury was severe enough to disrupt the endoneurial tube structure and its associated Schwann cells, multiple axonal sprouts will begin to migrate aimlessly throughout the damaged area into the epineurial, perineurial, or adjacent regions to form a stump neuroma.[27] If this occurs, it is unlikely that subsequent reinnervation of distal endorgans will occur.

Classification of Peripheral Nerve Injuries

The classification of peripheral nerve injuries was initially introduced by Seddon et al.[28] in 1943. Although this classification was generally accepted, it was rarely used because of its poor association with clinical usefulness. However, many of the terms currently used to describe the severity of nerve injury were first introduced by Seddon (Box 14-3).

Following the description of Seddon, Sunderland[29] developed one of the most widely used and recognized classifi-

cations of peripheral nerve injuries. The classification is clinically relevant, with each degree of injury suggesting a greater anatomic disruption—and thus an increasingly altered prognosis. A modified summary of the Sunderland Classification System is provided in Table 14-3.

▶ RISK FACTORS

Peripheral nerve injury following regional anesthetic techniques may be the result of several contributing factors (Box 14-1). Patient-, surgical-, and anesthetic-related risk factors have all been identified as potential etiologies.[30,31]

Patient Risk Factors

Patient risk factors most commonly associated with perioperative nerve injury include the male gender,[32] increasing age,[32] the extremes of body habitus,[32] diabetes mellitus,[8,32–37] and preexisting neurologic deficits (from several etiologies).[8,32–34,36,38–42] Preexisting neurologic deficits may include conditions such as diabetic neuropathy, chemotherapy-induced peripheral neuropathy, spinal stenosis, compressive radiculopathy, or multiple sclerosis (MS). Although MS is generally considered a disease of the *central* nervous system, patients with MS may be at increased risk of *peripheral* nerve lesions as well.[43] Many clinicians are unaware that subclinical neural compromise may be present within the PNS of patients with MS.[44] In fact, subclinical sensorimotor deficits have been identified in 45%[45] to 78%[46] of MS patients, with up to 43% having abnormalities in more than one peripheral nerve distribution. Finally, tobacco use[8,22,33,47–49] and hypertension[8] have also been implicated as contributors to peripheral nerve injury. Welch et al.[8] speculate that chronic hypertension may render nerves more susceptible to injury because of alterations in blood flow (i.e., microvascular changes) or a greater propensity for hemodynamic instability (i.e., hypoperfusion) during the perioperative period.

Regardless of the underlying etiology, the presence of chronic neural compromise secondary to mechanical (e.g., compression), ischemic (e.g., peripheral vascular disease), toxic (e.g., cisplatin chemotherapy), or metabolic (e.g., diabetes mellitus) derangements may theoretically place patients at increased risk of further neurologic injury.[50–52] Upton and McComas[50] were the first to describe the "Double-Crush" phenomenon, which suggests that patients with preexisting neural compromise may be more susceptible to injury at another site when exposed to a secondary insult (Fig. 14-2). Secondary insults may include a variety of concomitant patient, surgical, or anesthetic risk factors. Osterman[51] emphasized that not only are two low-grade insults along a peripheral nerve trunk worse than a single site, but that the damage of the dual injury far exceeds the expected additive damage caused by each isolated insult. It may be further postulated that the second "insult" need not be along the peripheral nerve trunk itself, but rather at any point along the neural transmission pathway. Therefore, the performance of neuraxial—as well as peripheral—techniques in patients with preexisting neurologic disorders may theoretically place them at increased risk of a "Double-Crush" phenomenon.

BOX 14-3 Terms Used to Classify Peripheral Nerve Injury

Neuropraxia: A minor contusion or compression of a peripheral nerve with the preservation of the axis cylinder. Minor edema within the cell body or focal disruption of the myelin sheath may result in a transient disruption of nerve conduction signaling. However, this generally recovers and resolves within days to weeks.

Axonotmesis: A more significant injury with breakdown of the axon and subsequent Wallerian degeneration. However, endoneurial tube structures and their associated Schwann cells are well preserved, thus allowing spontaneous regeneration and good functional recovery over time.

Neurotmesis: A severe injury secondary to an avulsion or crush injury with complete axonal transection. The axon, endoneurial tube structures, and associated Schwann cells are completely disrupted. The perineurium and epineurium are also disrupted to varying degrees. In general, significant functional recovery is unlikely.

TABLE 14-3 Sunderland Classification of Nerve Injury

DEGREE OF INJURY	AXONAL NERVE CONDUCTION	WALLERIAN DEGENERATION	ENDONEURIAL TUBE INTEGRITY	LOSS OF FUNCTION	RECOVER/TIME COURSE
Type I	Focally interrupted at the site of injury	No	Maintained	Variable; often motor > sensory	Complete restoration of function within days to weeks
Type II	Interrupted distally from the site of injury	Yes	Maintained	Transient loss of motor, sensory, and sympathetic function	Regeneration and functional recovery common within weeks to months
Type III	Interrupted distally from the site of injury	Yes	Disrupted with scarring of endoneurium	Prolonged motor, sensory, and sympathetic deficits	Partial regeneration possible; however complete return of function does not occur
Type IV	Interrupted distally from the site of injury	Yes	Disrupted; fascicle perineurium also disrupted	Severe loss of motor, sensory, and sympathetic function; cell-body mortality high	Deficits generally permanent; prognosis for significant return of function poor without surgery
Type V	Interrupted distally from the site of injury	Yes	Disrupted; external epineurium severed	Severe loss of motor, sensory, and sympathetic function; cell-body mortality high	Possibility of significant return of function remote, even with surgery

Adapted from Sunderland S. A classification of peripheral nerve injuries producing loss of function. *Brain* 1951;74:491–516.

Surgical Risk Factors

Surgical risk factors include direct intraoperative trauma or stretch,[30,53–55] vascular compromise,[56,57] perioperative inflammation or infection,[12,22] hematoma formation,[58] prolonged tourniquet ischemia,[9,59] or improperly applied casts or dressings. Horlocker et al.[12] examined the etiology of perioperative nerve injuries in 607 patients undergoing 1,614 blocks for upper extremity surgery. Surgical variables were believed to be the etiology in 55 (88.7%) of 62 neurologic complications identified. Direct surgical trauma or stretch occurred in 40 (73%) cases, inflammation or infection in 6 (11%) cases, hematoma or vascular compromise in 4 (7%) cases, cast irritation in 3 (5%) cases, and tourniquet ischemia in 2 (4%) cases. Interestingly, all complications involving motor deficits had a surgical cause. Fourteen patients (25%) required subsequent surgical intervention to restore nerve function.[12] Barrington et al.[11] have also demonstrated that the majority (90%) of postoperative neurologic deficits are from nonanesthesia-related etiologies.

Jacob et al.[9] examined patient, surgical, and anesthetic risk factors associated with perioperative nerve injury in 12,329 patients undergoing total knee arthroplasty. Bilateral surgical procedures and total tourniquet time were surgical factors associated with an increased risk of nerve injury.

For every 30-minute increment in tourniquet time, the risk of nerve injury increased by 28%.[9] Previous investigators have also demonstrated that the likelihood of postoperative neurologic dysfunction increases with prolonged tourniquet inflation times and that reperfusion intervals only modestly decrease the risk of nerve injury.[59]

Intraoperative mechanical forces such as surgical retraction, stretch, compression, and contusion are believed to be major contributors to perioperative nerve injury. However, when the clinical features of peripheral nerve injury cannot be explained by surgical trauma, intraoperative positioning, or regional anesthetic techniques, alternative etiologies must be considered. One such condition is postsurgical inflammatory neuropathy—an uncommon and under-appreciated cause of perioperative neurologic dysfunction. Although poorly understood, the condition is believed to be an idiopathic immune-mediated response to a physiologic stress such as a surgical procedure, a vaccination, or an infectious process.[22] The neuropathy may present with focal, multifocal, or diffuse neurologic deficits in the setting of negative radiographic imaging and normal ancillary serum testing. The onset of neurologic deficits following the surgical procedure is often delayed (i.e., the deficits are not immediately apparent after surgery) or in an anatomic distribution remote from the surgical site or regional anesthetic technique. Risk

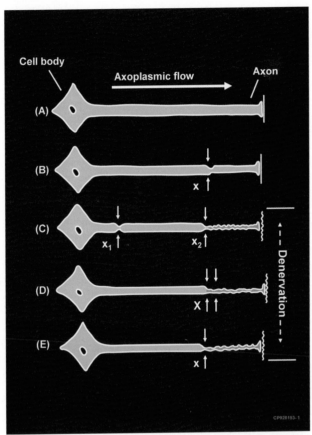

FIGURE 14-2. Neural lesions resulting in denervation. Axoplasmic flow is indicated by the degree of shading. Complete loss of axoplasmic flow results in denervation (**C, D, E**). **A:** Normal neuron. **B:** Mild neuronal injury at a single site (x) is insufficient to cause denervation distal to the insult. **C:** Mild neuronal injury at two separate sites (x_1 and x_2) may cause distal denervation (i.e., "Double Crush"). **D:** Severe neuronal injury at a single site (X) may also cause distal denervation. **E:** Axon with a diffuse, preexisting underlying disease process (toxic, metabolic, ischemic) may have impaired axonal flow throughout the neuron which may or may not be symptomatic, but predisposes the axon to distal denervation following a single minor neural insult at x (i.e., "Double Crush"). (By permission of Mayo Foundation for Medical Education and Research.)

factors for postsurgical inflammatory neuropathy include diabetes mellitus, malignancy, systemic infection, and a history of tobacco use.[22] Other potential triggers include recent blood transfusion or volatile anesthetic use, both of which are known to cause immune suppression.

Anesthetic Risk Factors

Regional anesthetic factors that may contribute directly or indirectly to perioperative nerve injury include needle- or catheter-induced mechanical trauma, ischemic nerve injury secondary to vasoconstrictors or neural edema, or chemical injury that may result from direct local anesthetic neurotoxicity.[30,60]

Mechanical Trauma: The Role of Needle Injury

Several authors have investigated the role of mechanical trauma, including the elicitation of paresthesias and the role of needle type, on peripheral nerve injury.[12,20,21,39,61–67]

Animal models have implicated needle gauge, type (long vs. short bevel), and bevel configuration as contributing to nerve injury.[61,65] Selander et al.[65] examined the role of needle trauma by piercing rabbit sciatic nerves, either isolated (*in vitro*) or *in situ*, using two different needle types. Both long- (14 degrees) and short-bevel (45 degrees) needles were examined. They found that neuronal injury occurred more frequently with long-beveled needles when compared to short-beveled ones (90% vs. 53%) in isolated (*in vitro*) nerve preparations. More pronounced fascicular sliding occurred *in situ*, resulting in a lower frequency of nerve injury with both needle types (long-bevel 47% vs. short-bevel 10%). While the overall frequency of nerve injury occurred less often when short-beveled needles were used, those injuries elicited were often as severe, if not more severe, than those seen with long-beveled needle injuries. Selander concluded that short-beveled needles significantly reduce the risk of fascicular injury and should therefore be used in clinical practice when performing PNB.

Scientific data from anatomic dissections and histologic findings may further support the notion that traumatic nerve injuries occur less often with short-beveled needles. Previous studies have shown that the much of the cross-sectional area of a peripheral nerve consists of connective tissue. This anatomic finding is particularly true with more distal peripheral nerves.[68–70] Because short-bevel needles are more likely to penetrate loose connective tissue than nerve fascicles protected by a dense fibrous perineural membrane,[71] one may speculate that short-bevel needles are "protective" against severe intrafascicular injury. This phenomenon may explain why select patients who receive an intraneural (but not intrafascicular) injection do not develop postoperative neurologic deficits.[72,73] In contrast to short-bevel needles, sharp needles have been found to penetrate cryopreserved cadaveric human sciatic nerves 3.2% of the time.[71]

Rice and McMahon[61] have also investigated the role of needle size and configuration on peripheral nerve injury in a rat model. Unlike Selander, who reported histologic findings within 2 hours of injury, Rice and McMahon examined the histologic, functional, and behavioral effects of nerve impalement 28 days following the traumatic event. They found that long-beveled needles in the parallel configuration produced less intraneural damage than transverse long-beveled or short-beveled needles immediately after injury and at 7 days. However, by 28 days, all injuries caused by long-beveled needles (parallel and transverse) were resolving, while those induced by short-beveled needles continued to display evidence of severe injury. Overall, nerve injury scores were also significantly lower for long-beveled needles 4 weeks following injury when compared to short bevels (Fig. 14-3). The authors concluded that when nerve fascicles are impaled by commercially available injection needles, lesions occur less frequently, are less severe, and are more rapidly repaired if they are induced by a long-beveled needle.

While these results appear to disagree with those of Selander's, two fundamental differences exist between the two studies. First, Selander et al. examined the immediate (2-hour) frequency of injury to the perineural membrane, which surrounds nerve fascicles, after nerve trunk impalement. Rice and McMahon examined the frequency, severity, and long-term (28 days) consequences of injury to fascicular

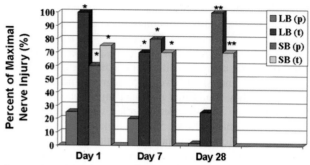

FIGURE 14-3. **Percent of maximal rat sciatic nerve injury as a function of time and needle bevel type and orientation.** Nerve injury is determined by the cumulative score of three graded components: intraneuronal disruption (graded 0–5), axonal degeneration (graded yes/no), and disorganized fiber regeneration (graded yes/no). Nerve lesions induced by short-bevel needles are more severe and take longer to repair than those induced by long-bevel needles. Nerve injury induced by short-bevel needles was often associated with persisting signs of injury 28 days after injury. LB(p), long-bevel needle in parallel configuration to nerve fibers; LB(t), long-bevel needle in transverse configuration to nerve fibers; SB(p), short-bevel needle in parallel configuration to nerve fibers; SB(t), short-bevel needle in transverse configuration to nerve fibers. *$p < 0.05$ versus LB(p) **$p < 0.05$ versus LB(p) and LB(t) (Reprinted with permission of Oxford University Press/*British Journal of Anaesthesia.*© The Board of Management and Trustees of the *British Journal of Anaesthesia.*)

contents after *in vivo* impalement of nerve fascicles. Second, different animal models were used by the two authors. Selander et al. used a rabbit sciatic nerve preparation, which is multifasciculated and often results in the sliding of nerve fascicles away from needle tips. They discussed the significance of this and postulated that it may have been a factor in the differing frequency of fascicular injury after the use of short- versus long-beveled needles. In contrast, Rice and McMahon used the rat sciatic nerve which consists of a single, large nerve fascicle at the level of the mid-thigh. Therefore, no fascicular sliding was possible, and neural (fascicular) penetration was ensured in all cases of impalement.

In summary, it appears from Selander's work that the likelihood of a traumatic insult may occur less frequently with short-beveled needles as a result of fascicular sliding that may occur within nerve trunks. However, when fascicular impalement does occur, both studies are in agreement that nerve injury may be more severe with short-bevel needles. In addition, Rice has demonstrated that neural repair may be accelerated and more organized with long-beveled injuries. Therefore, long-term consequences may be less of a concern when long-beveled needles are used. Furthermore, it has been suggested that sharper needles may be more comfortable for patients.[74] However, it must be emphasized that there are no confirmatory human studies to support—nor refute—the ability of various needle types and bevel configurations to impale human nerves within the clinical setting. Further clinical study is necessary before definitive recommendations can be made with regard to the optimal type and configuration of needles used during PNB.

Mechanical Trauma: The Role of Paresthesias

Traditionally, anesthesiologists would intentionally elicit a paresthesia during the performance of PNB to reliably localize neural structures. This may have originated, in part, from the long-established dictum "no paresthesia, no anesthesia."[75] Although the elicitation of a paresthesia may represent direct needle trauma, and theoretically increase the risk of neurologic injury, there are no prospective, randomized clinical studies that are able to definitively support nor refute these claims.[20,39,63,66,67,76,77] Selander et al.[20] performed one of the early prospective investigations examining the role of paresthesias and nerve injury. They reported a higher incidence of postoperative neurologic complications in patients where a paresthesia was intentionally sought during axillary blockade (2.8%) compared to those undergoing a perivascular technique (0.8%). While the difference was not found to be statistically significant, it should be noted that *unintentional* paresthesias were elicited and injected upon in patients within the perivascular group who experienced postoperative nerve injury. Winnie[78] argues that these results do in fact become statistically significant when groups are separated into those who actually experienced paresthesias versus those who did not. Overall, 40% of patients within the perivascular group reported unintentional paresthesias during the procedure, demonstrating the difficulty with standardization of technique and analysis of nerve injury. Postoperative neurologic deficits ranged from slight hypersensitivity to severe paresis and persisted from 2 weeks to >1 year. Interestingly, 67% of patients with injuries lasting >52 weeks had supplementation of their block following the initial regional technique. Theoretically, supplemental injections may significantly increase the risk of neural injury because of the absence of warning signs such as paresthesias when probing into a partially anesthetized plexus.

Urban and Urquhart[39] also performed a prospective investigation utilizing a variety of regional anesthetic approaches, including transarterial, paresthesia, and nerve stimulator techniques during brachial plexus blockade. The incidence of persistent postoperative paresthesias was 9% on the first day after surgery and 3% at 2 weeks in patients undergoing interscalene blockade. The majority of complaints consisted of hypoesthesia in the hand and resolved within 6 weeks in all but one patient (0.4%). The incidence of paresthesias at 2 weeks was significantly higher in those patients receiving bupivacaine compared to mepivacaine or lidocaine ($p = 0.013$). However, this observation was attributed to poor arm positioning during prolonged postoperative sensory anesthesia and not to local anesthetic toxicity. Patients undergoing axillary blockade had even higher complication rates. Paresthesias persisted into the first postoperative day in 19% of patients. These were not associated with the type of local anesthetic, the number of needle advances, anesthetic technique (paresthesia vs. transarterial), or the duration of tourniquet inflation. However, there was a significant increase in the incidence of acute postoperative dysesthesias in those patients who had preoperative neurologic symptoms within the extremity ($p = 0.02$). Only 5% of patients continued to experience new postoperative paresthesias at 2 weeks. Symptoms were confined to numbness and tingling within the fingers and forearm hyperesthesia. Once again, all but one patient (0.4%) had resolution of their symptoms by 4 weeks. Interestingly, a large percentage of patients in both groups (54% interscalene; 18% axillary) experienced a paresthesia on injection. In the axillary group, this occurred in many cases without an initial paresthesia during needle placement.

Investigations in which local anesthetic was *not* injected onto paresthesias have resulted in significantly lower neurologic complication rates than those described above.[63,67] Selander[63] examined the role of axillary catheter placement in providing prolonged or continuous brachial plexus anesthesia. During catheter placement, an unintentional paresthesia was obtained in 39% of patients. However, local anesthetic was never injected at the time of paresthesia elicitation. Following catheter placement and negative aspiration, local anesthetic was injected through the cannula with no report of pain or pressure paresthesias. Surprisingly, there were no neurologic sequelae (0%) postoperatively. Similarly, Stan et al.[67] report only a 0.2% incidence of neurologic complications in 996 patients undergoing transarterial axillary blockade. If an unintentional paresthesia was elicited during the performance of the block, the needle was redirected toward the artery with no injection of local anesthetic. Of the 119 (12%) patients in whom an unintentional paresthesia was elicited during the procedure, none reported a neurologic injury postoperatively. It is suspected that the two patients (0.2%) who did experience new sensory paresthesias postoperatively suffered unintentional mechanical trauma or intraneuronal injection during subsequent block supplementation.

Investigations such as those cited above appear to associate regional anesthesia-induced perioperative nerve injury with the injection of local anesthetic onto an elicited paresthesia. However, it has been argued that many of the studies condemning paresthesias have been performed in animal models in which nerve impalement occurs under direct vision.[79] Moore[79] suggests that a properly elicited paresthesia does not indicate that: (i) the bevel of the needle has punctured the epineurium; (ii) the nerve has been impaled; (iii) the neural fibers have been cut; or (iv) an intraneural injection will occur. He further emphasizes that no statistically significant clinical data have been published that demonstrate properly elicited paresthesias during regional blockade result in the temporary or permanent loss of neural function. Investigations by Winchell and Wolfe[66] and Pearce et al.[76] appear to support Moore's claim. Winchell and Wolfe[66] report only a 0.36% incidence of postoperative neurologic injury in 854 patients undergoing brachial plexus blockade. Of these, 835 (98%) experienced a paresthesia with subsequent injection of local anesthetic during the procedure. All postoperative neurologic sequelae involved diminished sensation within the distal extremity and had resolved within 7 months. Pearce et al.[76] prospectively examined the complication rates of four techniques (transarterial, paresthesia, transvenous, and tethering) used to identify the axillary neurovascular plexus. A paresthesia was elicited in 24% of patients during needle placement, and a pressure paresthesia occurred in 58% during local anesthetic injection. Overall, complications included mild acute local anesthetic toxicity (3.5%), axillary tenderness and bruising (9%), axillary hematoma (3%), and postoperative dysesthesias (12.5%). Interestingly, patients in whom the brachial plexus was identified using the transarterial technique had significantly more dysesthesias on the day following surgery when compared to all other groups. The authors postulate that subclinical hematoma formation, not paresthesias, may be contributing to the development of transient postoperative neurologic symptoms (PONSs).

Ischemic Injury: The Role of Epinephrine and Neural Edema

Epinephrine is a common adjuvant often added to local anesthetics during PNB. In a concentration of 1:200,000, epinephrine not only prolongs the duration of local anesthetic blockade, but also reduces the vascular uptake within the anesthetized area.[80] This adrenergic effect avoids the rapid redistribution of these drugs to the systemic circulation where they may cause potentially devastating toxic reactions. As a result, many authorities have recommended its use in procedures of neural blockade in tissues that do not have terminal arteries.

However, recent investigations have focused on the role of epinephrine and neural blood flow (NBF) in the pathogenesis of nerve fiber injury.[26,81–83] It has long been recognized that the functional integrity of peripheral nerves is highly dependent upon its microcirculation.[25] The blood supply to peripheral nerves consists of two sources: (i) an intrinsic supply of exchange vessels within the endoneurium and (ii) an extrinsic supply of larger, nonnutritive feeding vessels (Fig. 14-1). This extrinsic vasculature runs longitudinally along the nerve within the perineural space and crosses the perineurium to anastomose with the intrinsic circulation.[26] The epineurial circulation is a critical component of the overall neural circulation. Stripping the epineurium of this extrinsic vascular supply results in a 50% reduction in NBF and subsequent demyelination of intrinsic nerve fibers.[84] It is also this extrinsic circulation that is under adrenergic control and thus highly responsive to epinephrine-containing solutions.[85]

Myers and Heckman[26] examined the role of lidocaine, with or without epinephrine, in reducing NBF within rat sciatic nerve preparations. The topical application of 2% lidocaine resulted in a 39% reduction in NBF when compared to saline controls. The addition of epinephrine (1:200,000) to the local anesthetic resulted in an even greater reduction in NBF than 2% lidocaine alone (78% vs. 39%). Both values were significantly less than baseline and saline control values (Fig. 14-4). Differences between the 2% lidocaine and 2% lidocaine/epinephrine solutions were also statistically significant. As a result, it has been postulated that epi-

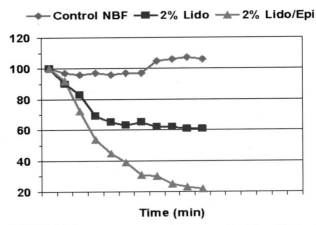

FIGURE 14-4. The effect of lidocaine on nerve blood flow. Effects of lidocaine 2% and lidocaine 2% with epinephrine on rat sciatic NBF. (Reprinted from Myers RR, Heckman HM. Effects of local anesthesia on nerve blood flow: studies using lidocaine with and without epinephrine. *Anesthesiology* 1989;71:757–762, with permission.)

nephrine may induce severe neural ischemia, resulting in potentially irreversible pathologic damage to nerve fibers and their supporting cellular structures. However, this risk of nerve injury may be limited to only those individuals with underlying toxic (e.g., chemotherapy) or metabolic (e.g., diabetes) neuropathies (Fig. 14-2E).[86] Under these clinical conditions, it may be prudent to minimize the concentration of epinephrine used during peripheral blockade. In contrast, the use of epinephrine and associated neural ischemia does *not* appear to be a concern in patients with normal underlying vascular and neuroanatomy.

Ischemic nerve injury may also occur following the intrafascicular injection of local anesthetics.[64,87] Selander and Sjostrand[87] demonstrated that intrafascicular injections may result in compressive nerve sheath pressures exceeding 600 mm Hg. This transient elevation in endoneurial fluid pressure may exceed capillary perfusion pressure for up to 15 minutes, interfering with the nerve's endoneurial microcirculation. Elevated pressures may also alter the permeability of the blood-nerve barrier and disrupt the internal milieu of the endoneurium. This results in axonal degeneration and pathologic damage to the peripheral nerve fibers, including Schwann cell injury and axonal dystrophy—particularly in nerves considered "at risk" from underlying toxic or metabolic abnormalities. Fibroblast proliferation has also been observed at the site of injury, contributing to late-occurring changes in perineural thickness and endoneurial fibrosis.[88] These changes may result in a delayed tissue reaction or scar formation and account for symptoms that develop days or even weeks following PNB.[10,12,19–21]

Chemical Injury: The Role of Local Anesthetic Toxicity

Clinical experience has demonstrated that local anesthetic use is overwhelmingly safe when administered correctly and in the recommended concentrations. However, when inappropriately high concentrations, prolonged exposure times (i.e., continuous infusions or epinephrine use), or intraneural injections are encountered, severe degenerative changes may occur, leading to long-lasting neurologic sequelae.[21,64,89,90] The clinical deficits encountered often implicate a mechanism of injury severe enough to produce loss of conduction in at least some nerve fiber populations. Nerve conduction deficits may result either from direct toxic or ischemic effects on the axon or Schwann cell[60] or from indirect effects that alter the permeability and microenvironment of the nerve.[91]

Several investigations have clearly demonstrated the acute toxic effects of local anesthetics within animal models.[92–94] Kalichman et al.[94] examined the relative neural toxicity of four different local anesthetics on the rat sciatic nerve *in vivo*. They injected 1 mL of various concentrations of either amide-linked (lidocaine, etidocaine) or ester-linked (2-chloroprocaine, procaine) local anesthetics onto exposed sciatic nerves. Test solutions were injected beneath the sheath of connective tissue separating the sciatic nerve from the overlying muscle. This method provides a well-defined perineural (extraneural) injection without the risk of physical trauma to the nerve. Nerve injury (axonal degeneration or demyelination), endoneural edema, and conduction abnormalities were all assessed 48 hours after local anesthetic administration. They found that all neurotoxic effects were concentration dependent, with the highest concentrations inducing the most severe nerve injury. Of the local anesthetics investigated,

etidocaine was found to have the highest toxicity, followed by lidocaine and 2-chloroprocaine, and then procaine. The order of potency for causing nerve injury was comparable to that for producing motor nerve conduction blockade. Therefore, the authors concluded that local anesthetic toxicity may in fact parallel anesthetic potency.

Interestingly, many of the acute (48-hour) histopathologic and functional findings described above do not appear to be present 10 to 14 days after local anesthetic exposure.[88,89,95] Gentili et al.[89] examined the neurotoxic effect of five local anesthetic agents (lidocaine, bupivacaine, mepivacaine, tetracaine, and procaine) on peripheral nerve tissue *in vivo*. Various concentrations, with and without epinephrine, were applied epineurally (extrafascicular) to exposed rat sciatic nerves. Microscopic examination after 10 days demonstrated no evidence of axonal injury. The internal architecture of all nerve fascicles was well maintained with a normal structure, independent of the local anesthetic used. Axonal and myelin sheath distribution was indistinguishable from that seen in saline controls. These findings suggest that the perineural (extrafascicular) application of commonly used local anesthetic agents does not result in significant histologic nerve damage 10 days following exposure. This includes both long- and short-acting agents, with and without epinephrine.

Additional investigations have reported similar findings after the topical application of bupivacaine (with and without epinephrine),[64,88,95] lidocaine,[88,95] tetracaine,[88] and 2-chloroprocaine.[88] In each of these investigations, the compound action potentials, as well as the *in vivo*, gross, and microscopic histologic examinations, were all normal 10 to 14 days following local anesthetic exposure. Therefore, it may be postulated that many of the acute (48-hour) histologic and functional toxic effects of local anesthetics may be transient in nature and fully reversible. In fact, the action of local anesthetics may be viewed as the expression of a limited and reversible toxic effect.[96]

Kroin et al.[90] examined the role of repeated perineural injections, as well as the effect of concentration and dose on lidocaine toxicity. They injected equipotent volumes of lidocaine 1%, 2%, or 4% around the sciatic nerves of rats three times daily for 3 days using two different catheter systems. The first system formed a 10-mm long, loosely fitting cuff around the sciatic nerve. This ensured that the injected volume would remain in contact with the sciatic nerve and prevent diffusion or dilution of the solution. The second catheter system simply had two slit openings and was positioned within 3 mm of the nerve. Functional assessment of the tibial nerve was conducted 48 hours after the last lidocaine treatment by measuring the twitch tension within the digital flexors of the paw. This was followed by microscopic and histologic examination of the nerve.

Two days after injection through the cuffed-catheter system, 4% lidocaine had reduced the toe tension twitch to nearly zero in all nerves; while the 1% and 2% solutions maintained the toe twitch at pretreatment levels. Histologically, 4% lidocaine caused the degeneration of approximately 25% of axons. This occurred both within the cuffed region and distally. The 1% and 2% lidocaine solutions induced less than a 10% degenerative change within the cuffed region only and were comparable to saline controls. Interestingly, these findings suggest that functional loss may precede any obvious histologic damage identified by microscopy.

All local anesthetic solutions injected through the slit-catheter system left the tibial nerves functionally and histologically intact. Only one of seven (14%) nerves treated with 4% lidocaine demonstrated a small amount of axonal degeneration. The authors attributed the severe neurotoxic effects seen within the cuffed-catheter animals to a prolonged exposure of a highly concentrated local anesthetic solution. Conversely, the slit-catheter system provided an extensive and rapid dilution of local anesthetic within the region surrounding the nerve, limiting neural exposure. The conclusion was that the perineural injection of 4% lidocaine is neurotoxic when not rapidly diluted and that lower concentrations of the same agent (1% and 2%) were innocuous to peripheral nerves regardless of the mode of application.

Finally, it has been suggested that regional anesthesia-induced perioperative nerve injury may be the result of a combined mechanical and chemical insult[21,64,89,97] (Fig. 14-5). Selander et al.[64] examined the role of intrafascicular injection versus topical application of local anesthetic agents using rabbit sciatic nerves *in vivo*. They found that

the topical application of 0.5% bupivacaine (with or without 1:200,000 epinephrine) as well as 1% bupivacaine did not result in axonal degeneration nor alter the permeability of endoneurial vessels 10 to 14 days following administration. In contrast, those animals receiving an intraneural injection of the same solutions demonstrated marked axonal degeneration and endoneurial edema. Interestingly, physiologic saline and 0.5% bupivacaine (without epinephrine) resulted in a similar degree of nerve injury, suggesting that these effects may be independent of the injected test solution and a result of injection trauma only. However, higher concentrations of bupivacaine (1%) and the addition of epinephrine (1:200,000) to lower concentrations of bupivacaine (0.5%) resulted in significantly more severe axonal injury than saline or bupivacaine (0.5%) alone. They concluded that neurologic injury following PNB may be multifactorial, involving traumatic, toxic, and ischemic variables. Furthermore, they suggested that local anesthetic toxicity may be greatly enhanced if administered in conjunction with neural (intrafascicular) trauma (Fig. 14-5).

Gentili et al.[89] also examined the role of intraneural injection versus topical application of local anesthetics on exposed rat sciatic nerves *in vivo*. They found that the topical administration of bupivacaine, mepivacaine, lidocaine, procaine, or tetracaine does not result in significant histologic nerve damage 10 days following application. In contrast, all of the local anesthetic agents caused some degree of axonal injury when administered intraneuronally. The degree of nerve damage varied with the agent, but often resulted in small petechial hemorrhages on the surface of the fascicle, thickening of the epineurial tissue, and significant myelin degeneration. Structural changes were noted as early as 1 hour after injection and progressed to severe neuronal injury at 10 days. Interestingly, in contrast to Selander's investigation,[64] Gentili et al. failed to demonstrate significant axonal injury following the intraneuronal injection of saline. As a result, the authors concluded that a combined mechanical and chemical insult must occur to induce significant neural injury. Postulated mechanisms of injury include a direct neurotoxic effect of the local anesthetic as well as an altered blood-nerve barrier resulting in endoneurial edema, elevated intrafascicular pressures, and an alteration in the chemical microenvironment. These mechanical, ischemic, and toxic changes may lead to severe and potentially irreversible axonal degeneration.[89]

Neural Localization: The Role of Nerve Stimulation

The use of nerve stimulation while performing regional anesthetic techniques was introduced by Greenblatt and Denson[98] in 1962. Advocates of the technique have reported several advantages, including (i) a high success rate; (ii) the ability to perform procedures on sedated or uncooperative patients; (iii) the avoidance of paresthesias and associated neurologic injury; and (iv) the avoidance of arterial puncture with subsequent vascular insufficiency or hematoma formation.[99–102] Many investigators claim that the proper use of a nerve stimulator avoids altogether the possibility of neuropathy from needle trauma.[78,103] However, there are no prospective, randomized clinical trials that clearly demonstrate nerve stimulator use to be associated with lower complication rates when compared to paresthesia, transarterial, or ultrasound-guided techniques (Chapter 17).

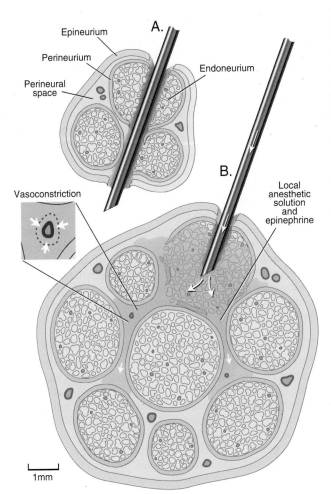

1mm

FIGURE 14-5. The multifactorial nature of peripheral nerve injury. Several factors may contribute to peripheral nerve injury. Actual injury may require a combination of factors. Direct needle trauma may result in full or partial transection of the nerve **(A)** or disruption of the nerve-blood barrier as a result of intrafascicular injection **(B)**. Once this barrier is breached, the nerve is exposed to possible chemical toxicity from local anesthetic and/or ischemia and/or reduced local anesthetic clearance from epinephrine.

Neurologic complication rates associated with nerve stimulator use range from 0%[99,102,104] to more than 8%.[39,77] However, within each of these investigations, there were no statistically significant differences between techniques (nerve stimulator, paresthesia, and transarterial) with regard to neurologic injury. Goldberg et al.[99] performed one of the early prospective, randomized studies comparing both the efficacy and the safety of various regional techniques during brachial plexus anesthesia. They randomized 59 patients scheduled for upper extremity surgery under axillary blockade to receive either a transarterial, single paresthesia or nerve stimulator technique. All three methods utilized an immobile needle technique while injecting 40 mL/70 kg of mepivacaine 1.5%. Success rates and the need for supplementation were not significantly different between groups. Importantly, there were no complications (0%) attributed to any of the anesthetic techniques postoperatively.

A more recent prospective, randomized comparison of mechanical paresthesia versus electrical stimulation in patients undergoing interscalene brachial plexus blockade found similar results.[77] Liguori et al.[77] randomized 218 patients undergoing interscalene blockade to either a paresthesia-seeking or peripheral nerve stimulation technique. Twenty-five (23%) patients in the nerve stimulation group experienced an unintentional paresthesia during needle placement. Success rates were similar between groups (paresthesia 96%; nerve stimulation 94%) as were the onset times for sensorimotor blockade. Patients in the nerve stimulation group received significantly more sedation and required a longer time to perform the block than patients receiving a paresthesia-seeking technique. There were no significant differences between groups with regard to the development of PONS. Overall, 11 (10.1%) patients in the nerve stimulation group and 10 (9.3%) patients in the paresthesia-seeking group experienced PONS that were likely anesthesia related. All neurologic deficits resolved within 12 months. The authors concluded that the choice of neural localization should be based upon the patient's and anesthesiologist's comfort and preference and not on concern for the development of PONS.[77]

Fanelli et al.[105] report a significantly higher neurologic complication rate during interscalene blockade with nerve stimulation when compared to axillary blockade using the same technique. Their prospective investigation demonstrated an overall neurologic complication rate of 1.3% within the first month following brachial plexus blockade. Neurologic injury occurred significantly more often after interscalene blockade than after axillary plexus blockade (4% vs. 1%; $p < 0.005$). Complete recovery of neurologic function was observed in all patients within 3 months (range 4–12 weeks). Among the variables that could be related to the development of postoperative neurologic dysfunction, only the type of nerve block (interscalene blockade) and tourniquet inflation pressure demonstrated univariate association with outcome. However, after performing multiple logistic regression, only tourniquet inflation pressures >400 mm Hg were found to be significant.[105]

Finally, many advocates of the nerve stimulator approach argue that this technique may be performed on heavily sedated, anesthetized, or uncooperative patients since it provides exact needle localization without the elicitation of a paresthesia. However, an investigation by Choyce et al.[106] has demonstrated that this may not be the case. In their study, the relationship between a subjective paresthesia and an objective motor response as elicited by a peripheral nerve stimulator was examined in patients undergoing axillary blockade. During their technique, a noninsulated stimulating needle was advanced until a paresthesia was elicited. At this point, the current on a nerve stimulator was gradually increased until an associated motor response was obtained. Interestingly, after acquiring a paresthesia, nearly 25% of patients required a current >0.5 mA to manifest a motor response, with 42% needing currents between 0.75 and 3.3 mA. The site of initial paresthesia matched the site of subsequent motor response in only 81% of cases. These worrisome findings suggest an inconsistency of elicited motor responses, despite the needle presumably being near the nerve.

Urmey and Stanton[107] also demonstrated that the use of a nerve stimulator does not replace a patient's ability to respond to the pain of needle trauma or intraneural injection. Interscalene blocks ($n = 30$) were performed on unpremedicated patients using the paresthesia technique with insulated (10 patients) and noninsulated (20 patients) needles. Paresthesias were elicited with the nerve stimulator power off. Upon elicitation of a paresthesia, the nerve stimulator was turned on, and the amperage slowly increased to a maximum of 1.0 mA. Only 30% of patients exhibited any motor response. Interestingly, there was no correlation between the site of the paresthesia and the associated motor response. These results further suggest that it is possible to have sensory nerve contact and not elicit a motor response, thereby challenging the argument that the use of a peripheral nerve stimulator protects heavily sedated or anesthetized patients from nerve injury.

Benumof[108] further emphasized this point by reporting four cases in which the performance of an interscalene blockade during general anesthesia with the aid of a nerve stimulator resulted in extensive permanent loss of bilateral cervical spinal cord function. In each case, magnetic resonance imaging (MRI) demonstrated evidence of severe central cord syrinx (cavitation) or hemorrhage, suggesting that intramedullary injection occurred during block placement. Therefore, the assumption that nerve stimulation allows clinicians to approximate neural structures without the risk of mechanical trauma or peripheral nerve injury does not appear to be valid.

Neural Localization: The Role of Ultrasound Guidance

Ultrasound-guided regional anesthesia is a commonly used method of neural localization. Reported benefits include a more rapid block onset time, increased success rates, prolonged duration of block, a reduction in the number of unintended vascular punctures and required needle manipulations, lower local anesthetic volumes, and shorter procedure times.[109–111] Advocates of the technique have also suggested that ultrasound guidance may decrease the rate of neurologic complications because of real-time needle visualization and the ability to safely approximate the needle relative to neural targets. However, despite these claims, the ability of ultrasound guidance to reduce the frequency of peripheral nerve injury remains unknown[111,112] (Chapter 17).

Anecdotal case reports and limited case series have shown that severe neurologic injury may still occur despite the use of ultrasound guidance.[43,113,114] Koff et al.[43] report a case of severe brachial plexopathy after an ultrasound-guided interscalene block in a patient with MS undergoing total shoulder arthroplasty. At 8 months postoperatively, the patient continued to have severe limitations with upper extremity range of motion and significant motor deficits. Cohen and Gray[113] describe an unrecognized intraneural injection in a patient undergoing an ultrasound-guided interscalene block for shoulder incision and drainage resulting in flaccid paralysis and a sensory deficit within the C5 and C6 nerve root distribution. The patient experienced a full neurologic recovery within 6 weeks. Finally, Reiss et al.[114] report a case of radial nerve denervation and severe brachial plexopathy at the level of the supraclavicular fossa in a patient undergoing an ultrasound-guided supraclavicular block for a left thumb arthroplasty and capsulodesis. Eight months after the injury, the patient remained disabled with a complete wrist-drop and the inability to use her hand. These and other reports within the literature suggest that despite "real-time needle visualization" during ultrasound guidance, catastrophic neurologic complications may still occur.

Fredrickson and Kilfoyle[109] have performed one of the few large, prospective investigations examining the frequency of neurologic complications after ultrasound-guided regional anesthesia. During a 3-year study period, 1,010 consecutive ultrasound-guided nerve blocks were performed on 911 patients. Both upper (interscalene, supraclavicular, infraclavicular) and lower (femoral, sciatic) extremity nerve blocks were performed. A follow-up telephone interview was performed 10 to 21 days after the block in all but 14 (1.5%) patients. Neurologic complications (from all causes) were reported in 8.2% of patients on day 10, 3.7% of patients at 1 month, and 0.6% of patients at 6 months. The regional technique could not be ruled out as a potential cause of injury in 33% of patients with persistent (>6 months) deficits. Interestingly, 12% of patients experienced a paresthesia during block placement despite the fact that real-time ultrasound guidance was used. Furthermore, patients experiencing a paresthesia had significantly higher rates of neurologic complications. The authors concluded that the rate of neurologic complications after ultrasound-guided regional anesthesia appears to be similar to more traditional techniques of neural localization (e.g., nerve stimulation).[109] These findings have been confirmed in subsequent prospective, randomized investigations as well.[6]

The ability of ultrasound-guided regional anesthesia to become the "Holy Grail" of regional anesthesia—providing neural blockade with rapid onset, long duration, and improved success without associated complications—has been discussed.[115] Although many advocates of ultrasound theorize that direct visualization of neural targets and needle advancement may decrease the frequency (and severity) of neurologic injury, current evidence does not support this claim.[111,112] Furthermore, speculation that ultrasound guidance can prevent needle-to-nerve contact, intraneural injection, or mechanical trauma has not been demonstrated in clinical practice.[72,73,113,116,117] In fact, the ability to visualize both the needle tip and relevant neural targets at all times has been shown to be difficult. Sites et al.[118] have demonstrated that failure to maintain needle visualization during advancement may occur in up to 43% of novices (<10 ultrasound-guided blocks) and 10% of experienced (>60 ultrasound-guided blocks) providers performing ultrasound-guided techniques.

Despite its potential advantages (e.g., more rapid block onset time, increased success rates, prolonged duration of block, fewer needle manipulations, lower local anesthetic volumes, shorter procedure times), clinicians must recognize the inherent limitations of ultrasound-guided technology in preventing peripheral nerve injury. Failure to appreciate the limitations of ultrasound may breed complacency and create an illusion of safety—factors that may actually *increase* the risk of nerve injury and adverse patient outcomes.[119]

▶ DIAGNOSTIC EVALUATION

Although most neurologic complications resolve completely within several days or weeks, significant neural injuries necessitate further neurologic consultation and investigation.[120] As a precursor to this assessment, it is imperative that preoperative neurologic deficits are clearly documented to allow the early diagnosis of new or worsening neurologic dysfunction postoperatively. Knowledge of the patient's baseline neurologic status prior to regional anesthesia is a critical element that is often missing—and impossible to recover—at the time of postoperative evaluation. Therefore, many experts suggest that a brief neurologic examination be performed prior to the performance of any regional anesthetic technique to document the presence of preexisting deficits.

The initial step in the postoperative diagnosis of peripheral nerve injury is the identification of neural dysfunction (Fig. 14-6).[120] Postoperative sensory or motor deficits do not necessarily infer injury and must first be distinguished from residual or prolonged local anesthetic effect. Historical features that are important to identify include: (i) the onset and severity of symptoms (timing relative to blockade); (ii) the type and quality of symptoms (sensory, motor, sympathetic); (iii) the clinical course of the deficits (constant, fluctuating, progressive); and (iv) the patient's past medical history (e.g., preexisting neurologic disorders, diabetes mellitus, prior chemotherapy, peripheral vascular disease). Similarly, surgical events such as intraoperative trauma or stretch, vascular injury, bleeding complications, or difficult exposure requiring extensive traction must be discussed with surgical colleagues.

Elements of the general physical examination are important to check routinely during postoperative rounds, even if a neurologic injury is not suspected.[121] Hematoma or ecchymosis at the site of injection with associated distal ischemia has clear implications. In addition, systemic manifestations of inadequate hemostasis or excessive anticoagulation may suggest a hemorrhagic complication compressing adjacent neural structures. Signs and symptoms of infection—including focal tenderness at the site of the regional technique—should prompt further evaluation for an infectious etiology. Finally, a detailed neurologic examination by a qualified neurologist or neurosurgeon should occur soon after the identification of an unexpected postoperative deficit. The goal of an examination is to identify if the process is affecting a single peripheral nerve, multiple peripheral nerves, the plexus, or the nerve roots.[120] The examination should also determine the severity of the deficits, which can be an important factor in long-term neurologic prognosis. Early neurologic consultation is important not only

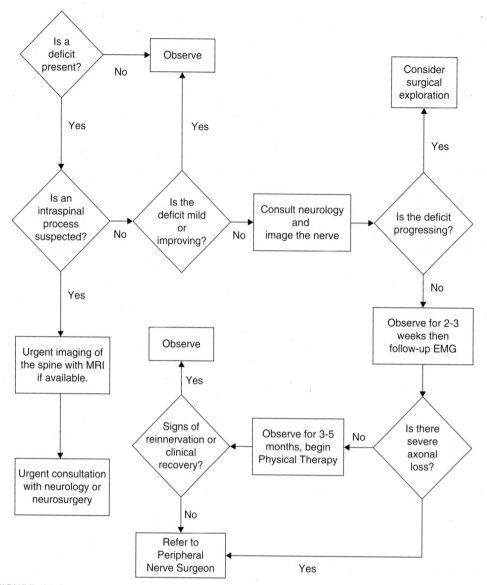

FIGURE 14-6. Evaluating and managing postoperative neurologic deficits. General recommendations outlining a diagnostic and management approach to postoperative neurologic deficits. (From Sorenson EJ. Neurological injuries associated with regional anesthesia. *Reg Anesth Pain Med* 2008;33:442–448.)

to document the degree of involvement, but to monitor the progression and/or resolution of symptoms, as well as to coordinate further evaluation. Early imaging techniques such as computed tomography or preferably MRI may be recommended to identify infectious or inflammatory disease processes, as well as expanding hematomas that may have immediate surgical implications.

Electrodiagnostic studies have also been used for decades to diagnose, and at times prognosticate, a wide variety of neurologic disorders. They may provide information on the preexisting status of the nerves, prognosis of the new lesion, and potentially the underlying pathology.[120] Sequential studies after a peripheral nerve injury may provide clinicians with an extensive foundation of knowledge (Box 14-4).[27] Nerve conduction studies, evoked potentials, and electromyography (EMG) are a few of the most common

---

BOX 14-4 Clinical Benefits of Electrodiagnostic Testing After Peripheral Nerve Injury

- Documentation of injury
- Localization of anatomic insult
- Defining the severity and mechanism of injury
- Follow recovery pattern(s)
- Develop prognosis
- Acquire objective data for impairment documentation
- Define underlying pathology
- Select optimal muscles for tendon transfer procedures (if applicable)

testing modalities. Each series of tests may provide an array of complementary information regarding nerve conductivity, axonal and myelin integrity, as well as muscle recruitment capabilities.

Sensory Nerve Conduction Studies

Sensory nerve conduction studies are used to assess the functional integrity of sensory nerve fibers. They measure the amplitude and velocity of somatosensory-induced sensory nerve action potentials (SNAPs). They can be performed orthodromically in the direction of normal nerve conduction, or antidromically in the distal part of major peripheral nerves. The primary goals of sensory nerve conduction studies are the assessment of: (i) the number of functioning axons (amplitude of SNAPs) and (ii) the state of myelin in these axons (conduction velocity of SNAPs). In patients with axonal degeneration neuropathies (e.g., injury after injection into a nerve fascicle or diabetic neuropathy), the primary feature is a markedly reduced sensory action potential amplitude. Under these circumstances, the conduction velocity may be slightly reduced, but only to the extent that the largest axons are gone. In contrast, demyelinating neuropathies (e.g., tourniquet compression or Guillain-Barré syndrome) generally cause profound abnormalities in conduction velocity, with or without alterations in action potential amplitude.[121]

Electromyography

EMG is capable of measuring and recording electrical activity within muscle. In patients with disease(s) of the motor unit, this electrical activity provides a guide to the pathological site of the underlying disorder. In neuropathic disease processes, the pattern of affected muscles also permits a lesion to be localized to the spinal cord, nerve roots, limb plexuses, or peripheral nerves. However, EMG findings are not pathognomonic of specific diseases, nor do they provide a definitive diagnosis of an underlying neuromuscular disorder. In general, EMG abnormalities can be divided into three discrete categories[121]:

1. *Excessive Response to Needle Insertion*: This usually takes the form of rhythmic trains of positive waves and are commonly seen in denervated muscle fibers or active myopathic processes.
2. *Abnormal Spontaneous Activity*: This occurs in the form of fasciculations or fibrillations. Fibrillations are rhythmic potentials emanating from denervated single-muscle fibers and are the hallmark of active or ongoing neuropathies. They appear 2 to 3 weeks after injury when degeneration of the axon progresses peripherally to cause destruction of the motor endplate. Fibrillation potentials are maximal 1 to 3 months after injury.
3. *Abnormal Recruitment*: As neurologic deficits progress, the number of motor axons in a given muscle decreases, resulting in a reduced number of motor unit action potentials for the level of voluntary effort. This is referred to as decreased recruitment, with the degree of reduction paralleling the severity of the lesion.

Despite their many applications, nerve conduction studies and EMG also have several limitations. Typically, only the large sensory and motor nerve fibers are evaluated, leaving the dysfunction of small unmyelinated fibers to go undetected. In addition, many abnormalities will not be noted on EMG immediately after injury, but rather require several weeks to evolve. Although it is often recommended to wait until the evidence of denervation has appeared before performing neurophysiologic testing (14–21 days), the acquisition of a baseline study (including evaluation of the contralateral extremity) immediately upon recognition of the neurologic deficit may be helpful in ruling out the underlying (subclinical) pathology or documenting a preexisting condition.[121]

▶ PREVENTION

The multitude of patient, surgical, and anesthetic risk factors (Box 14-1) that may contribute to peripheral nerve injury make the avoidance and prevention of these potentially devastating complications a complex and difficult challenge. The inability to influence patient and surgical risk factors forces clinicians to focus primarily on anesthesia-related causes. Although several anesthesia "risk factors" have been identified, many of these have been extrapolated from either *in vitro* laboratory studies or animal-based investigations. For example, evidence suggesting the relative "safety" of one needle-type versus another (sharp vs. blunt bevel)[61,65] and ischemic nerve insult secondary to local anesthetic additives[26] have *not* been validated in prospective, randomized clinical trials. Furthermore, general recommendations to avoid regional anesthetic techniques in asleep or heavily sedated patients, or the importance of avoiding pain with injection of local anesthetic, are based upon isolated case reports and limited case series.[52,122] No prospective, randomized clinical investigations have definitively demonstrated the superiority, or relative "safety," of these clinical practices.[52]

However, despite the absence of definitive clinical data, the importance of anesthetic-related risk factors should not be disregarded—or even minimized. Sufficient *in vitro* and *in situ* animal data—as well as limited clinical data—exist to warrant consideration when caring for patients at risk of perioperative nerve injury. Clinical goals should be to minimize the number of patient, surgical, and anesthetic "risk factors" any given patient is exposed to during an episode of care.[52] For example, the potential risks and benefits of performing a continuous peripheral nerve catheter technique in an elderly male patient with clinically significant spinal stenosis and diabetic neuropathy undergoing a lower extremity surgical procedure should be carefully considered. Under these circumstances, the introduction of multiple anesthetic risk factors (needle- or catheter-induced mechanical trauma, local anesthetic toxicity, and neural ischemia) in a patient with preexisting neural compromise (i.e., "Double-Crush" phenomenon) may not justify the potential benefit. However, if the clinical risk is deemed appropriate and/or warranted, clinical maneuvers such as reducing the local anesthetic dose or concentration, or minimizing the concentration of epinephrine additives, may be prudent.[52] Regardless, the potential risks and benefits of *all* anesthetic techniques should be discussed with patients in detail, so that an informed decision can be made with regard to their anesthetic care.

▶ TREATMENT AND REHABILITATION

The vast majority of perioperative nerve injuries are transient and self-limited neuropraxias.[120] For this reason, conservative measures (e.g., limb protection, physical rehabilitation, and range-of-motion exercises) and careful observation are appropriate during the initial phases of recovery. However, it is critically important that correctable causes of nerve injury (e.g., cast compression, hematoma formation, and neural impingement) are investigated and excluded during the immediate postoperative period. Patients presenting with neurologic deficits that cannot be explained by surgical trauma, intraoperative positioning, or regional anesthetic techniques should be evaluated by a neurologist for consideration of a peripheral nerve biopsy and initiation of immunotherapy if an inflammatory etiology is suspected or confirmed.[22] Neurologic referral and consultation is important to provide serial clinical and electrophysiologic examinations to monitor the progression and/or resolution of symptoms.[52,120] Under all circumstances, physical therapy should be instituted soon after the injury to maintain strength in the unaffected muscles, as well as joint range of motion. General recommendations for the management of postoperative neurologic deficits are outlined in Figure 14-6.[120]

Patients with persistent symptoms (3–5 months) or progressive neurologic deficits should undergo neurosurgical evaluation.[120] The goals of surgery may be threefold: (i) to halt the progression of sensorimotor deficits; (ii) to provide relief of pain and other neurologic symptoms; and (iii) to restore functional capacity. Surgical intervention and physical therapy may often accomplish these goals. However, the patient, their family, and the treating physician(s) must establish realistic expectations before a treatment plan is initiated. Furthermore, a frank discussion of associated complications—and worsening outcome—must also be discussed.

Early surgery intervention is rarely indicated in perioperative nerve injuries. Limited indications include the evacuation of a compressive hematoma, compartment syndrome, vascular injury (e.g., arteriovenous fistula, compressive pseudoaneurysm), iatrogenic neural impingement (e.g., unintentional suturing of neural structures), or intraoperative neural transection or laceration. Surgery within 72 hours is indicated under these conditions and is often critical in the treatment of clean, traumatic nerve injuries to facilitate the end-to-end anastomosis and repair of neural structures. In contrast, a bluntly transected or injured nerve is best repaired after a delay of several weeks. By that time, the extent of both proximal and distal neuromas will be obvious, allowing a complete resection back to healthy neural tissue and subsequent surgical repair.[123]

The majority of persistent perioperative nerve injuries do *not* result in the complete or partial transection of neural fibers. Rather, focal (i.e., needle- or catheter-induced mechanical trauma and intraneural injection) or diffuse (i.e., intraoperative trauma or stretch, tourniquet compression, ischemia, local anesthetic neurotoxicity) neural insults are more likely occur. Under these conditions, close observation with serial clinical and electrophysiologic examinations are recommended in contrast to early surgical intervention. Importantly, care must be taken in interpreting *subtle* suggestions of recovery—either clinical or electrophysiologic—as they do not necessarily predict effective or complete functional recovery. In these cases, waiting for more definitive signs of reinnervation over an extended period of time may in fact jeopardize neural integrity and compromise the overall likelihood of recovery. Therefore, in cases with clear early signs of spontaneous recovery, conservative nonoperative management can be continued.[120] However, in cases with no evidence of clinical or electrophysiologic recovery, surgical exploration and neurolysis should be considered. It is recommended that patients with focal lesions be surgically explored at 2 to 3 months, while those with more diffuse injuries explored at 3 to 5 months time.[123]

▶ SUMMARY

Peripheral nerve injuries are rare, though potentially catastrophic, perioperative complications. Patient, surgical, and anesthetic risk factors have all been identified as potential etiologies, with multiple factors commonly playing a role. The "Double-Crush" phenomenon has demonstrated that patients with several, concomitant risk factors may be at greatest risk of developing postoperative neurologic complications. Importantly, a comprehensive understanding of the complexities of perioperative nerve injury is critical to rapidly assess patients, identify potential etiologies, and intervene when appropriate during the immediate postoperative period. Although limited, appropriate preventative strategies include minimizing the number of risk factors a given patient is exposed to during an episode of care. Successful long-term management is highly dependent upon realistic patient and physician expectations, as well as an individualized, multidisciplinary therapeutic approach.

References

1. Neuhof H. Supraclavicular anesthetization of the brachial plexus. *JAMA* 1914;62:1629–1632.
2. Woolley EJ, Vandam LD. Neurological sequelae of brachial plexus nerve block. *Ann Surg* 1959;149:53–60.
3. Kulenkampff D, Persky MA. Brachial plexus anesthesia. Its indications, technic, and dangers. *Ann Surg* 1928;87:883.
4. Moberg E, Dhuner KG. Brachial plexus block analgesia with xylocaine. *J Bone Joint Surg Am* 1951; 33-A:884–888.
5. Auroy Y, Benhamou D, Bargues L, et al. Major complications of regional anesthesia in France: the SOS Regional Anesthesia Hotline Service. *Anesthesiology* 2002;97:1274–1280.
6. Liu SS, Zayas VM, Gordon MA, et al. A prospective, randomized, controlled trial comparing ultrasound versus nerve stimulator guidance for interscalene block for ambulatory shoulder surgery for postoperative neurological symptoms. *Anesth Analg* 2009;109:265–271.
7. Brull R, McCartney CJL, Chan VWS, et al. Neurological complications after regional anesthesia: contemporary estimates of risk. *Anesth Analg* 2007;104:965–974.
8. Welch MB, Brummett CM, Welch TD, et al. Perioperative peripheral nerve injuries: a retrospective study of 380,680 cases during a 10-year period at a single institution. *Anesthesiology* 2009;111:490–497.
9. Jacob AK, Mantilla CB, Sviggum HP, et al. Perioperative nerve injury after total knee arthroplasty: regional anesthesia risk during a 20-year cohort study. *Anesthesiology* 2011;114:311–317.
10. Auroy Y, Narchi P, Messiah A, et al. Serious complications related to regional anesthesia: results of a prospective survey in France. *Anesthesiology* 1997;87:479–486.

11. Barrington MJ, Watts SA, Gledhill SR, et al. Preliminary results of the Australasian Regional Anaesthesia Collaboration: a prospective audit of more than 7000 peripheral nerve and plexus blocks for neurologic and other complications. *Reg Anesth Pain Med* 2009;34:534–541.

12. Horlocker TT, Kufner RP, Bishop AT, et al. The risk of persistent paresthesia is not increased with repeated axillary block. *Anesth Analg* 1999;88:382–387.

13. Borgeat A, Blumenthal S, Lambert M, et al. The feasibility and complications of the continuous popliteal nerve block: a 1001-case survey. *Anesth Analg* 2006;103:229–233.

14. Borgeat A, Dullenkopf A, Ekatodramis G, et al. Evaluation of the lateral modified approach for continuous interscalene block after shoulder surgery. *Anesthesiology* 2003;99:436–442.

15. Capdevila X, Pirat P, Bringuier S, et al. Continuous peripheral nerve blocks in hospital wards after orthopedic surgery. *Anesthesiology* 2005;103:1035–1045.

16. Borgeat A, Ekatodramis G, Kalberer F, et al. Acute and nonacute complications associated with interscalene block and shoulder surgery: a prospective study. *Anesthesiology* 2001;95:875–880.

17. Bergman BD, Hebl JR, Kent J, et al. Neurologic complications of 405 consecutive continuous axillary catheters. *Anesth Analg* 2003;96:247–252.

18. Compere V, Rey N, Baert O, et al. Major complications after 400 continuous popliteal sciatic nerve blocks for post-operative analgesia. *Acta Anaesthesiol Scand* 2009;53:339–345.

19. Cheney FW, Domino KB, Caplan RA, et al. Nerve injury associated with anesthesia: a closed claims analysis. *Anesthesiology* 1999;90:1062–1069.

20. Selander D, Edshage S, Wolff T. Paresthesiae or no paresthesiae? Nerve lesions after axillary blocks. *Acta Anaesthesiol Scand* 1979;23:27–33.

21. Lofstrom B, Wennberg A, Wien L. Late disturbances in nerve function after block with local anaesthetic agents. An electroneurographic study. *Acta Anaesthesiol Scand* 1966;10:111–122.

22. Staff NP, Engelstad J, Klein CJ, et al. Post-surgical inflammatory neuropathy. *Brain* 2010;133:2866–2880.

23. Lee LA, Posner KL, Domino KB, et al. Injuries associated with regional anesthesia in the 1980s and 1990s: a closed claims analysis. *Anesthesiology* 2004;101:143–152.

24. Lee LA, Posner KL, Cheney FW, et al. Complications associated with eye blocks and peripheral nerve blocks. an american society of anesthesiologists closed claims analysis. *Reg Anesth Pain Med* 2008; 33:416–422.

25. Lundborg G. Ischemic nerve injury. Experimental studies on intraneural microvascular pathophysiology and nerve function in a limb subjected to temporary circulatory arrest. *Scand J Plast Reconstr Surg Suppl* 1970;6:3–113.

26. Myers RR, Heckman HM. Effects of local anesthesia on nerve blood flow: studies using lidocaine with and without epinephrine. *Anesthesiology* 1989;71:757–762.

27. Jobe M, Martinez S. Peripheral nerve injuries. In: Canale S, ed. *Campbell's Operative Orthopaedics*. 10th ed. Philadelphia, PA: Mosby, 2003.

28. Seddon HJ, Medawar PB, Smith H. Rate of regeneration of peripheral nerves in man. *J Physiol* 1943;102:191–215.

29. Sunderland S. A classification of peripheral nerve injuries producing loss of function. *Brain* 1951;74:491–516.

30. Neal JM, Hebl JR, Gerancher JC, et al. Brachial plexus anesthesia: essentials of our current understanding. *Reg Anesth Pain Med* 2002;27:402–428.

31. Neal JM, Gerancher JC, Hebl JR, et al. Upper extremity regional anesthesia: essentials of our current understanding, 2008. *Reg Anesth Pain Med* 2009;34:134–170.

32. Warner MA, Warner ME, Martin JT. Ulnar neuropathy. Incidence, outcome, and risk factors in sedated or anesthetized patients. *Anesthesiology* 1994;81:1332–1340.

33. Warner MA, Martin JT, Schroeder DR, et al. Lower-extremity motor neuropathy associated with surgery performed on patients in a lithotomy position. *Anesthesiology* 1994;81:6–12.

34. Hebl JR, Kopp SL, Schroeder DR, et al. Neurologic complications after neuraxial anesthesia or analgesia in patients with preexisting peripheral sensorimotor neuropathy or diabetic polyneuropathy. *Anesth Analg* 2006;103:1294–1299.

35. Gebhard RE, Nielsen KC, Pietrobon R, et al. Diabetes mellitus, independent of body mass index, is associated with a "higher success" rate for supraclavicular brachial plexus blocks. *Reg Anesth Pain Med* 2009;34:404–407.

36. Kalichman MW, Calcutt NA. Local anesthetic-induced conduction block and nerve fiber injury in streptozotocin-diabetic rats. *Anesthesiology* 1992;77:941–947.

37. Kroin JS, Buvanendran A, Williams DK, et al. Local anesthetic sciatic nerve block and nerve fiber damage in diabetic rats. *Reg Anesth Pain Med* 2010;35:343–350.

38. Dripps RD, Vandam LD. Exacerbation of pre-existing neurologic disease after spinal anesthesia. *N Engl J Med* 1956;255:843–849.

39. Urban MK, Urquhart B. Evaluation of brachial plexus anesthesia for upper extremity surgery. *Reg Anesth* 1994;19:175–182.

40. Moen V, Dahlgren N, Irestedt L. Severe neurological complications after central neuraxial blockades in Sweden 1990–1999. *Anesthesiology* 2004;101:950–959.

41. Hebl JR, Horlocker TT, Kopp SL, et al. Neuraxial blockade in patients with preexisting spinal stenosis, lumbar disk disease, or prior spine surgery: efficacy and neurologic complications. *Anesth Analg* 2010;111:1511–1519.

42. Horlocker TT, Cabanela ME, Wedel DJ. Does postoperative epidural analgesia increase the risk of peroneal nerve palsy after total knee arthroplasty? *Anesth Analg* 1994;79:495–500.

43. Koff MD, Cohen JA, McIntyre JJ, et al. Severe brachial plexopathy following an ultrasound guided single injection nerve block for total shoulder arthroplasty in a patient with multiple sclerosis. *Anesthesiology* 2008;108:325–328.

44. Hughes RAC. Peripheral neuropathy. *BMJ* 2002;324:466–469.

45. Sarova-Pinhas I, Achiron A, Gilad R, et al. Peripheral neuropathy in multiple sclerosis: a clinical and electrophysiologic study. *Acta Neurol Scand* 1995;91:234–238.

46. Pogorzelski R, Baniukiewicz E, Drozdowski W. Subclinical lesions of peripheral nervous system in multiple sclerosis patients. *Neurol Neurochir Pol* 2004;38:257–264.

47. Richardson JK, Jamieson SC. Cigarette smoking and ulnar mononeuropathy at the elbow. *Am J Phys Med Rehabil* 2004;83:730–734.

48. Mitchell BD, Hawthorne VM, Vinik AI. Cigarette smoking and neuropathy in diabetic patients. *Diabetes Care* 1990;13:434–437.

49. Faden A, Mendoza E, Flynn F. Subclinical neuropathy associated with chronic obstructive pulmonary disease: possible pathophysiologic role of smoking. *Arch Neurol* 1981;38:639–642.

50. Upton AR, McComas AJ. The double crush in nerve entrapment syndromes. *Lancet* 1973;2:359–362.

51. Osterman AL. The double crush syndrome. *Orthop Clin North Am* 1988;19:147–155.

52. Neal JM, Bernards CM, Hadzic A, et al. ASRA practice advisory on neurologic complications in regional anesthesia and pain medicine. *Reg Anesth Pain Med* 2008;33:404–415.

53. Lynch NM, Cofield RH, Silbert PL, et al. Neurologic complications after total shoulder arthroplasty. *J Shoulder Elbow Surg* 1996;5:53–61.

54. Hildebrand KA, Patterson SD, Regan WD, et al. Functional outcome of semiconstrained total elbow arthroplasty. *J Bone Joint Surg Am* 2000;82-A:1379–1386.

55. Cheng SL, Morrey BF. Treatment of the mobile, painful arthritic elbow by distraction interposition arthroplasty. *J Bone Joint Surg Br* 2000;82:233–238.

56. Benzel EC, Prejean CA, Hadden TA. Pulsatile dysesthesia and an axillary artery pseudoaneurysm associated with a penetrating axillary artery injury. *Surg Neurol* 1989;31:400–401.

57. Groh GI, Gainor BJ, Jeffries JT, et al. Pseudoaneurysm of the axillary artery with median-nerve deficit after axillary block anesthesia. A case report. *J Bone Joint Surg Am* 1990;72:1407–1408.

58. Ben-David B, Stahl S. Axillary block complicated by hematoma and radial nerve injury. *Reg Anesth Pain Med* 1999;24:264–266.

59. Horlocker TT, Hebl JR, Gali B, et al. Anesthetic, patient, and surgical risk factors for neurologic complications after prolonged total tourniquet time during total knee arthroplasty. *Anesth Analg* 2006;102:950–955.

60. Hogan QH. Pathophysiology of peripheral nerve injury during regional anesthesia. *Reg Anesth Pain Med* 2008;33:435–441.

61. Rice AS, McMahon SB. Peripheral nerve injury caused by injection needles used in regional anaesthesia: influence of bevel configuration, studied in a rat model. *Br J Anaesth* 1992;69: 433–438.

62. Moore DC. Complications of regional anesthesia. *Clin Anesth* 1969;2:218–251.

63. Selander D. Catheter technique in axillary plexus block. Presentation of a new method. *Acta Anaesthesiol Scand* 1977;21: 324–329.

64. Selander D, Brattsand R, Lundborg G, et al. Local anesthetics: importance of mode of application, concentration and adrenaline for the appearance of nerve lesions. An experimental study of axonal degeneration and barrier damage after intrafascicular injection or topical application of bupivacaine (Marcain). *Acta Anaesthesiol Scand* 1979;23:127–136.

65. Selander D, Dhuner KG, Lundborg G. Peripheral nerve injury due to injection needles used for regional anesthesia. An experimental study of the acute effects of needle point trauma. *Acta Anaesthesiol Scand* 1977;21:182–188.

66. Winchell SW, Wolfe R. The incidence of neuropathy following upper extremity nerve blocks. *Reg Anesth* 1985;10:12–15.

67. Stan TC, Krantz MA, Solomon DL, et al. The incidence of neurovascular complications following axillary brachial plexus block using a transarterial approach. A prospective study of 1,000 consecutive patients. *Reg Anesth* 1995;20:486–492.

68. Moayeri N, Bigeleisen PE, Groen GJ. Quantitative architecture of the brachial plexus and surrounding compartments, and their possible significance for plexus blocks. *Anesthesiology* 2008;108: 299–304.

69. Moayeri N, Groen GJ. Differences in quantitative architecture of sciatic nerve may explain differences in potential vulnerability to nerve injury, onset time, and minimum effective anesthetic volume. *Anesthesiology* 2009;111:1128–1134.

70. van Geffen GJ, Moayeri N, Bruhn J, et al. Correlation between ultrasound imaging, cross-sectional anatomy, and histology of the brachial plexus: a review. *Reg Anesth Pain Med* 2009;34:490–497.

71. Sala-Blanch X, Ribalta T, Rivas E, et al. Structural injury to the human sciatic nerve after intraneural needle insertion. *Reg Anesth Pain Med* 2009;34:201–205.

72. Bigeleisen PE. Nerve puncture and apparent intraneural injection during ultrasound-guided axillary block does not invariably result in neurologic injury. *Anesthesiology* 2006;105:779–783.

73. Robards C, Hadzic A, Somasundaram L, et al. Intraneural injection with low-current stimulation during popliteal sciatic nerve block. *Anesth Analg* 2009;109:673–677.

74. ANSI/ADA specification no. 54 for double-pointed parenteral, single use needles for dentistry. Council on Dental Materials, Instruments, and Equipment. *J Am Dent Assoc* 1986;113:952.

75. Moore DC. *Regional Block.* 4th ed. Springfield, IL: Charles C. Thomas, 1965.

76. Pearce H, Lindsay D, Leslie K. Axillary brachial plexus block in two hundred consecutive patients. *Anaesth Intensive Care* 1996;24:453–458.

77. Liguori GA, Zayas VM, YaDeau JT, et al. Nerve localization techniques for interscalene brachial plexus blockade: a prospective, randomized comparison of mechanical paresthesia versus electrical stimulation. *Anesth Analg* 2006;103:761–767.

78. Winnie AP. Does the transarterial technique of axillary block provide a higher success rate and a lower complication rate than a paresthesia technique? New evidence and old. *Reg Anesth* 1995;20:482–485.

79. Moore DC. "No paresthesias-no anesthesia," the nerve stimulator or neither? *Reg Anesth* 1997;22:388–390.

80. Fink BR, Aasheim GM, Levy BA. Neural pharmacokinetics of epinephrine. *Anesthesiology* 1978;48:263–266.

81. Myers RR, Mizisin AP, Powell HC, et al. Reduced nerve blood flow in hexachlorophene neuropathy: relationship to elevated endoneurial fluid pressure. *J Neuropathol Exp Neurol* 1982;41:391–399.

82. Myers RR, Powell HC. Galactose neuropathy: impact of chronic endoneurial edema on nerve blood flow. *Ann Neurol* 1984;16:587–594.

83. Tuck RR, Schmelzer JD, Low PA. Endoneurial blood flow and oxygen tension in the sciatic nerves of rats with experimental diabetic neuropathy. *Brain* 1984;107:935–950.

84. Rundquist I, Smith QR, Michel ME, et al. Sciatic nerve blood flow measured by laser Doppler flowmetry and [14C]iodoantipyrine. *Am J Physiol* 1985;248:H311–317.

85. Rechthand E, Hervonen A, Sato S, et al. Distribution of adrenergic innervation of blood vessels in peripheral nerve. *Brain Res* 1986;374:185–189.

86. Schneider U, Jund R, Nees S, et al. Differences in sensitivity to hyperglycemic hypoxia of isolated rat sensory and motor nerve fibers. *Ann Neurol* 1992;31:605–610.

87. Selander D, Sjostrand J. Longitudinal spread of intraneurally injected local anesthetics. An experimental study of the initial neural distribution following intraneural injections. *Acta Anaesthesiol Scand* 1978;22:622–634.

88. Myers RR, Kalichman MW, Reisner LS, et al. Neurotoxicity of local anesthetics: altered perineurial permeability, edema, and nerve fiber injury. *Anesthesiology* 1986;64:29–35.

89. Gentili F, Hudson AR, Hunter D, et al. Nerve injection injury with local anesthetic agents: a light and electron microscopic, fluorescent microscopic, and horseradish peroxidase study. *Neurosurgery* 1980;6:263–272.

90. Kroin JS, Penn RD, Levy FE, et al. Effect of repetitive lidocaine infusion on peripheral nerve. *Exp Neurol* 1986;94:166–173.

91. Kalichman MW. Physiologic mechanisms by which local anesthetics may cause injury to nerve and spinal cord. *Reg Anesth* 1993;18:448–452.

92. Kalichman MW, Powell HC, Myers RR. Pathology of local anesthetic-induced nerve injury. *Acta Neuropathol (Berl)* 1988;75:583–589.

93. Kalichman MW, Powell HC, Myers RR. Quantitative histologic analysis of local anesthetic-induced injury to rat sciatic nerve. *J Pharmacol Exp Ther* 1989;250:406–413.

94. Kalichman MW, Moorhouse DF, Powell HC, et al. Relative neural toxicity of local anesthetics. *J Neuropathol Exp Neurol* 1993;52:234–240.

95. Barsa J, Batra M, Fink BR, et al. A comparative in vivo study of local neurotoxicity of lidocaine, bupivacaine, 2-chloroprocaine, and a mixture of 2-chloroprocaine and bupivacaine. *Anesth Analg* 1982;61:961–967.

96. Selander D. Neurotoxicity of local anesthetics: animal data. *Reg Anesth* 1993;18:461–468.

97. Chambers WA. Peripheral nerve damage and regional anaesthesia. *Br J Anaesth* 1992;69:429–430.

98. Greenblatt GM, Denson JS. Needle nerve stimulatorlocator: nerve blocks with a new instrument for locating nerves. *Anesth Analg* 1962;41:599–602.

99. Goldberg ME, Gregg C, Larijani GE, et al. A comparison of three methods of axillary approach to brachial plexus blockade for upper extremity surgery. *Anesthesiology* 1987;66:814–816.

100. Eeckelaert JP, Filliers E, Alleman JJ, et al. Supraclavicular brachial plexus block with the aid of a nerve stimulator. *Acta Anaesthesiol Belg* 1984;35:5–17.

101. Baranowski AP, Pither CE. A comparison of three methods of axillary brachial plexus anaesthesia. *Anaesthesia* 1990;45: 362–365.

102. Davis WJ, Lennon RL, Wedel DJ. Brachial plexus anesthesia for outpatient surgical procedures on an upper extremity. *Mayo Clin Proc* 1991;66:470–473.

103. Gentili ME, Wargnier JP. Peripheral nerve damage and regional anaesthesia. *Br J Anaesth* 1993;70:594.

104. Carles M, Pulcini A, Macchi P, et al. An evaluation of the brachial plexus block at the humeral canal using a neurostimulator (1417 patients): the efficacy, safety, and predictive criteria of failure. *Anesth Analg* 2001;92:194–198.

105. Fanelli G, Casati A, Garancini P, et al. Nerve stimulator and multiple injection technique for upper and lower limb blockade: failure rate, patient acceptance, and neurologic complications. Study Group on Regional Anesthesia. *Anesth Analg* 1999;88:847–852.

106. Choyce A, Chan VW, Middleton WJ, et al. What is the relationship between paresthesia and nerve stimulation for axillary brachial plexus block? *Reg Anesth Pain Med* 2001;26:100–104.

107. Urmey WF, Stanton J. Inability to consistently elicit a motor response following sensory paresthesia during interscalene block administration. *Anesthesiology* 2002;96:552–554.

108. Benumof JL. Permanent loss of cervical spinal cord function associated with interscalene block performed under general anesthesia. *Anesthesiology* 2000;93:1541–1544.

109. Fredrickson MJ, Kilfoyle DH. Neurological complication analysis of 1000 ultrasound guided peripheral nerve blocks for elective orthopaedic surgery: a prospective study. *Anaesthesia* 2009;64:836–844.

110. Neal JM, Brull R, Chan VW, et al. The ASRA evidence-based medicine assessment of ultrasound-guided regional anesthesia and pain medicine: executive summary. *Reg Anesth Pain Med* 2010;35:S1–S9.

111. Liu SS, Ngeow JE, Yadeau JT. Ultrasound-guided regional anesthesia and analgesia: a qualitative systematic review. *Reg Anesth Pain Med* 2009;34:47–59.

112. Neal JM. Ultrasound-guided regional anesthesia and patient safety: an evidence-based analysis. *Reg Anesth Pain Med* 2010;35:S59–S67.

113. Cohen JM, Gray AT. Functional deficits after intraneural injection during interscalene block. *Reg Anesth Pain Med* 2010;35: 397–399.

114. Reiss W, Kurapati S, Shariat A, et al. Nerve injury complicating ultrasound/electrostimulation-guided supraclavicular brachial plexus block. *Reg Anesth Pain Med* 2010;35:400–401.

115. Horlocker TT, Wedel DJ. Ultrasound-guided regional anesthesia: in search of the holy grail. *Anesth Analg* 2007;104:1009–1011.

116. Russon K, Blanco R. Accidental intraneural injection into the musculocutaneous nerve visualized with ultrasound. *Anesth Analg* 2007;105:1504–1505.

117. Schafhalter-Zoppoth I, Zeitz ID, Gray AT. Inadvertent femoral nerve impalement and intraneural injection visualized by ultrasound. *Anesth Analg* 2004;99:627–628.

118. Sites BD, Spence BC, Gallagher JD, et al. Characterizing novice behavior associated with learning ultrasound-guided peripheral regional anesthesia. *Reg Anesth Pain Med* 2007;32:107–115.

119. Hebl JR. Ultrasound-guided regional anesthesia and the prevention of neurologic injury: fact or fiction? *Anesthesiology* 2008;108:186–188.

120. Sorenson EJ. Neurological injuries associated with regional anesthesia. *Reg Anesth Pain Med* 2008;33:442–448.

121. Hogan Q, Hendrix L, Jaradeh S. Evaluation of neurologic injury after regional anesthesia. In: Finucane BT, ed. *Complications of Regional Anesthesia.* 1st ed. Philadelphia, PA: Churchill Livingstone, 1999:271–291.

122. Bernards CM, Hadzic A, Suresh S, et al. Regional anesthesia in anesthetized or heavily sedated patients. *Reg Anesth Pain Med* 2008;33:449–460.

123. Spinner RJ, Kline DG. Surgery for peripheral nerve and brachial plexus injuries or other nerve lesions. *Muscle Nerve* 2000;23: 680–695.

15

Myotoxicity

Quinn H. Hogan

Muscle injury is not generally considered when discussing complications of regional anesthesia and pain medicine. Although it rarely manifests itself as a significant clinical injury, myotoxicity from local anesthetics does occur and can be debilitating. This chapter reviews how muscle injury may occur in the context of regional anesthetic techniques, its clinical significance, and how it may be prevented and treated.

▶ DEFINITION

The performance of regional anesthesia may cause muscle injury by several mechanisms. Ischemia from an occlusive tourniquet such as during an intravenous regional anesthetic may produce muscle damage, but only after 6 hours of inflation, which is typically longer than the duration of the anesthetic. Injury by ischemia may also follow either compartment syndrome from bleeding or direct occlusion of a vessel from needle damage.[1] However, the dominant mechanism by far is myotoxicity, which may be defined as the direct action of the local anesthetic agent on the muscle cell (myocyte) that initiates cellular process leading to the destruction of the cell.

▶ SCOPE OF THE PROBLEM

Local anesthetic solutions used in regional anesthesia are uniformly toxic to muscle tissue. Since most local anesthetic injections are in the immediate vicinity of muscle tissue, myotoxicity likely accompanies nearly all regional anesthetic blocks. Despite this predictable muscle damage, myotoxicity is only rarely a clinically important event.[2,3] Several factors may explain this. Only adult myocytes are damaged by local anesthetic, so basal lamina, vasculature, neural elements, and most importantly the immature myocytes (myoblasts) remain intact. This allows complete regeneration in 3 to 4 weeks.[4,5] In fact, it may be this destruction of old cells and the prompting of new growth that provides the therapeutic benefit in trigger point injection of local anesthetics for myofascial pain, possibly combined with the growth of new vessels.[6] Other factors concealing the muscle injury from clinical recognition may include postsurgical immobilization, injury sites too deep to examine, or lack of scrutiny as the pain and inflammation develop several days postinjection. Also, pain due to myotoxicity may be mistakenly attributed to the surgery. An exception to the generally low impact of local anesthetic myotoxicity is extraocular muscle damage, in which there is a growing recognition of extraocular muscle dysfunction after regional anesthesia for the eye. There are no large studies formally evaluating the incidence of local anesthetic injury of the extraocular muscles. However, many cases have been reported despite the apparent low frequency of this event, consequent to the common use of these injections.[7,8]

▶ PATHOPHYSIOLOGY

Within 5 minutes of injection of usual concentrations of any local anesthetic, muscle fibers appear hypercontracted.[9,10] Within 15 minutes, lytic degeneration of the muscle cell's sarcoplasmic reticulum (SR) and mitochondria is evident.[9,11] By 24 hours, the myocyte becomes edematous and necrotic. Inflammation ensues with phagocytosis of cellular debris and appearance of eosinophils,[12] and eventually fibers are regenerated from precursor cells (Fig. 15-1). Abnormal muscle fibers may be evident for months.[13] These changes happen predictably in all subjects.

The molecular mechanism of local anesthetic myotoxicity has not been fully elucidated, due to the diverse effects of local anesthetics on cellular homeostasis (Fig. 15-2). Local anesthetics irreversibly injure mature myocytes in culture, which eliminates denervation secondary to blockade of the action potential or neuromuscular junction as an etiologic possibility.[14] Tetrodotoxin, a local anesthetic without direct effects on intramuscular Ca^{2+}, is not myotoxic.[15] Therefore, inhibition of the sarcolemmal Na^+ channel also does not play a role.[16] Local anesthetics fail to elicit contractures, the earliest phase of local anesthetic myotoxicity, if SR accumulation of Ca^{2+} is prevented, which indicates that toxicity is not caused by direct action on the myofibrils.[17] Replication of local anesthetic myonecrosis with caffeine alone[16] points to pathologic efflux of intracellular Ca^{2+} from the SR of mature multinucleated myocytes as a key element in local anesthetic myotoxicity.

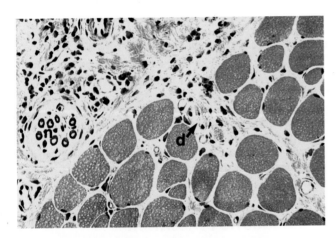

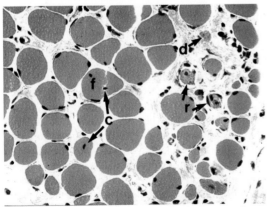

FIGURE 15-1. Histologic views (hematoxylin and eosin, ×125) of sternocleidomastoid muscle 54 days after bupivacaine injection. Myotoxic changes are evident, including eosinophilic infiltration (e), degenerating fibers (d), fiber splitting (f), fibers with central nuclei (c), and regenerating fibers (r). Nerves (n) and vessels (v) are not affected. (From Hogan Q, Dotson R, Erickson S, et al. Local anesthetic myotoxicity: a case and review. *Anesthesiology* 1994;80:942–947.)

Mature myocytes maintain a concentrated store of Ca^{2+} sequestered in the internal membrane system of the SR. Release of Ca^{2+} from SR via the Ca^{2+} release channels (also known as ryanodine receptors) triggers contraction of striated muscle. Local anesthetics cause a pathologic efflux of Ca^{2+} from the SR[18] essentially like malignant hyperthermia in miniature, producing contracture and cell destruction via activation of intracellular enzyme systems. There is some evidence that local anesthetics produce generalized permeability of the SR membrane.[17] Alternatively, other studies have shown a direct action of the anesthetic molecule on the Ca^{2+} release channel.[19] This action is complex and depends on drug concentration, pH, and Ca^{2+} loading status of the SR.[20–22]

Komai and Lokuta[23] demonstrated increased Ca^{2+} release channel activity in the presence of bupivacaine, whereas tetracaine caused inhibition. It is possible, therefore, that a general feature of local anesthetics, including tetracaine, procaine, benzocaine, and dibucaine, is a nonspecific action on sarcoplasmic membranes that causes Ca^{2+} release, whereas others such as bupivacaine,[23] lidocaine,[19] and prilocaine[19] have an additional direct action on the ryanodine receptor that accounts for their greater myotoxicity. Inhibition by local anesthetics of the Ca^{2+}-dependent ATPase of the SR, which transports Ca^{2+} back into intracellular stores following release, may be a further contributing factor,[24–27] and there is evidence that the plasma membrane pump that expels Ca^{2+} from the cell is also inhibited.[28] Interestingly, local anesthetic injury of primary sensory neurons may result from processes similar to that which damages muscle cells, specifically the triggering of pathologic discharge of Ca^{2+} from intracellular stores.[29]

Local anesthetics substantially affect mitochondrial bioenergetics. In the case of skeletal muscle, bupivacaine has been shown to dissipate the potential across the mitochondrial inner membrane, resulting in disrupted oxidative phosphorylation.[30,31] Because of the important role mitochondria play in regulating Ca^{2+} homeostasis, this mechanism may cause or interact with the features described above. Furthermore, events initiated in the mitochondria may trigger apoptosis, while depletion of Ca^{2+} stores may initiate SR stress, in which proteins that have been assembled but remain unfolded accumulate in the SR, which in turn may also mediate apoptosis. Thus, local anesthetics disrupt a broad set of homeostatic mechanisms, which individually or together lead to the destruction of the myocyte.[32]

▶ RISK FACTORS

While all local anesthetics tested produce myonecrosis, bupivacaine produces the most intense effect and procaine the least.[33] Recent studies confirm that ropivacaine also produces myotoxicity,[34] although less than bupivacaine at equipotent concentrations.[35,36] The myotoxicity that follows levobupivacaine administration has not been compared to other agents, but it would be expected to be high, since S-enantiomers show particular efficacy at releasing stored Ca^{2+} and disrupting cellular Ca^{2+} signaling.[31,37] The sensitivity of muscles is not uniform. Muscles composed of fibers that have high oxidative metabolism capacity are particularly sensitive, whereas those dependent on glycolytic

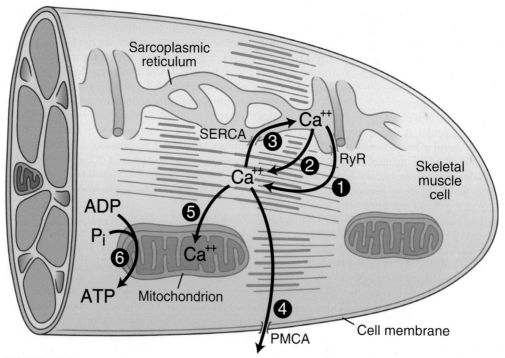

FIGURE 15-2. Cellular sites for local anesthetic myotoxicity. Upon exposure to local anesthetics, Ca^{2+} is released from the SR stores either through an action on the ryanodine receptor (also known as the Ca^{2+} release channel) (1) or directly on the SR membrane (2), causing elevated cytoplasmic Ca^{2+} levels. Additionally, local anesthetics may suppress the action of mechanisms that clear Ca^{2+} from the cytoplasm, both at the sarcoplasmic-endoplasmic Ca^{2+} ATP-ase (SERCA) (3) and the plasma membrane Ca^{2+} ATP-ase (PMCA) (4). Decrease in the mitochondrial inner membrane potential from local anesthetic exposure also interferes with Ca^{2+} uptake by the mitochondria (5) and reduces cellular energy production (6).

metabolism are resistant to bupivacaine toxicity.[30] The sensitivity to local anesthetic myotoxicity in rats is greater in young animals than in adults,[38] although there has been no examination of this distinction in humans.

The extent of damage is dose related[39,40] and is worse with serial administration.[41,42] Infusions lasting only 6-hour duration for femoral nerve blockade in pigs result in amplified damage compared to single injection, with the development of calcific deposits and scar formation.[36] Similarly, slow release of bupivacaine from microparticles shows that even subanesthetic concentrations produce myotoxicity if the duration of exposure is long.[43] Steroid[44] and epinephrine[45] in the injection amplify the muscle injury produced by local anesthetics. Injection outside a muscle, such as into the subcutaneous fat, produces damage to adjacent muscle,[9,46] but intramuscular injection results in maximal injury (Box 15-1). According to some reports,[47,48] hyaluronidase increases the myotoxicity of local anesthetics. However, these studies investigated effects on rat tibialis and rabbit orbicularis oculi muscles. In contrast, clinical reports indicate that the use of hyaluronidase for retrobulbar and peribulbar anesthesia may actually decrease the incidence of myotoxicity.[49,50]

DIAGNOSTIC EVALUATION

Pain and muscle tenderness that persists around the site of local anesthetic injection for more than a day may be the initial presentation of myotoxicity. Careful palpation and the provocation of pain by passive stretch or active contraction may confirm irritation in a muscle immediately adjacent to the site of injection. Symptoms may be maximal on the 3rd to 4th day after injection when the peak of the inflammatory response is expected. Magnetic resonance (MR) imaging as early as the day following injection may show swelling and altered signal intensity of the involved muscle (Fig. 15-3).[51] After approximately 4 weeks, electromyographic exam may show small, brief, polyphasic motor unit action potentials characteristic of myopathy. Although biopsy is rarely indicated, histologic exam is the definitive mode of diagnosis and would demonstrate cell lysis, inflammatory infiltrate, and eventual myocyte regeneration. Alternate diagnoses to consider include infection or hematoma.

The eyes are a very sensitive indicator of muscle dysfunction since the patient readily recognizes slight imbalances

---

BOX 15-1 Factors Potentiating Local Anesthetic Myotoxicity

- Bupivacaine > ropivacaine, lidocaine, prilocaine > tetracaine, procaine
- Dose related
- Direct intramuscular injection
- Serial or continuous administration, steroid, epinephrine

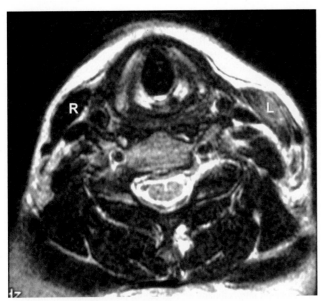

FIGURE 15-3. MRI of bupivacaine-induced myotoxicity. This axial image (T2-weighted fast spin-echo acquisition) at the level of the C6 vertebral body shows an enlarged left sternocleidomastoid muscle with increased signal intensity (L), compared to the normal right sternocleidomastoid muscle (R). (From Hogan Q, Dotson R, Erickson S, et al. Local anesthetic myotoxicity: a case and review. *Anesthesiology* 1994;80:942–947.)

in function after local anesthetic injection into or around the extraocular muscles. Diplopia, with or without blepharoptosis, has been described following successful cataract surgery[52–59] or scleral buckling[60] in recent reports. Patients typically describe diplopia immediately upon removal of the patch. Detailed exam shows an initial paresis and ultimately contracture of the muscles by scar.[59] There may also be an overaction phase attributable to a shortened muscle. Many of the reported injuries to muscle are probably due to local anesthetic toxicity, with an incidence of 0.25% after peribulbar and retrobulbar block,[61] compared to a zero incidence after general or topical anesthesia for cataract surgery. These cases have mostly had retrobulbar or peribulbar local anesthetic injection, although postoperative strabismus can also be the result of surgical trauma from suture placement, nerve palsy, or vascular accident.[53] The dysfunctional muscle is most often in the area of injection, and imaging has shown thickening of muscles at the sites most likely to be in the path of the blockade needle.[62] Needle trauma alone or with intramuscular injection of saline does not injure human extraocular muscles.[63]

It might be expected that muscle damage should be frequent since relatively large local anesthetic doses are deposited next to these small muscles, and experimental evidence in rats clearly shows massive damage to the extraocular muscles from retrobulbar injection of clinical concentrations of local anesthetics.[64,65] However, injury is rare in humans. This may be due to a species difference in which primate extraocular muscles are relatively resistant compared to rodents. Retrobulbar injection in monkeys produces only variable fiber degeneration on the surface of the muscles closest to the injection.[63] While this is sometimes extensive, most muscles are not affected. In another study in primates, relative resistance of the extraocular muscles to local anesthetic injury was

evident.[66] These authors reported greater damage of fibers with extensive SR and less injury in fibers with many mitochondria, which are a Ca^{2+} sink when cytoplasmic levels are high. Since extraocular muscles in general have many mitochondria, this may explain the evidently lower sensitivity of extraocular muscle to local anesthetics compared to other somatic muscles. Additionally, the fat of the orbital space may compete for local anesthetic molecules and reduce the concentration at the muscles. However, even in these two primate studies, myotoxicity was nonetheless identifiable after all injections. The main mechanism of clinically relevant human injury may be unintentional intramuscular injection, which produces a substantial injury. It remains to be determined, then, whether myotoxicity is rare in clinical situations or is common in humans and just not recognized.

▶ PREVENTION

Factors noted above that increase muscle injury caused by local anesthetic administration should be avoided when possible, including injection into the muscle itself, adding steroid or epinephrine to the injection, using large local anesthetic doses, and repeated injection. Muscle regeneration may be limited in the aged,[63] so precautions may be most important in these subjects. Certain patients may be poor candidates for blocks that risk muscle injury, including those with preexisting muscle compromise or ones in particular need of strength of the muscles near the injection, as in certain injections on athletes, laborers, or musicians.

Myotoxicity might be minimized during eye surgery by using techniques that avoid the extraocular muscles, such as injecting into the sub-Tenon (episcleral) space rather than retrobulbar or peribulbar.[67] However, local anesthetics injected into the episcleral (sub-Tenon's) space in volumes adequate to produce akinesia also enter the rectus muscles through their insertions into Tenon's fascia.[68] Enthusiasm for this block also rests on the belief that vascular and CNS complications will be less likely than with retrobulbar or peribulbar injection.[69] Comparative studies with enough cases to identify rare events have not yet been reported.

▶ TREATMENT

Specific treatment of myotoxic injury after local anesthetic injection is rarely necessary since muscle regeneration is usually prompt and complete. However, there are rare cases in which inflammation may persist for many weeks,[2] or permanent tissue loss results.[3] Therapies with potential benefit and little risk include avoidance of further myotoxic injections, immobilization, nonsteroidal anti-inflammatory agents, rehabilitation, and systemic steroids in selected cases. Initial findings indicate that specific approaches might be devised to interrupt the pathogenesis of local anesthetic myotoxicity. Mitochondrial structure and function is preserved in muscle exposed to bupivacaine when erythropoietin is coinjected,[70] and N-acetylcysteine prevents the generation of apoptotic mediators otherwise evoked by bupivacaine.[32] Thus, agents may be developed that will protect against muscle damage by local anesthetics.

► SUMMARY

Local anesthetic myotoxicity is largely a hidden problem. While the pharmacologic effect is highly predictable and muscle damage during neural blockade is probably a routine event, clinically important injury is only rarely recognized. It is not yet known whether local anesthetic myotoxicity produces substantial damage that is incorrectly attributed to other causes, or alternatively that muscle damage is very limited in extent in most subjects. This may be resolved in the future by advances in physiologic imaging, such as MR spectroscopy.[71]

References

1. Ott B, Neuberger L, Frey HP. Obliteration of the axillary artery after axillary block, *Anaesthesia* 1989;44:773–774.
2. Hogan Q, Dotson R, Erickson S, et al. Local anesthetic myotoxicity: a case and review. *Anesthesiology* 1994;80:942–947.
3. Parris WCV, Dettbarn WD. Muscle atrophy following bupivacaine trigger point injection. *Anesthesiol Rev* 1989;16:50–53.
4. Foster AH, Carlson BM. Myotoxicity of local anesthetics and regeneration of the damaged muscle fibers. *Anesth Analg* 1980;59:727–736.
5. Komorowski TE, Shepard B, Okland S, et al. An electron microscopic study of local anesthetic-induced skeletal muscle fiber degeneration and regeneration in the monkey. *J Orthop Res* 1990; 8:495–503.
6. Jejurikar SS, Welling TH, Zelenock JA, et al. Induction of angiogenesis by lidocaine and basic fibroblast growth factor: a model for *in vivo* retroviral-mediated gene therapy. *J Surg Res* 1997;67:137–146.
7. Rainin EA, Carlson BM. Postoperative diplopia and ptosis: a clinical hypothesis based on the myotoxicity of local anesthetics. *Arch Ophthalmol* 1985;103:1337–1339.
8. Salama H, Farr AK, Guyton DL. Anesthetic myotoxicity as a cause of restrictive strabismus after scleral buckling surgery. *Retina* 2000;20:478–482.
9. Benoit PW, Belt D. Destruction and regeneration of skeletal muscle after treatment with a local anesthetic, bupivacaine (Marcaine). *J Anat* 1970;107:547–556.
10. Hall-Craggs ECB. Early ultrastructural changes in skeletal muscle exposed to the local anesthetic bupivacaine (Marcaine). *Br J Exp Pathol* 1980;61:139–149.
11. Nonaka I, Takagi A, Ishiura S, et al. Pathophysiology of muscle fiber necrosis induced by bupivacaine hydrochloride (Marcaine). *Acta Neuropathol* 1983;60:167–174.
12. Pere P, Watanabe H, Pitkanen M, et al. Local myotoxicity of bupivacaine in rabbits after continuous supraclavicular brachial plexus block. *Reg Anesth* 1993;18:304–307.
13. Sadeh M, Czyzewski K, Stern L. Chronic myopathy induced by repeated bupivacaine injections. *J Neurol Sci* 1985;67:229–238.
14. Schultz E, Lipton BH. The effect of Marcaine on muscle and non-muscle cells in vitro. *Anat Rec* 1978;191:351–369.
15. Padera RF, Tse JY, Bellas E, et al. Tetrodotoxin for prolonged local anesthesia without myotoxicity. *Muscle Nerve* 2006;34:747–753.
16. Benoit PW, Yagiela JA, Fort NF. Pharmacological correlation between local anesthetic-induced myotoxicity and disturbances of intracellular calcium distribution. *Toxicol Appl Pharmacol* 1980;52:187–198.
17. Pike GK, Abramson JJ, Salama G. Effects of tetracaine and procaine on skinned muscle fibers depend on free calcium. *J Muscle Res Cell Motil* 1989;10:337–349.
18. Johnson PN, Inesi G. The effects of methylxanthines and local anesthetics on fragmented sarcoplasmic reticulum. *J Pharmacol Exp Ther* 1969;169:308–314.
19. Shoshan-Barmatz V, Zchut S. The interaction of local anesthetics with the ryanodine receptor of the sarcoplasmic reticulum. *J Membr Biol* 1993;133:171–181.
20. Xu L, Jones R, Meissner G. Effects of local anesthetics on single channel behavior of skeletal muscle calcium release channel. *J Gen Physiol* 1993;101:207–233.
21. Zahradnikova A, Palade P. Procaine effects on single sarcoplasmic reticulum Ca²⁺ release channels. *Biophys J* 1993;64:991–1003.
22. Gyorke S, Lukyanenko V, Gyorke I. Dual effects of tetracaine on spontaneous calcium release in rat ventricular myocytes. *J Physiol* 1997;500:297–309.
23. Komai H, Lokuta AJ. Interaction of bupivacaine and tetracaine with the sarcoplasmic reticulum Ca²⁺ release channel of skeletal and cardiac muscles. *Anesthesiology* 1999;90:835:43.
24. Takahashi SS. Local anesthetic bupivacaine alters function of sarcoplasmic reticulum and sarcolemmal vesicles from rabbit masseter muscle. *Pharmacol Toxicol* 1994;75:119–128.
25. Kutchai H, Mahaney JE, Geddis LM, et al. Hexanol and lidocaine affect the oligomeric state of the Ca-ATPase of sarcoplasmic reticulum. *Biochemistry* 1994;33:13208–13222.
26. Takara D, Sanchez GA, Alonso GL. Effect of carticaine on the sarcoplasmic reticulum Ca²⁺-adenosine triphosphatase. *Nauyn Schmiedebergs Arch Pharmacol* 2000;362:497–503.
27. Zink W, Graf BM, Sinner B, et al. Differential effects of bupivacaine on intracellular Ca²⁺ regulation: potential mechanisms of its myotoxicity. *Anesthesiology* 2002;97:710–716.
28. Garcia-Martin E, Gonzalez-Cabanillas S, Gutierrez-Merino C. Modulation of calcium fluxes across synaptosomal plasma membrane by local anesthetics. *J Neurochem* 1990;55:370–378.
29. Gold MS, Reichling DB, Hampl KF, et al. Lidocaine toxicity in primary afferent neurons from the rat. *J Pharmacol Exp Ther* 1998;285:413–421.
30. Irwin W, Fontaine E, Agnolucci L, et al. Bupivacaine myotoxicity is mediated by mitochondria. *J Biol Chem* 2002;277:12221–12227.
31. Nouette-Gaulain K, Sirvent P, Canal-Raffin M, et al. Effects of intermittent femoral nerve injections of bupivacaine, levobupivacaine, and ropivacaine on mitochondrial energy metabolism and intracellular calcium homeostasis in rat psoas muscle. *Anesthesiology* 2007;106:1026–1034.
32. Galbes O, Bourret A, Nouette-Gaulain K, et al. N-acetylcysteine protects against bupivacaine-induced myotoxicity caused by oxidative and sarcoplasmic reticulum stress n human skeletal myotubes. *Anesthesiology* 2010;113:560–569.
33. Foster AH, Carlson BM. Myotoxicity of local anesthetics and regeneration of the damaged muscle fibers. *Anesth Analg* 1980;59: 727–736.
34. Amanti E, Drampa F, Kouzi-Koliakos K, et al. Ropivacaine myotoxicity after single intramuscular injection in rats. *Eur J Anaesthesiol* 2006;23:130–135.
35. Zink W, Seif C, Bohl JRE, et al. The acute myotoxic effects of bupivacaine and ropivacaine after continuous peripheral nerve blockades. *Anesth Analg* 2003;97:1173–1179.
36. Zink W, Bohl JRE, Hacke N, et al. The long term myotoxic effects of bupivacaine and ropivacaine after continuous peripheral nerve blocks. *Anesth Analg* 2005;101:548–554.
37. Zink W, Missler G, Sinner B, et al. Differential effects of bupivacaine and ropivacaine enantiomers on intracellular Ca²⁺ regulation in murine skeletal muscle fibers. *Anesthesiology* 2005;102: 793–798.
38. Nouette-Gaulain K, Dadure C, Morau D, et al. Age-dependent bupivacaine-induced muscle toxicity during continuous peripheral nerve block in rats. *Anesthesiology* 2009;111:1120–1127.
39. Benoit PW, Belt WD. Some effects of local anesthetic agents on skeletal muscle. *Exp Neurol* 1972;34:264–278.
40. Zhang C, Phamonvaechavan P, Rajan A, et al. Concentration-dependent bupivacaine myotoxicity in rabbit extraocular muscle. *J AAPOS* 2010;14:323–327.
41. Kytta J, Heinon E, Rosenberg PH, et al. Effects of repeated bupivacaine administration on sciatic nerve and surrounding muscle tissue in rats. *Acta Anaesthesiol Scand* 1986;30:625–629.
42. Benoit PW. Microscarring in skeletal muscle after repeated exposures to lidocaine with epinephrine. *J Oral Surg* 1978;36:530–533.

43. Padera R, Bellas E, Tse JY, et al. Local myotoxicity from sustained release of bupivacaine from microparticles. *Anesthesiology* 2008;108:921–928.

44. Guttu RL, Page DG, Laskin DM. Delayed healing of muscle after injection of bupivacaine and steroid. *Ann Dent* 1990;49:5–8.

45. Benoit PW. Reversible skeletal muscle damage after administration of local anesthetics with and without epinephrine. *J Oral Surg* 1978;36:198–201.

46. Brun A. Effect of procaine, carbocain and xylocaine on cutaneous muscle in rabbits and mice. *Acta Anaesthesiol Scand* 1959;3:59–73.

47. Hall-Craggs ECB. Rapid degeneration and regeneration of a whole skeletal muscle following treatment with bupivacaine. *Exp Neurol* 1975;43:349–358.

48. McLoon LK, Wirtschafter J. Regional differences in the subacute response of rabbit orbicularis oculi to bupivacaine-induced myotoxicity as quantified with a neural cell adhesion molecule immunohistochemical marker. *Invest Ophthalmol Vis Sci* 1993;34:3450–3458.

49. Brown SM, Brooks SE, Mazow ML, et al. Cluster of diplopia cases after periocular anesthesia without hyaluronidase. *J Cataract Refract Surg* 1999;25:1245–1249.

50. Jehan FS, Hagan JC, Whittaker TJ, et al. Diplopia and ptosis following injection of local anesthesia without hyaluronidase. *J Cataract Refract Surg* 2001;27:1876–1879.

51. Taylor G, Devys JM, Heran F, et al. Early exploration of diplopia with magnetic resonance imaging after peribulbar anaesthesia. *Br J Anaesth* 2004;92:899–901.

52. Rainin EA, Carlson BM. Postoperative diplopia and ptosis: a clinical hypothesis based on the myotoxicity of local anesthetics. *Arch Ophthalmol* 1985;103:1337–1339.

53. Catalano RA, Nelson LA. Persistent strabismus presenting after cataract surgery. *Ophthalmology* 1987;94:491–494.

54. Hamed LM. Strabisumus presenting after cataract surgery. *Ophthalmology* 1991;98:247–252.

55. Grimmett MR, Lambert SR. Superior rectus muscle overaction after cataract extraction. *Am J Ophthalmol* 1992;114:72–80.

56. Esswein MB, von Noorden GK. Paresis of a vertical rectus muscled after cataract extraction. *Am J Ophthalmol* 1993;116:424–430.

57. Munoz M. Inferior rectus muscle overaction after cataract extraction. *Am J Ophthalmol* 1994;118:664–666.

58. Hunter DG, Lam GC, Guyton DL. Inferior oblique muscle injury from local anesthesia for cataract surgery. *Ophthalmology* 1995;102:501–509.

59. Capo H, Guyton DL. Ipsilateral hypertropia after cataract surgery. *Ophthalmology* 1996;103:721–730.

60. Salama H, Farr AK, Guyton DL. Anesthetic myotoxicity as a cause of restrictive strabismus after scleral buckling surgery. *Retina* 2000;20:478–482.

61. Gomez-Arnau JI, Yanguela J, Gonzales A, et al. Anaesthesia-related diplopia after cataract surgery. *Br J Anaesth* 2003;90:189–193.

62. Hamed LM, Mancuso A. Inferior rectus muscle contracture syndrome after retrobulbar anesthesia. *Ophthalmology* 1991;98:1506–1012.

63. Carlson BM, Emerick S, Komorowski TE, et al. Extraocular muscle regeneration in primates: local anesthetic-induced lesions. *Ophthalmology* 1992;99:582–589.

64. Carlson BM, Rainin EA. Rat extraocular muscle degeneration: repair of local anesthetic-induced damage. *Arch Ophthalmol* 1985;103:1373–1377.

65. Okland S, Komorowski TE, Carlson BM. Ultrastructure of mepivacaine-induced damage and regeneration in rat extraocular muscle. *Invest Ophthalmol Vis Sci* 1989;30:1643–1651.

66. Porter JD, Edney DP, McMahon EJ, et al. Extraocular myotoxicity of the retrobulbar anesthetic bupivacaine hydrochloride. *Invest Ophthalmol Vis Sci* 1988;29:163–174.

67. Steele MA, Lavrich JB, Nelson LB, et al. Sub-Tenon's infusion of local anesthetic for strabismus surgery. *Ophthalmic Surg* 1992;23:40–43.

68. Ripart J, Metge L, Prat-Pradal D, et al. Medial canthus single-injection episcleral (sub-Tenon anesthesia): computed tomography imaging. *Anesth Analg* 1998;87:42–45.

69. Ripart J, L'Hermite J, Charavel P, et al. Regional anesthesia for ophthalmic surgery performed by single episcleral (sub-Tenon) injection: a 802 cases experience. *Reg Anesth Pain Med* 1999;24:S59.

70. Nouette-Galain K, Bellance N, Prevost B, et al. Erythropoietin protects against local anesthetic myotoxicity during continuous regional analgesia. *Anesthesiology* 2009;110:648–659.

71. Newman RJ, Radda GK. The myotoxicity of bupivacaine, a 31P n.m.r. investigation. *Br J Pharmacol* 1983;79:395–399.

16

Pulmonary Complications

William F. Urmey

As anesthesiologists, it is important that we understand the basis of, and can therefore predict, the consistent physiologic changes that result from regional anesthesia. Neuraxial regional anesthetics, as well as brachial plexus techniques, have predictable effects on respiration. This chapter details the pathophysiology and management of the pulmonary complications that are associated with regional anesthetic techniques.

▶ DEFINITION

Neuraxial anesthesia has predictable significant effects on respiration. These changes include altered pulmonary function, chest wall mechanics, gas exchange, and ventilatory control. There have been comparatively few studies on the respiratory effects of neuraxial anesthesia. Indeed, some often-quoted reviews on "anesthesia" and respiration fail to even mention regional anesthesia.[1,2] Most of the respiratory changes associated with neuraxial anesthesia can be directly attributed to pharmacologic motor nerve blockade of respiratory musculature. In fact, neuraxial anesthesia provides a somewhat controllable experimental model for the reversible interruption of groups of respiratory muscles.

Although respiratory arrest or failure secondary to interscalene block has an extremely low incidence, the diaphragmatic paresis associated with this regional anesthetic technique results in very significant and predictable changes in respiration. Forced vital capacity (FVC) and forced expiratory volume in 1 second (FEV_1) are typically reduced by 20% to 40% within 15 minutes of interscalene block injection. The diminutions in lung volumes last 3 to 5 hours with mepivacaine interscalene block and more than 9 hours with bupivacaine.[3] Respiratory failure or arrest may also occur if the patient has preexisting respiratory disease,[4] but more typical etiologies of acute respiratory failure associated with peripheral nerve blocks are pneumothorax[5] or unintentional subarachnoid or epidural injection[6-9] (Chapter 18).

▶ SCOPE

Respiratory failure is an extremely rare complication of spinal or epidural anesthesia. Acute respiratory failure during neuraxial anesthesia is most often caused by total spinal anesthesia or massive epidural anesthesia or is secondary to the effects of opiates administered into the subarachnoid or epidural space. Respiratory failure in each case is usually secondary to cephalad distribution of the anesthetic agents. The predominant etiology is alteration of respiratory control secondary to direct effect on the medulla. The incidence of respiratory depression following epidural or subarachnoid opiate administration has been published and ranges between 0.07% and 0.90%.[10–16] The usual respiratory effects of neuraxial anesthesia are of negligible clinical concern in most patients (Chapters 19 and 20).

Since Urmey et al.[17] first reported that hemidiaphragmatic paresis with resultant respiratory impairment occurs with an incidence of 100% following interscalene block, numerous subsequent investigators have confirmed the consistency of this side effect.[18–21] Supraclavicular blocks, performed at more caudad levels than the interscalene approach, are associated with lower incidences of diaphragmatic paresis, although incidences up to 80% have been reported.[22] Despite a lower incidence of hemidiaphragmatic paresis,[23,24] significant alteration in respiration from supraclavicular block is variable. By contrast, most infraclavicular approaches do not have any significant effects on respiration.[25,26] However, a recent study found that the vertical infraclavicular block (VIB) approach was associated with a 26% incidence of hemidiaphragmatic paralysis.[27] In an original trial on the intersternocleidomastoid technique, Pham-Dang et al.[28] found an incidence of reversible phrenic nerve paresis of 60%.

Pneumothorax has been associated with brachial plexus block performed by either supraclavicular or infraclavicular approaches. Other regional anesthetic techniques have been associated with pneumothorax. These include intercostal block (0.07%–19% incidence),[29–32] paravertebral block (0.5% incidence),[33] and intrapleural block (2% incidence).[34]

The extremely rare complication of permanent or persistent phrenic nerve paralysis has been reported following interscalene brachial plexus block.[35–37] This presumably occurs as a result of direct trauma to the phrenic nerve by way of needle contact or intraneural injection (Box 16-1). This should be considered when performing techniques such as the intersternocleidomastoid technique,[28] which involves a more anterior insertion and may traverse the course of the phrenic nerve. A recent ultrasonographic analysis of the anatomic relationship of the phrenic nerve determined that the phrenic nerve was only 2 mm away from the C5 nerve root at the level of the cricoid cartilage (Fig. 16-1). As the phrenic nerve coursed more caudally in the neck, for every centimeter increase in caudal distance, the phrenic nerve added 3 mm separation (anteriorly) from the brachial plexus. Therefore, the phrenic nerve is more likely to be avoided by techniques performed below the conventional interscalene block as described by Winnie.[38]

▶ PATHOPHYSIOLOGY

Chest Wall Muscle Paralysis

Respiratory physiologists define the "chest wall" as the rib cage, abdomen, and diaphragm. If we understand the implications of paralyzing the abdominal muscles, rib cage muscles, and diaphragm, we should be able to predict and explain the changes that occur during neuraxial anesthesia. Studies of this nature have been performed on animals following selective sectioning of nerves supplying respiratory muscles[39–41] and on humans (either volunteers who relax groups of muscles[42,43] or on quadriplegic patients[44–46] with pathological denervation of respiratory muscles).

With more cephalad levels of epidural or spinal anesthesia, the chest wall muscles (rib cage and abdominal) are blocked, which in extreme cases may leave the diaphragm to work alone. This approximates the situation of the quadriplegic patient. Under routine neuraxial anesthesia, the main muscle of respiration, the diaphragm, remains unaffected and therefore pulmonary function is changed little. This is in contrast to other regional anesthetic techniques (e.g., interscalene block or intrapleural block), which affect the diaphragm by phrenic nerve paralysis and may therefore have more profound effects on pulmonary function and chest wall mechanics.[17,19,47] Nevertheless, rib cage muscular contraction and diaphragmatic contraction coordinate during normal breathing to move the rib cage in a homogenous manner.[46,48] If this coordination is interrupted by neuraxial block, chest wall deformation may occur and the characteristics of normal breathing will change.

Neuraxial Regional Anesthesia

Most clinical studies on normal patients receiving spinal or epidural anesthesia have found minimal effects on routine pulmonary function tests (PFTs).[49] This was confirmed in a study of 30 patients who received epidural anesthesia with 25 to 30 mL 2% lidocaine.[18] Epidural anesthesia to sensory levels averaging T5 to T6 caused mean diminution in FVC of just 176 mL ($p < 0.05$) and diminished peak expiratory flow rate of only 0.34 L/s ($p < 0.05$). Thus, although the effects of neuraxial anesthesia on the respiratory musculature and chest wall are indeed significant, routine PFTs are relatively insensitive in measuring the changes in respiratory system mechanics. This is because routine PFTs are dependent on lung mechanics and the chest wall muscle activity. In fact, FEV_1 is a more clinically useful measurement in the diagnosis of lung pathology based on its dependence on the lung. FEV_1 is reproducible despite variations in expiratory effort.

BOX 16-1 Respiratory Complications of Regional Anesthesia

Neuraxial regional anesthesia:

- Total spinal anesthesia
- Massive epidural anesthesia
- Cephalad spread of opioids

Brachial plexus regional anesthesia:

- Unintended neuraxial block
- Hemidiaphragmatic paresis
- Permanent phrenic nerve block

Pneumothorax

- Above-the-clavicle blocks
- Suprascapular nerve block
- Paravertebral blocks
- Intercostal nerve block

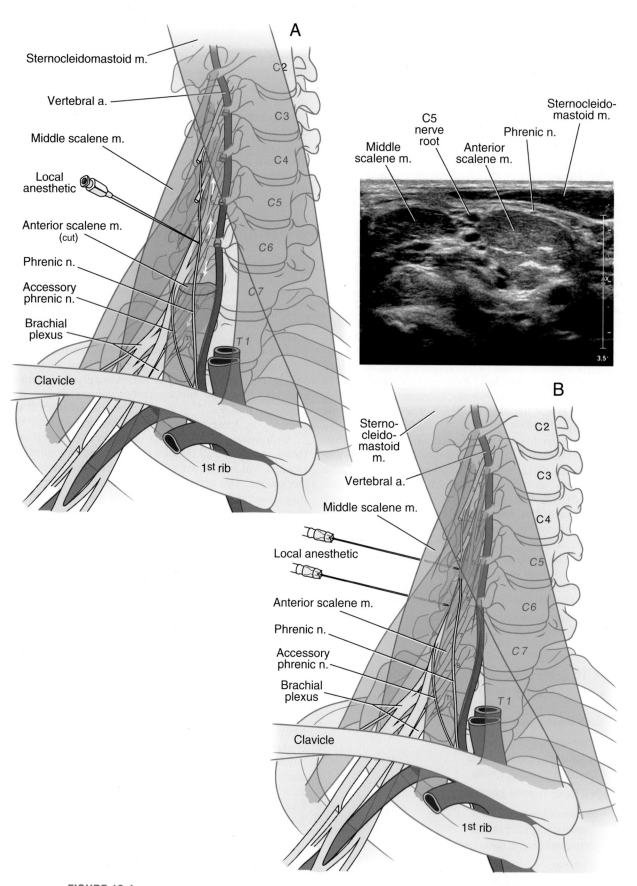

FIGURE 16-1. **Panel A: When a traditional paresthesia-seeking or peripheral nerve stimulation technique is used for interscalene block, the needle is placed at the C6 level.** The relatively large volumes of local anesthetic used during these techniques can spread to the cervical nerve roots, causing phrenic nerve anesthesia and hemidiaphragmatic paresis. The phrenic nerve's overlying position on the anterior scalene muscle also exposes it to possible local anesthetic actions or needle trauma. **Panel B:** When ultrasound guidance is used, local anesthetic is injected at the C5 level, where the phrenic nerve is within 2 mm of the C5 nerve root (**sonogram inset**). This is the purported mechanism for phrenic nerve anesthesia when using ultrasound guidance, despite the ability to use a relatively reduced volume of local anesthetic.

Conversely, FEV_1 or FVC is relatively insensitive for assessing alterations in respiratory muscle function and chest wall mechanics caused by neuraxial anesthesia. For instance, Sundberg et al.[50] found that high thoracic epidural anesthesia at levels of T1 to T5 had little effect on FVC, decreasing it by only 300 mL. Takasaki and Takahashi[51] found mean reductions in FVC after thoracic epidural anesthesia of 11%. Groeben et al.[52] similarly found that thoracic epidural anesthesia in patients with significant chronic obstructive pulmonary disease (COPD) resulted in only an 8% decrease in FVC and FEV_1. It must be kept in mind that, although abdominal or thoracic epidural analgesia may have a minor negative impact on respiratory function, the superior analgesia has resulted in improvement in FVC following general surgery or abdominal vascular surgery.[53]

Warner et al.[54] studied the effects of high epidural anesthesia (approximately a T1 sensory level) on the function of the human chest wall. They found that high epidural anesthesia abolished parasternal intercostal muscle activity while preserving scalene and diaphragmatic activity. High epidural levels decreased rib cage expansion, but paradoxical (inward) motion of the rib cage occurred in only one of six study subjects. High epidural anesthesia resulted in an increase in functional residual capacity (FRC), with a significant caudad displacement of the end expiratory position of the diaphragm. However, paradoxical respiration is markedly affected by the use of intravenous sedation in conjunction with neuraxial anesthesia. Significant decreases in percentage expansion of the rib cage and in pO_2 during propofol sedation during spinal anesthesia have been observed and attributed, in part, to upper airway obstruction.[55]

Despite sympathetic blockade, thoracic epidural anesthesia does not increase airway obstruction and only causes a small decrease in FEV_1.[52,56] Similarly, no significant decreases in spirometric tests were found during epidural anesthesia in parturients undergoing cesarean delivery. By contrast, Capdevila et al.[57] found that cervical epidural anesthesia had significant effects on breathing pattern, diaphragmatic function, and respiratory drive in healthy patients. Cervical epidural anesthesia was associated with decreased diaphragmatic excursion, diminution in maximal inspiratory pressure up to 40.5%, and reduction in FVC up to 26.3%. Similarly, Takasaki and Takahashi[51] found that cervical epidural anesthesia reduced FVC by a mean value of 28% and Michalek et al.[58] found approximately a 20% diminution in FEV_1 and FVC associated with cervical epidural sensory blockade from C2–C5. In a study of 324 patients undergoing carotid endarterectomy with cervical epidural anesthesia, 3 required intubation secondary to respiratory insufficiency.[59]

Respiratory System Mechanics

To understand the alterations in respiration that result from pharmacologic motor nerve blockade during epidural anesthesia, one must first appreciate the basic mechanics underlying normal chest wall motion and normal (nonparalyzed) respiratory muscle actions. These factors have been clarified through the work of Mead, De Troyer, and other respiratory physiologists. Goldman and Mead[43] first described the pressure-volume characteristics of the chest wall by using magnetometers to make indirect measurements of volume changes of the two major compartments

of the chest wall: (i) the rib cage (RC) and (ii) the abdomen-diaphragm (AB-Di). They measured the pressure driving these compartments by dividing the chest wall into three parts: (i) the RC, (ii) the AB, and (iii) the diaphragm. The following equations algebraically describe the transmural pressures across each part.

$$P_{RC} = P_{PL} - P_{BS} = P_{PL}$$
(at atmospheric pressure, $P_{BS} = 0$) $\qquad$ [16.1]

$$P_{ABW} = P_{AB} - P_{BS} = P_{AB} \qquad [16.2]$$

$$P_{DI} = P_{PL} - P_{AB} \qquad [16.3]$$

Here, P_{RC} = the transmural pressure driving the rib cage, P_{PL} = pleural pressure, P_{BS} = body surface pressure, P_{ABW} = pressure across the abdominal wall, P_{AB} = intraabdominal pressure, and P_{DI} = transdiaphragmatic pressure.

Although the active chest wall has mainly two degrees of freedom of motion,[41] the relaxed chest wall (all muscles voluntarily relaxed) has only one set of corresponding pressures and volumes. Thus, a "relaxation pressure-volume curve" could be generated for the voluntarily relaxed chest wall. Goldman and Mead noticed that quiet breathing followed this relaxed characteristic curve. To "stress the system" and make transmural driving pressure change, a large abdominal cuff was inflated to passively squeeze the abdomen of volunteers who relaxed their respiratory muscles. Each cm H_2O change in transdiaphragmatic pressure (P_{DI}) resulted in a decrease in pleural pressure (P_{PL}) of an equal magnitude. In addition, the increasing abdominal pressure expanded the rib cage. This can be understood algebraically by the examination of the following equations.

$$P_{RC} \text{ (isolated from diaphragm)} = P_{PL} - P_{DI} \qquad [16.4]$$

Substituting Equation 16.3 yields:

$$P_{RC} \text{ (isolated from diaphragm)} = P_{PL} - (P_{PL} - P_{AB}) \qquad [16.5]$$

$$P_{RC} \text{ (isolated from diaphragm)} = P_{AB} \qquad [16.6]$$

Thus, the pressure driving the rib cage in the absence of the diaphragm is intraabdominal pressure. Because diaphragmatic contraction increases the intraabdominal pressure (P_{AB}), Goldman and Mead[43] erroneously concluded that the diaphragm was the only active muscle during tidal breathing.

It later became evident from studies in quadriplegics[46] that true isolated diaphragmatic action expands only the lower rib cage (LRC). The upper rib cage (URC) is pulled inward by decreasing pleural pressure, which deforms the rib cage overall. This is similar to what had been described during high levels of spinal anesthesia by Eisele et al.[60] in 1968. They observed that during continuous spinal anesthesia to attain a T1 motor level, "the lower half of the chest moved out with inspiration while the upper half passively retracted."

Mead proposed a mechanism to explain these new findings by considering the diaphragm's geometry. The zone of apposition (Z_{ap}) allows for the direct application of P_{AB} to the

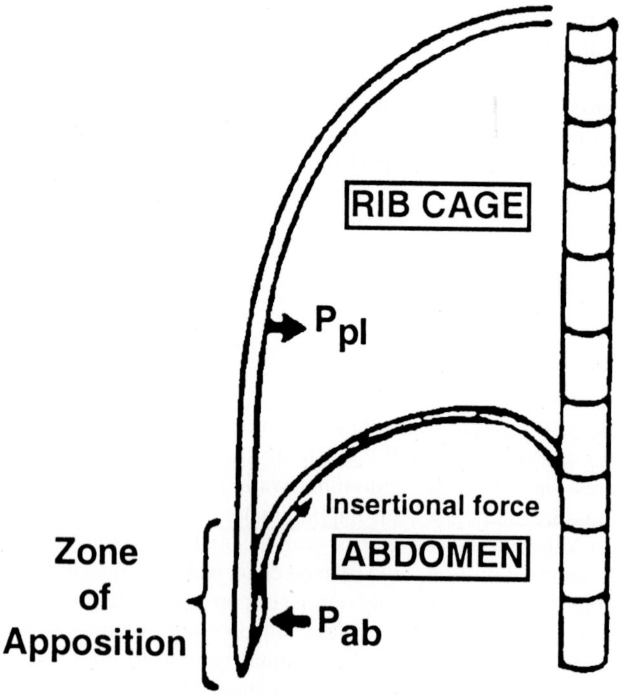

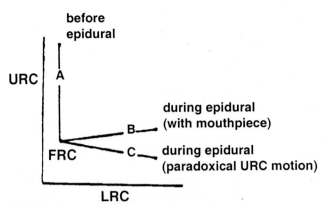

FIGURE 16-3. Upper rib cage (URC) and lower rib cage (LRC) expansion before and during epidural anesthesia. (FRC, functional residual capacity.) (Reproduced from Urmey W, Lambert D, Concepcion M. Routine spinal or epidural anesthesia causes rib cage distortion during spontaneous inspiration (abstract). *Anesthesiology* 1987;67:A538, with permission.)

FIGURE 16-2. Lateral schematic illustration of the chest wall. (P_{pl}, pleural pressure; P_{ab}, abdominal pressure.) (Adapted from Green N. *Physiology of Spinal Anesthesia, Pulmonary Ventilation and Hemodynamics.* Baltimore, MD: Williams & Wilkins, 1981.)

Both of these effects are only on the LRC. Decreasing pleural pressure passively sucks the URC inward in the absence of intercostal muscle function. This explains the characteristic deformation of the rib cage during epidural anesthesia, spinal anesthesia,[63,64] and quadriplegia (Fig. 16-3).

Diminished Cough Strength

Spinal or epidural anesthesia causes a level-dependent compromise in the ability to effectively cough. Unlike routine PFTs, the ability to cough effectively is dramatically and significantly affected by neuraxial anesthesia. In one study, 0.75% bupivacaine lumbar epidural anesthesia to levels of T3 to T4 caused an approximately 50% reduction in peak inspiratory pressure during cough (Fig. 16-4).[65] Egbert et al.[66] found a 53% reduction in intraabdominal pressure during cough in patients who had received spinal anesthesia. With ascending levels of neuraxial anesthesia, thoracoabdominal muscles are increasingly paralyzed.

inner rib cage wall such that increased P_{AB} by diaphragmatic contraction is directly applied to the inner RC wall through the Z_{ap}.[61] Urmey et al.[62] confirmed this theory in animal studies. Two components of diaphragmatic action on the LRC have thus been identified (Fig. 16-2):

- An insertional component, whereby the directional vector of diaphragm insertions and the mechanics of rib/vertebral articulations result in RC elevation and expansion
- An appositional component, whereby increases in P_{AB} are transmitted through the Z_{ap} to expand the rib cage

FIGURE 16-4. Reduction of cough strength as a function of time after epidural local anesthetic injection. (Reproduced with permission of Urmey WF. Case studies of regional anesthesia. In: *Complications of Regional Anesthesia.* New York, NY: Churchill-Livingstone, 1999.)

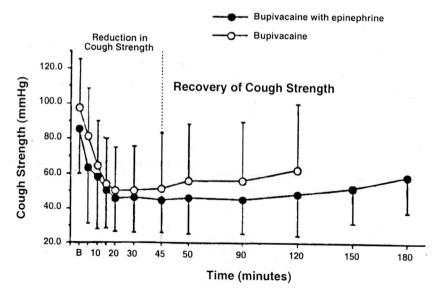

Pulmonary Gas Exchange

Pulmonary gas exchange during spinal or epidural anesthesia has not been adequately studied. The few existing clinical studies show a small reduction of approximately 10% to 20% in oxygen consumption and carbon dioxide production during neuraxial block. This is presumably due to muscle paralysis and immobility, resulting in decreased overall metabolism.[67] Changes in minute ventilation, alveolar/arterial oxygen partial pressure gradient, pulmonary dead space, or shunt are very small.[68] Distribution of ventilation was changed in patients who received spinal anesthesia when studied by nitrogen washout.[49,69] The chest wall mechanical and motion changes discussed in the preceding section are what cause the altered distribution of ventilation in the patient who receives neuraxial anesthesia.

Control of Ventilation

The few studies of the effects of neuraxial anesthesia on respiratory control have documented only small changes in minute ventilation, respiratory rate, and tidal volume. Arterial PCO_2 is maintained at normal levels during neuraxial blockade. Ventilation is, in fact, altered very little by neuraxial anesthesia. CO_2 response curves in unsedated patients with spinal anesthesia were characterized by a small increase in the response to a CO_2 challenge. This finding may have been secondary to anxiety and increased catecholamine levels. Changes in ventilatory control during spinal or epidural anesthesia are more likely to occur from the use of intravenously administered sedatives during regional anesthesia.

More important clinically are the effects of neuraxial opiates on ventilatory control. Respiratory arrest has been reported following intrathecal administration of sufentanil or fentanyl.[70–74] Special attention must be given to patients with sleep apnea[74] who receive neuraxial opiates. Intrathecal or epidural morphine leads to a well-documented dose-related inhibition of ventilation.[75]

In summary, the effects of neuraxial anesthesia can be attributed in large part to paralysis of abdominal and rib cage muscles. More cephalad levels of neuraxial anesthesia, therefore, have greater effects on respiratory physiology. Levels to T1 or above simulate quadriplegia (i.e., isolated diaphragmatic function). The effects of neuraxial anesthesia result largely in altered distribution of ventilation. These effects are much less significant than the respiratory effects of diaphragmatic paresis associated with brachial plexus blocks performed above the clavicle. Clinical neuraxial anesthesia usually results in minor changes in routine PFTs, tidal volume, respiratory control, and minute ventilation. Neuraxial anesthesia is usually a very safe option for the patient with preexisting pulmonary disease.

Brachial Plexus Regional Anesthesia

Originally, phrenic nerve paresis during interscalene block was attributed to the spread of local anesthetic to the nearby phrenic nerve in the neck[76] (Fig. 16-1). Diaphragmatic paresis is now known to occur via local anesthetic effects on the C3 to C5 cervical nerve roots before they form the phrenic nerve.[19] This is because drugs injected near the brachial plexus move freely into the cervical plexus above it.

Winnie et al.[77] demonstrated this by radiographic contrast-labeled local anesthetic injection. Sensory studies by Urmey and McDonald[19] and Urmey and Gloeggler[78] showed that dermatomal levels of C3 and C2 occur routinely. These levels occur despite the use of digital pressure.[79,80] The onset and offset of block of these cervical nerve roots correlate with the onset and offset of diaphragmatic dysfunction and changes in pulmonary function.

Consistent reductions in pulmonary function occur following interscalene block. Reductions of 20% to 40% in FEV_1 and FVC have been found in several studies,[19,20,78,81] but diminutions of more than 60% have also been observed in isolated cases.[78] These results are consistent with complete or near complete phrenic nerve paresis. The magnitude of the pulmonary function reductions are similar to those that have been reported following surgical phrenic nerve ablation[82] or complete phrenic nerve paralysis of a pathological etiology.[83] In a study of direct phrenic nerve infiltration with 1% mepivacaine in healthy volunteers, Gould et al.[84] demonstrated a 27% reduction in vital capacity.

▶ RISK FACTORS

Neuraxial Regional Anesthesia

Neuraxial anesthesia is rarely contraindicated on the basis of respiratory disease. Patients with pulmonary disease have not been documented to be at higher risk for respiratory complications than normal patients when receiving neuraxial anesthesia (lumbar spinal or epidural anesthesia). Spinal or epidural anesthesia does not adversely affect oxygenation during single lung ventilation and does not affect hypoxic pulmonary vasoconstriction. Neuraxial anesthesia does not cause bronchoconstriction, and it is safe to perform spinal or epidural anesthesia on asthmatic patients. Indeed, during epidural anesthesia in which epinephrine is added to the administered local anesthetic, bronchodilation may result.

Brachial Plexus Regional Anesthesia

Contralateral pneumonectomy and preexisting contralateral phrenic nerve paralysis are absolute contraindications to the performance of interscalene block. More relative contraindications include severe COPD and any disease of the respiratory system where a 25% diminution in vital capacity would not be tolerated. A reasonable contraindication for interscalene or supraclavicular block is an FVC < 1 L. Ankylosing spondylitis, a disease characterized by immobility of the rib cage, places a patient at increased risk of respiratory failure following interscalene block. This is because restriction of rib cage motion makes patients with ankylosing spondylitis more dependent on intact diaphragmatic function. Similarly, restriction from lateral positioning with the intact hemidiaphragm dependent on any positioning or strapping of the chest wall that inhibits contralateral rib cage expansion places a patient at increased risk. In fact, respiratory failure has been reported following extubation of a patient positioned in lateral decubitus position with the block side up and the intact hemidiaphragm dependent following interscalene block[4] (Box 16-2).

Patients who are very obese are more likely to develop areas of atelectasis or develop pulmonary complications, especially with prolonged or continuous brachial plexus block above the clavicle.[85]

DIAGNOSTIC EVALUATION

Hemidiaphragmatic paresis is an expected side effect of brachial plexus block performed above the clavicle. Dyspnea that develops after block administration is extremely rare in healthy patients. Importantly, associated pulmonary function changes are complete within 15 minutes of block administration. Therefore, changes are complete in the presence of the anesthesiologist. Patients having brachial plexus blocks above the clavicle should be monitored with pulse oximetry and should be administered supplemental oxygen. Capnography and equipment to assist or control ventilation should be immediately available. The duration of phrenic nerve block depends on the local anesthetic used and the dose administered. Phrenic, and therefore diaphragmatic, paralysis lasts 3 to 4 hours following mepivacaine interscalene block and >9 hours following bupivacaine block.

Fluoroscopy,[86] double exposure chest radiography,[87] and respiratory plethysmography have all been used to diagnose hemidiaphragmatic paresis. Ultrasonography is increasingly the method of choice to make this diagnosis. Ultrasonography and routine PFT can be used for preoperative assessment if preexisting pulmonary or diaphragmatic disease is suspected.

A chest radiograph may be obtained if pneumothorax is suspected (Box 16-3). However, a chest radiograph may

miss a small pneumothorax. An expiratory chest radiograph increases the ability to diagnose a pneumothorax. It should also be noted that a pneumothorax might take time to present clinically. In the absence of positive pressure ventilation, a pneumothorax may take 6 to 12 hours to become apparent on a radiograph. Pleuritic chest pain, diminished breath sounds to auscultation, or dyspnea may be associated with pneumothorax before it is evident on a chest radiograph. Treatment includes pulmonary consultation and thoracostomy, if indicated.

PREVENTION AND TREATMENT

The choice of anesthetic technique, and dosage and timing of local anesthetic administration during neuraxial block, may prevent unnecessarily high levels of blockade. The use of isobaric (plain) local anesthetic for subarachnoid injection limits intrathecal cephalad spread of the drug, thus preserving more chest wall muscle function. It is very rare to cause significant respiratory impairment by administration of an appropriate dose of isobaric local anesthetic for spinal anesthesia. For continuous neuraxial techniques, slow administration of the drug and partitioning the total dose over time decrease the possibility of a high spinal or a massive epidural. Careful monitoring of sensory level following neuraxial drug administration allows for prevention, earlier diagnosis, and treatment of respiratory impairment. Hyperbaric spinal anesthesia can be influenced to some degree by adjusting the patient's position. Despite the preventative measures outlined previously, undesired cephalad levels of neuraxial block with resulting respiratory muscle embarrassment may at times occur.

Dyspnea that develops during neuraxial anesthesia is most often due to anxiety secondary to ascending levels of respiratory muscle paralysis. High spinal or epidural anesthesia sufficient to cause respiratory failure must be ruled out. The patient's ability to speak is reassuring. A hand grip test is easy, rapid, and yields valuable information. A strong hand grip indicates that the brachial plexus is not significantly affected and therefore that the anesthetic level is caudad to the cervical level, indicating preservation of diaphragmatic function. The use of an anesthetic mask and a circuit with capnography allows for diagnosis of hypoventilation. Hypoxemia and decreased levels of arterial oxygen saturation are later signs of inadequate ventilation. Treatment may necessitate assistance by mask and positive pressure ventilation or endotracheal intubation and controlled ventilation.

Hemidiaphragmatic Paresis

The incidence of hemidiaphragmatic paresis is not decreased by decreasing the volume of local anesthetic to 20 mL[78] (Fig. 16-5). Nor is it prevented by the application of digital pressure immediately cephalad to the injection point.[79,80] The decreases in pulmonary function associated with (non-ultrasound-guided) blocks above the clavicle appear to be largely independent of the local anesthetic volume or concentration. Doses of 20 to 28 mL of 0.75% bupivacaine were found to result in pulmonary function decreases of 20% to 40% by Pere.[81] These decreases in pulmonary function as well as altered diaphragmatic motility persisted for at

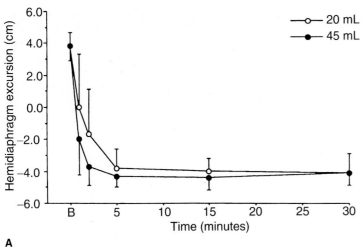

A

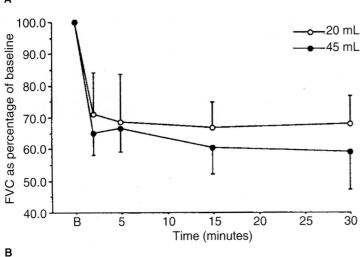

B

FIGURE 16-5. Hemidiaphragmatic excursion in centimeters and FVC with standard deviation is plotted as a function of time from interscalene block injection. Positive excursion values represent normal caudad motion and negative values represent paradoxical cephalad motion. There were no significant differences between 45- and 20-mL groups. (Reproduced from Urmey W, Gloeggler P. Pulmonary function changes during interscalene block: effects of decreasing local anesthetic injection volume. *Reg Anesth* 1993;18:244–249, with permission.)

least 24 hours when an infusion of 5 to 9 mL bupivacaine 0.125% was administered. A mean reduction in FVC of 32.0 ± 8.9% was found in a group of patients following a 20 mL injection of 1.5% mepivacaine for interscalene block.[78] Reducing the injection volume and concentration of bupivacaine to 10 mL of 0.25% bupivacaine provided analgesia with minimal effects on respiration.[88] Use of ropivacaine 0.5% was not found to diminish the alterations in pulmonary function during interscalene block. Infusions of 0.2% ropivacaine by interscalene catheter has been associated with significant diminutions in diaphragmatic motion and pulmonary function,[89] as well as lower lobe collapse.[90] Of interest, recent studies of brachial plexus blocks above the clavicle using extremely small local anesthetic volume and targeted ultrasound guidance have been consistent with an ability to avoid hemidiaphragmatic paresis. Although these low-volume blocks provided acceptable analgesia, the clinical practicality of these studies remains uncertain because general anesthesia often obscured the anesthetic attributes of the blocks.[91–93] Although less common, it is possible to cause phrenic paresis by brachial plexus block performed below the clavicle.[94,95] Approaches to the brachial plexus below the clavicle that are closest to the clavicle are most likely to cause diaphragmatic paresis. For example, a study of VIB was associated with a 20% incidence of diaphragmatic paresis.[27]

Dyspnea may be relieved by placing the patient in the sitting or upright position if tolerated. Sitting or beach-chair positioning optimizes diaphragmatic geometry, increases FRC, and lessens subjective symptoms.[19] Positive pressure ventilation may be needed in the rare patient. Assisted or controlled ventilation by facemask, laryngeal mask airway, or endotracheal intubation should be performed as clinically indicated. Dyspnea that develops during interscalene block may also be anxiety related.

Pneumothorax

Today, pneumothorax is a very rare complication of brachial plexus block. The possibility of pneumothorax depends on the brachial plexus technique. Traditional supraclavicular block by Kulenkampff's technique resulted in a 0.6% to 6% incidence of pneumothorax.[96] Modern supraclavicular blocks usually utilized ultrasonographic imaging, with the ability to identify the apex of the lung. Nevertheless, there have been cases of pneumothorax associated with ultrasound-guided supraclavicular block.[97,98] The lower components of the brachial plexus have an intimate anatomical relationship with the pleura and lung at the level that ultrasound-guided supraclavicular block is commonly performed. This can be readily appreciated by examining the sagittal MRI image illustrated in Figure 16-6. Interscalene block approaches the brachial

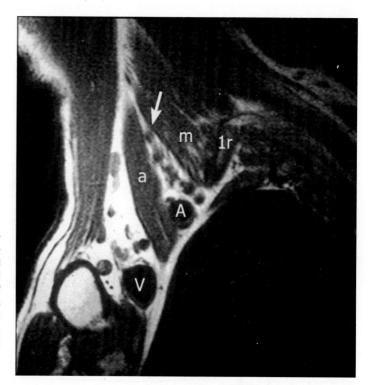

FIGURE 16-6. Sagittal magnetic resonance image of the brachial plexus nerve roots (indicated by *arrow*). The roots are surrounded by fat lying between the anterior (a) scalene and medial (m) scalene muscle. The first rib (1r) and subclavian artery (A) and vein (V) are labeled. The extremely close proximity to the apex of the lung to the lower brachial plexus should be appreciated. This intimate relationship underscores the need for extreme care when performing supraclavicular block and the necessity for maintaining a clear image of the needle tip throughout the procedure when using real-time ultrasonographic guidance. (Reproduced from Bowen et al. *Neuroimaging Clin N Am* 2004;14:59–85, with permission.)

plexus at a much higher point, at the level of the nerve roots. Winnie wrote that pneumothorax is "virtually impossible" as a result of interscalene block. In fact, if with the conventional approach, that is, the Winnie approach, interscalene block is performed correctly, with an appropriate needle (<4 cm), pneumothorax is impossible. If pneumothorax results from attempted interscalene block, it indicates that another approach (rather than an interscalene block) was made. However, when a catheter is advanced for continuous interscalene block, contact with the pleura is possible. In fact, reports of pneumothorax associated with interscalene catheters have been published.[99–101] The subclavian perivascular block and other approaches above the clavicle, including the plumb bob technique, were intended to help avoid pneumothorax. However, this complication is still a possibility with these approaches, including the intersternocleidomastoid approach. Franco and Vieira[102] published a series of 1,001 subclavian perivascular blocks using a nerve stimulator without encountering a pneumothorax. However, the patients were not systematically evaluated for pneumothorax.

The evolution of the infraclavicular block has been characterized by needle insertion sites more lateral to that of Raj's technique, an update of older techniques first published in 1973.[103] This has been followed by modifications of the technique by Sims[104] in 1977, Whiffler's[105] coracoid technique in 1981, and Grossi's[106] modification published in 2001. Each of these successive techniques diminished the possibility of pneumothorax. Pneumothorax following infraclavicular brachial plexus block has been reported when peripheral nerve stimulation was used to guide infraclavicular block.[107] The use of ultrasound guidance allows one to visualize the apex of the lung and may help to avoid this complication. By contrast to the commonly performed ultrasound-guided supraclavicular block, during infraclavicular block needle direction is sufficiently remote from the apex of the lung as

to make it nearly impossible to occur. The VIB has been shown to have a very real possibility of pneumothorax. The axillary approach completely avoids pneumothorax.

▶ SUMMARY

Of the commonly administered regional anesthetics, neuraxial blocks (such as spinal or epidural) or approaches to brachial plexus block above the clavicle have the most profound effects on respiration. The effects of neuraxial blockade are predicated by level-dependent blockade of abdominal and intercostal muscles. Increasing the level of abdominal/intercostal blockade causes a pattern of isolated diaphragmatic function. By contrast, cervical epidural anesthesia, interscalene block, and other supraclavicular approaches to brachial plexus block are associated with unilateral diaphragmatic paresis. Diaphragmatic paresis from brachial plexus block results in sizeable reductions in routine PFT, but the ability to cough effectively is largely preserved. Conversely, spinal or epidural anesthesia has minimal effects on PFT but significantly inhibits the ability to cough. More serious pulmonary complications associated with neuraxial block include respiratory arrest or failure from medullary effects associated with high levels of local anesthetic blockade or opiate action on the medulla (Chapter 19). Rare but serious complications from brachial plexus block are technique dependent and include pneumothorax and persistent phrenic nerve paresis. Visualization of the needle tip during ultrasound-guided supraclavicular block is critical to avoid pneumothorax. Attention to anatomy when performing interscalene block and more caudal approaches to the brachial plexus, along with the use of a nerve stimulator to detect diaphragmatic contractions, may help prevent persistent phrenic nerve injury. When performing regional anesthetic techniques, proper monitoring to diagnose effects on the respiratory system and the ability to immediately assist or control ventilation are mandatory.

References

1. Froese AB, Bryan AC. Effects of anesthesia and paralysis on diaphragmatic mechanics in man. *Anesthesiology* 1974;41:242–255.

2. Rehder K, Marsh H. Respiratory mechanics during anesthesia and mechanical ventilation. In: Fishman A, ed. *The Handbook of Physiology - Section 3: The Respiratory System*. Bethesda, MD: American Physiological Society, 1986:737–752.

3. Urmey W, Gloeggler P. Effects of bupivacaine 0.5% compared with mepivacaine 1.5% used for interscalene brachial plexus block (abstract). *Reg Anesth* 1992;17:13.

4. Gentili M, Lefoulon-Gourves M, Mamelle J, et al. Acute respiratory failure following interscalene block: complications of combined general and regional anesthesia (letter). *Reg Anesth* 1994;19:292–293.

5. Brown D, Cahill D, Bridenbaugh L. Supraclavicular nerve block: anatomic analysis of a method to prevent pneumothorax. *Anesth Analg* 1993;76:530–539.

6. Cook LB. Unsuspected extradural catheterization in an interscalene block. *Br J Anaesth* 1991;67:473–475.

7. Kumar A, Battit GE, Froese AB, et al. Bilateral cervical and thoracic epidural blockade complicating interscalene brachial plexus block: report of two cases. *Anesthesiology* 1971;35:650–652.

8. Ross S, Scarborough CD. Total spinal anesthesia following brachial-plexus block. *Anesthesiology* 1973;39:458.

9. Scammell SJ. Case report: inadvertent epidural anaesthesia as a complication of interscalene brachial plexus block. *Anaesth Intensive Care* 1979;7:56–57.

10. Mulroy MF. Monitoring opioids. *Reg Anesth* 1996;21:89–93.

11. Rawal N, Arner S, Gustafsson LL, et al. Present state of extradural and intrathecal opioid analgesia in Sweden. A nationwide follow-up survey. *Br J Anaesth* 1987;59:791–799.

12. de Leon-Casasola OA, Parker B, Lema MJ, et al. Postoperative epidural bupivacaine-morphine therapy. Experience with 4,227 surgical cancer patients. *Anesthesiology* 1994;81:368–375.

13. Scott DA, Beilby DS, McClymont C. Postoperative analgesia using epidural infusions of fentanyl with bupivacaine. A prospective analysis of 1,014 patients. *Anesthesiology* 1995;83:727–737.

14. Stenseth R, Sellevold O, Breivik H. Epidural morphine for postoperative pain: experience with 1085 patients. *Acta Anaesthesiol Scand* 1985;29:148–156.

15. Ready LB, Chadwick HS, Ross B. Age predicts effective epidural morphine dose after abdominal hysterectomy. *Anesth Analg* 1987;66:1215–1218.

16. Lubenow TR, Faber LP, McCarthy RJ, et al. Postthoracotomy pain management using continuous epidural analgesia in 1,324 patients. *Ann Thorac Surg* 1994;58:924–929; discussion 929–930.

17. Urmey W, Talts K, Sharrock N. One hundred percent incidence of hemidiaphragmatic paresis associated with interscalene brachial plexus anesthesia as diagnosed by ultrasonography. *Anesth Analg* 1991;72:498–503.

18. Urmey W, McDonald M. Changes in pulmonary function tests (PFT) during high-dose epidural anesthesia (abstract). *Anesthesiology* 1990;73:A1154.

19. Urmey W, McDonald M. Hemidiaphragmatic paresis during interscalene brachial plexus block: effects on pulmonary function and chest wall mechanics. *Anesth Analg* 1992;74:352–357.

20. Pere P, Pitkanen M, Rosenberg PH, et al. Effect of continuous interscalene brachial plexus block on diaphragm motion and on ventilatory function. *Acta Anaesthesiol Scand* 1992;36:53–57.

21. Casati A, Fanelli G, Cedrati V, et al. Pulmonary function changes after interscalene brachial plexus anesthesia with 0.5% and 0.75% ropivacaine: a double-blinded comparison with 2% mepivacaine. *Anesth Analg* 1999;88:587–592.

22. Knoblanche GE. The incidence and aetiology of phrenic nerve blockade associated with supraclavicular brachial plexus block. *Anaesth Intensive Care* 1979;7:346–349.

23. Neal JM, Moore JM, Kopacz DJ, et al. Quantitative analysis of respiratory, motor, and sensory function after supraclavicular block. *Anesth Analg* 1998;86:1239–1244.

24. Mak PH, Irwin MG, Ooi CG, et al. Incidence of diaphragmatic paralysis following supraclavicular brachial plexus block and its effect on pulmonary function. *Anaesthesia* 2001;56:352–356.

25. Dullenkopf A, Blumenthal S, Theodorou P, et al. Diaphragmatic excursion and respiratory function after the modified Raj technique of the infraclavicular plexus block. *Reg Anesth Pain Med* 2004;29:110–114.

26. Rodriguez J, Barcena M, Rodriguez V, et al. Infraclavicular brachial plexus block effects on respiratory function and extent of the block. *Reg Anesth Pain Med* 1998;23:564–568.

27. Rettig HC, Gielen MJ, Boersma E, et al. Vertical infraclavicular block of the brachial plexus: effects on hemidiaphragmatic movement and ventilatory function. *Reg Anesth Pain Med* 2005;30:529–535.

28. Pham-Dang C, Gunst JP, Gouin F, et al. A novel supraclavicular approach to brachial plexus block. *Anesth Analg* 1997;85:111–116.

29. Shanti CM, Carlin AM, Tyburski JG. Incidence of pneumothorax from intercostal nerve block for analgesia in rib fractures. *J Trauma* 2001;51:536–539.

30. Bartlett R. Bilateral intercostal nerve block for upper abdominal surgery. *Surg Gynecol Obstet* 1940;71:194–197.

31. Moore DC. Intercostal nerve block for postoperative somatic pain following surgery of thorax and upper abdomen. *Br J Anaesth* 1975;47 suppl:284–286.

32. McCleery R, Zollinger R, Lenahan N. A clinical study of the effect of intercostal nerve block with Nupercaine in oil following upper abdominal surgery. *Surg Gynecol Obstet* 1948;86:680–686.

33. Lonnqvist PA, MacKenzie J, Soni AK, et al. Paravertebral blockade. Failure rate and complications. *Anaesthesia* 1995;50:813–815.

34. Stromskag KE, Minor B, Steen PA. Side effects and complications related to interpleural analgesia: an update. *Acta Anaesthesiol Scand* 1990;34:473–477.

35. Robaux S, Bouaziz H, Boisseau N, et al. Persistent phrenic nerve paralysis following interscalene brachial plexus block. *Anesthesiology* 2001;95:1519–1521.

36. Bashein G, Robertson HT, Kennedy WF Jr. Persistent phrenic nerve paresis following interscalene brachial plexus block. *Anesthesiology* 1985;63:102–104.

37. Ediale KR, Myung CR, Neuman GG. Prolonged hemidiaphragmatic paralysis following interscalene brachial plexus block. *J Clin Anesth* 2004;16:573–575.

38. Winnie AP. Interscalene brachial plexus block. *Anesth Analg* 1970;49:455–466.

39. De Troyer A, Kelly S. Chest wall mechanics in dogs with acute diaphragm paralysis. *J Appl Physiol* 1982;53:373–379.

40. De Troyer A, Kelly S, Zin WA. Mechanical action of the intercostal muscles on the ribs. *Science* 1983;220:87–88.

41. De Troyer A, Sampson M, Sigrist S, et al. How the abdominal muscles act on the rib cage. *J Appl Physiol* 1983;54:465–469.

42. Konno K, Mead J. Measurement of the separate volume changes of rib cage and abdomen during breathing. *J Appl Physiol* 1967;22:407–422.

43. Goldman MD, Mead J. Mechanical interaction between the diaphragm and rib cage. *J Appl Physiol* 1973;35:197–204.

44. Estenne M, De Troyer A. Relationship between respiratory muscle electromyogram and rib cage motion in tetraplegia. *Am Rev Respir Dis* 1985;132:53–59.

45. De Troyer A, Heilporn A. Respiratory mechanics in quadriplegia. The respiratory function of the intercostal muscles. *Am Rev Respir Dis* 1980;122:591–600.

46. Urmey W, Loring S, Mead J, et al. Upper and lower rib cage deformation during breathing in quadriplegics. *J Appl Physiol* 1986;60:618–622.

47. Kowalski SE, Bradley BD, Greengrass RA, et al. Effects of inter-pleural bupivacaine (0.5%) on canine diaphragmatic function. *Anesth Analg* 1992;75:400–404.

48. De Troyer A, Estenne M. Coordination between rib cage muscles and diaphragm during quiet breathing in humans. *J Appl Physiol* 1984;57:899–906.

49. Greene N. *Physiology of Spinal Anesthesia, Pulmonary Ventilation and Hemodynamics*. Baltimore, MD: Williams & Wilkins, 1981.

50. Sundberg A, Wattwil M, Arvill A. Respiratory effects of high thoracic epidural anaesthesia. *Acta Anaesthesiol Scand* 1986;30:215–217.

51. Takasaki M, Takahashi T. Respiratory function during cervical and thoracic extradural analgesia in patients with normal lungs. *Br J Anaesth* 1980;52:1271–1276.

52. Groeben H, Schafer B, Pavlakovic G, et al. Lung function under high thoracic segmental epidural anesthesia with ropivacaine or bupivacaine in patients with severe obstructive pulmonary disease undergoing breast surgery. *Anesthesiology* 2002;96:536–541.

53. Manikian B, Cantineau JP, Bertrand M, et al. Improvement of diaphragmatic function by a thoracic extradural block after upper abdominal surgery. *Anesthesiology* 1988;68:379–386.

54. Warner DO, Warner MA, Ritman EL. Human chest wall function during epidural anesthesia. *Anesthesiology* 1996;85:761–773.

55. Yamakage M, Kamada Y, Toriyabe M, et al. Changes in respiratory pattern and arterial blood gases during sedation with propofol or midazolam in spinal anesthesia. *J Clin Anesth* 1999;11:375–379.

56. Tenling A, Joachimsson PO, Tyden H, et al. Thoracic epidural analgesia as an adjunct to general anaesthesia for cardiac surgery. Effects on pulmonary mechanics. *Acta Anaesthesiol Scand* 2000;44:1071–1076.

57. Capdevila X, Biboulet P, Rubenovitch J, et al. The effects of cervical epidural anesthesia with bupivacaine on pulmonary function in conscious patients. *Anesth Analg* 1998;86:1033–1038.

58. Michalek P, David I, Adamec M, et al. Cervical epidural anesthesia for combined neck and upper extremity procedure: a pilot study. *Anesth Analg* 2004;99:1833–1836, table of contents.

59. Bonnet F, Derosier JP, Pluskwa F, et al. Cervical epidural anaesthesia for carotid artery surgery. *Can J Anaesth* 1990;37:353–358.

60. Eisele J, Trenchard D, Burki N, et al. The effect of chest wall block on respiratory sensation and control in man. *Clin Sci* 1968;35:23–33.

61. Mead J. Functional significance of the area of apposition of diaphragm to rib cage [proceedings]. *Am Rev Respir Dis* 1979;119:31–32.

62. Urmey WF, De Troyer A, Kelly KB, et al. Pleural pressure increases during inspiration in the zone of apposition of diaphragm to rib cage. *J Appl Physiol* 1988;65:2207–2212.

63. Pascucci RC, Hershenson MB, Sethna NF, et al. Chest wall motion of infants during spinal anesthesia. *J Appl Physiol* 1990;68:2087–2091.

64. Urmey W, Lambert D, Concepcion M. Routine spinal or epidural anesthesia causes rib cage distortion during spontaneous inspiration (abstract). *Anesthesiology* 1987;67:A538.

65. Mineo R, Sharrock N, Castellano P, et al. Effect of adding epinephrine to epidural bupivacaine assessed by thoraco-abdominal muscle strength (abstract). *Reg Anesth* 1990;15:70.

66. Egbert LD, Tamersoy K, Deas TC. Pulmonary function during spinal anesthesia: the mechanism of cough depression. *Anesthesiology* 1961;22:882–885.

67. Steinbrook RA. Respiratory effects of spinal anesthesia. *Int Anesthesiol Clin* 1989;27:40–45.

68. Steinbrook RA, Topulos GP, Concepcion M. Ventilatory responses to hypercapnia during tetracaine spinal anesthesia. *J Clin Anesth* 1988;1:75–80.

69. Hedenstierna G, Lofstrom J. Effect of anaesthesia on respiratory function after major lower extremity surgery. A comparison between bupivacaine spinal analgesia with low-dose morphine and general anaesthesia. *Acta Anaesthesiol Scand* 1985;29:55–60.

70. Cornish PB. Respiratory arrest after spinal anesthesia with lidocaine and fentanyl. *Anesth Analg* 1997;84:1387–1388.

71. Ferouz F, Norris MC, Leighton BL. Risk of respiratory arrest after intrathecal sufentanil. *Anesth Analg* 1997;85:1088–1090.

72. Liu SS, Neal JM, Pollock JE, et al. Respiratory depression with addition of fentanyl to spinal anesthesia. *Anesth Analg* 1997;85:1416–1417.

73. Lu JK, Schafer PG, Gardner TL, et al. The dose-response pharmacology of intrathecal sufentanil in female volunteers. *Anesth Analg* 1997;85:372–379.

74. Ostermeier AM, Roizen MF, Hautkappe M, et al. Three sudden postoperative respiratory arrests associated with epidural opioids in patients with sleep apnea. *Anesth Analg* 1997;85:452–460.

75. Bailey PL, Rhondeau S, Schafer PG, et al. Dose-response pharmacology of intrathecal morphine in human volunteers. *Anesthesiology* 1993;79:49–59; discussion 25A.

76. Shaw W. Paralysis of the phrenic nerve during brachial plexus anesthesia. *Anesthesiology* 1949;10:627–628.

77. Winnie AP, Radonjic R, Akkinemi S, et al. Factors influencing the distribution of local anesthetics in the brachial plexus sheath. *Anesth Analg* 1979;58:225–234.

78. Urmey W, Gloeggler P. Pulmonary function changes during inter-scalene block: effects of decreasing local anesthetic injection volume. *Reg Anesth* 1993;18:244–249.

79. Urmey W, Grossi P, Sharrock N, et al. Digital pressure during interscalene block is clinically ineffective in preventing anesthetic spread to the cervical plexus. *Anesth Analg* 1996;83:366–370.

80. Sala-Blanch X, Lazaro JR, Correa J, et al. Phrenic nerve block caused by interscalene brachial plexus block: effects of digital pressure and a low volume of local anesthetic. *Reg Anesth Pain Med* 1999;24:231–235.

81. Pere P. The effect of continuous interscalene brachial plexus block with 0.125% bupivacaine plus fentanyl on diaphragmatic motility and ventilatory function. *Reg Anesth* 1993;18:93–97.

82. Fackler CD, Perret GE, Bedell GN. Effect of unilateral phrenic nerve section on lung function. *J Appl Physiol* 1967;23:923–926.

83. Arborelius Jr M, Lilja B, Senyk J. Regional and total lung function studies in patients with hemidiaphragmatic paralysis. *Respiration* 1975;32:253–264.

84. Gould L, Kaplan S, McElhinney AJ, et al. A method for the production of hemidiaphragmatic paralysis. Its application to the study of lung function in normal man. *Am Rev Respir Dis* 1967;96:812–814.

85. Erickson JM, Louis DS, Naughton NN. Symptomatic phrenic nerve palsy after supraclavicular block in an obese man. *Orthopedics* 2009;32:368.

86. Kreitzer SM, Feldman NT, Saunders NA, et al. Bilateral diaphragmatic paralysis with hypercapnic respiratory failure. A physiologic assessment. *Am J Med* 1978;65:89–95.

87. Hickey R, Ramamurthy S. The diagnosis of phrenic nerve block on chest x-ray by a double-exposure technique. *Anesthesiology* 1989;70:704–707.

88. al-Kaisy AA, Chan VW, Perlas A. Respiratory effects of low-dose bupivacaine interscalene block. *Br J Anaesth* 1999;82:217–220.

89. Borgeat A, Perschak H, Bird P, et al. Patient-controlled interscalene analgesia with ropivacaine 0.2% versus patient-controlled intravenous analgesia after major shoulder surgery: effects on diaphragmatic and respiratory function. *Anesthesiology* 2000;92:102–108.

90. Sardesai AM, Chakrabarti AJ, Denny NM. Lower lobe collapse during continuous interscalene brachial plexus local anesthesia at home. *Reg Anesth Pain Med* 2004;29:65–68.

91. Renes SH, Spoormans HH, Gielen MJ, et al. Hemidiaphragmatic paresis can be avoided in ultrasound-guided supraclavicular brachial plexus block. *Reg Anesth Pain Med* 2009;34:595–599.

92. Renes SH, Rettig HC, Gielen MJ, et al. Ultrasound-guided low-dose interscalene brachial plexus block reduces the incidence of hemidiaphragmatic paresis. *Reg Anesth Pain Med* 2009;34:498–502.

93. Renes SH, van Geffen GJ, Rettig HC, et al. Minimum effective volume of local anesthetic for shoulder analgesia by ultrasound-guided block at root C7 with assessment of pulmonary function. *Reg Anesth Pain Med* 2010;35:529–534.

94. Gentili ME, Deleuze A, Estebe JP, et al. Severe respiratory failure after infraclavicular block with 0.75% ropivacaine: a case report. *J Clin Anesth* 2002;14:459–461.

95. Stadlmeyer W, Neubauer J, Finkl RO, et al. Unilateral phrenic nerve paralysis after vertical infraclavicular plexus block. *Anaesthesist* 2000;49:1030–1033.

96. Winnie AP. *Plexus Anesthesia, Perivascular Techniques of Brachial Plexus Block.* Philadelphia, PA: WB Saunders, 1990.

97. Bhatia A, Lai J, Chan VW, et al. Case report: pneumothorax as a complication of the ultrasound-guided supraclavicular approach for brachial plexus block. *Anesth Analg* 2010;111:817–819.

98. Le V, Moore R, Wang D. Pneumothorax after an ultrasound-guided supraclavicular block (abstract). *Reg Anesth Pain Med* 2010;35:S165.

99. Borgeat A, Ekatodramis G, Kalberer F, et al. Acute and nonacute complications associated with interscalene block and shoulder surgery: a prospective study. *Anesthesiology* 2001;95:875–880.

100. Bryan NA, Swenson JD, Greis PE, et al. Indwelling interscalene catheter use in an outpatient setting for shoulder surgery: technique, efficacy, and complications. *J Shoulder Elbow Surg* 2007;16:388–395.

101. Jenkins CR, Karmakar MK. An unusual complication of interscalene brachial plexus catheterization: delayed catheter migration. *Br J Anaesth* 2005;95:535–537.

102. Franco C, Vieira Z. 1,001 subclavian perivascular brachial plexus blocks. Success with a nerve stimulator. *Reg Anesth Pain Med* 2000;25:41–46.

103. Raj PP, Montgomery SJ, Nettles D, et al. Infraclavicular brachial plexus block—a new approach. *Anesth Analg* 1973;52:897–904.

104. Sims JK. A modification of landmarks for infraclavicular approach to brachial plexus block. *Anesth Analg* 1977;56:554–555.

105. Whiffler K. Coracoid block–a safe and easy technique. *Br J Anaesth* 1981;53:845–848.

106. Grossi P. Brachial plexus block. The anesthetic line is a guide for new approaches. *Minerva Anestesiol* 2001;67:45–49.

107. Sanchez HB, Mariano ER, Abrams R, et al. Pneumothorax following infraclavicular brachial plexus block for hand surgery. *Orthopedics* 2008;31:709.

17

The Role of Nerve Localization Techniques in Safety

Joseph M. Neal

Ultrasound-guided regional anesthesia (UGRA) is a major technological advance in the subspecialty, not unlike the advent of peripheral nerve stimulation (PNS) nearly four decades ago. These technologies, along with the traditional but decidedly less technical paresthesia-seeking method, are at their core techniques for accurately localizing neural structures prior to injection of local anesthetic or other drugs. With each new nerve localization tool comes the understandable hope that peripheral nerve blocks will become not only more efficient, but also safer.

This chapter seeks to examine the contribution of nerve localization tools to patient safety by considering their effect on five major complications of regional anesthesia—postoperative neurologic symptoms (PONS), local anesthetic systemic toxicity (LAST), hemidiaphragmatic paresis (HDP), pneumothorax, and perineuraxial injury[1] (Table 17-1). The chapter also considers the effects of nerve localization techniques on certain minor side effects, such as unintended anesthesia of the recurrent laryngeal nerve

or cervicothoracic sympathetic trunk. The focus will be on two contemporary nerve localization techniques—PNS and UGRA. Data for paresthesia-seeking techniques will be considered when applicable, recognizing that comparative complication data for this modality are limited.[2] There are also insufficient data to comment on the safety effects of nerve localization choice for neuraxial[3] and truncal blocks.[4] Similarly, ultrasound versus other forms of imaging for interventional pain medicine will not be discussed because of insufficient comparative literature.[5]

▶ DEFINITION

This chapter defines permanent nerve injury as a neural deficit that remains 1 year after block placement, a definition that is generally agreed upon by neurologists. Injuries <1 year in duration are referred to as PONS, which describes early and delayed neural symptoms that usually

TABLE 17-1 Strength of Evidence—the Effect of Ultrasound Guidance on Patient Safety

Peripheral Nerve Injury (III)

- Proving statistical differences in nerve injury as a function of nerve localization technique is likely futile
- Underpowered results from randomized clinical trials (RCTs) and large case series find no difference in surrogate markers of nerve injury, such as paresthesia during or immediately after block placement, or temporary postoperative neurologic symptoms
- Ultrasound-guided regional anesthesia (UGRA) appears to be associated with a frequency of perioperative nerve injury similar to historical reports of nerve injury after peripheral nerve stimulation (PNS)

Local Anesthetic Systemic Toxicity (Ia and III)

- Compared to PNS, UGRA lowers the risk of unintended vascular puncture, a surrogate outcome for local anesthetic systemic toxicity (*Ia*)
- The weight of conflicting evidence is that UGRA does not affect the incidence of local anesthetic-induced seizures (*III*)

Hemidiaphragmatic Paresis (Ia and IV)

- RCTs confirm the ability of low-volume UGRA to reduce (but not eliminate) the incidence and severity of hemidiaphragmatic paresis (HDP) using the interscalene approach. The incidence of HDP is nearly 0% using the supraclavicular approach with ultrasound guidance (*Ia*)
- No RCTs or case reports address whether or not patients at risk of pulmonary compromise can undergo above the clavicle regional anesthetic block. Because HDP can still occur unpredictably, caution remains warranted in any patient unable to withstand a 25%–30% diminution of pulmonary function (*IV*)

Pneumothorax (III)

- No adequately powered studies directly address the risk of pneumothorax with UGRA
- Pneumothorax has occurred despite the use of UGRA (*III*)

Unintended Destinations of Local Anesthetic (IV)

- For upper extremity block, no studies report the effect of ultrasound guidance on perineuraxial spread of local anesthetic. Few studies report the incidence of unintended anesthesia of the recurrent laryngeal nerve or the cervicothoracic sympathetic trunk
- Although lower local anesthetic volumes facilitated by ultrasound use may reduce these effects, there are no supporting data to confirm or refute this theory (*IV*)

Levels of evidence: Ia, evidence from meta-analysis; III, evidence from well-designed, nonexperimental descriptive studies such as comparative studies or case reports; IV, expert opinion.
Table modified from Neal JM. Ultrasound-guided regional anesthesia and patient safety: an evidence-based analysis. *Reg Anesth Pain Med* 2010;35:S59–S67, with permission from the American Society of Regional Anesthesia and Pain Medicine.

are transient. Although early after nerve injury PONS can serve as a surrogate marker for permanent nerve injury, the rate of conversion from PONS to permanent injury is unknown. LAST refers to any central nervous system (CNS) or cardiac manifestation of local anesthetic toxicity, but this chapter focuses only on the most serious complications—seizure and/or cardiac arrest.

▶ POSTOPERATIVE NEUROLOGICAL SYMPTOMS

Scope

The incidence of regional anesthesia-associated peripheral nerve injury is difficult to define and is significantly influenced by the time elapsed since block placement. Because permanent block-related injury is extremely rare, most studies report surrogate PONS metrics, for example, persistent

paresthesia or transient sensory and/or motor dysfunction. In the first 24 hours after peripheral nerve block, PONS may be present in up to 19% of patients. Over the ensuing weeks and months, these symptoms typically resolve, with well over 99% no longer present at 1 year.[2,6] The large French surveillance studies of the late 1990s/early 2000s reported that neurologic injury was still present at 6 months in 1.4[7] to 1.9[8] per 10,000 patients (95% confidence interval [95% CI] 0.5–4.8/10,000).[8] Data are much less robust for defining the incidence of permanent injury. In a review of neurologic complications published between 1995 and 2005, only one permanent injury was reported in 65,092 blocks.[9]

Pathophysiology

The pathophysiology of peripheral nerve injury is discussed in detail in Chapter 14. Recent research has vastly expanded and indeed changed our understanding of needle-to-nerve proximity and the postulated mechanisms of injury. This section aims to review the pathophysiology of peripheral nerve injury as it relates specifically to nerve localization technique.

The generally accepted mechanism of regional anesthesia-associated peripheral nerve injury posits the concept that needle damage to a nerve's structural integrity mechanically injures the nerve and/or disrupts the nerve-blood barrier, which in turn allows local anesthetic to contact denuded fascicles and result in neurotoxicity. Prior to ultrasound's contributions as a powerful research tool for studying nerve injury, most experts presumed that any needle breach of the nerve's structural integrity was capable of causing injury.[10] Despite previous animal studies that clearly demonstrate the perineurium is the most important physical barrier between local anesthetic and nerve axons, much clinical literature fails to differentiate between a needle that penetrates only the epineurium versus one that disrupts the perineurium, thereby gaining access to the nerve fascicles. In these descriptions, needle penetration into a nerve is referred to generically as "intraneural injection" without regard to what component of the nerve's architecture is breached. With the advent of ultrasound, two observations quickly became apparent. First, PNS- and paresthesia-seeking needles penetrate the epineurium and come to lie within the nerve's connective tissue much more frequently than clinicians had suspected previously.[11] Second, this breach is rarely associated with injury. In animal experiments, histologic and functional injury

occurs only when the needle is intentionally (and often with great difficulty) placed within the perineurium to disrupt the fascicular architecture. In summary, peripheral nerve injury theory presumes that needle disruption of the nerve's intraperineurial architecture is a prelude to at least some forms of neural injury. If this is indeed the case, then nerve localization techniques that avoid potentially harmful needle-to-perineurium contact should reduce the risk of nerve injury.

Within this framework of nerve injury pathophysiology, we can now examine the theoretical contributions of the various nerve localization techniques. Ultrasound-assisted animal and human studies have improved our understanding of PNS-guided needle-to-nerve contact. These studies consistently report that stimulating needles can be extraneural or subepineurial at a wide range of stimulating currents. For instance, an axillary block study reported that paresthesia was only 38% sensitive, and motor response 75% sensitive (≤0.5 mA), for confirming (using ultrasound visualization) needle-to-nerve contact.[12] A similar 83% motor block sensitivity (0.2–0.5 mA) was reported for popliteal sciatic nerve block.[13] For the supraclavicular approach, a human study documented subepineurial placement of a block needle when the stimulating current was ≤0.2 mA, but could not distinguish extraneural from intraneural needle placement between >0.2 and ≤0.5 mA.[14] Animal studies confirm this absence of consistency between electrical current and actual needle position,[15] suggesting that PNS is a fallible descriptor of needle-to-nerve relationship (Fig. 17-1). For ultrasound-guided

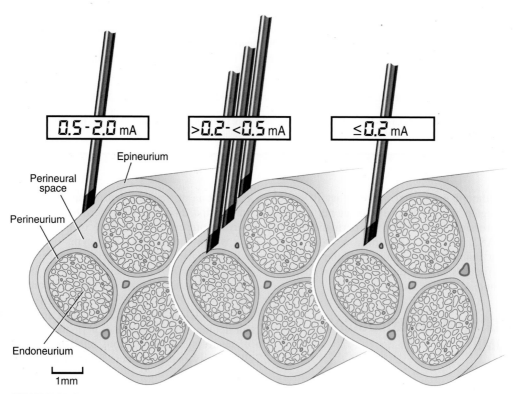

FIGURE 17-1. PNS has limited sensitivity for accurately indicating needle placement within a nerve. At ≤0.2 mA, the needle is reliably intraneural, that is, subepineurial, but may be inside or outside the perineurium. Between 0.2 and ≥0.5 mA, the needle could reside at any location within the nerve or be completely extraneural. Figure created using human supraclavicular nerve block data as reported by Bigeleisen et al.[14] and human popliteal sciatic nerve block data as reported by Robards et al.[13] (Modified with permission from *Anesthesiology* and *Anesthesia and Analgesia*.)

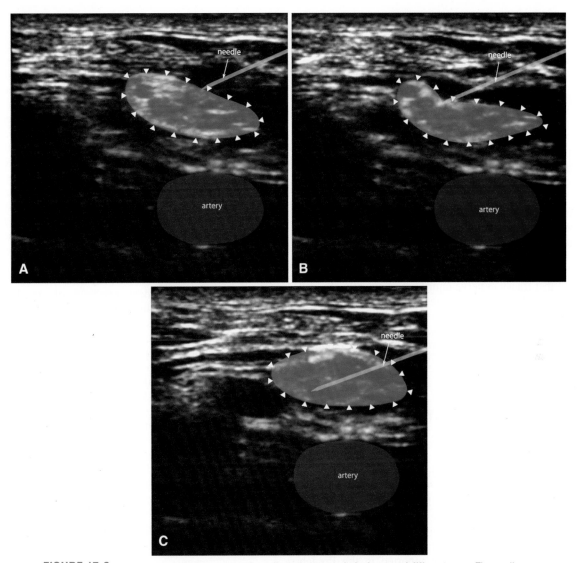

FIGURE 17-2. **Ultrasound guidance can reveal needle-to-nerve proximity in several different ways.** The needle can be seen to indent the nerve (B) or actually penetrate the nerve (C). If the needle is intraneural, the nerve can be observed to swell during injection of local anesthetic. Figure created using human supraclavicular nerve block sonograms as reported by Bigeleisen et al.[14] (Modified with permission from *Anesthesiology.*)

localization techniques, studies show that needle tips can be observed to touch and indent nerves[14] or herald subepineurial placement by observing nerve swelling upon injection of local anesthetic[14–18] (Fig. 17-2). However, nerve swelling has not been correlated with actual nerve injury,[18] suggesting that ultrasound may more accurately depict needle-to-nerve contact as compared with PNS, but that the relationship of needle contact to actual injury remains unknown. Therefore, neither PNS nor UGRA is entirely sensitive or a specific tool for determining needle-to-nerve contact in a manner that predictably recognizes or prevents peripheral nerve injury.

Effect of Nerve Localization Technique

Although studies regarding PONS as a function of nerve localization technique are limited, several suggest that there is no difference in the incidence of significant injury. A study that compared paresthesia-seeking and PNS techniques for interscalene block found no difference in the incidence of

paresthesia (9.3% vs. 10.1%, respectively).[19] A study that compared PNS to UGRA for interscalene block found no difference in PONS at 4- to 6-week follow-up (7% vs. 6%, respectively).[20] In the Australasian Regional Anaesthesia Collaboration study of over 7,000 nerve blocks,[21] the incidence of transient (up to 60 days follow-up) PONS was not statistically different between those patients who underwent regional anesthesia using either PNS or UGRA localization techniques. Although historical comparisons are problematic, it is interesting that the frequency of early and late PONS (4/10,000) is nearly identical to the frequency of nerve injury reported a decade earlier from the French surveillance study, in which nearly all patients underwent PNS-directed block.[7,8,22] A slightly smaller quality assurance study[23] also found no statistical difference in the incidence of early neurologic symptoms between PNS and UGRA. That UGRA is not completely protective against transient or permanent peripheral nerve injury has been demonstrated by several case reports of injuries despite its use.[24–26]

In summary, it is unlikely that an adequately powered study to differentiate the effect of nerve localization procedure on late postoperative symptoms, much less permanent injury, will ever be completed[27] (Box 17-1). The few studies that use the surrogate PONS markers lend no convincing argument that transient nerve injury is significantly affected by localization technique. To date, there are no studies that focus on those patients most at risk for peripheral nerve injury, such as those with diabetes or chemotherapy-induced neuropathy. These groups may prove to be a better model to study the relative safety effects of various nerve localization techniques.

► LOCAL ANESTHETIC SYSTEMIC TOXICITY

Scope

Similar to nerve injury, the incidence of LAST largely depends on how it is defined. Early markers of local anesthetic vascular uptake, such as CNS excitation and hemodynamic changes, may occur as frequently as 1/1,000 patients.[28] However, life-threatening toxicity from seizures or cardiac arrest is exceedingly rare.[29] The rate of peripheral nerve block-related seizure reported in the French surveillance studies was 7.5/10,000 patients (95% CI, 3.9–11.2/10,000), and no patient in 21,278 blocks experienced a LAST-associated cardiac arrest.[8] Unintentional vascular puncture, as diagnosed by aspiration, hematoma formation, or direct observation with ultrasound, is a surrogate marker for LAST. While vascular puncture is clearly a precursor to more serious complications, there are no data to accurately define how often it is linked to clinically apparent LAST.

Pathophysiology

The pathophysiology of LAST relates to nerve localization technique in one of two ways. First, immediate LAST implies inadequate detection of intravascular injection, which the localization technique should identify ideally prior to injecting significant amounts of local anesthetic. There are no universally recognized signs of blood vessel entry when using PNS. Conversely, UGRA offers the possibility of either avoiding vascular puncture or halting further injection if local anesthetic cannot be observed surrounding the target tissue. Second, UGRA enables the use of smaller volumes, which might temper toxicity by limiting the availability of local anesthetic for tissue uptake.

Effect of Nerve Localization Technique

Evidence that nerve localization technique influences the occurrence of LAST is equivocal. Individual studies and a meta-analysis[30] provide strong evidence that the use of ultrasound significantly reduces the incidence of unintentional vascular puncture as compared with PNS techniques. However, it is less clear whether this surrogate outcome equates to a reduction in the true outcomes of seizure and/or cardiac arrest. The Australasian Collaboration found no difference in the incidence of serious LAST events between UGRA and PNS techniques.[21] In this study, the 0.98/1,000 incidence of LAST is remarkably similar to the 0.8/1,000 incidence previously reported for PNS.[7] The Pittsburgh quality assurance study showed a statistically significant advantage ($p = 0.044$) to UGRA over PNS with regard to the incidence of seizure, but the absence of an epinephrine test dose could have influenced the incidence of LAST in either group.[23]

Ultrasound guidance consistently achieves comparable anesthesia using smaller local anesthetic volumes. For adult doses, this reduction in volume is statistically significant, but may still be capable of causing a serious episode of LAST. For instance, ultrasound facilitates the reduction of mean volume from 26 mL using PNS to 15 mL (95% CI, 7–23) during femoral nerve block,[31] yet even 15 mL of a potent local anesthetic could be problematic if injected intravascularly, particularly in patients at increased risk for LAST, for example, cardiac disease or extremes of age.[32] The ability to anesthetize a target nerve using less local anesthetic may be most useful in pediatrics, where their smaller size places children at increased risk for LAST.[32] No studies have directly evaluated LAST in pediatric patients, although as with adults, the risk of unintentional vascular puncture is reduced by the use of ultrasound.[33] Importantly, UGRA has been linked to faster absorption and higher plasma concentrations of local anesthetic in children, which suggests that using the lowest volume possible in these populations is not just advantageous, but warranted.[34]

► HEMIDIAPHRAGMATIC PARESIS

Scope

When PNS techniques are used for interscalene blocks, the incidence of HDP approaches 100%.[35] When local anesthetic is deposited distally along the brachial plexus, the incidence of HDP drops to approximately 50% at the supraclavicular approach[36] and nears 0% with the most lateral infraclavicular approaches.[2] The incidence of HDP is significantly less with UGRA techniques—13% to 45% for the interscalene approach[37,38] and 95% CI 0% to 14% for the supraclavicular approach.[39]

Pathophysiology

With PNS techniques, local anesthetic conduction block of the phrenic nerve can occur directly as it courses atop the anterior scalene muscle, or from the spread to the C3-C5 nerve roots within the prevertebral fascial compartment.[35,40] Both of these mechanisms imply a volume effect, particularly as the local anesthetic is placed distal along the brachial plexus, that is, more distant from the affected nerve roots. Conversely, ultrasound-guided approaches allow for brachial plexus anesthesia with smaller volumes of local anesthetic. Although this likely limits local anesthetic spread within the prevertebral fascial plane, the phrenic nerve nevertheless lies within 2 mm of the C5 nerve root at the level where a block needle is typically directed during an ultrasound-assisted interscalene approach.[41]

Effect of Nerve Localization Technique

The incidence of HDP is clearly reduced by using UGRA instead of PNS. This finding is likely volume related. In studies of interscalene[37,38] and supraclavicular[39] brachial plexus blocks, the incidence and severity of HDP is reduced when UGRA is utilized. Some investigators have reported reducing the incidence of HDP associated with the interscalene approach to 45% using 5 mL ropivacaine 0.5% (C5-C6 level)[38] or 13% using 10 mL ropivacaine 0.75% (C7 level),[37] while other investigators have reported no change in incidence using 10 or 20 mL ropivacaine 0.5% at the cricoid level.[42] For the supraclavicular approach, the diaphragm is even less affected and HDP has been reported as 0%, 95% CI 0% to 14% using 20 mL ropivacaine 0.75%,[39] or 1%, 95% CI 0.4% to 2.3% using 33 ± 8 mL.[43] Despite these impressive results, the practical significance of the reduced incidence of HDP is questionable, since it is never completely eliminated at the interscalene approach. Since HDP is neither completely eliminated nor is it possible to predict individual patient response, we cannot know with certainty when it is safe to administer a low-volume interscalene block to those individuals most at risk for significant HDP, that is, a patient unable to withstand a 30% reduction in pulmonary function.[27]

▶ PNEUMOTHORAX

Scope

The precise incidence of pneumothorax is unknown, but is certainly well less than the 0.5% to 6% reported decades ago using the classic approaches to the supraclavicular portion of the brachial plexus.[2] Based on projections from recent studies of ultrasound-guided supraclavicular block, the upper limit 95% CI for pneumothorax is 0.5%.[27]

Effect of Nerve Localization Technique

Patients who undergo above the clavicle and medial infraclavicular approaches to the brachial plexus are at risk for pneumothorax from a needle penetrating the pleura. Although the pleura is easily identifiable using ultrasound, case reports have nevertheless documented pneumothoraces during supraclavicular[44] and infraclavicular[45] blocks. There are no direct comparisons of UGRA to PNS for this complication.

▶ UNINTENDED DESTINATIONS OF LOCAL ANESTHETICS

Scope

Local anesthetic may be deposited within or spread to the neuraxis during interscalene block. This event is so rare as

to defy accurate incidence reporting. Other unintended destinations of local anesthetic are better defined. Involvement of the recurrent laryngeal nerve occurs in 1.3% of supraclavicular and 10% of cervical paravertebral blocks using traditional PNS techniques. Anesthesia of the cervicothoracic sympathetic trunk, which manifests as Horner's syndrome, occurs in 20% to 90% of supraclavicular and 40% of cervical paravertebral blocks using traditional high-volume, PNS-directed techniques.[2]

Pathophysiology

Neuraxial anesthesia after placement of an interscalene block is caused by either overly deep placement of a medially directed block needle (toward the spinal cord or its meningeal coverings) or by local anesthetic deposition into a long dural root sleeve (Fig. 18-1). Medially directed PNS- or paresthesia-guided needles are described using the Winnie[46] technique. Conversely, the modified lateral technique of Borgeat[47] relies on a presumably safer superficial needle approach (Chapter 18). Ultrasound-guided interscalene blocks also use a superficial lateral-to-medial needle approach that should theoretically avoid proximity with the neuraxis and all but the longest dural root sleeves.

Hoarseness is directly related to the proximity of the recurrent laryngeal and vagus nerves to the neural components of the brachial plexus. Similarly, the proximity of the cervicothoracic sympathetic trunk to the C8 and T1 nerve roots explains the occurrence of Horner's syndrome. Although it is reasonable to postulate that these unintended effects of local anesthetic may in part relate to the injected volume, there is no evidence that the 20 to 40 mL volumes used with conventional PNS approaches differentially affect the incidence of recurrent laryngeal or cervicothoracic trunk anesthesia.[2] Theoretically, the smaller volumes used with UGRA techniques may reduce the incidence of these nuisance side effects. However, this may not be the case if the effect is related less to the volume and more to the spread along tissue planes.

The Effect of Nerve Localization Technique

With regard to local anesthetic spread to the recurrent laryngeal nerve or the cervicothoracic sympathetic trunk, there are no direct comparisons of these side effects as a function of nerve localization technique. Ultrasound studies that report these side effects suggest that the incidence may be lower than that observed with PNS techniques, most likely secondary to smaller injected volumes of local anesthetic.

▶ PREVENTION

Of the previously discussed regional anesthesia complications, it appears that only the incidence of HDP can be reduced considerably by the use of UGRA compared with PNS. Even then, ultrasound does not completely prevent the complication. Therefore, there is no compelling evidence that one's choice of nerve localization technique can reliably prevent peripheral nerve injury, LAST, HDP, pneumothorax, or complications arising from unintended spread of local anesthetic.

One aspect of prevention is avoiding overconfidence in a technique's ability to confer an advantage that has yet to be proven. In this paragraph, the author offers his opinion regarding a proposed advantage of UGRA—specifically, intentional intraneural injection (presumably, subepineurial but extraperineurial) for the purpose of improving qualities of neural blockade such as onset and duration. Unintentional intraneural injection at one institution occurred in 17% (95% CI 12%–22%) of patients undergoing ultrasound-guided interscalene and supraclavicular block.[48] Clinical observations in a small number of patients have documented intraneural injection without evidence of subsequent injury,[13,14,17,48,49] which has led some respected investigators to suggest that intentional intraneural injection may be advantageous.[50,51] I and others[24,52,53] have challenged this suggestion based on two main arguments: (i) the incidence of peripheral nerve injury is so small as to prohibit conclusions based on a very small number of published reports of apparently harmless intraneural injections and (ii) the spatial resolution of contemporary ultrasound machines is insufficient to distinguish intra- versus extrafascicular needle placement.[54] It is thus my opinion that the unknown and probably limited benefits of intentional subepineurial injection are likely less than its unknown but potentially serious risks.[52]

▶ SUMMARY

There is no compelling evidence that nerve localization technique, particularly UGRA or PNS, significantly affects the incidence of major complications such as PONS, LAST, pneumothorax, or unintended destinations of local anesthetic. The two localization techniques are different with regard to the incidence and severity of HDP, with ultrasound guidance providing superior results. However, even this advantage is limited by the absence of total effectiveness in all patients and the unpredictable nature of its effect (Table 17-1).

References

1. Neal JM, Brull R, Chan VWS, et al. The ASRA evidence-based medicine assessment of ultrasound-guided regional anesthesia and pain medicine: executive summary. *Reg Anesth Pain Med* 2010;35:S1–S9.
2. Neal JM, Gerancher JC, Hebl JR, et al. Upper extremity regional anesthesia. Essentials of our current understanding, 2008. *Reg Anesth Pain Med* 2009;34:134–170.
3. Perlas A. Evidence for the use of ultrasound in neuraxial blocks. *Reg Anesth Pain Med* 2010;35:S43–S46.
4. Abrahams M, Horn J-L, Noles LM, et al. Evidence-based medicine: ultrasound guidance for truncal blocks. *Reg Anesth Pain Med* 2010;35:S36–S42.
5. Narouze SN. Ultrasound-guided interventional procedures in pain medicine: evidence-based medicine. *Reg Anesth Pain Med* 2010;35:S55–S58.
6. Neal JM, Bernards CM, Hadzic A, et al. ASRA Practice Advisory on neurologic complications in regional anesthesia and pain medicine. *Reg Anesth Pain Med* 2008;33:404–422.
7. Auroy Y, Benhamou D, Bargues L, et al. Major complications of regional anesthesia in France. The SOS regional anesthesia hotline service. *Anesthesiology* 2002;97:1274–1280.
8. Auroy Y, Narchi P, Messiah A, et al. Serious complications related to regional anesthesia. Results of a prospective survey in France. *Anesthesiology* 1997;87:479–486.
9. Brull R, McCartney CJL, Chan VWS, et al. Neurological complications after regional anesthesia: contemporary estimates of risk. *Anesth Analg* 2007;104:965–974.
10. Hogan QH. Pathophysiology of peripheral nerve injury during regional anesthesia. *Reg Anesth Pain Med* 2008;33:435–441.
11. Sala-Blanch X, Ribalta T, Rivas E, et al. Structural injury to the human sciatic nerve after intraneural needle insertion. *Reg Anesth Pain Med* 2009;34:201–205.
12. Perlas A, Niazi A, McCartney C, et al. The sensitivity of motor reponses to nerve stimulation and paresthesia for nerve localization as evaluated by ultrasound. *Reg Anesth Pain Med* 2006;31:445–450.
13. Robards C, Hadzic A, Somasundaram L, et al. Intraneural injection with low-current stimulation during popliteal sciatic nerve block. *Anesth Analg* 2009;109:673–677.
14. Bigeleisen PE, Moayeri N, Groen GJ. Extraneural versus intraneural stimulation thresholds during ultrasound-guided supraclavicular block. *Anesthesiology* 2009;110:1235–1243.
15. Chan VW, Brull R, McCartney CJ, et al. An ultrasonic and histologic study of intraneural injection and electrical stimulation in pigs. *Anesth Analg* 2007;104:1281–1284.
16. Altermatt FR, Cummings TJ, Auten KM, et al. Ultrasonographic appearance of intraneural injections in the porcine model. *Reg Anesth Pain Med* 2010;35:203–206.
17. Bigeleisen PE. Nerve puncture and apparent intraneural injection during ultrasound-guided axillary block does not invariably result in neurologic injury. *Anesthesiology* 2006;105:779–783.
18. Lupu CM, Kiehl T-R, Chan VWS, et al. Nerve expansion seen on ultrasound predicts histological but not functional nerve injury following intraneural injection in pigs. *Reg Anesth Pain Med* 2010;35:132–139.
19. Liguori GA, Zayas VM, YaDeau JT, et al. Nerve localization techniques for interscalene brachial plexus blockade: a prospective, randomized comparison of mechanical paresthesia versus electrical stimulation. *Anesth Analg* 2006;103:761–777.
20. Liu SS, Zayas VM, Gordon MA, et al. A prospective, randomized, controlled trial comparing ultrasound versus nerve stimulator guidance for interscalene block for ambulatory shoulder surgery for posoperative neurological symptoms. *Anesth Analg* 2009;109:265–271.
21. Barrington MJ, Watts SA, Gledhill SR, et al. Preliminary results of the Australasian Regional Anaesthesia Collaboration. A prospective audit of over 7000 peripheral nerve and plexus blocks for neurological and other complications. *Reg Anesth Pain Med* 2009;34:534–541.
22. Benhamou D, Auroy Y, Amalberti R. Safety during regional anesthesia: what do we know and how can we improve our practice? (editorial). *Reg Anesth Pain Med* 2010;35:1–3.
23. Orebaugh SL, Williams BA, Vallejo M, et al. Adverse outcomes associated with stimulator-based peripheral nerve blocks with versus without ultrasound visualization. *Reg Anesth Pain Med* 2009;34:251–255.
24. Cohen JM, Gray AT. Functional deficits after intraneural injection during interscalene block. *Reg Anesth Pain Med* 2010;35:397–399.
25. Koff MD, Cohen JA, McIntyre JJ, et al. Severe brachial plexopathy after an ultrasound-guided single-injection nerve block for total shoulder arthroplasty in a patient with multiple sclerosis. *Anesthesiology* 2008;108:325–328.
26. Reiss W, Kurapati S, Shariat A, et al. Nerve injury complicating ultrasound/electrostimulation-guided supraclavicular brachial plexus block. *Reg Anesth Pain Med* 2010;35:400–401.
27. Neal JM. Ultrasound-guided regional anesthesia and patient safety: an evidence-based analysis. *Reg Anesth Pain Med* 2010;35:S59–S67.
28. Mulroy MF, Hejtmanek MR. Prevention of local anesthetic systemic toxicity. *Reg Anesth Pain Med* 2010;35:177–180.
29. Neal JM, Bernards CM, Butterworth JF, et al. ASRA practice advisory on local anesthetic systemic toxicity. *Reg Anesth Pain Med* 2010;35:152–161.

30. Abrahams MS, Aziz MF, Fu RF, et al. Ultrasound guidance compared with electrical neurostimulation for peripheral nerve block: a systematic review and meta-analysis of randomized controlled trials. *Br J Anaesth* 2009;102:408–417.

31. Casati A, Baciarello M, Di Cianni S, et al. Effects of ultrasound guidance on the minimum effective anaesthetic volume required to block the femoral nerve. *Br J Anaesth* 2007;98:823–827.

32. Di Gregorio G, Neal JM, Rosenquist RW, et al. Clinical presentation of local anesthetic systemic toxicity: a review of published cases, 1979–2009. *Reg Anesth Pain Med* 2010;35:181–187.

33. Tsui BC, Pillay JJ. Evidence-based medicine: assessment of ultrasound imaging for regional anesthesia in infants, children and adolescents. *Reg Anesth Pain Med* 2010;35:S47–S54.

34. Weintraud M, Lundblad M, Kettner S, et al. Ultrasound versus landmark-based technique for ilioinguinal-iliohypogastric nerve blockade in children: the implications on plasma levels of ropivacaine. *Anesth Analg* 2009;108:1488–1492.

35. Urmey WF, Talts KH, Sharrock NE. One hundred percent incidence of hemidiaphragmatic paresis associated with interscalene brachial plexus anesthesia as diagnosed by ultrasonography. *Anesth Analg* 1991;72:498–503.

36. Neal JM, Moore JM, Kopacz DJ, et al. Quantitative analysis of respiratory, motor, and sensory function after supraclavicular block. *Anesth Analg* 1998;86:1239–1244.

37. Renes SH, Rettig HC, Gielen MJ, et al. Ultrasound-guided low-dose interscalene brachial plexus block reduces the incidence of hemidiaphragmatic paresis. *Reg Anesth Pain Med* 2009;34:498–502.

38. Riazi S, Carmichael N, Awad I, et al. Effect of local anaesthetic volume (20 vs 5 ml) on the efficacy and respiratory consequences of ultrasound-guided interscalene brachial plexus block. *Br J Anaesth* 2008;101:549–556.

39. Renes SH, Spoormans HH, Gielen MJ, et al. Hemidiaphragmatic paresis can be avoided in ultrasound-guided supraclavicular brachial plexus block. *Reg Anesth Pain Med* 2009;34:595–599.

40. Urmey W, McDonald M. Hemidiaphragmatic paresis during interscalene brachial plexus block: effects on pulmonary function and chest wall mechanics. *Anesth Analg* 1992;74:352–357.

41. Kessler J, Schafhalter-Zoppoth I, Gray AT. An ultrasound study of the phrenic nerve in the posterior cervical triangle: implications for the interscalene brachial plexus block. *Reg Anesth Pain Med* 2008;33:545–550.

42. Sinha SK, Abrams JH, Barnett JT, et al. Decreasing the local anesthetic volume from 20 to 10 mL for ultrasound-guided interscalene block at the cricoid level does not reduce the incidence of hemidiaphragmatic paresis. *Reg Anesth Pain Med* 2011;36:17–20.

43. Perlas A, Lobo G, Lo N, et al. Ultrasound-guided supraclavicular block. Outcome of 510 consecutive cases. *Reg Anesth Pain Med* 2009;34:171–176.

44. Bhatia A, Lai J, Chan VWS, et al. Pneumothorax as a complication of the ultrasound-guided supraclavicular approach for brachial plexus block. *Anesth Analg* 2010;111:817–819.

45. Koscielniak-Nielsen Z, Rasmussen H, Hesselbjerg L. Pneumothorax after an ultrasound-guided lateral sagittal infraclavicular block. *Acta Anaesthesiol Scand* 2008;52:1176.

46. Winnie AP. Interscalene brachial plexus block. *Anesth Analg* 1970;49:455–466.

47. Borgeat A, Dullenkopf A, Ekatodramis G, et al. Evaluation of the lateral modified approach for continuous interscalene block after shoulder surgery. *Anesthesiology* 2003;99:436–442.

48. Liu SS, YaDeau JT, Shaw PM, et al. Incidence of unintentional intraneural injection and postoperative neurological complications with ultrasound-guided interscalene and supraclavicular nerve blocks. *Anaesthesia* 2011;66:168–174.

49. Sala-Blanch X, Lopez AM, Carazo J, et al. Intraneural injection during nerve stimulator-guided sciatic nerve block at the popliteal fossa. *Br J Anaesth* 2009;102:855–861.

50. Bigeleisen PE, Chelly J. An unsubstantiated condemnation of intra-neural injection. *Reg Anesth Pain Med* 2011;36:95.

51. Rosenblatt MA, Bigeleisen PE. Ultrasound-guided intraneural injection: a powerful tool for regional anesthesia. In: Bigeleisen PE, ed. *Ultrasound-Guided Regional Anesthesia and Pain Medicine.* Philadelphia, PA: Wolters Kluwer/Lippincott Williams & Wilkins, 2010.

52. Neal JM, Wedel DJ. Ultrasound guidance and peripheral nerve injury. Is our vision as sharp as we think it is? *Reg Anesth Pain Med* 2010;35:335–337.

53. Reiss W, Kurapati S, Shariat A, et al. Reply to Drs. Bigeleisen and Chelly. *Reg Anesth Pain Med* 2011;36:88–99.

54. Silvestri E, Martinoli C, Derchi LE, et al. Echotexture of peripheral nerves: correlation between US and histologic findings and criteria to differentiate tendons. *Radiology* 1995;197:291–296.

Unintended Destinations of Local Anesthetics

Alain Borgeat and José Aguirre

Local anesthetics used for peripheral nerve blockade are occasionally injected directly into or spread into tissues where their actions are either unintended or unwelcome. The vascular system is a frequent unintended destination, and intravascular placement of sufficient local anesthetic mass results in systemic toxicity. Unintended placement of local anesthetic and/or needle injury may also affect hollow organs such as the bladder, rectum, or vagina during the classic technique for an obturator nerve block. This chapter highlights other unintended destinations of local anesthetics, particularly those related to blocks placed in the neck region or in close proximity to the neuraxis.

▶ DEFINITION

Unintended neuraxial anesthesia is one of the most severe complications that can occur during performance of a peripheral or plexus block (Box 18-1). The interscalene approach to the brachial plexus is a classic example of how local anesthetic can be unintentionally injected into the epidural, subdural, or subarachnoid spaces, thereby resulting in high spinal or massive epidural anesthesia. As one moves caudad along the neuraxis, unintended subarachnoid or epidural injection may also occur during paravertebral or psoas compartment blocks.

Systemic local anesthetic toxicity is fully discussed in Chapter 7. There is, however, an aspect of proximal brachial plexus block that deserves further emphasis with regard to intravascular injection. Because these blocks occur in close proximity to arteries that directly supply the brain, unintentional injection of even extremely small amounts of local anesthetic into the vertebral, carotid, or subclavian artery (followed by retrograde flow into the carotid or vertebrals) can result in the rapid development of seizures. Indeed, vertebral artery injection of 2.5 mg of bupivacaine has caused a convulsion during performance of an interscalene block.

Less serious than intra-arterial injection or direct injection near the neuraxis is the soft tissue spread of local anesthetics to anatomic structures near the intended neural target. These side effects occur most commonly during proximal approaches to the brachial plexus, such as with interscalene or supraclavicular blocks. Unintended spread

BOX 18-1 Unintended Destinations of Local Anesthetic

- Soft tissue spread: cervicothoracic sympathetic chain, vagus or recurrent laryngeal nerve
- Intravascular injection or vascular uptake from adjacent tissues
- Hollow viscus perforation with local anesthetic deposition and/or needle trauma

BOX 18-2 Plexus Blocks and Neuraxial Anesthesia: Pathways to the Spinal Cord

- Injection through the intervertebral foramen, leading to epidural, subdural, or subarachnoid placement
- Retrograde local anesthetic migration via the intervertebral foramen into the epidural space
- Injection into the dural root sleeve
- Distal intrafascicular injection with retrograde migration to the spinal cord

to the cervicothoracic sympathetic chain results in Horner's syndrome (characterized by ptosis, miosis, and anhydrosis), whereas local anesthetic may also affect the nearby vagus or recurrent laryngeal nerves, causing hoarseness.

► SCOPE

The incidence of unintended neuraxis involvement from interscalene block is not well defined. Epidural and spinal extension have been reported in isolated case reports,[1-6] wherein the vast majority occur with Winnie's technique and some with the posterior approach (i.e., the cervical paravertebral block). For the psoas compartment approaches, Macaire et al.[7] reported a retrospective study including 4,319 blocks performed by 42 teams. Spinal extension occurred in 0.6% of blocks, whereas epidural diffusion varied from 1% to 10% according to each team.

Minor problems such as Horner's syndrome occur in 12% to 75% of brachial plexus blocks using the interscalene or especially the supraclavicular approach.[8] Recurrent laryngeal nerve block occurs more frequently on the right side, and its incidence varies from 6% to 12% with interscalene block, or 1.3% with supraclavicular block.[8] Horner's syndrome and hoarseness may occur concurrently.

► PATHOPHYSIOLOGY

Neuraxial Placement

Various mechanisms may be implicated in the occurrence of total spinal or high epidural anesthesia following interscalene block (Box 18-2). Direct injection into the subdural (or epidural) space may be the consequence of incorrect needle placement through an intervertebral foramen. A perineural or intraneural injection may lead to a secondary migration of the drug into the subdural space.[8] Selander and Sjostrand[9] demonstrated that 20% of endoneural sciatic nerve injections reached the spinal cord. In their rabbit model, endoneural (intrafascicular) injections were associated with high pressure (300–750 mm Hg) and caused a rapid spread of radioisotope-labeled local anesthetic over long distances within the fascicle. This study showed that the fascicle is not just a grouping of nerve fibers but a conduit connecting the peripheral nervous system with the central nervous system

(CNS). Finally, long dural root sleeves have been shown in autopsy studies to extend as far as 3 to 5 cm beyond the intervertebral foramen. Placement of a needle into an abnormally long dural root sleeve[10] may therefore provide another explanation for the unintended transfer of local anesthetic into the intrathecal space[11] (Fig. 18-1).

Unintended neuraxial injection or spread of local anesthetic consequent to psoas compartment or paravertebral block may follow a similar pathway as described previously. Direct intrafascicular injection or injection via the intervertebral foramen or dural root sleeve is possible, as is retrograde local anesthetic spread into the epidural space.

Soft Tissue Spread

The stellate ganglion and recurrent laryngeal nerve lie in close proximity to the brachial plexus in the lower neck. The stellate ganglion is positioned anteriorly and between the transverse process of C7 and the first rib and lies behind the vertebral artery (Fig. 18-2). The right recurrent laryngeal nerve leaves the vagus as it crosses the subclavian artery, loops under it, and ascends in the tracheoesophageal groove. On the left side, it leaves the vagus as it crosses the aortic arch, loops under the arch, and ascends in the tracheoesophageal groove (Fig. 18-3). These structures may be easily affected during interscalene block, particularly if the Winnie or posterior approaches are performed.

► RISK FACTORS

Unintended epidural or spinal extension after interscalene block may be more likely to occur if the Winnie technique is used, because of the medial angulation of the needle coupled with excessive depth of needle placement. This point was highlighted by Sardasai et al.[12] who nicely demonstrated that the approach angle of the technique is the one that matches most closely with the angle of the spinal nerve as it exits the intervertebral foramen. The posterior approach may also present increased risk if the needle is angulated too far medially.

Concerning the psoas compartment block, the landmarks suggested by Capdevila et al.[13] for minimizing the risk of epidural (spinal) spread are recommended. As opposed to

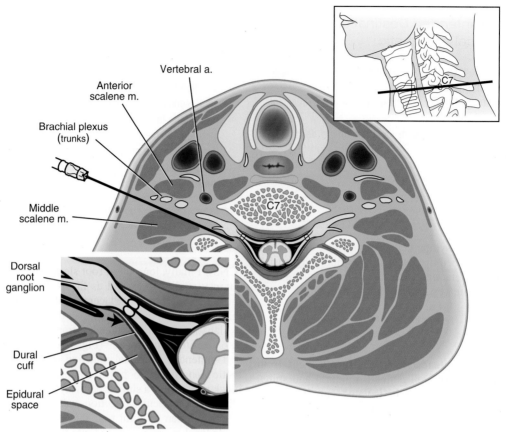

FIGURE 18-1. **Axial section of the left neck. Note the proximity of the brachial plexus to the dorsal nerve root ganglia (needle).** The spinal nerve root cuff is medial to the ganglia. Note also the proximity of the epidural space, the subarachnoid space, and the vertebral artery. (Drawing based on cryomicrotome section by Quinn H. Hogan, M.D. Modified from Neal JM, Hebl JR, Gerancher JC, et al. Brachial plexus anesthesia: essentials of our current understanding. *Reg Anesth Pain Med* 2002;27:402–428, with permission.)

the Winnie et al. technique of lumbar plexus block,[14] which directs the needle at a slightly medial inclination, the Capdevila approach directs the needle at right angles to the skin in all planes. The Capdevila technique also relies on identifying the transverse process as a fixed landmark, from which the needle should not be advanced more than 2 cm. Finally, a contraction of the abductor muscles should not be accepted as an adequate motor response, because it indicates an overly medial position of the needle. The previously described maneuvers are designed to avoid the neuraxis and thus limit the chance of central injection or spread of local anesthetic during psoas compartment block.

▶ DIAGNOSTIC EVALUATION

Neuraxial Injection

Unintended injection or spread of local anesthetic into the neuraxis manifests CNS symptoms that range from the inability to speak to unconsciousness and the rapid development of bilateral flaccid paralysis. Careful observation of symptom presentation may allow the anesthesiologist to distinguish among epidural, subdural, and subarachnoid

involvement (Table 18-1). Total spinal anesthesia, the most dramatic and rapidly progressing example of accidental neuraxial injection of local anesthetic, classically presents with dilated pupils, apnea, flaccid paralysis, and hypotension/bradycardia. Bilaterally dilated nonreactive pupils are frequently observed and are consistent with loss of parasympathetic efferent activity from the Edinger-Westphal nucleus. This sign demonstrates that some amount of local anesthetic has entered the cranial cerebrospinal fluid. The occurrence of apnea is typical, but not universal. The development of bradycardia, hypotension, and occasionally ventricular arrhythmias is explained either by cervicothoracic spinal anesthesia with blockade of the cardioaccelerator fibers (T1-T4) or by the migration of local anesthetic into the medullary region of the CNS.

In contrast to total spinal anesthesia from subarachnoid injection of local anesthetic, the appearance of signs and symptoms of epidural or subdural anesthesia is more progressive in nature. Because the epidural space does not extend into the cranium, medullary signs and symptoms such as dilated pupils do not occur. In the case of subdural injection, the clinical picture develops more slowly than with subarachnoid injection and is typically asymmetrical in distribution.

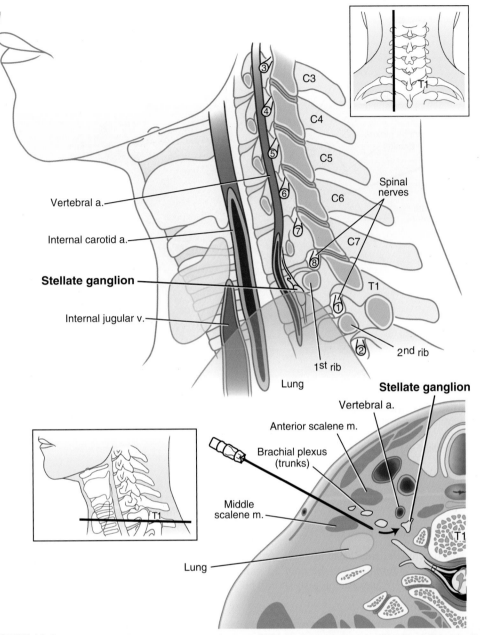

FIGURE 18-2. Parasagittal section of the neck demonstrating how local anesthetic may affect the stellate ganglia during the performance of an interscalene block. Note the proximity of the stellate ganglia to the C8 and T1 nerve roots. The jugular vein and internal carotid artery are seen in longitudinal section. (Drawing based on cryomicrotome section by Quinn H. Hogan, M.D. Modified from Neal JM, Hebl JR, Gerancher JC, et al. Brachial plexus anesthesia: essentials of our current understanding. *Reg Anesth Pain Med* 2002;27:402–428, with permission.)

The clinical signs and symptoms of neuraxis block after a psoas compartment block are more or less similar to those seen with epidural or subdural injection. Lower limb blockade and hypotension will typically appear first, followed by local anesthetic induced effects on the CNS.

Intravascular Injection

Although intra-arterial injection typically results in immediate seizure and loss of consciousness, it can at times be difficult to differentiate these complications from neuraxial injections. Hypotension and bradycardia may also occur due to local anesthetic induced myocardial depression. Intravascular injection or rapid blood reabsorption of local anesthetics should always be considered with the occurrence of both CNS toxicity and hemodynamic instability. However, the appearance of paralysis or motor weakness is not consistent with local anesthetic systemic toxicity. In contrast, the time course of symptoms from local anesthetic toxicity from tissue absorption during brachial plexus blocks is delayed, and their appearance is, in the majority of cases, much more progressive (one specific symptom appearing after the other).

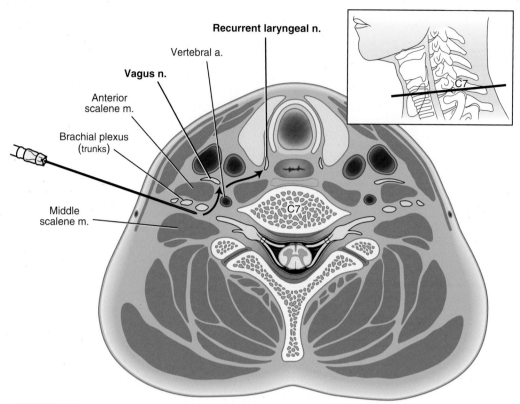

FIGURE 18-3. **Axial section of the neck.** Arrows demonstrate the ease with which local anesthetic administered during interscalene block can affect the vagus and recurrent laryngeal nerves. (Drawing based on cryomicrotome section by Quinn H. Hogan, M.D. Modified from Neal JM, Hebl JR, Gerancher JC, et al. Brachial plexus anesthesia: essentials of our current understanding. *Reg Anesth Pain Med* 2002;27:402–428, with permission.)

▶ PREVENTION

Neuraxial or Intravascular Placement

Preventing unintended neuraxial anesthesia involves several precautions. Because the C6 foramen may be only 23 mm from the skin in some patients,[15] anesthesiologists should be particularly mindful of excessively deep needle placement using the interscalene approach. Furthermore, the approach chosen for performing an interscalene block may influence the potential for certain complications. Neuraxial placement has only been described with the use of the Winnie technique or the posterior approach. To date, no case has been linked to the modified lateral technique.[16,17] The use of ultrasound

TABLE 18-1 Differential Diagnosis of Neuraxial Anesthesia Following Interscalene Block

PHYSICAL SIGNS	NEURAXIAL DESTINATION		
	SUBARACHNOID	SUBDURAL	EPIDURAL
Onset	Rapid (5 min)	Delayed (10–15 min)	Progressive (15–20 min)
Pupils	Dilated bilaterally	Comparable to subarachnoid, but less consistent because of asymmetrical distribution	Not dilated
Apnea	Yes		
Hemodynamic changes	Hypotension, bradycardia, ventricular arrhythmias		Variable hypotension, bradycardia, ventricular arrhythmias

guidance, similar to the modified lateral technique, allows for a more superficial needle approach to interscalene block and therefore might also be expected to reduce the frequency of these complications, but there are no data to substantiate this theory (Fig. 18-4). The advantages and disadvantages of each technique are outlined in Table 18-2. High-pressure injection has been shown to favor epidural spread during lumbar plexus block.[18] Whether this observation might be valid during interscalene block is not known. Anatomically, the two blocks are very different. The lumbar plexus is performed in a space that has a low compliance while the space surrounding the trunks of the brachial plexus has a high compliance. Moreover, estimation of resistance is difficult to appreciate when the LA is injected through a catheter.

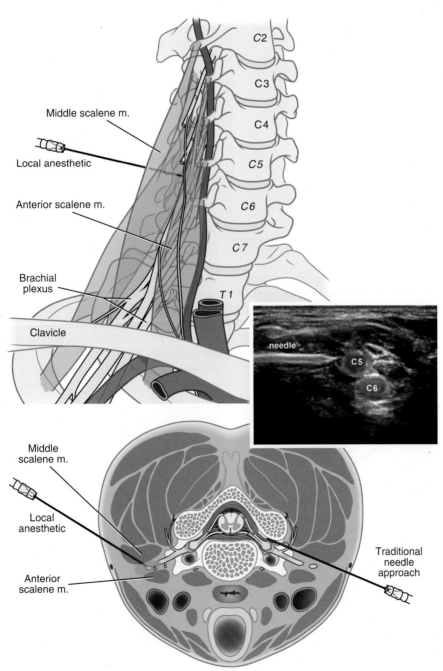

FIGURE 18-4. In theory, the use of ultrasound guidance may reduce the chance of unintended neuraxial anesthesia or neuraxial needle damage during the performance of interscalene block. As shown in the top panel and the left side of the bottom panel, ultrasound guidance facilitates a trans-middle scalene muscle, lateral-to-medial approach to the brachial plexus at the C5 level (sonogram inset). Thus the needle path is superficial to the neuraxis. Compare this to the traditional Winnie technique (right side of bottom panel) wherein the needle path is more directly toward the neuraxis.

TABLE 18-2 Interscalene Block: Advantages and Disadvantages of Common Techniques[a]			
	WINNIE	POSTERIOR (CERVICAL PARAVERTEBRAL)	MODIFIED LATERAL
Subarachnoid injection	++	++	−
Epidural injection	++	++	−
Vertebral artery injection	+	+	−
Intravenous injection	+	+	+
Pneumothorax	+	+	+
Discomfort	+	++	+
Ease of catheter placement	−	+	++

[a]Based on the author's experience.
Key: + likely, ++ more likely, − unlikely.

The first and basic precautions for minimizing unintended local anesthetic spread or deposition are to administer the drug slowly and to repeat aspiration. However, despite the strict application of incremental injection and aspiration, intravascular or neuraxial drug administration is always possible. As previously noted, the choice of interscalene approach has implications for this complication. Winnie's approach (medial, posterior, slightly caudad) directs the needle toward the spine and therefore increases the risk of injection through an intervertebral foramen, particularly if the needle is directed too horizontally (Fig. 18-5B). Because the posterior approach is a paravertebral block, it carries the risk of puncturing a dural cuff that accompanies a nerve distal to the intervertebral foramen. The modified lateral approach, which keeps the needle away from spinal structures, is most likely the safest technique for avoiding this complication (Fig. 18-5A).

Threading a perineural catheter more than 2 to 3 cm past the tip of the needle does not offer any advantage, but may present increased risk. For instance, by threading the catheter too far, the anesthesiologist may no longer control its position (i.e., interscalene catheters may be placed within the pleura).

A final but very important precaution is to perform interscalene blocks only in awake or lightly sedated patients (Chapter 10). This allows the patient to report a painful paresthesia (signifying injection too close to a nerve root) and/or pain upon injection (possibly signifying intraneural injection). Further, a minimally sedated patient facilitates early recognition of and prompt response to early signs of local anesthetic systemic toxicity. The same precautions are valid for the psoas compartment block.

Soft Tissue Spread

Cervicothoracic sympathetic or recurrent laryngeal block is unpredictable, and thus prevention is difficult. The use of the modified lateral technique, or the more needle-superficial ultrasound-guided approaches should theoretically decrease their incidence (due to the more lateral position of the needle), but to date no prospective study has addressed this issue. As with unintended neuraxial spread, ultrasound per se is unlikely to prevent soft tissue spread, but rather any advantage is more likely secondary to the more superficial

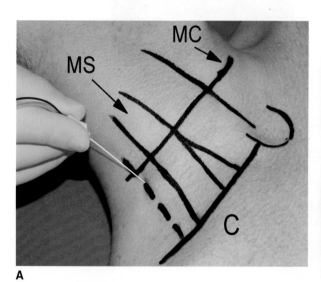

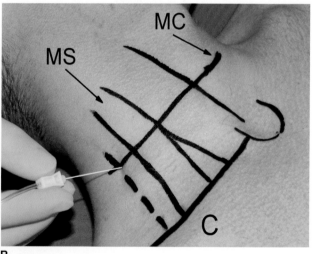

FIGURE 18-5. Winnie's vs. modified lateral interscalene techniques. **A: Modified lateral interscalene approach.** The needle is inserted toward the plane of the interscalene space at an angle of 45 to 60 degrees. The needle is thus directed away from the neuraxis. **B: Winnie technique.** The needle is directed medially, caudally, and slightly posterior (toward the transverse process of C6). This technique tends to direct the needle close to the neuraxis. (MC, cricothyroid membrane; MS, clavicular head of the sternocleidomastoid; C, clavicle; dotted line, interscalene groove.)

needle trajectory. Similarly, there is no literature to support the reduction of injected local anesthetic volume as a means of significantly lowering the incidence of these side effects.

▶ TREATMENT

Neuraxial Placement

Regardless of whether the local anesthetic has been injected into or spread into the subarachnoid or the epidural space, the first step is to immediately discontinue drug injection. Further management includes assisted manual or mechanical ventilation with 100% oxygen. In the case of subarachnoid injection, tracheal intubation is not always mandatory. Manual ventilation is often sufficient in cases of epidural injection. Patient-related factors such as mental status, administered drugs, and surgical conditions should be considered. Volume expansion may be necessary to prevent hemodynamic instability and atropine, ephedrine, or epinephrine to correct bradycardia or hypotension. As with any episode of spinal hypotension and bradycardia, the absence of rapid symptom resolution is an indication for epinephrine and aggressive resuscitation. Last, the patient should be monitored until the block resolves.

Soft Tissue Spread

There is no specific treatment for Horner's syndrome and hoarseness. The patient needs to receive complete information and reassurance that symptoms will resolve once the local anesthetic dissipates.

▶ SUMMARY

Unintended destinations of local anesthetics after proximal brachial plexus, paravertebral, or psoas compartment blocks occur infrequently, but may have serious consequences. The anesthesiologist must be vigilant that unintended epidural or spinal anesthesia may occur after performance of these blocks. Avoiding known risk factors and using careful block technique should reduce the incidence of these complications.

References

1. Tetzlaff JE, Yoon HJ, O'Hara J, et al. Alkalinization of mepivacaine accelerates onset of interscalene block for shoulder surgery. *Reg Anesth* 1990;15:242–244.
2. Mahoudeau G, Gaertner E, Launoy A, et al. Interscalenic block: accidental catheterization of the epidural space. *Ann Fr Anesth Reanim* 1995;14:438–441.
3. Dutton RP, Eckhardt WF III, Sunder N. Total spinal anesthesia after interscalene blockade of the brachial plexus. *Anesthesiology* 1994;80:939–941.
4. Passannante AN. Spinal anesthesia and permanent neurologic deficit after interscalene block. *Anesth Analg* 1996;82:873–874.
5. Norris D, Klahsen A, Milne B. Delayed bilateral spinal anaesthesia following interscalene brachial plexus block. *Can J Anaesth* 1996;43:303–305.
6. Iocolano CF. Total spinal anesthesia after an interscalene block. *J Perianesth Nurs* 1997;12:163–168:quiz 169–70.
7. Macaire P, Gaertner E, Choquet O. Le bloc du plexus lombaire est-il dangereux? In: SFAR, ed. *Évaluation et traitement de la douleur.* Paris, France: Elsevier, 2002:37–50.
8. Neal JM, Hebl JR, Gerancher JC, et al. Brachial plexus anesthesia: essentials of our current understanding. *Reg Anesth Pain Med* 2002;27:402–428.
9. Selander D, Sjostrand J. Longitudinal spread of intraneurally injected local anesthetics: an experimental study of the initial neural distribution following intraneural injections. *Acta Anaesthesiol Scand* 1978;22:622–634.
10. Evans PJ, Lloyd JW, Wood GJ. Accidental intrathecal injection of bupivacaine and dextran. *Anaesthesia* 1981;36:685–687.
11. Kowalewski R, Schurch B, Hodler J, et al. Persistent paraplegia after an aqueous 7.5% phenol solution to the anterior motor root for intercostal neurolysis: a case report. *Arch Phys Med Rehabil* 2002;83:283–285.
12. Sardesai AM, Patel R, Denny MN, et al. Interscalene plexus block: can the risk of entering the spinal canal be reduced. *Anesthesiology* 2006;105:9–13.
13. Capdevila X, Macaire P, Dadure C, et al. Continuous psoas compartment block for postoperative analgesia after total hip arthroplasty: new landmarks, technical guidelines, and clinical evaluation. *Anesth Analg* 2002;94:1606–1613.
14. Winnie AP, Ramamurthy S, Durrani Z. The inguinal paravascular technic of lumbar plexus anesthesia: the "3-in-1 block." *Anesth Analg* 1973;52:989–996.
15. Lombard TP, Couper JL. Bilateral spread of analgesia following interscalene brachial plexus block. *Anesthesiology* 1983;58:472–473.
16. Borgeat A, Dullenkopf A, Ekatodramis G, et al. Evaluation of the lateral modified approach for continuous interscalene block after shoulder surgery. *Anesthesiology* 2003;99:436–442.
17. Long TR, Wass CT, Burkle CM. Perioperative interscalene blockade: an overview of its history and current clinical use. *J Clin Anesth* 2002;14:546–556.
18. Gadsden JC, Lindenmuth DM, Hadzic A, et al. Lumbar plexus block using high-pressure injection leads to contralateral and epidural spread. *Anesthesiology* 2008;109:683–688.

SECTION II

Pain Medicine

COMPLICATIONS OF ACUTE PAIN MANAGEMENT

19

Complications Associated with Systemic Opioids and Patient-controlled Analgesia

Jane C. Ballantyne and Thomas H. Scott

Opioids have long been the preferred treatment for moderate to severe acute pain. This is because other analgesics do not offer equal efficacy, nor can they be titrated to effect. Nonopioid analgesics have a ceiling effect related to efficacy, side effects, or both and are used for mild to moderate pain or as opioid adjuncts. Opioids, on the other hand, can generally be safely titrated to achieve satisfactory analgesia even for severe pain. The only means of attaining similarly reliable analgesia comes from neural blockade, but neural blockade has limited indications and does not entirely displace opioids as the best analgesic for moderate to severe acute pain. Complications and adverse sequelae of long-term opioid therapy and neuraxial opioid therapy are described elsewhere in this book. Here, the focus is on complications of systemic opioid use in the acute pain setting.

Opioid effects are well known and are listed in Box 19-1. Side effects such as nausea and pruritus interfere with treatment success. Nausea is typically controlled with antiemetics, changing the opioid, or opioid dose reduction. Adjunctive ketamine, dexmedetomidine, and regional nerve blocks may also reduce opioid-related nausea and pruritis. While H1 histamine receptor antagonists are commonly used to treat opioid-induced pruritus, there is little clinical or pathophysiological basis supporting their routine use in the treatment of this side effect. Opioid-induced pruritis may be managed with μ-opioid receptor antagonists (naloxone), mixed opioid receptor agonists/antagonists (nalbuphene), 5-HT3 antagonists (ondansetron), dopamine D2 agonists (droperidol), and propofol.[1] Other opioid effects can be helpful or not, depending on the circumstance. For example, euphoria is helpful during the treatment of severe, acute, or cancer pain, but can also trigger a confusional state in vulnerable individuals (the elderly and patients on other psychotropic medications). Sedation may be helpful during periods of acute distress, but harmful if it contributes to respiratory depression. During the treatment of acute pain, two opioid effects produce potentially serious complications: respiratory depression and bowel slowing. Respiratory depression can cause hypoxia and hypercarbia and even death. It is the only opioid effect that is likely to cause immediate death, and it is the primary reason for cautious dose selection when prescribing opioids for acute pain. Bowel slowing worsens ileus or causes constipation. Because of their importance in acute pain management, opioid-induced respiratory depression and bowel slowing are highlighted in this chapter.

► RESPIRATORY DEPRESSION

Definition

Respiratory depression is most often defined as bradypnea or reduced respiratory rate. However, one of the difficulties of determining rates of respiratory depression is that there is no clear definition in the literature. It has been variously defined in different studies as hypoxia, hypoxemia, hypercarbia, hypercarbemia, or bradypnea.[2,3]

Scope

Respiratory depression is a well-known and widely recognized opioid effect, and the literature does not help establish a rate for the effect. The effect is dose dependent and highly sensitive to risk factors. Respiratory depression is more likely to occur during acute rather than chronic pain treatment because (i) patients are often opioid naive and (ii) other respiratory depressant drugs (hypnotics and anxiolytics) are often used concomitantly. Some degree of respiratory depression is an inevitable consequence of opioid use in opioid naive patients even at low doses. Mild respiratory depression may warrant supplementary oxygen, but is otherwise clinically unimportant. Serious respiratory depression can cause hypoxic brain injury, even death, making it the most serious adverse effect of acute opioid therapy. The effect can usually be avoided by using safe dosing protocols and appropriate monitoring.

Proposed Mechanism

The brain-stem rostral ventrolateral medulla is thought to be the main target for opioid respiratory depressant effects (Fig. 19-1). The area is the chief generator of respiratory rhythm.[4–6] Exogenous opioids may reach this area from the systemic circulation, after crossing the blood-brain barrier, or from cerebrospinal fluid (CSF) in the case of neuraxial administration.

Risk Factors

Respiratory depression is more likely to occur in opioid naive patients and is therefore a particular risk in acute pain treatment. Opioid respiratory depressant effects are exacerbated by concomitant use of sedative drugs (hypnotics, anesthetics, and anxiolytics), with which they have a powerful synergistic effect. The risk of respiratory depression is also increased in the very young, the elderly, and the infirm.[7] In neonates and infants, the immaturity of the nervous system (together with poor clearance) accounts for the increased sensitivity. In the elderly, increased sensitivity occurs chiefly because of poor clearance. In sick patients, a number of factors could contribute, including baseline mental status deterioration, poor clearance, and general debilitation. Other conditions associated with special risk are neuromuscular disorders, including myasthenia gravis, chronic lung disease, and sleep apnea.

Diagnostic Evaluation

Rapid-onset apnea can occur in two situations: (i) immediately after an intravenous (IV) injection of a high opioid dose, particularly of lipophilic opioids such as fentanyl or (ii) sometime after a neuraxial injection, typically of intrathecal morphine. More commonly, there is a progressive decrease in the respiratory rate before apnea occurs, and early intervention can prevent serious progression toward hypoxia or apnea. It is more important to monitor respiratory rate than oxygenation because hypoxia may not arise until

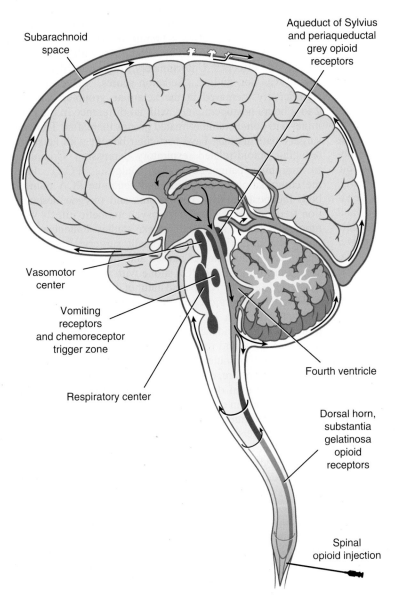

Subarachnoid space

Aqueduct of Sylvius and periaqueductal grey opioid receptors

Vasomotor center

Vomiting receptors and chemoreceptor trigger zone

Respiratory center

Fourth ventricle

Dorsal horn, substantia gelatinosa opioid receptors

Spinal opioid injection

FIGURE 19-1. **CSF flow diagram showing targets for spinal opioids.** Drugs injected into the epidural space or intrathecal space will tend to accumulate in CSF at the level of injection. The accumulation of hydrophilic drugs such as morphine will tend to be greater than that of lipophilic drugs such as fentanyl. Slowly diffusing drugs such as morphine will be subject to bulk flow of CSF and will tend to move cephalically toward the ventricular system in the brain. Bulk CSF flow varies markedly from patient to patient. If drug does reach the ventricular system, notably the fourth ventricle, it is likely to cause respiratory depression (and possibly nausea) because the respiratory center and chemoreceptor trigger zone are at the base of the fourth ventricle. Slowly diffusing drugs will likely provide a good spread of analgesia, as the drug will spread widely to the opioid receptors concentrated in the substantia gelatinosa of the dorsal horn.

late in the course of respiratory depression. Pulse oximetry serves as a useful signal for hypoxia, but is less useful as an early warning. It should be possible to preempt hypoxia by responding to decreases in respiratory rate. Practical methods for monitoring respiratory rate are direct observation and respiratory monitoring. Respiratory monitors use sensors that detect chest wall movement. Present-day multichannel monitors often incorporate respiratory monitors and use the electrocardiogram electrodes to sense the chest wall movement. Monitors that use dedicated sensors are more reliable and are sometimes used for neonates and infants in whom chest wall excursions are smaller and more sensitivity is required. Capnography can also be used to detect respiratory rate and hypercarbia, but is not usually practical for nonintubated awake patients. All monitoring equipment is subject to error, and thus the most reliable method is direct observation. During periods of high risk (e.g., early in the course of treatment), the respiratory rate should always be directly observed, even when respiratory monitors and pulse oximetry are used.

Prevention

Three approaches can be used to minimize serious complications of respiratory depression:

1. Use of safe dosing protocols, and appropriate adjustment when risk factors are present
2. Careful monitoring of respiratory depression and early intervention
3. Use of opioid-sparing analgesia regimes

Intervention

Opioid antagonists can be used to reverse opioid-induced respiratory depression, but there are drawbacks. Even small doses may reverse analgesia, so that well-controlled pain becomes agonizing. The effects of the agonist often outlive those of the antagonist, and thus there is a risk of recurrence of respiratory depression once the antagonist wears off. One recommended regime for naloxone is 0.4 mg diluted into 10 mL saline, giving 1 mL per dose while observing effects. Before giving naloxone, simple strategies such as shaking the patient, reminding them to breathe, talking to them, or otherwise stimulating them can be tried. Other analeptics such as physostigmine or flumazenil can successfully reverse respiratory depression without reversing analgesia, especially after anesthesia.

Opioid Sparing

The concept of opioid sparing began with the recognition that surgical outcome could be improved by reestablishing normal physiological function as early as possible after surgery. This meant getting patients out of bed early, removing feeding tubes and urinary catheters early, feeding early, encouraging coughing and deep breathing, and early resumption of normal activities. Many opioid effects run counter to these goals, particularly sedation and bowel effects. Opioid-sparing strategies include epidural analgesia, nerve blocks, dexmedetomidine, ketamine, and nonsteroidal anti-inflammatory drugs (NSAIDs).

There is robust evidence that, relative to IV opioids, continuous epidural analgesia has superior analgesic efficacy while reducing postoperative respiratory depression and recovery of bowel function (Table 19-1).[8–16] Epidural analgesia is effective because it uses low-dose (if any) opioid in the epidural space, which in turn has limited systemic absorption. Spinal analgesia is thus maximized, whereas undesirable systemic effects such as respiratory depression, sedation, nausea, and bowel slowing are minimized. Extended-release epidural morphine may be an exception to this principle, with one recent meta-analysis showing more respiratory depression compared with parenteral opioids.[17]

Ketamine is an *NMDA* (*N*-methyl-D-aspartic acid) receptor antagonist that functions clinically as a dissociative anesthetic with analgesic properties. Its principal negative side effects are dose-dependent psychomimetic symptoms, specifically vivid dreams, hallucinations, and delirium. Subanesthetic doses of ketamine given perioperatively consistently reduce the total dose of opioid for postoperative pain.[18–25] In contrast, single dose of pre-incision ketamine has little clinical benefit with respect to opioid sparing in the first two postoperative days and opioid-related side effects.[26,27]

A 2005 Cochrane review found that 27 of 37 included trials showed that perioperative ketamine reduced 24-hour opioid dose as well as nausea and vomiting, with minimal or absent side effects.[28] Unfortunately, respiratory depression *per se* was not studied. "Sedation scores," however, were significantly increased in the ketamine group in the first 2 to 4 hours postoperatively, with no difference in the ketamine- and non–ketamine-treated groups thereafter. Thoracic surgery patients may have particular benefit with ketamine reducing opioid-related respiratory depression. Compared to morphine patient-controlled analgesia (PCA) alone, the combination of morphine and ketamine PCA reduced both the postoperative pain scores and oxygen desaturation frequency.[18–20] No adverse psychomimetic effects were reported from the ketamine in these studies. Patients undergoing abdominal[22,23,29] and orthopedic surgery[21,24] also have shown lower incidence of nausea and improved pain scores compared to morphine PCA alone with minimal ketamine-related side effects. A separate audit of 1,026 patients from a wide variety of surgical populations who received morphine and ketamine in a 1:1 weight ratio for postoperative pain found that the incidence of vivid dreams and/or hallucinations was 6.2% and respiratory depression (bradypnea, RR < 8/min for 10 minutes) was 1.2%.[30] Subanesthetic doses of ketamine, therefore, constitute a safe and effective means of reducing the total opioid dose and opioid-induced respiratory depression in certain patient populations.

Dexmedetomidine and clonidine are centrally acting alpha-2 adrenergic receptor agonists used in anesthetic practice for their sedative and analgesic properties. These drugs tend to produce bradycardia and hypotension, which can be therapeutic. At high dose, or in sensitive individuals (e.g., neonates and children), respiratory depression can occur secondary to central nervous system (CNS) depression.[31–34] With appropriate dosing, the agents typically produce sedation, amnesia, and mild analgesia with minimal respiratory depression.[35] Dexmedetomidine is given intravenously, whereas clonidine is often given neuraxially, but may also be given orally, transdermally, or intraarticularly. In terms of opioid sparing, IV dexmedetomidine has two major roles, first as an adjunct sedative/analgesic during procedural

---

TABLE 19-1 Key Studies Validating the Ability of Epidural Analgesia to Reduce Respiratory Depression

STUDY	TYPE	*N*	TREATMENT	MEASURED	REDUCED	STATISTICAL SIGNIFICANCE
Rodgers (2000)	Meta-analysis	9,559	Regional vs. no regional	Respiratory depression (bradypnea)	Y	0.5% vs. 0.8%, $p < 0.001$
Park (2001)	Large trial, aortic subgroup only	374	Epidural vs. no epidural	Respiratory failure[a]	Y	14% vs. 28%, $p < 0.01$
Rigg (2002)	Large trial	915	Epidural vs. no epidural	Respiratory failure[b]	Y	23% vs. 30%, $p = 0.02$

Note: All control group patients received systemic opioid for postoperative analgesia.

[a]Respiratory failure is defined here as the need for intubation and mechanical ventilation for more than 24 h postoperatively or the need for reintubation and mechanical ventilation after 1 h postoperatively.

[b]Respiratory failure is defined here as the need for ventilation beyond 1 h after surgery or reintubation; $PaO_2 \leq 50$ mm Hg; or $PaCO_2 \, \varepsilon \, 50$ mm Hg.

sedation and second as an adjunct analgesic for the treatment of perioperative pain. Opioid sparing during the immediate postoperative period after pre-induction or intraoperative dexmedetomidine has been demonstrated in multiple trials, although the effect does not persist into the first postoperative day.[36–43] There may also be a role for postoperative dexmedetomidine. For example, a randomized controlled trial of 100 women undergoing total abdominal hysterectomy, dexmedetomidine (5 µg/mL)/morphine (1 mg/mL) PCA was superior to morphine PCA alone for postoperative analgesia with respect to pain scores, opioid use, nausea, and vomiting, with no difference in respiratory depression or sedation and lower heart rate and mean blood pressure.[44] Like dexmedetomidine, clonidine has been shown to enhance analgesia and reduce opioid doses in the perioperative period when given neuraxially,[31,45–48] orally,[49] and intraarticularly.[50,51] Data on clonidine reducing opioid-related side effects are more limited. Overall, the alpha-2 receptor agonists do appear to have useful analgesic and opioid-sparing effects, although as with many sedating drugs used as adjuncts to opioids, their ability to reduce opioid-induced respiratory depression *per se* may be less certain.

NSAIDs have also been studied as opioid-sparing analgesic adjuncts. Without question, NSAIDs reduce to the total dose of narcotic required for pain relief.[52–58] With respect to reducing respiratory depression, however, the literature is more equivocal with only selected trials showing decreased rates of respiratory depression.[52,54,56,58]

Peripheral nerve blocks, like epidural analgesia, offer excellent treatment of acute pain with minimal to no opioid supplementation. Numerous studies have demonstrated that peripheral nerve blockade is an effective means of opioid sparing following extremity surgery[59–61] and certain types of abdominal surgery, specifically open appendectomy, cesarean section, and hysterectomy.[62–64] Unfortunately, peripheral nerve blocks are not an option for many types of abdominal and thoracic surgery. Even for surgery on the upper and lower extremities, catheters frequently become dislodged requiring replacement or opioid supplementation, thus limiting their benefit with frequent reliance on opioids for acute postoperative pain. Nonetheless, a recent meta-analysis of femoral nerve blocks for knee arthroscopy with 10 studies and 1,016 patients showed that even a single-shot femoral nerve block significantly reduced nausea, postoperative pain scores at 24 and 48 hours and 12- and 24-hour postoperative morphine consumption.[61] There was no difference in sedation scores between parenteral opioids alone, single-shot femoral nerve block, and continuous femoral nerve blockade. Thus, where feasible, peripheral nerve blockade may be a useful option to reduce opioid consumption for postoperative analgesia. Their ability to reduce opioid-related respiratory complications, however, remains unproven.

Summary

Respiratory depression is a potentially dangerous opioid effect that is especially likely to occur during systemic opioid treatment of acute pain. The use of safe dosing protocols, knowledge of risk factors, use of appropriate monitoring, early intervention, and use of opioid-sparing techniques can help minimize related complications.

BOX 19-2 Causes of Opioid Dosing Errors

- Failure to follow recommended dosing protocol
- Lack of knowledge of risk factors, failure to recognize existence of risk, and/or failure to adjust dose according to risk
- Calculation errors
- Misreading orders
- Lack of familiarity with treatment
- Pharmacy errors

▶ OVERDOSE

Scope

The chief reason for avoiding overdose is to avoid respiratory depression. Dosing errors arise for a number of reasons (Box 19-2). Most dosing errors are human errors; some are system errors. The introduction of standardized protocols and especially the use of computerized systems with coding for ordering, distributing, and delivering medications has markedly reduced both human and system medication errors.[65,66]

Prevention

A question that must arise is whether the use of PCA can reduce the incidence of respiratory depression by reducing the likelihood of inappropriate dosing. PCA does have intrinsic safety in that small and frequent doses are used and the patient controls dosing (Fig. 19-2). Provided dosing parameters are set correctly and the method is used correctly (i.e., without being overridden by anyone other than the patient), patients are unlikely to receive an overdose because they will usually stop activating the pump when they are obtunded. Conventional methods are thought to be less safe because larger doses are given less often. Slow

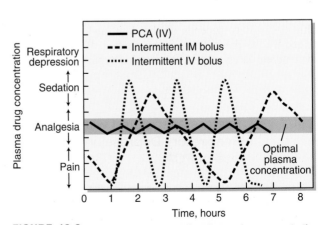

FIGURE 19-2. Relationship between the plasma drug concentration and pharmacologic effect of opioid analgesics over time when administered using various methods: PCA (patient-controlled analgesia), IV (intravenous), and IM (intramuscular).

absorption from intramuscular (IM) or subcutaneous (SC) deposit sites makes IM and SC administration safer than IV administration during conventional dosing, but it is still possible to absorb suprathreshold doses after the onset of obtundation.

Despite the theoretical advantage of PCA in terms of safety and avoidance of overdose, there is little support in the literature for superior safety. Two meta-analyses, one published in 1993[67] and the other in 2001,[68] failed to show any superiority for PCA in terms of adverse effects. Fifteen trials (787 patients) were included in the first analysis and 32 trials (2,072 patients) in the second. The first meta-analysis was able to show convincingly that patients prefer PCA to conventional analgesia and that PCA has slightly better analgesic efficacy. The mean difference in satisfaction was 42% ($p = 0.02$), whereas the mean difference in pain score on a scale of 0 to 100 was 5.6 ($p = 0.006$). However, there was no difference in opioid usage, adverse effects (including respiratory depression), or length of hospital stay. Most recently, in 2006, a systematic Cochrane review of patient-controlled IV opioids versus conventional, as needed IV opioid analgesia, confirmed the findings of the previous two meta-analyses.[69] Despite the passing of almost 20 years, and the addition of 38 trials (3,074 patients) to the first meta-analysis, the results of the third analysis differ very little from either the first or the second. Thus, patients' preference for PCA was confirmed, as was slightly better analgesic efficacy. There was no difference in adverse effects (including respiratory depression), and no convincing evidence of a difference in surgical outcome. A Canadian review of 1,600 charts of patients receiving PCA after surgery found eight cases of respiratory depression.[70] Factors associated with respiratory depression (Box 19-3) were the use of a background infusion (in addition to patient-controlled boluses), concomitant use of sedatives, and a history of sleep apnea. None of the cases were due to operator error or equipment malfunction.

Summary

PCA would seem to be a safer mode of delivery for opioids for acute and postoperative pain. However, the literature does not support the contention that PCA is safer, although clearly patients prefer it to conventional methods. It may be difficult to show differences in safety because ultimately safety depends on the dose, and dose is determined by the prescriber, not the method. If, for example, the inherent safety of patient control is bypassed by running a background infusion PCA safety may be compromised. Despite this consideration, present evidence does not support superior safety of PCA.

▶ BOWEL EFFECTS

Definition

Opioids are constipating during chronic use, or they prolong ileus.

Scope

Constipation and prolongation of ileus can be serious medical problems with potentially serious sequelae. The problem of constipation differs from that of prolonged ileus in several respects. Constipation tends to occur in the setting of chronic opioid use. Untreated constipation can eventually cause fecal impaction, possibly requiring surgical intervention. Fecal impaction may also cause bowel rupture. Impaction can usually be avoided by using a bowel regime during continuous opioid treatment.

Ileus tends to occur in surgical patients, or after trauma, particularly when there has been bowel injury or the bowel has been manipulated. In surgical patients, the bowel is often empty (after oral bowel preparation regimens) and the problem is one of bowel standstill and inability to tolerate oral intake. Delay in resumption of normal feeding after surgery has many adverse effects. Insulin, glucocorticoid, and growth hormone responses do not return to normal until feeding is resumed. Bowel motility cannot return to normal until the gut is presented with fluid or food, and a vicious cycle is set up of worsening bowel wall paralysis and fluid and food intolerance. Ileus is a common reason for delayed recovery and prolonged hospital stay after surgery, and these are associated with worse surgical outcomes.[71]

Pathophysiology

Opioids increase the tone of bowel luminal musculature, thereby interfering with normal gastrointestinal motility, delaying content transit, and increasing time for fluid absorption.[72–74] They also stimulate sphincters, including the sphincter of Oddi and the pylorus.[75–76] These effects are mediated by opioid receptors, mainly μ and κ receptors, which are plentiful in the gut's myenteric plexus.[77]

Risk Factors

Any factors that cause complete or partial bowel obstruction can increase the risk of opioid-induced constipation or prolonged ileus. Such factors include intraabdominal masses, adhesions, diverticulae, volvulus, and intussusception. Certain opioids may be more likely than others to produce sphincter spasm, and morphine has traditionally been implicated. This was based on early studies that measured biliary pressures, but later endoscopic studies showed that all opioids constrict sphincters, and it is likely that there are no clinically important differences among them.[78,79]

BOX 19-3 Factors Associated with Respiratory Depression During Use of PCA

- Use of background (basal) infusions in addition to patient-controlled boluses
- Concomitant use of sedatives
- History of sleep apnea

Bowel effects are dose related, and thus high doses also pose extra risk.

Diagnostic Evaluation

Diagnostic evaluation includes history, physical examination, and if necessary abdominal imaging. Silent abdomen is characteristic of ileus, whereas tinkering bowel sounds are characteristic of bowel obstruction. Straight abdominal x-ray (KUB) can be used to identify copious feces indicative of constipation and/or loops of air indicative of ileus or obstruction.

Prevention

Constipation can usually be avoided by placing opioid-treated patients on a bowel regimen consisting of a stimulating laxative (e.g., a sennoside-containing preparation) and a stool softener such as docusate. During postoperative pain treatment, however, opioids prolong ileus rather than produce constipation, and ileus should not be treated with laxatives. Although postoperative ileus cannot be prevented, certain interventions can help minimize the prolongation of ileus by opioids. These include changing the route of administration, use of oral antagonists, and opioid sparing.

Route of Administration

Oral administration of opioid agonists is likely to worsen opioid bowel effects through direct action on the bowel mucosa. Parenteral administration should therefore be continued until there is complete recovery and full diet is reestablished. Transdermal fentanyl is sometimes helpful. The neuraxial route is also preferred (see material following).

Peripheral Opioid Antagonists

The opioid antagonists naloxone and naltrexone have been used orally in low dose and can improve bowel motility without unduly compromising analgesia. More recently, methylnaltrexone and alvimopan (opioid antagonists with limited absorption and ability to cross the blood-brain barrier) have shown success in treating opioid-induced constipation (methylnaltrexone)[80-82] and postoperative ileus (alvimopan).[81,83-85] In 2008, both agents were approved by the FDA for treatment of inpatients with opioid-induced bowel dysfunction. In the case of methylnaltrexone it is for opioid-related bowel dysfunction refractory to laxatives in the setting of critical illness. Alvimopan has been approved for the treatment and prevention of postoperative ileus.[86] The FDA has issued a black box warning concerning a possible increased incidence of myocardial infarction in patients receiving alvimopan.

Opioid Sparing

Epidural analgesia is the most effective opioid-sparing technique in terms of minimizing the deleterious effect of opioids on the bowel in postoperative patients, as it is in minimizing respiratory depressant effects. In addition to opioid sparing (lower plasma opioid levels and selective spinal opioid analgesia), neuraxial local anesthetics have other benefits. They contribute by blocking visceral sympathetics, leaving the stimulating parasympathetics unopposed. Several published trials specifically assessing ileus confirm that epidural analgesia compared to systemic opioid therapy reduces the length of ileus, in turn reducing the length of hospital stay.[87-91]

Studies also confirm the opioid-sparing effect of NSAIDs,[54-57] but does this opioid-sparing effect confer any benefit in terms of ileus? A limited number of studies demonstrate accelerated recovery in association with less nausea and sedation, improved mobility, and earlier return of bowel function[53,92-94] but others fail to show any benefit in terms of recovery.[54,56,95,96] Overall, the literature is equivocal about whether opioid sparing by NSAIDs promotes rapid recovery in general or in terms of bowel recovery.

Data are very limited regarding the use of ketamine, dexmedetomidine, clonidine, and nerve blocks to hasten the recovery of bowel function following abdominal surgery. Comparing the effect of PCA with ketamine and morphine to morphine alone, one prospective randomized trial confirmed the opioid-sparing effects, but failed to show accelerated recovery of bowel function in the ketamine group.[29] Another study found reduced nausea, vomiting, and pruritus with combined postoperative ketamine/morphine compared with morphine alone, but late recovery of bowel function was not reported.[23] There is some limited data to support epidural clonidine in accelerating the recovery of bowel function postoperatively. One small randomized trial of 40 patients used pre-medication with epidural clonidine and postoperative patient-controlled epidural analgesia (PCEA) with morphine and clonidine compared with morphine and ropivacaine only for postoperative pain and showed lower total morphine dose, improved pain scores, and faster recovery of bowel function over the 72-hour postoperative period.[97] Intraoperative dexmedetomidine in bariatric surgery patients failed to improve rates of postoperative bowel recovery, though there was less nausea and vomiting in the dexmedetomidine group.[38,39] While the transversus abdominis block reduced opioid usage, nausea, vomiting, and pruritus, it has not been shown to accelerate the recovery of bowel function or reduce ileus.[62-64] These results are too limited to advocate routine usage of any of these opioid-sparing strategies for the purpose of accelerating the recovery of bowel function.

Summary

Although opioid bowel effects are not as immediately dangerous as respiratory depression, opioid-sparing strategies are aimed primarily at improving bowel mobility so as to reduce ileus and consequent delays in recovery. While peripheral opioid antagonists are a promising new option for the prevention and treatment of opioid-induced bowel dysfunction, limited clinical experience, coupled with a possible increased incidence of myocardial infarction (alvimopan), argues for some caution with these agents. The use of epidural analgesia is the most time-tested and effective way to reduce the adverse opioid effects on the bowel and is recommended especially for bowel surgery (unless contraindicated).

▶ BEHAVIORAL ISSUES

Fear of addiction has been, and in some cases remains, a reason caregivers and patients are hesitant about using opioids. A 1980 landmark report by Porter and Jick[98] did much to counteract these fears. This report stated that only 4 of 11,882 patients treated with opioids in Boston hospitals developed a problem with addiction. Guidelines have strongly supported liberal opioid use during acute pain treatment and emphasized that addiction is not likely to occur.[99,100] Clinical experience over the years since the Porter and Jick report confirms that addiction almost never develops when opioids are used *de novo* for acute pain.

Behavioral issues may arise, however, when patients have a history of past or present substance abuse. Control of acute pain can be especially problematic when it is opioids that are abused. Pain is difficult to control in those with opioid tolerance, and it is difficult to then interpret opioid-seeking behavior. These difficulties often lead to undertreatment of pain in this population. A policy of generous but structured dosing with careful monitoring works best. As is the case with other patients, opioid-sparing strategies are helpful in terms of optimizing pain relief while minimizing opioid usage. One should always try to ascertain the extent of current drug usage so that a plan to replace normal dosage can be incorporated into the acute pain management plan. It is important to obtain a history of "recreational drug use" both past and present. The information may be unreliable, but should at least be sought. Ascertain if the patient could be in withdrawal, and if so, treat the withdrawal. Alpha-2 agonists such as clonidine may be useful because they provide analgesia and reverse symptoms of withdrawal. Benzodiazepines and/or neuroleptics and general supportive measures may also be helpful. Large doses of opioids may be needed to avoid withdrawal and treat pain. Even patients who abuse substances such as alcohol, cocaine, or marijuana may exhibit some degree of cross-tolerance with opioids, thus requiring higher than normal opioid doses. Patients on methadone maintenance should continue their pre-admission dose, or this can be converted to an alternative opioid and/or mode of delivery and additional opioid prescribed as needed.[101] PCA is an effective modality for drug abusers in that it provides an element of control and lessens the anxiety associated with trying to obtain additional medication. It is not necessary or helpful to address the behavioral issues until after the acute pain episode, although it is helpful to work closely with addiction specialists, including psychiatrists and social workers, to prepare the patients for discharge and possible rehabilitation.

▶ UNDERTREATED PAIN

Scope

Although this chapter has focused on complications related to opioid overuse, it should not be forgotten that opioid underuse also causes complications. In many circumstances, there is no alternative to opioid treatment for severe pain, especially when there are contraindications to alternative or opioid-sparing strategies. Recent reports, studies, and position statements suggest that many types of pain (including postoperative pain) are undertreated.[100,102–109] Undertreatment of pain may be due as much to patients' and physicians' attitudes about opioids and opioid regulations as to their fear of medical complications.[110–112]

Pathophysiology

The goal of improving surgical outcome by encouraging rapid return of normal physiological function can be hampered by inadequate pain control as much as by the opioid adverse effects already described. Normal function cannot be restored when patients cannot cough sufficiently to clear secretions, comply with incentive spirometry to minimize atelectasis, or get out of bed and walk to encourage venous return and bowel activity. The benefits of optimal analgesia are confirmed by countless trials that have demonstrated improved surgical outcome in association with good pain control.[55,113]

In addition to the benefits of pain relief in terms of surgical outcome, there is also a growing body of preclinical evidence that unchecked pain produces CNS changes that are potentially deleterious. These changes have the net effect of increasing pain sensitivity.[114–118] It is not yet clear if the changes have clinical significance in terms of postoperative pain or its transition into chronic pain. Pain treatment with opioids or neural blockade attenuates metabolic stress responses, although the clinical relevance of these effects is unclear.[119,120] Untreated pain may have damaging psychological consequences, which is another reason pain control should be optimal.[121,122]

Diagnostic Evaluation

The only satisfactory way of assessing pain is by regular measurement, either asking patients to rate their pain level on a simple verbal scale or using a visual scale. Pain measurement, documentation, and treatment have now been mandated by the Joint Commission on Accreditation of Healthcare Organizations (JCAHO).[123] Pain is usually charted as the "fifth vital sign" in patients' charts and medical records. It is regrettable that such steps are necessary, but they have gone a long way toward increasing the awareness of pain's existence and the need to treat it.

▶ SUMMARY

We have recently emerged from a period when opioids were regrettably underused in the treatment of pain, largely because of unfounded fears about addiction and physician censure. Pain advocacy has been successful in reestablishing opioids as humane and appropriate treatment for acute (and cancer) pain. There is often no substitute for opioids when treating severe pain, so we must be prepared to use them. At the same time, there are complications that may arise during opioid treatment, and these must be appreciated. Strategies for minimizing complications are summarized in Box 19-4. Opioid pain treatment involves titrating to maximize efficacy while minimizing adverse effects, utilizing nonopioid treatments to reduce opioid requirements, and treating adverse effects with appropriate countermeasures.

BOX 19-4 Avoiding Complications of Systemic Opioid Treatment for Acute Pain

- Avoid complications of undertreated pain by using opioids appropriately.
- Fear of addiction is largely unwarranted in the acute pain setting and should not compromise opioid use.
- Undertreated pain is best identified using regular and formal pain assessments.
- Opioid-sparing strategies (including use of epidurals and NSAIDs) reduce opioid requirement and risk.
- Use standard dosing protocols and adjust according to known risks.
- Monitoring for respiratory depression is especially important early in the course of treatment.
- Observation is the most reliable and effective monitor.
- Early recognition and intervention can abort serious consequences of respiratory depression.

References

1. Ganesh A, Maxwell LG. Pathophysiology and management of opioid-induced pruritus. *Drugs* 2007;67(16):2323–2333.
2. Ko S, Goldstein DH, VanDenKerkhof EG. Definitions of "respiratory depression" with intrathecal morphine postoperative analgesia: a review of the literature. *Can J Anaesth* 2003;50(7):679–688.
3. Cousins MJ, Mather LE. Intrathecal and epidural administration of opioids. *Anesthesiology* 1984;61(3):276–310.
4. Takita K, Herlenius EA, Lindahl SG, et al. Actions of opioids on respiratory activity via activation of brainstem mu-, delta- and kappa-receptors; an in vitro study. *Brain Res* 1997;778(1):233–241.
5. Takeda S, Eriksson LI, Yamamoto Y, et al. Opioid action on respiratory neuron activity of the isolated respiratory network in newborn rats. *Anesthesiology* 2001;95(3):740–749.
6. Tabatabai M, Kitahata LM, Collins JG. Disruption of the rhythmic activity of the medullary inspiratory neurons and phrenic nerve by fentanyl and reversal with nalbuphine. *Anesthesiology* 1989;70(3):489–495.
7. Cepeda MS, Farrar JT, Baumgarten M, et al. Side effects of opioids during short-term administration: effect of age, gender, and race. *Clin Pharmacol Ther* 2003;74(2):102–112.
8. Rodgers A, Walker N, Schug S, et al. Reduction of postoperative mortality and morbidity with epidural or spinal anaesthesia: results from overview of randomised trials. *BMJ* 2000;321(7275):1493.
9. Park WY, Thompson JS, Lee KK. Effect of epidural anesthesia and analgesia on perioperative outcome: a randomized, controlled Veterans Affairs cooperative study. *Ann Surg* 2001;234(4):560–569.
10. Rigg JR, Jamrozik K, Myles PS, et al. Epidural anaesthesia and analgesia and outcome of major surgery: a randomised trial. *Lancet* 2002;359(9314):1276–1282.
11. American Society of Anesthesiologists Task Force on Neuraxial Opioids, Horlocker TT, Burton AW, et al. Practice guidelines for the prevention, detection, and management of respiratory depression associated with neuraxial opioid administration. *Anesthesiology* 2009;110(2):218–230.
12. Werawatganon T, Charuluxanun S. Patient controlled intravenous opioid analgesia versus continuous epidural analgesia for pain after intra-abdominal surgery. *Cochrane Database Syst Rev* 2005;(1):004088.
13. Zingg U, Miskovic D, Hamel CT, et al. Influence of thoracic epidural analgesia on postoperative pain relief and ileus after laparoscopic colorectal resection: benefit with epidural analgesia. *Surg Endosc* 2009;23(2):276–282.
14. Gendall KA, Kennedy RR, Watson AJ, et al. The effect of epidural analgesia on postoperative outcome after colorectal surgery. *Colorectal Dis* 2007;9(7):584–598.
15. Marret E, Remy C, Bonnet F, et al. Meta-analysis of epidural analgesia versus parenteral opioid analgesia after colorectal surgery. *Br J Surg* 2007;94(6):665–673.
16. Nakayoshi T, Kawasaki N, Suzuki Y, et al. Epidural administration of morphine facilitates time of appearance of first gastric interdigestive migrating complex in dogs with paralytic ileus after open abdominal surgery. *J Gastrointest Surg* 2007;11(5):648–654.
17. Sumida S, Lesley MR, Hanna MN, et al. Meta-analysis of the effect of extended-release epidural morphine versus intravenous patient-controlled analgesia on respiratory depression. *J Opioid Manag* 2009;5(5):301–305.
18. Atangana R, Ngowe Ngowe M, Binam F, et al. Morphine versus morphine-ketamine association in the management of post operative pain in thoracic surgery. *Acta Anaesthesiol Belg* 2007;58(2):125–127.
19. Carstensen M, Moller AM. Adding ketamine to morphine for intravenous patient-controlled analgesia for acute postoperative pain: a qualitative review of randomized trials. *Br J Anaesth* 2010;104(4):401–406.
20. Nesher N, Ekstein MP, Paz Y, et al. Morphine with adjuvant ketamine vs higher dose of morphine alone for immediate post-thoracotomy analgesia. *Chest* 2009;136(1):245–252.
21. Remerand F, Le Tendre C, Baud A, et al. The early and delayed analgesic effects of ketamine after total hip arthroplasty: a prospective, randomized, controlled, double-blind study. *Anesth Analg* 2009;109(6):1963–1971.
22. Zakine J, Samarcq D, Lorne E, et al. Postoperative ketamine administration decreases morphine consumption in major abdominal surgery: a prospective, randomized, double-blind, controlled study. *Anesth Analg* 2008;106(6):1856–1861.
23. Sami Mebazaa M, Mestiri T, Kaabi B, et al. Clinical benefits related to the combination of ketamine with morphine for patient controlled analgesia after major abdominal surgery. *Tunis Med* 2008;86(5):435–440.
24. Adam F, Chauvin M, Du Manoir B, et al. Small-dose ketamine infusion improves postoperative analgesia and rehabilitation after total knee arthroplasty. *Anesth Analg* 2005;100(2):475–480.
25. Michelet P, Guervilly C, Helaine A, et al. Adding ketamine to morphine for patient-controlled analgesia after thoracic surgery: influence on morphine consumption, respiratory function, and nocturnal desaturation. *Br J Anaesth* 2007;99(3):396–403.
26. Dullenkopf A, Muller R, Dillmann F, et al. An intraoperative pre-incision single dose of intravenous ketamine does not have an effect on postoperative analgesic requirements under clinical conditions. *Anaesth Intensive Care* 2009;37(5):753–757.
27. Abu-Shahwan I. Ketamine does not reduce postoperative morphine consumption after tonsillectomy in children. *Clin J Pain* 2008;24(5):395–398.
28. Bell RF, Dahl JB, Moore RA, et al. Peri-operative ketamine for acute post-operative pain: a quantitative and qualitative systematic review (Cochrane review). *Acta Anaesthesiol Scand* 2005;49(10):1405–1428.
29. McKay WP, Donais P. Bowel function after bowel surgery: morphine with ketamine or placebo; a randomized controlled trial pilot study. *Acta Anaesthesiol Scand* 2007;51(9):1166–1171.

30. Sveticic G, Eichenberger U, Curatolo M. Safety of mixture of morphine with ketamine for postoperative patient-controlled analgesia: an audit with 1026 patients. *Acta Anaesthesiol Scand* 2005;49(6):870–875.

31. Hansen TG, Henneberg SW. Caudal clonidine in neonates and small infants and respiratory depression. *Paediatr Anaesth* 2004;14(6):529–530.

32. Garg R. Be vigilant during use of intrathecal clonidine in former preterm infants. *Paediatr Anaesth* 2009;19(1):58.

33. Aouad MT, Moukaddem FH, Akel SR, et al. Respiratory failure in a former preterm infant following high spinal anesthesia with bupivacaine and clonidine. *Paediatr Anaesth* 2008;18(10): 1000–1001.

34. Luebbe N, Walz R, Walz K, et al. Clonidine prolongs fentanyl-induced ventilatory depression. *Eur J Anaesthesiol* 1998;15(3): 292–296.

35. Bailey PL, Sperry RJ, Johnson GK, et al. Respiratory effects of clonidine alone and combined with morphine, in humans. *Anesthesiology* 1991;74(1):43–48.

36. Olutoye OA, Glover CD, Diefenderfer JW, et al. The effect of intraoperative dexmedetomidine on postoperative analgesia and sedation in pediatric patients undergoing tonsillectomy and adenoidectomy. *Anesth Analg* 2010;111(2):490–495.

37. Sadhasivam S, Boat A, Mahmoud M. Comparison of patient-controlled analgesia with and without dexmedetomidine following spine surgery in children. *J Clin Anesth* 2009;21(7):493–501.

38. Tufanogullari B, White PF, Peixoto MP, et al. Dexmedetomidine infusion during laparoscopic bariatric surgery: the effect on recovery outcome variables. *Anesth Analg* 2008;106(6):1741–1748.

39. Bakhamees HS, El-Halafawy YM, El-Kerdawy HM, et al. Effects of dexmedetomidine in morbidly obese patients undergoing laparoscopic gastric bypass. *Middle East J Anesthesiol* 2007;19(3): 537–551.

40. Arain SR, Ruehlow RM, Uhrich TD, et al. The efficacy of dexmedetomidine versus morphine for postoperative analgesia after major inpatient surgery. *Anesth Analg* 2004;98(1):153–158.

41. Gomez-Vazquez ME, Hernandez-Salazar E, Hernandez-Jimenez A, et al. Clinical analgesic efficacy and side effects of dexmedetomidine in the early postoperative period after arthroscopic knee surgery. *J Clin Anesth* 2007;19(8):576–582.

42. Gurbet A, Basagan-Mogol E, Turker G, et al. Intraoperative infusion of dexmedetomidine reduces perioperative analgesic requirements. *Can J Anaesth* 2006;53(7):646–652.

43. Unlugenc H, Gunduz M, Guler T, et al. The effect of pre-anaesthetic administration of intravenous dexmedetomidine on postoperative pain in patients receiving patient-controlled morphine. *Eur J Anaesthesiol* 2005;22(5):386–391.

44. Lin TF, Yeh YC, Lin FS, et al. Effect of combining dexmedetomidine and morphine for intravenous patient-controlled analgesia. *Br J Anaesth* 2009;102(1):117–122.

45. Tripi PA, Palmer JS, Thomas S, et al. Clonidine increases duration of bupivacaine caudal analgesia for ureteroneocystostomy: a double-blind prospective trial. *J Urol* 2005;174(3):1081–1083.

46. Paech MJ, Pavy TJ, Orlikowski CE, et al. Postcesarean analgesia with spinal morphine, clonidine, or their combination. *Anesth Analg* 2004;98(5):1460–1466.

47. Sites BD, Beach M, Biggs R, et al. Intrathecal clonidine added to a bupivacaine-morphine spinal anesthetic improves postoperative analgesia for total knee arthroplasty. *Anesth Analg* 2003;96(4):1083–1088.

48. Paech MJ, Pavy TJ, Orlikowski CE, et al. Postoperative epidural infusion: a randomized, double-blind, dose-finding trial of clonidine in combination with bupivacaine and fentanyl. *Anesth Analg* 1997;84(6):1323–1328.

49. Goyagi T, Tanaka M, Nishikawa T. Oral clonidine premedication enhances postoperative analgesia by epidural morphine. *Anesth Analg* 1999;89(6):1487–1491.

50. Tran KM, Ganley TJ, Wells L, et al. Intraarticular bupivacaine-clonidine-morphine versus femoral-sciatic nerve block in pediatric patients undergoing anterior cruciate ligament reconstruction. *Anesth Analg* 2005;101(5):1304–1310.

51. Joshi W, Reuben SS, Kilaru PR, et al. Postoperative analgesia for outpatient arthroscopic knee surgery with intraarticular clonidine and/or morphine. *Anesth Analg* 2000;90(5):1102–1106.

52. Gillies GW, Kenny GN, Bullingham RE, et al. The morphine sparing effect of ketorolac tromethamine. A study of a new, parenteral non-steroidal anti-inflammatory agent after abdominal surgery. *Anaesthesia* 1987;42(7):727–731.

53. Chen JY, Ko TL, Wen YR, et al. Opioid-sparing effects of ketorolac and its correlation with the recovery of postoperative bowel function in colorectal surgery patients: a prospective randomized double-blinded study. *Clin J Pain* 2009;25(6):485–489.

54. Moote C. Efficacy of nonsteroidal anti-inflammatory drugs in the management of postoperative pain. *Drugs* 1992;44(suppl 5): 14–29.

55. Kehlet H. Multimodal approach to control postoperative pathophysiology and rehabilitation. *Br J Anaesth* 1997;78(5): 606–617.

56. Ballantyne JC. Use of nonsteroidal antiinflammatory drugs for acute pain management. *Probl Anesth* 1998;10(1):606–617.

57. Ballantyne JC, Ulmer JF, Marenholz D. Acute Pain Management. ACHPR Guideline Technical Report. 1995.

58. Hodsman NB, Burns J, Blyth A, et al. The morphine sparing effects of diclofenac sodium following abdominal surgery. *Anaesthesia* 1987;42(9):1005–1008.

59. Fredrickson MJ, Ball CM, Dalgleish AJ. Analgesic effectiveness of a continuous versus single-injection interscalene block for minor arthroscopic shoulder surgery. *Reg Anesth Pain Med* 2010;35(1):28–33.

60. Hogan MV, Grant RE, Lee Jr L. Analgesia for total hip and knee arthroplasty: a review of lumbar plexus, femoral, and sciatic nerve blocks. *Am J Orthop* (Belle Mead NJ) 2009;38(8): E129–E133.

61. Paul JE, Arya A, Hurlburt L, et al. Femoral nerve block improves analgesia outcomes after total knee arthroplasty: a meta-analysis of randomized controlled trials. *Anesthesiology* 2010;113(5): 1144–1162.

62. McDonnell JG, Curley G, Carney J, et al. The analgesic efficacy of transversus abdominis plane block after cesarean delivery: a randomized controlled trial. *Anesth Analg* 2008;106(1):186–191, table of contents.

63. Carney J, McDonnell JG, Ochana A, et al. The transversus abdominis plane block provides effective postoperative analgesia in patients undergoing total abdominal hysterectomy. *Anesth Analg* 2008;107(6):2056–2060.

64. Petersen PL, Mathiesen O, Torup H, et al. The transversus abdominis plane block: a valuable option for postoperative analgesia? A topical review. *Acta Anaesthesiol Scand* 2010;54: 529–535.

65. Hantson P, Vanbinst R, Wallemacq P. Accidental methadone overdose in an opiate-naive elderly patient. *Intensive Care Med* 2003;29(11):2105.

66. Khan FA, Hoda MQ. Drug related critical incidents. *Anaesthesia* 2005;60(1):48–52.

67. Ballantyne JC, Carr DB, Chalmers TC, et al. Postoperative patient-controlled analgesia: meta-analyses of initial randomized control trials. *J Clin Anesth* 1993;5(3):182–193.

68. Walder B, Schafer M, Henzi I, et al. Efficacy and safety of patient-controlled opioid analgesia for acute postoperative pain. A quantitative systematic review. *Acta Anaesthesiol Scand* 2001; 45(7):795–804.

69. Hudcova J, McNicol E, Quah C, et al. Patient controlled opioid analgesia versus conventional opioid analgesia for postoperative pain. *Cochrane Database Syst Rev* 2006;(4):CD003348.

70. Etches RC. Respiratory depression associated with patient-controlled analgesia: a review of eight cases. *Can J Anaesth* 1994;41(2):125–132.

71. Miedema BW, Johnson JO. Methods for decreasing postoperative gut dysmotility. *Lancet Oncol* 2003;4(6):365–372.

72. Murphy DB, Sutton JA, Prescott LF, et al. Opioid-induced delay in gastric emptying: a peripheral mechanism in humans. *Anesthesiology* 1997;87(4):765–770.

73. Thorn SE, Wattwil M, Lindberg G, et al. Systemic and central effects of morphine on gastroduodenal motility. *Acta Anaesthesiol Scand* 1996;40(2):177–186.

74. De Schepper HU, Cremonini F, Park MI, et al. Opioids and the gut: pharmacology and current clinical experience. *Neurogastroenterol Motil* 2004;16(4):383–394.

75. Vieira ZE, Zsigmond EK, Duarate B, et al. Evaluation of fentanyl and sufentanil on the diameter of the common bile duct by ultrasonography in man: a double blind, placebo controlled study. *Int J Clin Pharmacol Ther* 1994;32(6):274–277.

76. Radnay PA, Duncalf D, Novakovic M, et al. Common bile duct pressure changes after fentanyl, morphine, meperidine, butorphanol, and naloxone. *Anesth Analg* 1984;63(4):441–444.

77. Kurz A, Sessler DI. Opioid-induced bowel dysfunction: pathophysiology and potential new therapies. *Drugs* 2003;63(7):649–671.

78. Lee F, Cundiff D. Meperidine vs morphine in pancreatitis and cholecystitis. *Arch Intern Med* 1998;158(21):2399.

79. Thompson DR. Narcotic analgesic effects on the sphincter of Oddi: a review of the data and therapeutic implications in treating pancreatitis. *Am J Gastroenterol* 2001;96(4):1266–1272.

80. Yuan CS, Foss JF. Oral methylnaltrexone for opioid-induced constipation. *JAMA* 2000;284(11):1383–1384.

81. McNicol ED, Boyce D, Schumann R, et al. Mu-opioid antagonists for opioid-induced bowel dysfunction. *Cochrane Database Syst Rev* 2008;(2):CD006332.

82. Thomas J, Karver S, Cooney GA, et al. Methylnaltrexone for opioid-induced constipation in advanced illness. *N Engl J Med* 2008;358(22):2332–2343.

83. Liu SS, Hodgson PS, Carpenter RL, et al. ADL 8–2698, a trans-3,4-dimethyl-4-(3-hydroxyphenyl) piperidine, prevents gastrointestinal effects of intravenous morphine without affecting analgesia. *Clin Pharmacol Ther* 2001;69(1):66–71.

84. Schmidt WK. Alvimopan* (ADL 8–2698) is a novel peripheral opioid antagonist. *Am J Surg* 2001;182(5A suppl):27S–38S.

85. Taguchi A, Sharma N, Saleem RM, et al. Selective postoperative inhibition of gastrointestinal opioid receptors. *N Engl J Med* 2001;345(13):935–940.

86. Becker G, Blum HE. Novel opioid antagonists for opioid-induced bowel dysfunction and postoperative ileus. *Lancet* 2009;373 (9670):1198–1206.

87. de Leon-Casasola OA, Karabella D, Lema MJ. Bowel function recovery after radical hysterectomies: thoracic epidural bupivacaine-morphine versus intravenous patient-controlled analgesia with morphine: a pilot study. *J Clin Anesth* 1996;8(2):87–92.

88. Steinbrook RA. Epidural anesthesia and gastrointestinal motility. *Anesth Analg* 1998;86(4):837–844.

89. Stevens RA, Mikat-Stevens M, Flanigan R, et al. Does the choice of anesthetic technique affect the recovery of bowel function after radical prostatectomy? *Urology* 1998;52(2):213–218.

90. Williams BA, DeRiso BM, Figallo CM, et al. Benchmarking the perioperative process: III. Effects of regional anesthesia clinical pathway techniques on process efficiency and recovery profiles in ambulatory orthopedic surgery. *J Clin Anesth* 1998;10(7):570–578.

91. Jorgensen H, Wetterslev J, Moiniche S, et al. Epidural local anaesthetics versus opioid-based analgesic regimens on postoperative gastrointestinal paralysis, PONV and pain after abdominal surgery. *Cochrane Database Syst Rev* 2000;(4):001893.

92. Reasbeck PG, Rice ML, Reasbeck JC. Double-blind controlled trial of indomethacin as an adjunct to narcotic analgesia after major abdominal surgery. *Lancet* 1982;2(8290):115–118.

93. Grass JA, Sakima NT, Valley M, et al. Assessment of ketorolac as an adjuvant to fentanyl patient-controlled epidural analgesia after radical retropubic prostatectomy. *Anesthesiology* 1993;78(4):642–648.

94. Schlachta CM, Burpee SE, Fernandez C, et al. Optimizing recovery after laparoscopic colon surgery (ORAL-CS): effect of intravenous ketorolac on length of hospital stay. *Surg Endosc* 2007;21(12):2212–2219.

95. Thind P, Sigsgaard T. The analgesic effect of indomethacin in the early post-operative period following abdominal surgery. A double-blind controlled study. *Acta Chir Scand* 1988;154(1):9–12.

96. Higgins MS, Givogre JL, Marco AP, et al. Recovery from outpatient laparoscopic tubal ligation is not improved by preoperative administration of ketorolac or ibuprofen. *Anesth Analg* 1994;79(2):274–280.

97. Wu CT, Jao SW, Borel CO, et al. The effect of epidural clonidine on perioperative cytokine response, postoperative pain, and bowel function in patients undergoing colorectal surgery. *Anesth Analg* 2004;99(2):502–509.

98. Porter J, Jick H. Addiction rare in patients treated with narcotics. *N Engl J Med* 1980;302(2):123.

99. National Guideline Clearinghouse │ Assessment and management of pain. Available at: http://www.guideline.gov/content.aspx?id=11507&search=acute+pain. Accessed November 4, 2010.

100. American Pain Society Quality of Care Committee. Quality improvement guidelines for the treatment of acute pain and cancer pain. *JAMA* 1995;274(23):1874–1880.

101. Mitra S, Sinatra RS. Perioperative management of acute pain in the opioid-dependent patient. *Anesthesiology* 2004;101(1):212–227.

102. Marks RM, Sachar EJ. Undertreatment of medical inpatients with narcotic analgesics. *Ann Intern Med* 1973;78(2):173–181.

103. Donovan M, Dillon P, McGuire L. Incidence and characteristics of pain in a sample of medical-surgical inpatients. *Pain* 1987;30(1):69–78.

104. Abbott FV, Gray-Donald K, Sewitch MJ, et al. The prevalence of pain in hospitalized patients and resolution over six months. *Pain* 1992;50(1):15–28.

105. Gu X, Belgrade MJ. Pain in hospitalized patients with medical illnesses. *J Pain Symptom Manage* 1993;8(1):17–21.

106. Carr DB, Miaskowski C, Dedrick SC, et al. Management of perioperative pain in hospitalized patients: a national survey. *J Clin Anesth* 1998;10(1):77–85.

107. Carr DB, Goudas LC. Acute pain. *Lancet* 1999;353(9169):2051–2058.

108. Drayer RA, Henderson J, Reidenberg M. Barriers to better pain control in hospitalized patients. *J Pain Symptom Manage* 1999;17(6):434–440.

109. Oden R. Acute postoperative pain: incidence, severity, and the etiology of inadequate treatment. *Anesthesiol Clin North Am* 1989;7:1–15.

110. Bostrom M. Summary of the Mayday Fund Survey: public attitudes about pain and analgesics. *J Pain Symptom Manage* 1997;13(3):166–168.

111. Stieg RL, Lippe P, Shepard TA. Roadblocks to effective pain treatment. *Med Clin North Am* 1999;83(3):809–821.

112. Gilson AM, Maurer MA, Joranson DE. State medical board members' beliefs about pain, addiction, and diversion and abuse: a changing regulatory environment. *J Pain* 2007;8(9):682–691.

113. Ballantyne JC, Carwood C. Optimal postoperative analgesia. In: Fleisher LA, ed. *Evidence Based Practice of Anesthesiology.* Philadelphia, PA: W B Saunders Company, 2004:449–457.

114. Price DD, Mao J, Mayer DJ. Central mechanisms of normal and abnormal pain states. In: Fields HL, Liebeskine JC, eds. *Progress in Pain Research and Management*. Seattle, WA: IASP Press, 1994:61–84.

115. Woolf CJ. Evidence for a central component of post-injury pain hypersensitivity. *Nature* 1983;306(5944):686–688.

116. Ji RR, Woolf CJ. Neuronal plasticity and signal transduction in nociceptive neurons: implications for the initiation and maintenance of pathological pain. *Neurobiol Dis* 2001;8(1):1–10.

117. Ma QP, Allchorne AJ, Woolf CJ. Morphine, the NMDA receptor antagonist MK801 and the tachykinin NK1 receptor antagonist RP67580 attenuate the development of inflammation-induced progressive tactile hypersensitivity. *Pain* 1998;77(1):49–57.

118. Coderre TJ, Katz J, Vaccarino AL, et al. Contribution of central neuroplasticity to pathological pain: review of clinical and experimental evidence. *Pain* 1993;52(3):259–285.

119. Liu S, Carpenter RL, Neal JM. Epidural anesthesia and analgesia. Their role in postoperative outcome. *Anesthesiology* 1995;82(6):1474–1506.

120. Hall GM, Ali W. The stress response and its modification by regional anaesthesia. *Anaesthesia* 1998;53(suppl 2):10–12.

121. Tasmuth T, Estlanderb AM, Kalso E. Effect of present pain and mood on the memory of past postoperative pain in women treated surgically for breast cancer. *Pain* 1996;68(2–3):343–347.

122. Desbiens NA, Wu AW, Alzola C, et al. Pain during hospitalization is associated with continued pain six months later in survivors of serious illness. The SUPPORT Investigators. Study to Understand Prognoses and Preferences for Outcomes and Risks of Treatments. *Am J Med* 1997;102(3):269–276.

123. Approaches to Pain Management, Second Edition (PDF book) – Joint Commission Resources. Available at: http://www.jcrinc.com/e-books/EBAPM10/2213/. Accessed November 3, 2010.

20

Complications Associated with Continuous Epidural Analgesia

Christopher L. Wu and Jean-Pierre P. Ouanes

Postoperative epidural analgesia is a relatively safe and efficacious method for controlling postoperative pain. Systematic analysis of available randomized and nonrandomized data indicates that compared with systemic opioids epidural analgesia provides significantly superior analgesia in the postoperative period[1,2] (Table 20-1). In addition, perioperative epidural analgesia may confer some physiologic benefits. Some data suggest that epidural analgesia may be associated with improvements in postoperative morbidity and possibly mortality,[3–6] although the effect on outcomes may vary depending on many factors, including the congruency of the catheter placement in relationship to the incisional site, the analgesic agent administered (opioid vs. local anesthetic), and the duration of epidural analgesia[7]. Postoperative epidural analgesia may also be associated with improvements in patient-oriented outcomes such as patient satisfaction and quality of life.[8,9]

Despite the potential benefits of continuous epidural analgesia for postoperative pain management, there are risks and complications associated with the use of this technique. The majority of these complications (e.g., nausea, vomiting, itching, urinary retention, motor block, catheter failure) are not life threatening but may be bothersome for the patient, decrease patient satisfaction and quality of recovery, or even delay postoperative convalescence. Other complications are much less common (e.g., intravascular or intrathecal migration), and some can result in permanent and devastating injuries (e.g., epidural hematoma or abscess).

In general, complications from continuous epidural analgesia can be categorized as medication related or catheter related. Medication-related complications include nausea, vomiting, pruritus, motor block, hypotension, and respiratory depression. Catheter-related complications include catheter failure/dislodgement, intrathecal or intravascular migration, and epidural hematoma or abscess. Many of the rare but devastating complications that may be associated with continuous epidural analgesia are described in greater detail in other chapters (Chapter 4, *Bleeding Complications*; Chapter 5, *Infectious Complications*; Chapter 7, *Local Anesthetic Systemic Toxicity*; and Chapter 11, *Local Anesthetic Neurotoxicity and Cauda Equina*). In this chapter, we focus on some of the more common medication- and catheter-related side effects and complications associated with continuous epidural analgesia.

▶ MEDICATION-RELATED COMPLICATIONS

Although many agents may be used for postoperative epidural analgesia, the two most common agents administered for continuous epidural analgesia are opioids and local anesthetics. As would be expected, there are differences in the incidences of side effects between epidurally administered opioids and local anesthetic. Opioids and local anesthetic are typically administered in tandem, as this combination may provide at least additive if not synergistic analgesia while minimizing the incidence of complications from each agent. Although the optimal epidural local anesthetic-opioid combinations are unknown, bupivacaine, ropivacaine, or levobupivacaine (≤0.125% bupivacaine or levobupivacaine, or ≤0.2% ropivacaine) are the local anesthetics typically chosen due to their differential and preferential clinical sensory-motor blockade[10–12]. A lipophilic opioid such as fentanyl (2–5 µg/mL) or sufentanil (0.5–1 µg/mL) is commonly used to allow for rapid titration of analgesia, especially if patient-controlled analgesia is chosen,[13–15] although a hydrophilic opioid (morphine 0.05–0.1 mg/mL or hydromorphone 0.01–0.05 mg/mL) added to a local anesthetic will also provide effective postoperative analgesia.[13,15] However, both opioids and local anesthetics may be used as the sole agent to provide continuous epidural analgesia. It should be noted that there may be a wide range of incidences quoted for each complication, which may reflect the variability in how each complication is defined (and thus recorded) in different studies.

TABLE 20-1 Large Trials or Systematic Reviews of Postoperative Epidural Analgesia					
STUDY	TYPE OF SUBJECTS	NUMBER OF SUBJECTS/TRIAL	STUDY DESIGN	ANALGESIC EVIDENCE[a]	SOLUTION
Block, 2003	MIX	6,698 S	META	1a	MIX
Brodner, 2000	MIX	6,349 S	OBS	2b	MIX
Broekema, 1996	MIX	614 S	OBS	2b	0.125% BUP 1 µg/mL SUF
Burstal, 1998	MIX	1,062 S	OBS	2b	MIX
Cashman, 2004	MIX	165 T	SYST	2a	MIX
De Leon-Casasola, 1994	CAN	4,227 S	OBS	2b	0.05/0.1% BUP 0.01% MOR
Dolin, 2002	MIX	165 T	SYST	2a	MIX
Flisberg, 2003	MIX	1,670 S	OBS	2b	0.25% BUP
Liu, 2010	ORTHO	3,736 S	OBS	1b	MIX
Liu, 1998	MIX	1,030 S	OBS	2b	0.05% BUP 4 µg/mL FEN
Lubenow, 1994	THOR	1,324 S	OBS	2b	MIX

TABLE 20-1 Large Trials or Systematic Reviews of Postoperative Epidural Analgesia (Continued)

STUDY	TYPE OF SUBJECTS	NUMBER OF SUBJECTS/TRIAL	STUDY DESIGN	ANALGESIC EVIDENCE[a]	SOLUTION
Marret, 2007	COLO	806 S	META	1a	MIX
Ready, 1999	MIX	25,000 S	OBS	2b	MIX
Rygnestad, 1997	MIX	2,000 S	OBS	2b	0.25% BUP 0.04 mg/mL MOR
Scherer, 1993	MIX	1,071 S	OBS	2b	0.375% BUP
Scott, 1995	MIX	1,014 S	OBS	2b	0.1% BUP 1–10 µg/mL FEN
Tan, 2010	MIX	928 S	OBS	1b	0.125% BUP + 2µg/mL FEN
Tanaka, 1993	ABD	40,010S	OBS	2b	MIX
Werawatganon, 2005	ABD	711 S	SYS	1a	MIX
Wheatley, 2001	MIX	n/a	SYST	2a	MIX
Wigfull, 2001	MIX	1,057 S	OBS	2b	0.1% BUP 5 µg/mL FEN
Wu, 2005	MIX	50 T	META	1a	MIX

ABD (abdominal), BUP (bupivacaine), CAN (cancer), COLO (colorectal), FEN (fentanyl), META (meta-analysis), MIX (mixed), n/a (not available), MOR (morphine), OBS (observational study), S (subjects), SUF (sufentanil), SYST (systematic review), T (trials), and THOR (thoracic).

[a]Level of evidence based on recommendation from the Oxford Centre for Evidence-based Medicine Levels of Evidence (2001) (http://www.cebm.net/index.aspx?o=1025; accessed December 22, 2010).

Block BM, Liu SS, Rowlingson AJ, et al. Efficacy of postoperative epidural analgesia: a meta-analysis. *JAMA* 2003;290:2455–2463.

Brodner G, Mertes N, Buerkle H, et al. Acute pain management: analysis, implications and consequences after prospective experience with 6349 surgical patients. *Eur J Anaesthesiol* 2000;17:566–575.

Broekema AA, Gielen MJ, Hennis PJ. Postoperative analgesia with continuous epidural sufentanil and bupivacaine: a prospective study in 614 patients. *Anesth Analg* 1996;82:754–759.

Burstal R, Wegener F, Hayes C, et al. Epidural analgesia: prospective audit of 1062 patients. *Anaesth Intensive Care* 1998;26:165–172.

Cashman JN, Dolin SJ. Respiratory and haemodynamic effects of acute postoperative pain management: evidence from published data. *Br J Anaesth* 2004;93:212–223.

de Leon-Casasola OA, Parker B, Lema MJ, et al. Postoperative epidural bupivacaine-morphine therapy. Experience with 4,227 surgical cancer patients. *Anesthesiology* 1994;81:368–375.

Dolin SJ, Cashman JN, Bland JM. Effectiveness of acute postoperative pain management: I. Evidence from published data. *Br J Anaesth* 2002;89:409–423.

Flisberg P, Rudin A, Linner R, et al. Pain relief and safety after major surgery. A prospective study of epidural and intravenous analgesia in 2696 patients. *Acta Anaesthesiol Scand* 2003;47:457–465.

Liu SS, Bieltz M, Wukovits B et al. Prospective survey of patient-controlled epidural analgesia with bupivacaine and hydromorphone in 3736 postoperative orthopedic patients. *Reg Anesth Pain Med* 2010;35:351–354.

Liu SS, Allen HW, Olsson GL. Patient-controlled epidural analgesia with bupivacaine and fentanyl on hospital wards: prospective experience with 1,030 surgical patients. *Anesthesiology* 1998;88:688–695.

Lubenow TR, Faber LP, McCarthy RJ, et al. Postthoracotomy pain management using continuous epidural analgesia in 1,324 patients. *Ann Thorac Surg* 1994;58:924–929.

Marret E, Remy C, Bonnet F. Meta-analysis of epidural analgesia versus parenteral opioid analgesia after colorectal surgery. *Br J Anaesth* 2007;94:665–673.

Ready LB. Acute pain: lessons learned from 25,000 patients. *Reg Anesth Pain Med* 1999;24:499–505.

Rygnestad T, Borchgrevink PC, Eide E. Postoperative epidural infusion of morphine and bupivacaine is safe on surgical wards. Organisation of the treatment, effects and side-effects in 2000 consecutive patients. *Acta Anaesthesiol Scand* 1997;41:868–876.

Scherer R, Schmutzler M, Giebler R, et al. Complications related to thoracic epidural analgesia: a prospective study in 1071 surgical patients. *Acta Anaesthesiol Scand* 1993;37:370–374.

Scott DA, Beilby DS, McClymont C. Postoperative analgesia using epidural infusions of fentanyl with bupivacaine. A prospective analysis of 1,014 patients. *Anesthesiology* 1995;83:727–737.

Tan T, Wilson D, Walsh A, et al. Audit of a ward-based patient-controlled epidural analgesia service in Ireland. *Ir J Med Sci* 2011;180:417–421

Tanaka K, Watanabe R, Harada T, et al. Extensive application of epidural anesthesia and analgesia in a university hospital: incidence of complications related to technique. *Reg Anesth* 1993;18:34–38.

Werawatganon T, Charuluxanun S. Patient controlled intravenous opioid analgesia versus continuous epidural analgesia for pain after intra-abdominal surgery. *Cochrane Database Syst Rev* 2005;(1):CD004088.

Wheatley RG, Schug SA, Watson D. Safety and efficacy of postoperative epidural analgesia. *Br J Anaesth* 2001;87:47–61.

Wigfull J, Welchew E. Survey of 1057 patients receiving postoperative patient-controlled epidural analgesia. *Anaesthesia* 2001;56:70–75.

Wu CL, Cohen SR, Richman JM, et al. Efficacy of postoperative patient-controlled and continuous infusion epidural analgesia versus intravenous patient-controlled analgesia with opioids: a meta-analysis. *Anesthesiology* 2005;103:1079–1088.

Complications Associated with Epidural Administration of Opioids

When opioids are used as a solo agent for continuous postoperative epidural infusions, they offer several advantages over continuous local anesthetic epidural infusions in that they do not generally cause motor block or hypotension.[14] Epidural opioid infusions, however, may be associated with nausea, vomiting, pruritus, and respiratory depression (Fig. 20-1). These side effects are similar to those seen with systemic administration of opioids. Although lipophilic agents such as fentanyl and sufentanil may be used for continuous epidural infusions, the analgesic site of action for continuous epidural infusions of lipophilic opioids appears to be systemic rather than spinal,[16–18] as randomized controlled trials indicate no differences in plasma concentrations, side effects, or pain scores between those randomized to receive either intravenous or epidural infusion of fentanyl.[16,17] On the other hand, there may be more utility in administering a continuous epidural infusion of a hydrophilic opioid such as morphine or hydromorphone, where the analgesic site of action is primarily spinal,[15] which may be particularly useful in situations where epidural catheter insertion is not congruent with the site of surgery or when local anesthetic-related side effects (e.g., hypotension, motor block) interfere with the efficacy of postoperative epidural analgesia. Although a single dose or intermittent boluses of a hydrophilic opioid may be administered epidurally for effective postoperative analgesia, use of a continuous infusion may result in superior analgesia with fewer side effects[15,19] and may provide superior analgesia compared to traditional "as-needed" administration of systemic opioids.[20,21]

Nausea and Vomiting

Scope of the Problem. Postoperative nausea and vomiting (PONV) associated with continuous epidural analgesia is relatively common, with an overall incidence for continuous epidural analgesia ranging from 3% to 60%

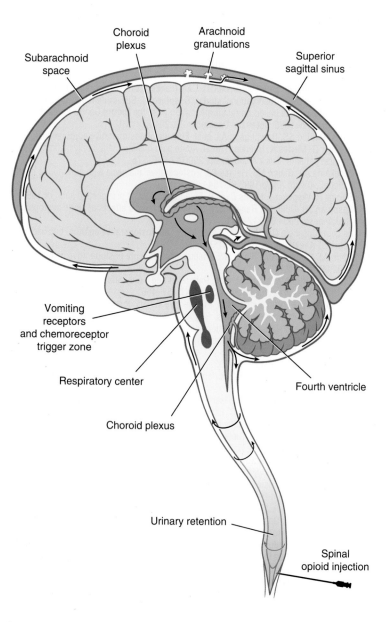

FIGURE 20-1. Anatomic sites of opioid action following neuraxial administration. Opioid administered along the neuraxis reaches the CSF, either directly during intrathecal administration or after diffusion from the epidural space through the dura and into the CSF. Within the CSF, the opioid circulates to more rostral centers within the CNS. Binding to specific receptors produces predictable opioid-related effects. Analgesia results from binding to specific receptors within the dorsal horn of the spinal cord and higher centers within the brain stem, notably the periaqueductal gray matter. Nausea and vomiting result from binding to receptors within the floor of the fourth ventricle, termed the chemoreceptor trigger zone. Binding to specific receptors within the vasomotor and respiratory centers located in the medulla oblongata produces the characteristic increase in vagal tone and respiratory depression associated with opioids.

(Table 20-2 and Box 20-1). A meta-analysis of randomized trials examining continuous epidural analgesia indicated that continuous epidural analgesia solutions consisting of a local anesthetic-based regimen (with or without opioid) appeared to generally have a lower incidence of PONV compared with an opioid-only regimen (i.e., up to 42% PONV with a local anesthetic-based solution vs. up to 60% PONV with opioids alone).[1] The selection of opioid appears to influence the incidence of PONV associated with continuous epidural analgesia, as the use of fentanyl (either alone or in combination with a local anesthetic) is associated with a lower incidence of PONV than continuous epidural infusions containing

---

BOX 20-1 Incidence of Nausea and Vomiting During Epidural Analgesia

- Infusions of opioid alone > combined opioid + local anesthetic infusions
- Morphine > fentanyl
- Continuous infusion > single-shot epidural injections (cumulative incidence)

TABLE 20-2 Overall Incidence of Side Effects and Complications of Continuous Postoperative Epidural Analgesia[a]

STUDY	PONV	PRURITUS	HYPOTENSION	MOTOR BLOCK	RESPIRATORY DEPRESSION
Block, 2003	5%–60%	2%–38%	1%–14%	1%–7%	n/a
Brodner, 2000	0%–11.9%	n/a	n/a	0.9%–50.1%	0%
Broekema, 1996	7.8%	14.9%	2%	6.5%	0.4%
Burstal, 1998	2.8%	2.4%	2.9%	8.4%	0.24%
Cashman, 2004	n/a	n/a	5.5%	n/a	0.1%
De Leon-Casasola, 1994	22%	22%	3%	n/a	0.07%
Flisberg, 2003	3.2%	4.4%	6.0%	3.4%	0.04%
Liu, 2010	30%	15%	10%	n/a	0%
Liu, 1999	14.8%	16.7%	6.8%	2%	0.3%
Lubenow, 1994	11.2%	14.1%	4.3%	1.1%	0.07%
Popping, 2008	25.4%	22.9%	5.0%	n/a	n/a
Ready, 1999	n/a	n/a	8%–11%	2%–51%	n/a
Rygnestad, 1997	18.6%	n/a	0.7%	3.5%	0.15%
Scherer, 1993	n/a	n/a	n/a	n/a	0.1%
Scott, 1995	3.1%	10.2%	6.6%	3%	0.4%
Tan, 2010	0.5%	0.1%	2.2%	1.7%	0%
Wheatley, 2001	n/a	n/a	0.7%–3%	0.1%–3%	0.24%–1.6%
Wigfull, 2001	n/a	1.8%	4.3%	0.1%	0.2%
Wu, 2005	21.8%–30.3%	28.3%–42.8%	n/a	3.2%–28.3%	n/a

[a]Complications as defined by the articles referenced. A range is given for systematic reviews. For multiple entries from individual studies (e.g., measured incidence of PONV for each POD), the highest incidence recorded is provided.
N (nausea); V (vomiting).

morphine.[20–24] In addition, the cumulative incidence of PONV may be higher in those receiving continuous infusions of opioids rather than a single-shot dose (45%–80% vs. 20%–50%).[22,23,25,26]

Pathophysiology. PONV from neuraxial opioids is related to the activation of the chemoreceptor trigger zone and area postrema in the medulla resulting from the cephalad migration of opioid within the cerebrospinal fluid.[27] Based on both clinical and experimental data, the incidence of PONV from neuraxial opioids appears to be dose dependent.[28–31]

Prevention and Treatment. Although a variety of agents (including naloxone, droperidol, metaclopramide, dexamethasone, and transdermal scopolamine) may be used to treat PONV, the majority of trials have examined these agents for the prevention and treatment of PONV associated with primarily single-shot neuraxial opioids, not continuous epidural infusions of opioids[25,26,32,33] (Box 20-2). One of the few studies to examine an intervention for PONV after continuous epidural analgesia with morphine was performed by Nakata et al., in which 120 patients undergoing thoracic or abdominal surgery received an intraoperative epidural injection of 2 mg morphine followed by a postoperative continuous epidural infusion of 4 mg/d of morphine.[26] Patients were randomized to receive saline, a single intraoperative dose of intravenous droperidol (2.5 mg), a postoperative continuous epidural droperidol infusion (2.5 mg/d), or a single intraoperative dose of intravenous droperidol (2.5 mg) followed by a postoperative continuous epidural infusion of droperidol (2.5 mg/d). Both intravenous and epidural droperidol significantly reduced the frequency and severity of PONV induced by continuous epidural morphine.[26]

Other randomized controlled trials have examined various interventions for the prevention and treatment of PONV resulting from a single-shot administration of opioid (e.g., spinal morphine for postoperative analgesia after cesarean delivery). All of the agents (serotonin receptor antagonists, dexamethasone, droperidol, metoclopramide, scopolamine transdermal) examined appear to be relatively efficacious in preventing or treating PONV associated with neuraxial opioids, although the data supporting the efficacy of each agent are somewhat equivocal. Dexamethasone (5 mg intravenously) appears to have the most consistent benefit for PONV associated with single-shot neuraxial opioids, with at least six randomized controlled trials supporting its benefit in the prevention of PONV associated with neuraxial opioids.[25,34–38] The patients in these studies were females undergoing a variety of gynecologic and obstetric procedures. However, two other studies[39,40] did not demonstrate a benefit of dexamethasone for PONV associated with neuraxial opioids. Droperidol and transdermal scopolamine also appear to be efficacious in reducing PONV associated with neuraxial opioids,[35,41–43] although these agents may not be commonly used in part due to some safety concerns (droperidol) or side effects (transdermal scopolamine).[44,45] Finally, the efficacy of serotonin receptor antagonists (e.g., ondansteron, tropisetron) on PONV associated with neuraxial opioids is equivocal, with some randomized controlled trials demonstrating a beneficial effect in reducing the incidence of PONV[39,46] while other studies showing no benefit.[36,47]

Pruritus

Scope of the Problem. Pruritus is a relatively common side effect from continuous epidural analgesia, especially for those analgesic regimens containing opioids[1] (Box 20-3). The overall incidence of pruritus for continuous epidural analgesia ranges from 2% to 38% (Table 20-2), although a meta-analysis indicated that continuous epidural analgesic solutions consisting of an opioid alone (incidence of ~7%–38%) will result in a higher incidence of pruritus than an epidural regimen containing a local anesthetic and opioid (incidence reported at ~2%).[1] Using fentanyl instead of morphine in the epidural analgesic solution appears to be generally associated with a lower incidence of pruritus.[22,24,48] The higher incidence of pruritus with continuous infusions of epidural opioids (which may be as high as 60% to 100% compared with a lower incidence of ~15%–18% with epidural local anesthetic administration or systemic opioids[48–50]) is similar to that seen with single-shot intrathecal opioid (typically morphine).

Pathophysiology. The etiology of neuraxial opioid-induced pruritus is unclear, although there are several theories. One postulated mechanism includes the presence of an "itch" center, similar to the emesis center for PONV.[51] Experimental studies suggest that this itch center may be located in the medullary dorsal horn or lower medulla that includes the trigeminal nucleus.[51,52] It does appear that the μ-opioid receptor may in part mediate neuraxial opioid-induced pruritus possibly via opioid antagonism of central inhibitory neurotransmitters (e.g., gamma-aminobutyric acid and glycine).[51,53] In addition, other receptors (especially the serotonin receptors) may play a role in neuraxial opioid-induced pruritus.[51] Peripheral histamine release does not appear to be an important etiology of neuraxial induced opioid pruritus. Clinical and experimental data suggest that there is a dose-dependent relationship between the incidence of pruritus and the dose of neuraxial opioid.[54–57]

BOX 20-2 Treatments with Proven Benefit for Nausea and Vomiting Associated with Epidural Analgesia

- Intravenous dexamethasone
- Intravenous droperidol
- Transdermal scopolamine
- Equivocal: ondansetron/tropisetron (serotonin receptor antagonists)

BOX 20-3 Incidence of Pruritus Associated with Epidural Analgesia

- Opioid alone > opioid + local anesthetic
- Morphine > fentanyl
- Continuous infusion ≅ single shot

BOX 20-4 Treatments with Proven Benefit for Pruritus Associated with Epidural Analgesia

- Naloxone
- Nalbuphine
- Low-dose propofol (nonobstetric patients)

BOX 20-5 Incidence of Respiratory Depression Associated with Epidural Analgesia

- Respiratory depression requiring naloxone administration occurs in <1% of patients receiving epidural analgesia.
- The incidence of respiratory depression associated with neuraxial administration of opioids appears to be similar to that following systemic administration of opioids.

However, a quantitative systematic review seems to indicate otherwise.[50]

Prevention and Treatment. A variety of agents have been used for the prevention and treatment of neuraxial opioid-induced pruritus, although the vast majority of studies have evaluated these agents primarily after a single-shot intrathecal dose of opioid (typically morphine) and not with continuous epidural infusions of opioid (Box 20-4). These agents include opioid antagonists, propofol, droperidol, and serotonin receptor antagonists. A systematic review indicated that both pure opioid antagonists (e.g., naloxone) and opioid agonist-antagonists (e.g., nalbuphine) were efficacious in the prevention of neuraxial opioid-induced pruritus. However, the higher doses of these agents (e.g., >2 µg/kg/h of naloxone)—which were more efficacious in preventing neuraxial opioid-induced pruritus—also decreased the quality of analgesia.[50] A randomized trial comparing nalbuphine (40 mg intravenous dose) to placebo indicated that nalbuphine was efficacious in preventing pruritus but was associated with increased drowsiness.[51] An interesting option for the prevention and treatment of neuraxial opioid-induced pruritus is propofol in subhypnotic doses. Randomized data in nonobstetric patients indicate that propofol is efficacious in preventing (10 mg bolus followed by 30 mg over 24 hours) and treating (10-mg bolus) neuraxial opioid-induced pruritus.[58,59] However, randomized controlled trials in obstetric patients do not confirm these benefits of subhypnotic doses of propofol.[60,61] Finally, because of the possible involvement of the serotonin receptor in mediating neuraxial opioid-induced pruritus, there have been several randomized controlled trials examining the efficacy of serotonin receptor antagonists (e.g., ondansetron) for the prevention or treatment of the incidence or severity of pruritus.[46,62–68] Two systematic reviews provide somewhat conflicting results, with an earlier systematic review suggesting that serotonin receptor antagonists significantly reduced the odds of pruritus (number needed to treat = 6) and intensity/treatment requests for pruritus[69] while a more recent meta-analysis indicated that serotonin receptor antagonists were ineffective in reducing the incidence of pruritus in patients undergoing Cesarean section, although the severity and need for treatment were improved with serotonin receptor antagonists.[70]

Respiratory Depression

Scope of the Problem. A relatively uncommon but potentially life-threatening complication of single-shot or continuous epidural infusion of neuraxial opioids is respiratory depression (Box 20-5). The incidence of neuraxial opioid-related respiratory depression may in part depend on the wide variety of definitions for respiratory depression used in individual trials (e.g., need for naloxone, ventilatory frequency, oxygen saturation below a predetermined level, or $PaCO_2$ above a predetermined level).[71] However, large-scale trials indicate that the overall incidence (typically based on the use of naloxone) appears to be <1% (Table 20-2). The incidence of respiratory depression associated with neuraxial administration of opioids is dose dependent and typically ranges from 0.04% to 1.6% (Table 20-2). A systematic review of 165 trials (which included a total of 50,642 patients with epidural analgesia) noted a mean incidence of respiratory depression necessitating naloxone use of only 0.1% (95% confidence interval [CI] of 0.1%–0.2%).[71] When used appropriately, neuraxial opioids (either as a single-shot or continuous infusion) do not appear to have a higher incidence of respiratory depression than that seen with systemic administration of opioids.[71,72] In fact, in one systematic review, the mean incidence of respiratory depression (necessitating naloxone use) for epidural analgesia (0.1% with 95% CI of 0.1%–0.2%) was significantly lower than that from intravenous patient-controlled analgesia with opioids (1.9% with 95% CI of 1.9%–2.0%).[71] Although the necessity of intensive care–like monitoring for patients who receive neuraxial opioids is controversial, many large-scale trials have demonstrated the relative safety (incidence of respiratory depression <0.9%) of this technique on regular surgical wards.[73–76]

Pathophysiology. The mechanism of neuraxial opioid-related respiratory depression is related to the interaction of the neuraxial opioid (whether it be systematically via absorption into the vasculature [i.e., early respiratory depression] or spinally via cephalad spread through the cerebrospinal fluid [i.e., delayed respiratory depression]) with the opioid receptors in ventral respiratory group in the brain stem, although the exact sites for opioid-induced effects on respiration have not yet been elucidated.[77,78] Although neuraxial administration of lipophilic opioids (e.g., fentanyl, sufentanil) may be associated with early respiratory depression due to the relatively greater systemic absorption, lipophilic opioids are generally considered to have a lower incidence of delayed respiratory depression than hydrophilic opioids (e.g., morphine, hydromorphone).[79–81] Delayed respiratory depression with neuraxial administration of hydrophilic opioids is generally related to the cephalad spread of opioid in the cerebrospinal fluid, which typically occurs within 12 hours following injection.[82]

Risk Factors. Although the risk factors for neuraxial opioid-related respiratory depression have not been clearly

BOX 20-6 Risk Factors for Neuraxial Opioid-induced Respiratory Depression

- Increasing age
- Increasing dose
- Concomitant use of systemic opioids or sedatives
- Presence of comorbidities (e.g., chronic pulmonary disease, obstructive sleep apnea)
- Thoracic surgery

elucidated, some identified risk factors include increasing dose, increasing age, concomitant use of systemic opioids or sedatives, and possibly prolonged or extensive surgery, presence of comorbidities, and thoracic surgery[82] (Box 20-6). In addition, more recent data suggest that the use of extended-release epidural morphine may be associated with significantly higher odds of respiratory depression compared to intravenous patient-controlled analgesia with opioids.[83]

Prevention and Treatment. It is important to note that typical clinical assessments, such as respiratory rate, may not reliably predict a patient's ventilatory status or impending respiratory depression.[28] There are no large-scale randomized controlled trials specifically examining various interventions for the treatment or prevention of neuraxial opioid-related respiratory depression. However, treatment with an opioid antagonist such as naloxone (0.1–0.4 mg intravenous boluses followed by a continuous infusion at 0.5–5 µg/kg/h if needed as the clinical duration of action is relatively short compared to the respiratory depressant effect of neuraxial opioids) and airway management if necessary is generally effective in treating neuraxial opioid-related respiratory depression.[13,18] Guidelines for the prevention, detection, and treatment of respiratory depression associated with neuraxial opioid administration have recently been published.[84]

Summary of Opioid-related Complications

Neuraxial opioids are a valuable analgesic option for postoperative pain management. The majority of side effects (e.g., pruritus, nausea, vomiting) are generally not life threatening but occur relatively frequently and can occasionally be bothersome for the patient. Severe respiratory depression is a far less common but potentially life-threatening side effect of neuraxial opioids. Judicious use (i.e., identifying the presence of risk factors) of neuraxial opioids would theoretically decrease the chance of neuraxial opioid-related respiratory depression.

Complications Associated with Epidural Administration of Local Anesthetics

Although continuous epidural infusions of a local anesthetic/opioid combination are most commonly used for postoperative pain management, epidural infusions of local anesthetic alone may also be used for postoperative analgesia but generally are not as effective in controlling pain and may be associated with a higher failure rate (from regression of sensory block and inadequate analgesia) and higher incidence of motor block and hypotension compared with the local anesthetic/opioid combinations.[14,85,86] Continuous epidural infusions of local anesthetic alone may be necessary in situations where epidural opioid-related side effects (e.g., nausea, vomiting, pruritus) are unbearable for the patient or in certain clinical situations (e.g., severe obstructive sleep apnea) where there may be a theoretical concern about the respiratory depressant effects from systemic absorption of a lipophilic agent, although the indications or contraindications for neuraxial opioids in these situations are unclear.

Hypotension

Scope of the Problem. Postoperative hypotension may occur with continuous epidural analgesia and is more common in those receiving a local anesthetic-based solution. Unlike opioids, local anesthetics administered neuraxially or used in an epidural analgesic regimen may block sympathetic fibers, which may contribute to postoperative hypotension. Systematic analysis of randomized trials indicates that continuous epidural analgesia with a local anesthetic-based solution results in a higher incidence of postoperative hypotension than a continuous epidural infusion of opioid alone (8%–14% with local anesthetics vs. 0%–1% with opioids).[1] Although there is a wide range (0.7%–14%) of postoperative hypotension reported with continuous epidural analgesia (Table 20-2), one of the largest systematic reviews (which examined studies incorporating 20,370 patients) reported a mean incidence of hypotension of 5.5% (95% CI of 3.2%–9.3%) by all definitions of hypotension (according to the definition provided in the individual studies).[71] This result was similar (5.6% with a 95% CI of 3.0%–10.2%) to that seen when hypotension was defined as a blood pressure below a predetermined level (e.g., systolic arterial pressure below 100 mm Hg).[71] Another large systematic review found the incidence of hypotension to be in the range of 0.7%–3%, although two large studies of patient-controlled analgesia with a local anesthetic-based solution reported incidences of hypotension of 4.3% and 6.8%.[14,87,88]

Pathophysiology. Hypotension from postoperative epidural analgesia is presumably due to the local anesthetic-induced sympathetic blockade, which results primarily in a decrease in systemic vascular resistance. Lumbar epidural catheter placement might theoretically result in less hypotension than placement in the thoracic region, in that a high thoracic sympathetic block might also attenuate the normal cardiac compensatory mechanism (increase in heart rate).

Prevention and Treatment. There are no large-scale randomized controlled trials specifically examining various interventions for the treatment or prevention of postoperative hypotension associated with continuous epidural analgesia (Box 20-7). If the patient does not have critical or life-threatening hypotension, treatment strategies may include decreasing the overall dose of local anesthetic (by decreasing either the rate or concentration), switching to an opioid-only epidural regimen (in that it is unlikely that neuraxial opioid administration *per se* would contribute to postoperative hypotension), or employing fluid administration and/or vasopressors.[13,14] It is important to consider other

BOX 20-7 Treatment Strategies for Hypotension Associated with Epidural Analgesia

- Ensure that hypotension does not cause life-threatening consequences (e.g., cerebral or cardiac hypoperfusion).
- Consider other etiologies first (e.g., ongoing surgical blood loss).
- Decrease the overall dose of local anesthetic by decreasing the rate and/or concentration.
- Switch to an epidural solution containing opioid alone.
- Administer fluids.
- Administer vasopressors.

BOX 20-8 Risk Factors for Appearance or Persistence of Motor Block During Continuous Epidural Analgesia

- Use of local anesthetic based solution rather than solution containing opioid alone
- Higher concentration of local anesthetic
- Lumbar (rather than thoracic) epidural catheter location

possible etiologies of postoperative hypotension before automatically attributing the cause of the hypotension to the epidural analgesic regimen.

Motor Block

Scope of the Problem. Unlike continuous epidural analgesia with opioids alone, use of local anesthetics for postoperative epidural analgesia may result in lower extremity motor block due to local anesthetic inhibition of motor fibers. Although there is a wide range reported for the incidence of motor block with epidural analgesia due in part to the differences in definitions for motor block (e.g., patient complaint of motor block, inability to ambulate, predetermined Bromage score), a meta-analysis of randomized controlled trials indicated that the incidence of motor block with postoperative epidural analgesia ranged from 1% to 7%.[1,87] Many large-scale observational trials report a slightly lower incidence of motor block, generally ranging from approximately 1% to 3% (Table 20-2.)

Pathophysiology. Lower extremity motor block from epidural administration of local anesthetic is presumably the result of the local anesthetic blocking the motor fibers from the spinal nerve exiting through the epidural space. Use of more potent or higher concentrations of local anesthetics may be associated with a higher overall dosage of local anesthetic administered into the epidural space, which may result in a higher incidence of motor blockade. As discussed in the subsequent section, the actual location of epidural catheter placement may influence the degree of motor block, as lumbar catheter placement would theoretically result in greater delivery of local anesthetic to motor fibers of the lower extremity, which may also result in a higher incidence of motor blockade.

Risk Factors. Risk factors for the development of motor block from continuous epidural analgesia appear to be use of a local anesthetic-based (rather than opioid alone) solution, a higher concentration of local anesthetic, or lumbar (rather than thoracic) epidural catheter placement (Box 20-8).[88–91] For instance, randomized trials of different concentrations of local anesthetics suggest that a higher concentration of local anesthetic is associated with a higher incidence of motor block.[89–91] Due to the segmental nature of epidural blockade by continuous epidural analgesia, it is not surprising that

lumbar rather than thoracic placement of an epidural catheter is likely to result in a higher incidence of motor block.[88]

Prevention and Treatment. There are no large-scale randomized controlled trials specifically examining various interventions for the treatment or prevention of motor block associated with continuous epidural analgesia (Box 20-9). One of the most obvious things a clinician can do to prevent motor block for surgical procedures in the abdominal or thoracic region is to insert the epidural catheter in a location congruent to the incisional dermatome (i.e., catheter-incision congruent epidural analgesia), although this may not be helpful if the surgical site (i.e., lower extremity) necessitates a lumbar placement of the epidural catheter. In terms of treatment of mild to moderate motor block associated with continuous epidural analgesia, changing the epidural analgesic regimen to a lower concentration of local anesthetic or even eliminating the local anesthetic and continuing with an opioid-only epidural regimen may decrease the incidence or severity of motor block.[89–91] The clinician should be aware of the potential dangers if the patient has a complete or persistent motor block, in that etiologies other than a relative excess of local anesthetic (i.e., epidural hematoma, epidural abscess, intrathecal catheter migration) may be the cause of the motor block, especially if the patient is receiving a low-dose/low-concentration local anesthetic-based epidural regimen.[14] Although stopping the continuous epidural infusion may result in improvement or resolution of the motor block or neurologic exam within 4 to 6 hours, persistent or increasing motor block should be promptly evaluated and other etiologies considered (e.g., epidural hematoma, epidural abscess, or intrathecal catheter migration), with appropriate medical consultation initiated if necessary.[14]

BOX 20-9 Prevention and Management of Motor Block During Continuous Epidural Analgesia

- Reduce the incidence by placing a thoracic epidural catheter for surgical incisions involving the thoracic dermatomes.
- Decrease or eliminate the local anesthetic in the epidural solution.
- Suspect other etiologies (e.g., epidural hematoma, epidural abscess, or intrathecal catheter migration) if persistent or complete motor block appears despite reduction or elimination of local anesthetic infusion.

Summary of Local Anesthetic-related Complications

Epidural administration of a local anesthetic-based solution is the cornerstone of effective postoperative epidural analgesia. However, epidural local anesthetic may be associated with a number of side effects (e.g., hypotension, motor block), which may decrease the overall analgesic efficacy of this technique. Although these side effects are generally not life threatening and are easily treated, one must recognize that the differential diagnosis for these side effects includes more insidious etiologies (e.g., epidural hematoma, shock), which should be considered during evaluation and treatment of the patient.

▶ EPIDURAL CATHETER-RELATED COMPLICATIONS

In addition to medication-related side effects and complications, the epidural catheter itself may be associated with postoperative complications. Some of the more serious complications are described elsewhere in this book (Chapter 4, *Bleeding Complications*; Chapter 5, *Infectious Complications*); however, it should be noted that guidelines and

practices advisories have been recently published for local anesthetic toxicity[92] and the use of regional anesthesia in patients receiving antithrombotic or thrombolytic therapy.[93] Despite being taped to the skin after insertion, epidural catheters may migrate out of the epidural space or into the intrathecal or intravascular spaces. Epidural catheters that are "fixed" to the skin by adhesive dressings or even by tunneling or sutures may occasionally exhibit both outward and inward movement of >2 cm.[94–96] Movement of the epidural catheter outside its intended location may result in catheter-related side effects and complications.

Intrathecal Catheter Migration

Scope of the Problem

One of the relatively uncommon catheter-related complications is migration of the epidural catheter from the epidural space into the intrathecal space. There is little data on the overall incidence of this occurrence. However, several large-scale observational trials indicate that the incidence ranges from 0% to 0.18% (Table 20-3).

Risk Factors

It is unclear what risk factors might increase the incidence of intrathecal migration of the epidural catheter. For instance,

TABLE 20-3 Incidence of Catheter Failure, Intrathecal Migration, or Intravascular Migration

CATHETER-RELATED STUDY	COMPLICATIONS/FAILURE[a]	INTRATHECAL MIGRATION	INTRAVASCULAR MIGRATION
Brodner, 2000	3.2%–5.6%	n/a	n/a
Burstal, 1998	13%	0.09%	0.28%
De Leon-Casasola, 1994	1.6%	0%	0%
Dolin, 2002	5.7%	n/a	n/a
Liu, 1999	12%	0.1%	0%
Lubenow, 1994	6.2%	n/a	n/a
Popping, 2008	7%	n/a	n/a
Ready, 1991	5.0%	0.2%	0.2%
Ready, 1999	17%	n/a	n/a
Scherer, 1993	n/a	0%	n/a
Scott, 1995	18.7%	0.1%	n/a
Tanaka, 1993	4.1%	n/a	0.67%
Wheatley, 2001	n/a	0.15%–0.18%	0.18%
Wigfull, 2001	14.5%	n/a	n/a
Range	1.6%–18.7%	0%–0.2%	0.18%–0.67%

[a]Incidence of dislodgement was recorded if available.

different catheter stiffnesses may result in a differential ability to penetrate human tissue such as the dura mater or even blood vessels.

Mechanism

There are two main types of epidural catheters, with one being a stiffer nylon/polyurethane-based epidural catheter and the other being a more flexible coil-reinforced epidural catheter.[97,98] Nylon/polyurethane catheters have a bending stiffness twice as high as that of coil-reinforced catheters (i.e., coil-reinforced catheters are more flexible).[98] On the other hand, wire-styletted nylon/polyurethane-based epidural catheters had a 23- to 90-fold greater bending stiffness than that of the nonstyletted nylon/polyurethane-based epidural catheters (i.e., nonstyletted catheters are more flexible).[98] Although the clinical importance of these findings is unclear, one might speculate that "stiffer" epidural catheters may have a higher incidence of intrathecal or intravascular insertion or migration despite the fact that there are no large-scale trials to confirm this.[97] In a nonrandomized trial comparing 1,352 parturients who received a coil-reinforced flexible epidural catheter for labor analgesia with 1,260 parturients who received a stiffer nylon/polyurethane-based epidural catheter, the catheter perforated the dura mater in 0.4% of cases with both catheters.[99] In addition, one might speculate that using a combined spinal-epidural technique might increase the risk of intrathecal migration of the epidural catheter. However, a study using a human cadaveric model indicated that neither a 19-gauge Arrow Flex Tip Plus (Arrow International Inc., Reading, MI, USA) single-port catheter (i.e., flexible) nor a 20-gauge Portex (Sims Portex, Hythe, Kent, UK) three-port closed-end tip catheter (i.e., nonflexible) was able to pass through the hole created by a single 25-gauge Whitacre spinal needle puncture (0 of 90 attempts for each).[100] Neither catheter penetrated the intact dura in this model.[100]

The reason migration of the epidural catheter from the epidural space into the intrathecal space is important is that the analgesic dose for the epidural space is approximately 10 times that for the intrathecal space.[101] This may result in a relative overdose of either local anesthetic or opioid, causing an excessive motor-sensory block, hypotension, or respiratory depression.

Diagnosis, Prevention, and Treatment

Although there are no large-scale randomized controlled trials specifically examining various interventions for the treatment or prevention of intrathecal catheter migration (as would be expected from the relatively low incidence of this complication), the clinician should be aware of the possible presenting signs and differential diagnosis, which also includes several potentially devastating diagnoses such as epidural hematoma and epidural abscess, both of which may also present with excessive or complete motor block. Lack of aspiration of cerebrospinal fluid from a suspected epidural catheter does not preclude the catheter from being intrathecal. If intrathecal migration of the epidural catheter has indeed occurred, stopping the continuous epidural infusion will result in improvement or resolution of the motor block with normalization of the neurologic exam within 4 to 6 hours. However, if persistent or increasing motor block should occur, other etiologies should be considered

(e.g., epidural hematoma, epidural abscess) and appropriate medical consultation initiated.

Intravascular Catheter Migration

Scope of the Problem

Another relatively uncommon catheter-related complication is the migration of the epidural catheter from the epidural space into a blood vessel, such as epidural veins. Several large-scale observational trials indicate that the incidence ranges from 0% to 0.67% (Table 20-3). This is similar to the intravascular migration rate (0.25%) reported in a large-scale cohort study of 19,259 neuraxial blocks for labor analgesia.[102]

Risk Factors and Mechanism

It is unclear what risk factors might increase the incidence of intravascular migration of the epidural catheter. Theoretically, the different catheter stiffnesses of the stiffer nylon/polyurethane-based epidural catheter and the more flexible coil-reinforced epidural catheter may result in a different incidence of epidural vein cannulation or intravascular catheter migration.[97] Although there is no large-scale data on the incidence of intravascular migration between different epidural catheter types, there are some data on accidental venous cannulation. In a nonrandomized trial of 2,612 parturients, the incidence of epidural venipuncture was 1.1% with a more flexible coil-reinforced epidural catheter versus 5.7% with a stiffer nylon/polyurethane-based epidural catheter ($p < .0001$).[99] In another study of 222 attempts at epidural placement in parturients requesting epidural analgesia for labor, the incidence of epidural venipuncture was 0% with a more flexible coil-reinforced epidural catheter versus 10% with a stiffer nylon/polyurethane-based epidural catheter ($p < .0001$).[97] These overall rates of accidental venous puncture (~3.3%–5%)[97,99] are similar to that (3%) reported in a large prospective observational study of 10,995 parturients who received epidural analgesia for labor.[103]

Diagnosis, Prevention, and Treatment

In instances where intravascular migration of the epidural catheter has occurred, the patient may present with inadequate analgesia (in that the analgesic agents are not being infused into the epidural space). Theoretically, systemic local anesthetic toxicity (as marked by signs and symptoms of tinnitus, perioral numbness, or even seizures or cardiac events) could occur as the local anesthetic is being infused into the vasculature. With appropriate dosing of the epidural regimen, it is unlikely the plasma concentrations of local anesthetics would reach toxic levels. Certainly, one potentially dangerous situation where the catheter has migrated intravascularly is if the clinician were to administer a large unfractionated dose of local anesthetic to a patient with severe postoperative pain (as would be expected for an epidural catheter that is not in the proper space). The clinician should aspirate the epidural catheter for blood and consider re-test dosing the epidural catheter (e.g., 3 ml of 1.5% lidocaine with 1:200,000 epinephrine) before administering the local anesthetic bolus in fractionated doses. There are no large-scale randomized controlled trials specifically examining various interventions for the treatment or prevention of the intravascular migration of the epidural catheter. In general, once intravascular migration of the epidural catheter has been identified, it is advisable to remove the epidural catheter from the patient and consider replacing it in a different location. Local anesthetic toxicity is more likely to result from this type of bolus than from the infusion of the local anesthetic-based analgesic regimen into the epidural vein. It should be noted that in patients with local anesthetic toxicity, only 60% exhibited the classic pattern of presentation while in the remainder of cases, there was an abnormal presentation of local anesthetic toxicity including cases where the symptoms were substantially delayed after the injection of local anesthetic.[104] Physicians should be familiar with the proper diagnosis and treatment (e.g., airway management, oxygenation, ventilation, basic life support, and lipid infusion) of local anesthetic toxicity when it occurs.[105]

Early Dislodgement or Catheter Failure

Scope of the Problem

Although systematic analysis of available data indicates that epidural analgesia does provide superior pain control compared with systemic opioids in the postoperative period,[1,106] a certain percentage of epidural catheters will fail through either actual premature dislodgement or removal due to side effects (as discussed earlier in this chapter). The incidence of premature removal or dislodgement of an epidural catheter may be surprisingly high. Some large-scale observation studies report a failure rate of as high as 14.5% to 18.7%, although a systematic review of 165 trials noted that actual premature epidural catheter dislodgement was only 5.7% (95% CI of 4.0%–7.4%)[2]. These failure rates are similar (~5%–7%) to those reported for labor epidurals.[102,103]

Prevention

The premature removal of epidural catheter decreases the overall analgesic efficacy of this technique. Even when secured to the skin (typically by adhesive tape/dressings or occasionally by suturing or tunneling[94]), epidural catheters can move relative to the site of insertion. Epidural catheters have been shown to move a clinically significant amount with reference to the skin regardless of body habitus as patients change positions, with some epidural catheters possibly being pulled partially out of the epidural space.[106] To prevent the epidural catheter from being pulled out of the epidural space, the authors of one study advocated that multiorificed epidural catheters be inserted at least 4 cm into the epidural space and that patients be in the sitting upright or lateral position while securing the catheter to the skin.[106] A randomized trial of 102 patients noted that a clamp device may significantly decrease epidural catheter movement.[96] Another randomized trial noted that a clear adhesive occlusive dressing with additional filter-shoulder fixation was significantly more efficacious in preventing epidural catheter movement.[95]

Summary of Epidural Catheter-related Complications

In general, epidural analgesia provides effective pain control. Occasionally, catheter-related complications occur when the epidural catheter is not in the proper location, which can decrease the overall effectiveness. Epidural catheter dislodgement probably occurs more frequently than previously realized. Other complications are much less frequent but potentially more ominous (e.g., local anesthetic toxicity with intravascular migration), especially in that other diagnoses (e.g., epidural hematoma) may have a similar clinical presentation (e.g., intrathecal migration).

▶ OTHER COMPLICATIONS ASSOCIATED WITH CONTINUOUS EPIDURAL ANALGESIA

Other complications associated with continuous epidural analgesia include urinary retention and pressure sores of the heel and other areas.

Urinary Retention

Scope of the Problem

Urinary retention may be associated with both epidural opioids and local anesthetics. The precise incidence of urinary retention associated with continuous epidural analgesia with either opioids or local anesthetics is unclear because patients who undergo major surgical procedures are often routinely catheterized. The incidence of urinary retention seen with neuraxially administered opioids may be as high as 70% to 80%,[28, 57] which is higher than opioids given parenterally (~18%).[49,57] The use of continuous epidural administration of local anesthetics may also be associated with a relatively high incidence of urinary retention, with a reported rate of approximately 10% to 30%.[107,108]

Pathophysiology

Urinary retention associated with neuraxial administration of opioids or local anesthetics is related to interference of detrusor contractility and decreased sensation of urgency. With the use of neuraxial opioids, the decreased bladder function is caused by a dose-dependent suppression of detrusor contractility and decreased sensation of urgency resulting from activation of the opioid receptors in the spinal cord.[27,109] Although some data indicate that neuraxial opioid-induced urinary retention does not appear to be dependent on opioid dose,[28,57,110] some recent experimental data suggest that a dose-dependent suppression of detrusor activity occurs with a dose-dependent recovery time.[109]

Treatment

Urinary retention associated with neuraxial administration of opioids may be treated with the use of low-dose naloxone. However, analgesia may be reversed with naloxone infusion.[111] Continuous epidural analgesia with local anesthetics causes a clinically significant disturbance of bladder function due to the interruption of the micturition reflex, with bladder function impaired until the block has regressed to the third sacral segment.[112] Thus, a higher dose of continuous epidural analgesia (either via higher infusion rates or concentration of local anesthetics) may be associated with a greater extent of sensory-motor block and higher incidence of urinary retention.[108]

Pressure Ulcerations

Scope of the Problem

Another complication associated with continuous epidural analgesia is the occurrence of pressure sores, typically of the heel. Although the precise incidence of this complication is unknown, several case reports of this complication associated with continuous epidural analgesia have been reported.[113–119]

Risk Factors

The risk factors for the development of pressure sores associated with epidural analgesia have not been fully elucidated. However, some factors reported include the presence of motor block or restricted movement of the legs, or patient-related characteristics such as elderly, emaciated/debilitated, unconscious, bedridden, or those with metastatic cancer.[115,119] It is unclear whether intraoperative or postoperative factors predominate, but pressure sores may occur as soon as the first postoperative day.[115,119]

Prevention

Whether routine assessment for such problems should be a part of routine monitoring in patients receiving continuous epidural analgesia is controversial. Interventions that have been reported (but not proven) to prevent pressure sores include the use of pressure-relieving mattresses and heel pads, avoidance of hypotension and motor/sensory block, and turning patients with motor block on a regular basis.[115]

► SUMMARY

Continuous epidural analgesia is a common and efficacious method of postoperative pain management. Like any other technique, there are risks, side effects, and complications associated with continuous epidural analgesia, some of which are rare but devastating. The vast majority of side effects and complications are bothersome for the patient but rarely life threatening. Clinicians should evaluate the use of continuous epidural analgesia on an individual basis, assessing both the benefits and the risks of this technique for each particular patient and surgical intervention.

References

1. Block BM, Liu SS, Rowlingson AJ, et al. Efficacy of postoperative epidural analgesia: a meta-analysis. *JAMA* 2003;290:2455–2463.
2. Dolin SJ, Cashman JN, Bland JM. Effectiveness of acute postoperative pain management: I. Evidence from published data. *Br J Anaesth* 2002;89:409–423.
3. Wu CL, Hurley RW, Anderson GF, et al. Effect of postoperative epidural analgesia on morbidity and mortality following surgery in medicare patients. *Reg Anesth Pain Med* 2004;29:525–533.
4. Ballantyne JC, Carr DB, deFerranti S, et al. The comparative effects of postoperative analgesic therapies on pulmonary outcome: cumulative meta-analyses of randomized, controlled trials. *Anesth Analg* 1998;86:598–612.
5. Beattie WS, Badner NH, Choi P. Epidural analgesia reduces postoperative myocardial infarction: a meta-analysis. *Anesth Analg* 2001;93:853–858.
6. Rodgers A, Walker N, Schug S, et al. Reduction of postoperative mortality and morbidity with epidural or spinal anaesthesia: results from overview of randomised trials. *BMJ* 2000;321:1493.
7. Wu CL, Fleisher LA. Outcomes research in regional anesthesia and analgesia. *Anesth Analg* 2000;91:1232–1242.
8. Wu CL, Richman JM. Postoperative pain and quality of recovery. *Curr Opin Anaesthesiol* 2004;17:455–460.
9. Carli F, Mayo N, Klubien K, et al. Epidural analgesia enhances functional exercise capacity and health-related quality of life after colonic surgery: results of a randomized trial. *Anesthesiology* 2002;97:540–549.
10. Stevens RA, Bray JG, Artuso JD, et al. Differential epidural block. *Reg Anesth* 1994;17:22–25.
11. White JL, Stevens RA, Beardsley D, et al. Differential epidural block: does the choice of local anesthetic matter? *Reg Anesth* 1994;19:335–338.
12. Zaric D, Nydahl PA, Philipson L, et al. The effect of continuous lumbar epidural infusion of ropivacaine (0.1%, 0.2%, and 0.3%) and 0.25% bupivacaine on sensory and motor block in volunteers: a double-blind study. *Reg Anesth* 1996;21:14–25.
13. Grass JA. Epidural analgesia. *Probl Anesth* 1998;10:445.
14. Wheatley RG, Schug SA, Watson D. Safety and efficacy of postoperative epidural analgesia. *Br J Anaesth* 2001;87:47–61.
15. de Leon-Casasola OA, Lema MJ. Postoperative epidural opioid analgesia: what are the choices? *Anesth Analg* 1996;83:867–875.
16. Loper KA, Ready LB, Downey M, et al. Epidural and intravenous fentanyl infusions are clinically equivalent after knee surgery. *Anesth Analg* 1990;70:72–75.
17. Sandler AN, Stringer D, Panos L, et al. A randomized, double-blind comparison of lumbar epidural and intravenous fentanyl infusions for postthoracotomy pain relief. Analgesic, pharmacokinetic, and respiratory effects. *Anesthesiology* 1992;77:626–634.
18. Guinard JP, Mavrocordatos P, Chiolero R, et al. A randomized comparison of intravenous versus lumbar and thoracic epidural fentanyl for analgesia after thoracotomy. *Anesthesiology* 1992;77:1108–1115.
19. Rauck RL, Raj PP, Knarr DC, et al. Comparison of the efficacy of epidural morphine given by intermittent injection or continuous infusion for the management of postoperative pain. *Reg Anesth* 1994;19:316–324.
20. Loper KA, Ready LB. Epidural morphine after anterior cruciate ligament repair: a comparison with patient-controlled intravenous morphine. *Anesth Analg* 1989;68:350–352.
21. Malviya S, Pandit UA, Merkel S, et al. A comparison of continuous epidural infusion and intermittent intravenous bolus doses of morphine in children undergoing selective dorsal rhizotomy. *Reg Anesth Pain Med* 1999;24:438–443.
22. Gedney JA, Liu EH. Side-effects of epidural infusions of opioid bupivacaine mixtures. *Anaesthesia* 1998;53:1148–1155.
23. White MJ, Berghausen EJ, Dumont SW, et al. Side effects during continuous epidural infusion of morphine and fentanyl. *Can J Anaesth* 1992;39:576–582.
24. Ozalp G, Guner F, Kuru N, et al. Postoperative patient-controlled epidural analgesia with opioid bupivacaine mixtures. *Can J Anaesth* 1998;45:938–942.
25. Tzeng JI, Hsing CH, Chu CC, et al. Low-dose dexamethasone reduces nausea and vomiting after epidural morphine: a comparison of metoclopramide with saline. *J Clin Anesth* 2002;14:19–23.
26. Nakata K, Mammoto T, Kita T, et al. Continuous epidural, not intravenous, droperidol inhibits pruritus, nausea, and vomiting during epidural morphine analgesia. *J Clin Anesth* 2002;14:121–125.
27. Chaney MA. Side effects of intrathecal and epidural opioids. *Can J Anaesth* 1995;42:891–903.
28. Bailey PL, Rhondeau S, Schafer PG, et al. Dose-response pharmacology of intrathecal morphine in human volunteers. *Anesthesiology* 1993;79:49–59.
29. Kelly MC, Carabine UA, Mirakhur RK. Intrathecal diamorphine for analgesia after caesarean section: a dose finding study and assessment of side-effects. *Anaesthesia* 1998;53:231–237.

30. Milner AR, Bogod DG, Harwood RJ. Intrathecal administration of morphine for elective Caesarean section: a comparison between 0.1 mg and 0.2 mg. *Anaesthesia* 1996;51:871–873.

31. Kirson LE, Goldman JM, Slover RB. Low-dose intrathecal morphine for postoperative pain control in patients undergoing transurethral resection of the prostate. *Anesthesiology* 1989;71:192–195.

32. Choi JH, Lee J, Choi JH, et al. Epidural naloxone reduces pruritus and nausea without affecting analgesia by epidural morphine in bupivacaine. *Can J Anaesth* 2000;47:33–37.

33. Moscovici R, Prego G, Schwartz M, et al. Epidural scopolamine administration in preventing nausea after epidural morphine. *J Clin Anesth* 1995;7:474–476.

34. Ho ST, Wang JJ, Tzeng JI, et al. Dexamethasone for preventing nausea and vomiting associated with epidural morphine: a dose-ranging study. *Anesth Analg* 2001;92:745–748.

35. Tzeng JI, Wang JJ, Ho ST, et al. Dexamethasone for prophylaxis of nausea and vomiting after epidural morphine for postcaesarean section analgesia: comparison of droperidol and saline. *Br J Anaesth* 2000;85:865–868.

36. Wang JJ, Tzeng JI, Ho ST, et al. The prophylactic effect of tropisetron on epidural morphine-related nausea and vomiting: a comparison of dexamethasone with saline. *Anesth Analg* 2002;94:749–753.

37. Wang JJ, Ho ST, Wong CS, et al. Dexamethasone prophylaxis of nausea and vomiting after epidural morphine for post-cesarean analgesia. *Can J Anaesth* 2001;48:185–190.

38. Wang JJ, Ho ST, Liu YH, et al. Dexamethasone decreases epidural morphine-related nausea and vomiting. *Anesth Analg* 1999;89:117–120.

39. Szarvas S, Chellapuri RS, Harmon DC, et al. A comparison of dexamethasone, ondansetron, and dexamethasone plus ondansetron as prophylactic antiemetic and antipruritic therapy in patients receiving intrathecal morphine for major orthopedic surgery. *Anesth Analg* 2003;97:259–263.

40. Nortcliffe SA, Shah J, Buggy DJ. Prevention of postoperative nausea and vomiting after spinal morphine for Caesarean section: comparison of cyclizine, dexamethasone and placebo. *Br J Anaesth* 2003;90:665–670.

41. Ben-David B, DeMeo PJ, Lucyk C, et al. Minidose lidocaine-fentanyl spinal anesthesia in ambulatory surgery: prophylactic nalbuphine versus nalbuphine plus droperidol. *Anesth Analg* 2002;95:1596–1600.

42. Kotelko DM, Rottman RL, Wright WC, et al. Transdermal scopolamine decreases nausea and vomiting following cesarean section in patients receiving epidural morphine. *Anesthesiology* 1989;71:675–678.

43. Loper KA, Ready LB, Dorman BH. Prophylactic transdermal scopolamine patches reduce nausea in postoperative patients receiving epidural morphine. *Anesth Analg* 1989;68:144–146.

44. Shafer SL. Safety of patients reason for FDA black box warning on droperidol. *Anesth Analg* 2004;98:551–552.

45. Kranke P, Morin AM, Roewer N, et al. The efficacy and safety of transdermal scopolamine for the prevention of postoperative nausea and vomiting: a quantitative systematic review. *Anesth Analg* 2002;95:133–143.

46. Yazigi A, Chalhoub V, Madi-Jebara S, et al. Prophylactic ondansetron is effective in the treatment of nausea and vomiting but not on pruritus after cesarean delivery with intrathecal sufentanil-morphine. *J Clin Anesth* 2002;14:183–186.

47. Pitkanen MT, Numminen MK, Tuominen MK, et al. Comparison of metoclopramide and ondansetron for the prevention of nausea and vomiting after intrathecal morphine. *Eur J Anaesthesiol* 1997;14:172–177.

48. Bucklin BA, Chestnut DH, Hawkins JL. Intrathecal opioids versus epidural local anesthetics for labor analgesia: a meta-analysis. *Reg Anesth Pain Med* 2002;27:23–30.

49. Walder B, Schafer M, Henzi I, et al. Efficacy and safety of patient-controlled opioid analgesia for acute postoperative pain: a quantitative systematic review. *Acta Anaesthesiol Scand* 2001;45:795–804.

50. Kjellberg F, Tramer MR. Pharmacological control of opioid-induced pruritus: a quantitative systematic review of randomized trials. *Eur J Anaesthesiol* 2001;18:346–357.

51. Szarvas S, Harmon D, Murphy D. Neuraxial opioid-induced pruritus: a review. *J Clin Anesth* 2003;15:234–239.

52. Thomas DA, Williams GM, Iwata K, et al. The medullary dorsal horn: a site of action of morphine in producing facial scratching in monkeys. *Anesthesiology* 1993;79:548–554.

53. Krajnik M, Zylicz Z. Understanding pruritus in systemic disease. *J Pain Symp Manage* 2001;21:151–168.

54. Ko MC, Naughton NN. An experimental itch model in monkeys: characterization of intrathecal morphine-induced scratching and antinociception. *Anesthesiology* 2000;92:795–805.

55. Stocks GM, Hallworth SP, Fernando R, et al. Minimum local analgesic dose of intrathecal bupivacaine in labor and the effect of intrathecal fentanyl. *Anesthesiology* 2001;94:593–598.

56. Herman NL, Choi KC, Affleck PJ, et al. Analgesia, pruritus, and ventilation exhibit a dose-response relationship in parturients receiving intrathecal fentanyl during labor. *Anesth Analg* 1999;89:378–383.

57. Slappendel R, Weber EW, Dirksen R, et al. Optimization of the dose of intrathecal morphine in total hip surgery: a dose-finding study. *Anesth Analg* 1999;88:822–826.

58. Torn K, Tuominen M, Tarkkila P, et al. Effects of sub-hypnotic doses of propofol on the side effects of intrathecal morphine. *Br J Anaesth* 1994;73:411–412.

59. Borgeat A, Wilder-Smith OH, Saiah M, et al. Subhypnotic doses of propofol relieve pruritus induced by epidural and intrathecal morphine. *Anesthesiology* 1992;76:510–512.

60. Beilin Y, Bernstein HH, Zucker-Pinchoff B, et al. Subhypnotic doses of propofol do not relieve pruritus induced by intrathecal morphine after cesarean section. *Anesth Analg* 1998;86:310–313.

61. Warwick JP, Kearns CF, Scott WE. The effect of subhypnotic doses of propofol on the incidence of pruritus after intrathecal morphine for caesarean section. *Anaesthesia* 1997;52:270–275.

62. Wells J, Paech MJ, Evans SF. Intrathecal fentanyl-induced pruritus during labour: the effect of prophylactic ondansetron. *Int J Obstet Anesth* 2004;13:35–39.

63. Waxler B, Mondragon SA, Patel SN, et al. Prophylactic ondansetron does not reduce the incidence of itching induced by intrathecal sufentanil. *Can J Anaesth* 2004;51:685–689.

64. Tzeng JI, Chu KS, Ho ST, et al. Prophylactic iv ondansetron reduces nausea, vomiting and pruritus following epidural morphine for postoperative pain control. *Can J Anaesth* 2003;50:1023–1026.

65. Korhonen AM, Valanne JV, Jokela RM, et al. Ondansetron does not prevent pruritus induced by low-dose intrathecal fentanyl. *Acta Anaesthesiol Scand* 2003;47:1292–1297.

66. Gurkan Y, Toker K. Prophylactic ondansetron reduces the incidence of intrathecal fentanyl-induced pruritus. *Anesth Analg* 2002;95:1763–1766.

67. Charuluxananan S, Somboonviboon W, Kyokong O, et al. Ondansetron for treatment of intrathecal morphine-induced pruritus after cesarean delivery. *Reg Anesth Pain Med* 2000;25:535–539.

68. Kyriakides K, Hussain SK, Hobbs GJ. Management of opioid-induced pruritus: a role for 5-HT3 antagonists? *Br J Anaesth* 1999;82:439–441.

69. George RB, Allen TK, Habib AS. Serotonin receptor antagonists for the prevention and treatment of pruritus, nausea, and vomiting in women undergoing cesarean delivery with intrathecal morphine: a systematic review and meta-analysis. *Anesth Analg* 2009;109:174–82.

70. Bonnet MP, Marret E, Josserand J, and Mercier FJ (2008). Effect of prophylactic 5-HT3 receptor antagonists on pruritus induced by neuraxial opioids: a quantitative systematic review. *Br J Anaesth* 2009;101:311319.

71. Cashman JN, Dolin SJ. Respiratory and haemodynamic effects of acute postoperative pain management: evidence from published data. *Br J Anaesth* 2004;93:212–223.

72. Etches RC. Respiratory depression associated with patient-controlled analgesia: a review of eight cases. *Can J Anaesth* 1994;41:125–132.

73. de Leon-Casasola OA, Parker B, Lema MJ, et al. Postoperative epidural bupivacaine-morphine therapy: experience with 4,227 surgical cancer patients. *Anesthesiology* 1994;81:368–375.

74. Ready LB, Loper KA, Nessly M, et al. Postoperative epidural morphine is safe on surgical wards. *Anesthesiology* 1991;75:452–456.

75. Stenseth R, Sellevold O, Breivik H. Epidural morphine for postoperative pain: experience with 1085 patients. *Acta Anaesthesiol Scand* 1985;29:148–156.

76. Rygnestad T, Borchgrevink PC, Eide E. Postoperative epidural infusion of morphine and bupivacaine is safe on surgical wards: organisation of the treatment, effects and side-effects in 2000 consecutive patients. *Acta Anaesthesiol Scand* 1997;41:868–876.

77. Takita K, Herlenius EA, Lindahl SG, et al. Actions of opioids on respiratory activity via activation of brainstem mu-, delta- and kappa-receptors; an in vitro study. *Brain Res* 1997;778:233–241.

78. Shook JE, Watkins WD, Camporesi EM. Differential roles of opioid receptors in respiration, respiratory disease, and opiate-induced respiratory depression. *Am Rev Respir Dis* 1990;42:895–909.

79. Swenson JD, Owen J, Lamoreaux W, et al. The effect of distance from injection site to the brainstem using spinal sufentanil. *Reg Anesth Pain Med* 2001;26:306.

80. Norris MC, Fogel ST, Holtmann B. Intrathecal sufentanil (5 vs. 10 microg) for labor analgesia: efficacy and side effects. *Reg Anesth Pain Med* 1998;23:252–257.

81. Katsiris S, Williams S, Leighton BL, et al. Respiratory arrest following intrathecal injection of sufentanil and bupivacaine in a parturient. *Can J Anaesth* 1998;45:880–883.

82. Mulroy MF. Monitoring opioids. *Reg Anesth* 1996;21 (6 suppl):89–93.

83. Sumida S, Lesley MR, Hanna MN, et al. Meta-analysis of the effect of extended-release epidural morphine versus intravenous patient-controlled analgesia on respiratory depression. *J Opioid Manag* 2009;5:301–305.

84. American Society of Anesthesiologists Task Force on Neuraxial Opioids, Horlocker TT, Burton AW, Connis RT, et al. Practice guidelines for the prevention, detection, and management of respiratory depression associated with neuraxial opioid administration. *Anesthesiology* 2009;110:218–230.

85. Kopacz DJ, Sharrock NE, Allen HW. A comparison of levobupivacaine 0.125%, fentanyl 4 microg/mL, or their combination for patient-controlled epidural analgesia after major orthopedic surgery. *Anesth Analg* 1999;89:1497–1503.

86. Scott DA, Beilby DS, McClymont C. Postoperative analgesia using epidural infusions of fentanyl with bupivacaine: a prospective analysis of 1,014 patients. *Anesthesiology* 1995;83:727–737.

87. Wigfull J, Welchew E. Survey of 1057 patients receiving postoperative patient-controlled epidural analgesia. *Anaesthesia* 2001;56:70–75.

88. Liu SS, Allen HW, Olsson GL. Patient-controlled epidural analgesia with bupivacaine and fentanyl on hospital wards: prospective experience with 1,030 surgical patients. *Anesthesiology* 1998;88:688–695.

89. Liu SS, Moore JM, Luo AM, et al. Comparison of three solutions of ropivacaine/fentanyl for postoperative patient-controlled epidural analgesia. *Anesthesiology* 1999;90:727–733.

90. Hodgson PS, Liu SS. A comparison of ropivacaine with fentanyl to bupivacaine with fentanyl for postoperative patient-controlled epidural analgesia. *Anesth Analg* 2001;92:1024–1028.

91. Scott DA, Beilby DS, McClymont C. Postoperative analgesia using epidural infusions of fentanyl with bupivacaine: a prospective analysis of 1,014 patients. *Anesthesiology* 1995;83:727–737.

92. Neal JM, Bernards CM, Butterworth JF 4th, et al. ASRA practice advisory on local anesthetic systemic toxicity. *Reg Anesth Pain Med* 2010;35:152–161.

93. Horlocker TT, Wedel DJ, Rowlinson JC, et al. Regional anesthesia in the patient receiving antithrombotic or thrombolytic therapy: American Society of Regional Anesthesia and Pain Medicine Evidence-Based Guidelines (Third Edition). *Reg Anesth Pain Med* 2010;35:64–101.

94. Chadwick VL, Jones M, Poulton B, et al. Epidural catheter migration: a comparison of tunnelling against a new technique of catheter fixation. *Anaesth Intensive Care* 2003;31:518–522.

95. Burns SM, Cowa CM, Barclay PM, et al. Intrapartum epidural catheter migration: a comparative study of three dressing applications. *Br J Anaesth* 2001;86:565–567.

96. Clark MX, O'Hare K, Gorringe J, et al. The effect of the Lockit epidural catheter clamp on epidural migration: a controlled trial. *Anaesthesia* 2001;56:865–870.

97. Banwell BR, Morley-Forster P, Krause R. Decreased incidence of complications in parturients with the arrow (FlexTip Plus) epidural catheter. *Can J Anaesth* 1998;45:370–372.

98. Eckmann DM. Variations in epidural catheter manufacture: implications for bending and stiffness. *Reg Anesth Pain Med* 2003;28:37–42.

99. Jaime F, Mandell GL, Vallejo MC, et al. Uniport soft-tip, open-ended catheters versus multiport firm-tipped close-ended catheters for epidural labor analgesia: a quality assurance study. *J Clin Anesth* 2000;12:89–93.

100. Angle PJ, Kronberg JE, Thompson DE, et al. Epidural catheter penetration of human dural tissue: in vitro investigation. *Anesthesiology* 2004;100:1491–1496.

101. Mercadante S. Neuraxial techniques for cancer pain: an opinion about unresolved therapeutic dilemmas. *Reg Anesth Pain Med* 1999;24:74–83.

102. Pan PH, Bogard TD, Owen MD. Incidence and characteristics of failures in obstetric neuraxial analgesia and anesthesia: a retrospective analysis of 19,259 deliveries. *Int J Obstet Anesth* 2004;13: 227–233.

103. Paech MJ, Godkin R, Webster S. Complications of obstetric epidural analgesia and anaesthesia: a prospective analysis of 10,995 cases. *Int J Obstet Anesth* 1998;7:5–11.

104. Di Gregorio G, Neal JM, Rosenquist RW, et al. Clinical presentation of local anesthetic systemic toxicity: a review of published cases, 1979 to 2009. *Reg Anesth Pain Med* 2010;35: 181–187.

105. Weinberg GL. Treatment of local anesthetic systemic toxicity (LAST). *Reg Anesth Pain Med* 2010;35:188–193.

106. Hamilton CL, Riley ET, Cohen SE. Changes in the position of epidural catheters associated with patient movement. *Anesthesiology* 1997;86:778–784.

107. Curatolo M, Petersen-Felix S, Scaramozzino P, et al. Epidural fentanyl, adrenaline and clonidine as adjuvants to local anaesthetics for surgical analgesia: meta-analyses of analgesia and side-effects. *Acta Anaesthesiol Scand* 1998;42:910–920.

108. Turner G, Blake D, Buckland M, et al. Continuous extradural infusion of ropivacaine for prevention of postoperative pain after major orthopaedic surgery. *Br J Anaesth* 1996;76:606–610.

109. Kuipers PW, Kamphuis ET, van Venrooij GE, et al. Intrathecal opioids and lower urinary tract function: a urodynamic evaluation. *Anesthesiology* 2004;100:1497–1503.

110. O'Riordan JA, Hopkins PM, Ravenscroft A, et al. Patient-controlled analgesia and urinary retention following lower limb joint replacement: prospective audit and logistic regression analysis. *Eur J Anaesthesiol* 2000;17:431–435.

111. Wang J, Pennefather S, Russell G. Low-dose naloxone in the treatment of urinary retention during extradural fentanyl causes excessive reversal of analgesia. *Br J Anaesth* 1998;80: 565–566.

112. Kamphuis ET, Ionescu TI, Kuipers PW, et al. Recovery of storage and emptying functions of the urinary bladder after spinal anesthesia with lidocaine and with bupivacaine in men. *Anesthesiology* 1998;88:310–316.

113. Cherng CH, Wong CS. Pressure sore induced by epidural catheter in a patient receiving postoperative pain control. *Reg Anesth Pain Med* 2003;28:580.

114. Alfirevic A, Argalious M, Tetzlaff JE. Pressure sore as a complication of labor epidural analgesia. *Anesth Analg* 2004;98: 1783–1784.

115. Shah JL. Lesson of the week: postoperative pressure sores after epidural anaesthesia. *BMJ* 2000;321:941–942.

116. Alexander R. Pressure sore following low-dose epidural infusion. *Anaesthesia* 2000;5:709–710.

117. Punt CD, van Neer PA, de Lange S. Pressure sores as a possible complication of epidural analgesia. *Anesth Analg* 1991;73: 657–659.

118. Pither CE, Hartrick CJ, Raj PP. Heel sores in association with prolonged epidural analgesia. *Anesthesiology* 1985;63:459.

119. Smet IG, Vercauteren MP, De Jongh RF, et al. Pressure sores as a complication of patient-controlled epidural analgesia after cesarean delivery. *Case report. Reg Anesth* 1996;21:338–341.

21

Continuous Peripheral Nerve Blocks

Brian M. Ilfeld and Matthew T. Charous

A perineural local anesthetic infusion—also called a continuous peripheral nerve block (CPNB)—may be used to improve postoperative analgesia. This technique involves the percutaneous insertion of a catheter directly adjacent to the peripheral nerve(s) supplying the surgical site. Infusing local anesthetic via the perineural catheter then provides potent, site-specific analgesia. This method was first described in 1946 using a cork to stabilize a needle placed adjacent to the brachial plexus divisions to provide a "continuous" supraclavicular block.[1] However, recent advances in needle technology, placement techniques (e.g., ultrasound), catheter design, and infusion pump mechanics have allowed practitioners to more easily provide continuous blocks. While evidence accumulates that continuous blocks provide multiple benefits, complications involving this technique do occur. This chapter reviews these possible complications, describes steps to minimize their occurrence, and details appropriate management when they do occur.

▶ DEFINITION OF THE PROBLEM

Complications related to continuous perineural local anesthetic infusion can take many forms, which in turn may occur during various stages of patient care. The major stages during which complications occur include: during catheter placement, during local anesthetic infusion, following infusion, and during ambulatory infusion.

▶ SCOPE OF THE PROBLEM

Unfortunately, the relatively recent widespread use of perineural local anesthetic infusion and lack of large clinical studies make evaluating the incidence of related complications problematic. One of the largest prospective investigations to date involving 700 patients receiving an interscalene perineural infusion following shoulder surgery suggested that the incidence of related complications was very low—at least as low as single-injection techniques.[2] Additional studies involving other catheter sites suggest a similar incidence of complications.[3–6]

► CAUSATION AND MANAGEMENT

Many of the complications that occur during catheter placement result from the needle used to place the catheter and are therefore similar (or identical) to complications of single-injection peripheral nerve blocks. Issues related specifically to perineural catheters are highlighted below, and readers are referred to Chapters 14 to 18 for thorough discussions on complications common to single-injection peripheral nerve blocks.

Complications During Catheter Placement

Inaccurate Catheter Placement

Inaccurate catheter placement may occur in a substantial number of cases. There are multiple techniques and equipment available for catheter insertion. One common insertion technique involves giving a bolus of local anesthetic via the needle to provide the initial surgical block, followed by the introduction of a catheter.[7–9] Using this technique, it is possible to provide a successful surgical block, but inaccurate catheter placement.[5,8–12] The inadequate perineural infusion will not be detected until after surgical block resolution, hours after placement. The incidence of this complication is presumably dependent upon many factors, including the experience of the practitioner, equipment and technique, as well as patient factors such as body habitus.[13,14] While the use of ultrasound guidance might, at first, appear to decrease the risk of this complication, it is often difficult to visualize the catheter tip location relative to the target nerve[8]; and techniques such as air injection may give a false-positive or false-negative result.[15,16] The reported range of what has been called "secondary block failure" is 0% to 40% (Box 21-1).[5,8,11,17] In an effort to decrease the chances of an unidentified misplacement, investigators have first inserted the catheter and then injected the initial local anesthetic via the catheter.[2,18–21] If a surgical block does not develop, the catheter may be replaced. Unfortunately, this technique decreases the incidence of surgical block and is best reserved for providing solely postoperative analgesia.[8]

However, even using this bolus-via-catheter technique, practitioners must wait 5 to 15 minutes for surgical block onset to determine if the catheter must be replaced. In an attempt to further improve catheter-placement success rates and decrease insertion time, "stimulating" catheters have been developed that deliver current to the catheter tip.[22–25] This design provides feedback on the positional relationship of the catheter tip to the target nerve prior to local anesthetic dosing.[18–20] There are data suggesting that stimulating catheters may be placed, on average, closer to the target nerve/plexus compared with nonstimulating devices.[26–28] However, it remains unclear if clinical benefits are provided compared with nonstimulating catheters.[29–32] In addition, stimulating catheters may take far more time to insert, on average, than nonstimulating catheters, especially when ultrasound is utilized.[9,33–36] The optimal placement techniques and equipment for perineural catheter placement have yet to be determined and require further investigation.[8,37]

Vascular Puncture

While puncturing a vessel is certainly a well-known complication of single-injection peripheral nerve blocks, this may be a more significant occurrence when placing a perineural catheter since the needle gauge is often larger to allow for endoluminal catheter insertion. The incidence of this complication is reportedly between 0% and 11% and most likely is influenced significantly by such variables as the anatomic block location, placement technique (e.g., ultrasound), and needle/catheter design.[3,6,17,19,38,39] Indirect evidence for the latter case was recently described by investigators who experienced no needle vascular punctures out of 76 infraclavicular catheters placed using the coracoid technique.[40,41] However, these same investigators using the identical coracoid approach reported an 11% incidence of needle vascular puncture using a different needle/catheter set.[19] Initial evidence suggests that vascular puncture can be reduced dramatically with the use of ultrasound, but definitive data have yet to be published.[8,9,33–36,42–44] Should vascular puncture occur, removal of the needle/catheter is indicated, direct pressure should be applied to the site, and distal vascular compromise ruled out. Prolonged Horner's syndrome due to neck hematoma is a rare complication but has been reported.[45] While a hematoma may require weeks for resolution (months for a Horner's syndrome), practitioners and patients should be reassured with the multiple case reports of complete neural recovery following hematoma resolution.[38,45–47] In some extraordinary cases, surgical incision and drainage may be necessary.[48]

If vascular puncture does occur, it is still possible to successfully place a perineural catheter using a nerve stimulator and insulated needle following a period of direct pressure, although a resulting hematoma will conduct electrical current and may decrease the ability to stimulate the target nerve with subsequent attempts.[19] Use of ultrasound guidance will render this issue mute.[8] Of note, clinically significant hematoma formation has been reported in patients with a psoas compartment catheter who received low molecular weight heparin for anticoagulation.[46,47] These occurrences have led some practitioners to manage patients with a psoas compartment catheter in much the same way as those having neuraxial block when thromboprophylaxis is ordered,[46] although others have questioned this practice.[49] The Third American Society of Regional

---

BOX 21-1 Secondary Block Failure

Initial bolus injection of local anesthetic via the needle or perineural catheter can produce an adequate primary block, but mask an improperly positioned catheter. This results in secondary block failure as the dense primary block dissipates, but the more dilute local anesthetic infusion fails to elicit an adequate analgesic block.

Anesthesia consensus statement on neuraxial anesthesia and anticoagulation now explicitly recommends that the same precautions as neuraxial techniques be exercised for deep procedures such as posterior lumbar plexus blocks/catheters—specifically, that any catheter be removed prior to administration of various anticoagulants at certain doses (e.g., enoxaparin 30 mg twice daily).[50] While "deep procedures" is not defined, presumably this subset includes psoas compartment, high sciatic, and possibly infraclavicular catheter insertion.

Intravascular Local Anesthetic Injection

Even if the bolus of local anesthetic for initial surgical block placement is given via the catheter, practitioners should be cautioned that intravascular injection with subsequent toxicity is possible.[51] As with all single-injection techniques, gentle aspiration should be performed prior to local anesthetic injection; repeated aspiration between divided doses of local anesthetic is warranted; and many, if not most, investigators have included epinephrine as an intravascular marker with all local anesthetic boluses.[52] Use of ultrasound does not preclude this complication, although it may decrease its incidence.[53] When a bolus is given via the needle, subsequent unintentional intravascular catheter insertion is still possible.[40,51] Therefore, investigators have recommended injecting a "test dose" containing epinephrine via the catheter prior to local anesthetic infusion initiation.[54] Practitioners should be aware of the signs, symptoms, and treatment for local anesthetic toxicity (Chapter 7).[52,55,56]

Perineuraxis Injection

When placing a catheter near the neuraxis as with the psoas compartment, interscalene, and paravertebral locations, it is possible to cannulate the epidural[57–61] or intrathecal[62] spaces. Injection of local anesthetic is potentially catastrophic and may result in unconsciousness and extreme hypotension requiring aggressive resuscitation.[63] In an effort to avoid intrathecal injection, gentle aspiration for cerebrospinal fluid should be conducted prior to local anesthetic injection. As with intravascular catheter placement, it is possible to accurately inject the initial bolus of local anesthetic via the needle, followed by cannulation of the epidural,[57] intrathecal,[62] and even intrapleural spaces with the catheter.[64] Therefore, a "test dose" containing local anesthetic should be injected via the catheter prior to local anesthetic infusion.[10,40,62,65,66] Obviously, a misplaced catheter should be removed and the patient observed for related complications.[62] Practitioners should be aware of the signs, symptoms, and treatment for intrathecal, epidural, or intrapleural local anesthetic injection and have appropriate resuscitation equipment immediately available (Chapter 18).[63] Of note, when working close to the neuraxis, it is possible to get epidural local anesthetic spread even with an accurately placed perineural catheter, resulting in a sympathectomy and possible hypotension.[39,59,67,68] Additionally, some practitioners recommend placing a perineural catheter only a small distance past the needle tip in an effort to ensure that the catheter does not migrate further than the desired target.[60,61,69] And while ultrasound guidance may render this complication a past relic, practitioners are urged to remain mindful of this possibility, at least until many years of further experience are gained with this relatively new modality.[8]

Nerve Injury

Nerve injury is a recognized complication following the placement of both single-injection and CPNBs, presumably related to needle trauma and/or subsequent local anesthetic/adjuvant neurotoxicity.[70] While one might assume that the larger gauge of most needles designed for catheter placement would increase the risk of nerve injury, the extremely limited evidence suggests otherwise.[2] In one prospective study of 521 patients with an interscalene block or catheter for shoulder surgery, 11% of patients with a continuous block reported either paresthesia, dysesthesia, or pain not related to surgery after 10 days, compared with 17% in the single-injection group (difference not statistically significant).[38] All but one of these cases resolved over the following 9 months. Another prospective study examined 1,398 CPNBs in 849 orthopedic patients.[6] Thirteen of these patients (0.9%) presented with neurologic deficits following catheter discontinuation; symptoms were transient in twelve of these patients. Examination of the one permanent nerve injury revealed a retroperitoneal hematoma in a patient with a continuous femoral nerve catheter for a total knee replacement. The origin of the hematoma was believed to be from injury to the femoral artery, though direct diagnosis could not be made.[6]

While the true incidence of neural injury is most probably related to the needle/catheter design, anatomic block location, and subsequent infusate selection, practitioners may be reassured that the current available evidence suggests that placing a perineural catheter during a regional nerve block does not appear to increase the risk of neural injury (Box 21-2).[2,4,38] The use of ultrasound guidance may decrease the risk of nerve injury,[44,71] but to date there are no data supporting this proposition, and nerve injury following ultrasound-guided peripheral nerve block does occur.[72–74] The identification and treatment of suspected neural injuries following catheter placement does not differ from single-injection techniques (other than possible catheter removal), and readers are referred to Chapter 14 for a thorough discussion regarding these important topics.[75]

Complications During Infusion

Dislodgement

One of the most common complications during perineural infusion is simply unintentional catheter dislodgement.[5,10,23,40,66,76,77] The reported incidence of dislodgement varies greatly between 0% and 30% and is most likely related to the anatomical location, equipment type, and technique used to secure the catheter.[17,77–79] Every effort to optimally secure the catheter must be made to maximize patient benefits. Measures have included the use of sterile liquid

---

BOX 21-2 Clinical Caveat

Limited data suggest that the placement of perineural catheters does not increase the incidence of perioperative nerve injury beyond that seen with single-injection peripheral nerve block techniques.

adhesive (e.g., benzoin), sterile tape (e.g., "Steri-Strips"), securing of the catheter-hub connection with either tape or specifically designed devices (e.g., "Statlock"), subcutaneous tunneling of the catheter,[22,80] and the use of 2-octyl cyanoacrylate glue.[81] Using a combination of these maneuvers,[18–20,82] investigators have reported a catheter retention rate of 95% to 100% for 6 to 27 days of infusion.[83,84]

Infection

While catheter site bacterial colonization is relatively common,[85,86] clinically relevant infection is not.[6,38,86–88] In one study involving 211 femoral catheters that were removed and cultured after 48 hours, 57% were positive for bacterial colonization.[85] Three patients (1.5%) had transitory signs of systemic bacteremia that were noted and resolved following catheter removal, and nine other patients (4%) had discomfort at the insertion site. However, ultrasound of the insertion site and the psoas muscle revealed no abscesses. In a retrospective study of 405 axillary catheters, the incidence of infection was 0.25%.[89] In prospective investigations of interscalene[38] and posterior popliteal[4] catheters involving over 800 patients, no infections were identified. In a subsequent study of interscalene catheters by the same authors, six patients (0.8%) out of 700 developed signs and symptoms of catheter site infection after 3 to 4 days.[2]

Three large series illustrate the low incidence of infection.[5,6,90] These series consisted of 1,398, 3,491, and 2,285 catheters, respectively, and revealed inflammation in 0.6%, 4.2%, and 4.2%, self-resolving infection in 0.2%, 2.4%, and 3.2%, and infection requiring surgical intervention in 0%, 0.8%, and 0.9%, respectively.[5,6,90] In addition, there is one case report of a psoas abscess following 4 days of femoral perineural infusion.[91] In these few cases, all infections completely resolved within 10 days.[91] Overall, the relatively rare incidence of infection may be related to local anesthetics' bactericidal and static properties.[61] However, major infectious complications do occur. These range from a nonsurgical abscess to florid sepsis requiring a prolonged intensive care unit admission.[48,92–94] With adequate medical treatment, all of these cases resolved, and there has never been a published case of permanent injury due to a perineural catheter infection.

Risk factors for perineural catheter-related infection include an intensive care unit admission, duration of catheter use >48 hours, absence of antibiotic prophylaxis, axillary and femoral sites, and frequent dressing changes.[88,95] Signs and symptoms of catheter site infection are similar to those of infection of any foreign body: local erythema, induration, purulent exudate, localized discomfort, as well as signs and symptoms of bacteremia. Treatment should include catheter removal, with the tip of the catheter sent for bacteriologic examination to help guide antibiotic therapy.[85] Ultrasonography is useful to help rule out an abscess requiring surgical drainage.[2] The available evidence suggests that clinically relevant catheter site infection is a very rare occurrence, and that with adequate treatment does not result in lasting impairment.[2,4,38,85,89,91] Limiting catheter use to 3 days will decrease the incidence of this complication, and practitioners should balance the need for analgesia with the risk of infection.[86,96] However, strict sterile catheter insertion technique is probably the most important factor in reducing the incidence of catheter site infection.[97]

Catheter Migration

While there are case reports of initially misplaced catheters, spontaneous migration into adjacent anatomic structures following a documented correct placement has not been described,[98] but remains a theoretical risk.[51,58,62,64,99] Possible complications include intravascular or interpleural migration resulting in local anesthetic toxicity and epidural/intrathecal migration when using an interscalene, intersternomastoid, paravertebral, or psoas compartment catheter. An early symptom may include a decrease in analgesia accompanied by signs of epidural/intrathecal anesthesia. Of note, it is possible to accidentally position the catheter tip in the epidural space (and presumably other structures) following partial catheter withdrawl.[57] Therefore, a test dose containing both local anesthetic and epinephrine should follow any catheter repositioning.[57,100]

Repeated large boluses of bupivacaine have resulted in myonecrosis in both animal models[101,102] and patients,[99,103] suggesting that intramuscular migration may have pathologic consequences (Chapter 15).[104] In minipigs, a bolus of bupivacaine followed by 6 hours of infusion resulted in severe tissue damage, whereas ropivacaine induced fiber injury of a significantly smaller extent.[105] Furthermore, bupivacaine results in far more muscle fiber apoptosis than ropivacaine in an animal model.[105–107] Although muscle injury has not been reported following a continuous perineural local anesthetic basal infusion (as opposed to repeated large boluses) in humans, practitioners may want to consider avoiding bupivacaine when using a catheter that is specifically placed into a muscle belly (e.g., a posterior lumbar plexus catheter placed using a nerve stimulator and insulated needle inserted into the psoas muscle).[59,67,108]

Signs and symptoms of myonecrosis include muscle tenderness, intensification of pain with stretch, pain relief with shortening, elevated serum levels of muscle-type creatine kinase, inflammatory or necrotic myopathy on electromyography, increased protein, blood flow, and edema in T1-weighted magnetic resonance imaging.[104] An abrupt decrease in surgical site analgesia accompanied by an increase in pain in the area of the catheter tip is suggestive of myonecrosis and warrants catheter removal.[104]

Delayed Local Anesthetic Toxicity

All practitioners using continuous block techniques should consider systemic local anesthetic toxicity due to a postoperative perineural infusion. The maximum safe doses for the long-acting local anesthetics as well as the incidence of systemic toxicity are unknown. There have been cases of patients reporting early symptoms of toxicity, such as perioral numbness, that resolved with infusion termination.[89,109] However, two subjects participating in placebo-controlled studies have reported early symptoms of toxicity that resolved upon infusion discontinuation, and each of these patients was subsequently found to have been receiving normal saline (unpublished data, Ilfeld et al. 2001). Investigators have reported successful analgesia and blood concentrations well below toxic levels using the following schedule with dilute (e.g., 0.125%–0.2%) long-acting local anesthetics (e.g., bupivacaine or ropivacaine) in patients free of renal or hepatic disease: basal rate of 5 to 10 mL/h, bolus volume of 2 to 5 mL, and lockout duration of 20 to 60 minutes.[77,84,87,109–118] Of particular importance is a prospective investigation of long-term (1–4 weeks) perineural ropivacaine 0.2% infusion that reported no evidence of local anesthetic toxicity, even though 2 of 15 subjects had serum plasma levels of ropivacaine in the toxic range.[84] Interestingly, the duration of the ropivacaine infusion was not correlated with the free concentration of local anesthetic.[84]

As a preventative measure, practitioners should consider reviewing the signs and symptoms of local anesthetic toxicity with patients receiving continuous nerve blocks. In addition, providing patients with the ability to self-administer bolus doses decreases local anesthetic consumption.[18-20,119-126] Finally, some investigators have utilized elastomeric pumps that provide "bolus-only" dosing when the patient releases a clamp on the tubing connecting the pump and catheter.[127-129] The patient is instructed to re-clamp the tubing after a specified period of time.[127,128] If a patient forgets to re-clamp the tubing, it is possible for the entire contents of the local anesthetic reservoir to be administered in under an hour. This potentially devastating scenario has been reported, although no apparent morbidity has yet occurred.[129] While the safety of this method may be demonstrated in the future, practitioners should consider the relative risks and benefits now that multiple pumps are available providing *controlled* bolus dosing.[120,130-133]

Nerve Injury

Continuous nerve blocks differ from single-injection blocks in that a catheter remains *in situ* and a larger total dose of local anesthetic may be delivered, albeit over a greater duration of time.[134] There is limited evidence that this increased exposure to local anesthetic may have negative consequences.[102] In an animal model, repeated boluses of 0.5% bupivacaine over 3 days led to a marked degree of disruption and vacuolization of myelin sheaths.[102] However, a 3-hour *infusion* of bupivacaine resulted in only minor injury to muscle tissue.[102] Furthermore, the prospective clinical evidence from human subjects suggests that the incidence of neural injury from a perineural catheter and ropivacaine (0.2%) infusion is no higher than following single-injection regional blocks.[38,89] There are two case reports of interscalene perineural catheters possibly resulting in brachial plexus irritation.[135] In both of these cases, repeated boluses of 0.25% bupivacaine had been injected over a period of days, and patient discomfort ceased upon removal of the catheters.[135]

In one case of prolonged sensory and motor deficit following a continuous femoral nerve block, postoperative electrophysiologic testing suggested subclinical polyneuropathy that was unknown preoperatively.[136] Long-term follow-up of this patient revealed complete sensorimotor recovery of the quadriceps muscles.[136] There is also evidence that in diabetes, the risk of local anesthetic-induced nerve injury is increased.[137,138] The identification and treatment of suspected neural injuries following catheter placement does not differ from single-injection techniques (apart from catheter removal),[139] and readers are referred to Chapter 14 for a thorough discussion regarding these important topics.[75]

Falls

Although pain fiber inhibition is the primary aim of CPNBs in the perioperative setting, local anesthetics affect other afferent and efferent nerve fibers.[140] Consequently, perineural infusion induces muscular weakness,[141] particularly concerning during perineural infusion involving the femoral nerve since ambulation is depended upon a functioning quadriceps femoris muscle. One meta-analysis of three randomized, double-masked, placebo-controlled studies found evidence that perineural infusion involving the femoral nerve does increase the risk of falling.[142] The risk of falling must be minimized, given that a fall may be catastrophic in many patients, especially the elderly.[143,144] Unfortunately, decreasing the concentration of perineural local anesthetic often results in not only less muscle weakness, but analgesia as well.[145] Alternatively, retaining the total delivered dose by increasing the delivered volume while decreasing the local anesthetic concentration has little effect on either sensory or motor block.[146] Practitioners should consider interventions that may decrease the risk of falls, such as minimizing the dose/mass of local anesthetic[146]; providing limited-volume patient-controlled bolus doses that allow for a decreased basal dose without compromising analgesia in some[19,147]—but not all—cases[18]; utilizing a knee immobilizer and walker/crutches during ambulation,[148] and educating physical therapists, nurses, and surgeons of possible CPNB-induced muscle weakness and necessary fall precautions.

Complications Following Infusion

Catheter Knotting and Retention

Multiple cases of catheter retention have been published,[19,149-152] and one retrospective study of nearly 6,000 catheters reported an incidence of 0.13%.[153] The most common etiology is knot formation below the skin or fascia and has been reported in fascia iliaca,[149] femoral,[150] psoas compartment,[151] and sciatic catheters.[152] Occasionally, a case requires surgical exploration for catheter removal.[150,151] However, removal of a knotted fascia iliaca catheter has been achieved using simple hip flexion,[149] or a relatively noninvasive technique involving fluoroscopy.[153] In all reported cases of knot formation, the catheter had been advanced more than 5 cm past the needle tip. Advancing the catheter more than 3 to 5 cm is often attempted in an effort to decrease the risk of dislodgement, or to "thread" the catheter tip toward the lumbar plexus when using the femoral or fascia iliaca insertion points.[6,12,95,121,123,153-158] Unfortunately, this practice probably increases the risk of a retained catheter due to a knot formed under the skin or fascia iliaca.[149,153] Retention rates of 95% to 100% have been reported using a maximum distance of 5 cm,[10,18-20,40,41,66,159] and—in the absence of using a catheter-over-wire Seldinger technique[121,123,157,158]—the catheter tip rarely reaches the lumbar plexus following a femoral insertion even when the catheter is advanced 15 to 20 cm.[154] Therefore, although there is no consensus regarding the optimal distance of catheter insertion, the available data suggest that insertion >5 cm is unnecessary and most probably increases the risk of catheter knotting.[149]

In an unusual case, a posterior lumbar plexus catheter tip was adhered to surgical tissue after intraoperative inadvertent coagulation forceps contact by the surgeon.[160] Catheter retention has also occurred when the metallic tip of a stimulating catheter became "caught" on underlying tissue.[19] Infraclavicular catheter insertion and postoperative infusion were uneventful, and the complication was discovered only after attempts at removal resulted in severe pain. Fluoroscopy did not reveal a knot, and the catheter was extracted surgically under general anesthesia. The overall incidence of this unusual complication is unknown, but of more than 10,000 stimulating catheters placed by one investigator, there was only one incidence of a retained catheter (Andre Boezaart, MD, *personal communication,* May 2003). Because the etiology of this complication remains unknown, steps for prevention are, at best, speculative. However, it should be noted that increased forward force placed on the catheter during insertion might increase the risk of the metallic end getting caught on surrounding tissue, and a paresthesia during catheter removal should be viewed as a warning sign.

Catheter Shearing or Breaking

It is possible to "shear off" a segment of catheter if, following insertion past the needle tip, the catheter itself is withdrawn back into the needle.[6] Therefore, this maneuver should only be attempted when using needle/catheter combinations that have been specifically designed for catheter withdrawal. And when using specifically designed needle/catheter combinations—such as with some stimulating catheters—catheter withdrawal should cease with any resistance, and the needle itself retracted until the catheter resistance resolves.[6,18–20,159,161] In one reported case, a 6-cm femoral catheter fragment was sheared off and remained *in situ* for 1 week, causing persistent pain of the ipsilateral groin, thigh, and knee.[162] Despite an embedded radio-opaque strip, the catheter fragment could not be visualized with plain radiographs. However, a computerized tomographic scan did localize the fragment and the femoral nerve neuralgia resolved in the week following surgical extraction of the fragment.[162] In an additional case, an axillary catheter fragment was diagnosed with ultrasonography and surgically extracted.[89] Practitioners should be reassured that in all of the case reports of retained catheters/fragments, no patient has experienced persistent symptoms following removal.[19,89,162] Finally, practitioners should document successful catheter tip extraction following catheter removal.[82]

Complications of Ambulatory Infusion

Outpatients may theoretically experience the same level of analgesia previously afforded only to those remaining hospitalized by combining the perineural catheter with a portable infusion pump.[82] However, complications that could be managed routinely within the hospital may take longer to identify or be more difficult to manage in medically unsupervised patients at home.[163] Because not all patients desire, or are capable of accepting, the extra responsibility that comes with the catheter and pump system, *appropriate patient selection is crucial for safe ambulatory local anesthetic infusion* (Box 21-3).[82]

Medical Complications

Related to this, investigators often exclude patients with known hepatic or renal insufficiency in an effort to avoid local anesthetic toxicity.[10,40,66,110] For infusions that may affect the phrenic nerve and ipsilateral diaphragm function (e.g., interscalene or cervical paravertebral catheters), patients with heart or lung disease are often excluded since continuous interscalene local anesthetic infusions have been shown to cause frequent ipsilateral diaphragm paralysis.[164]

> **BOX 21-3** Key Concepts for Successful Ambulatory Infusion Strategies
>
> - Appropriate patient selection—medically, psychologically, and with appropriate support systems—is crucial
> - Physician availability throughout ambulatory perineural catheter use
> - Understandable and specific verbal and written instructions
> - Thorough understanding of equipment, particularly portable infusion pumps

---

Although the effect on overall pulmonary function may be minimal for relatively healthy patients,[165] a case of clinically relevant lower lobe collapse in a patient with an interscalene infusion at home has occurred.[166] Conservative application of this technique is warranted until additional investigation of hospitalized, medically supervised, patients documents its safety.[167] In an effort to decrease complications, investigators have suggested that patients be contacted by telephone daily,[10,40,54,66,128] while others have provided twice-daily home nursing visits in addition to telephone calls.[168,169]

Patient Instruction

Since some degree of postoperative cognitive dysfunction is common following surgery[170] investigators often require patients to have a "caretaker" at least through the first postoperative night.[10,18–20,40,41,66] Whether a caretaker for one night or for the entire duration of infusion is necessary remains unresolved.[163] Although currently uninvestigated, there is consensus among investigators that both verbal and written instructions may decrease complications and should be provided, along with contact numbers for health care providers who are available throughout the infusion duration.[40,98,128,169] If catheter removal will be performed by the patient or caretaker, instructions provided over the telephone by a health care provider may help to avoid complications,[171] although multiple centers provide only written instructions for catheter extraction.[172,173] In one case in which instruction was not provided, a patient cut the catheter close to the skin, complicating removal and requiring extraction in the emergency room.[18]

Following a single-injection nerve block for ambulatory surgery, discharge with an insensate extremity results in minimal complications.[174] However, whether or not patients should weight bear with a CPNB of the lower extremity remains unexamined. Therefore, conservative management may be optimal and some investigators have recommended that patients avoid using their surgical limb for weight bearing.[20,66,175] This is usually accomplished with the use of crutches, and the patient's ability to utilize these aids without difficulty must be demonstrated prior to discharge. Protecting the surgical extremity must be emphasized, and any removable brace or splint should remain in place, except during physical therapy sessions.[82] The risk of falling with a femoral or posterior lumbar plexus local anesthetic infusion must be addressed as well (see above for discussion).[142]

Infusion Pump Malfunction

Multiple small, portable infusion pumps are currently available, and many factors must be taken into account when determining the optimal device for a given clinical situation.[82,130–133,176] A malfunctioning infusion pump is a challenging complication during ambulatory infusion since the pump is not easily replaced as is possible for hospitalized patients. There are little published data regarding the failure rates or reliability of the various pump models.[82,177,178] There are electronic pumps that have been noted to infuse without an erroneous alarm for over 10,000 cumulative hours of clinical use.[18–20,159] And while the nonelectronic pumps cannot trigger audible alarms, which are an irritant to both patients and health care providers,[168,179,180] there is also no warning if a catheter occlusion or pump malfunction occurs.[66]

▶ SUMMARY

There is a large and growing body of evidence that CPNBs provide a multitude of clinical benefits. However, because of the relatively recent evolution of modern techniques, illuminating data are often unavailable. Future prospective investigation is required to determine the optimal insertion technique(s) using ultrasound guidance; the true incidence of complications associated with perineural infusion; and the necessary procedures to minimize their incidence and optimize diagnostic evaluation and subsequent management.

References

1. Ansbro FP. A method of continuous brachial plexus block. *Am J Surg* 1946;71:716–722.
2. Borgeat A, Dullenkopf A, Ekatodramis G, et al. Evaluation of the lateral modified approach for continuous interscalene block after shoulder surgery. *Anesthesiology* 2003;99:436–442.
3. Borgeat A, Ekatodramis G, Dumont C. An evaluation of the infraclavicular block via a modified approach of the Raj technique. *Anesth Analg* 2001;93:436–441.
4. Borgeat A, Blumenthal S, Karovic D, et al. Clinical evaluation of a modified posterior anatomical approach to performing the popliteal block. *Reg Anesth Pain Med* 2004;29:290–296.
5. Neuburger M, Breitbarth J, Reisig F, et al. Complications and adverse events in continuous peripheral regional anesthesia. Results of investigations on 3,491 catheters. *Anaesthesist* 2006;55:33–40.
6. Wiegel M, Gottschaldt U, Hennebach R, et al. Complications and adverse effects associated with continuous peripheral nerve blocks in orthopedic patients. *Anesth Analg* 2007;104:1578–1582.
7. Grant SA, Nielsen KC, Greengrass RA, et al. Continuous peripheral nerve block for ambulatory surgery. *Reg Anesth Pain Med* 2001;26:209–214.
8. Ilfeld BM, Fredrickson MJ, Mariano ER. Ultrasound-guided perineural catheter insertion: three approaches but few illuminating data. *Reg Anesth Pain Med* 2010;35:123–126.
9. Mariano ER, Loland VJ, Sandhu NS, et al. Comparative efficacy of ultrasound-guided and stimulating popliteal-sciatic perineural catheters for postoperative analgesia. *Can J Anaesth* 2010;57:919–926.
10. Ilfeld BM, Morey TE, Wright TW, et al. Continuous interscalene brachial plexus block for postoperative pain control at home: a randomized, double-blinded, placebo-controlled study. *Anesth Analg* 2003;96:1089–1095.
11. Salinas FV. Location, location, location: continuous peripheral nerve blocks and stimulating catheters. *Reg Anesth Pain Med* 2003;28:79–82.
12. Ganapathy S, Wasserman RA, Watson JT, et al. Modified continuous femoral three-in-one block for postoperative pain after total knee arthroplasty. *Anesth Analg* 1999;89:1197–1202.
13. Nielsen KC, Guller U, Steele SM, et al. Influence of obesity on surgical regional anesthesia in the ambulatory setting: an analysis of 9,038 blocks. *Anesthesiology* 2005;102:181–187.
14. Coleman MM, Chan VW. Continuous interscalene brachial plexus block. *Can J Anaesth* 1999;46:209–214.
15. Sandhu NS, Capan LM. Ultrasound-guided infraclavicular brachial plexus block. *Br J Anaesth* 2002;89:254–259.
16. Swenson JD, Davis JJ, DeCou JA. A novel approach for assessing catheter position after ultrasound-guided placement of continuous interscalene block. *Anesth Analg* 2008;106:1015–1016.
17. Klein SM, Grant SA, Greengrass RA, et al. Interscalene brachial plexus block with a continuous catheter insertion system and a disposable infusion pump. *Anesth Analg* 2000;91:1473–1478.
18. Ilfeld BM, Morey TE, Wright TW, et al. Interscalene perineural ropivacaine infusion: a comparison of two dosing regimens for postoperative analgesia. *Reg Anesth Pain Med* 2004;29:9–16.
19. Ilfeld BM, Morey TE, Enneking FK. Infraclavicular perineural local anesthetic infusion: a comparison of three dosing regimens for postoperative analgesia. *Anesthesiology* 2004;100:395–402.
20. Ilfeld BM, Thannikary LJ, Morey TE, et al. Popliteal sciatic perineural local anesthetic infusion: a comparison of three dosing regimens for postoperative analgesia. *Anesthesiology* 2004;101:970–977.
21. Pham-Dang C, Kick O, Collet T, et al. Continuous peripheral nerve blocks with stimulating catheters. *Reg Anesth Pain Med* 2003;28:83–88.
22. Boezaart AP, de Beer JF, du Toit C, et al. A new technique of continuous interscalene nerve block. *Can J Anaesth* 1999;46:275–281.
23. Sutherland ID. Continuous sciatic nerve infusion: expanded case report describing a new approach. *Reg Anesth Pain Med* 1998;23:496–501.
24. Kick O, Blanche E, Pham-Dang C, et al. A new stimulating stylet for immediate control of catheter tip position in continuous peripheral nerve blocks. *Anesth Analg* 1999;89:533–534.
25. Copeland SJ, Laxton MA. A new stimulating catheter for continuous peripheral nerve blocks. *Reg Anesth Pain Med* 2001;26:589–590.
26. Salinas FV, Neal JM, Sueda LA, et al. Prospective comparison of continuous femoral nerve block with nonstimulating catheter placement versus stimulating catheter-guided perineural placement in volunteers. *Reg Anesth Pain Med* 2004;29:212–220.
27. Casati A, Fanelli G, Koscielniak-Nielsen Z, et al. Using stimulating catheters for continuous sciatic nerve block shortens onset time of surgical block and minimizes postoperative consumption of pain medication after halux valgus repair as compared with conventional nonstimulating catheters. *Anesth Analg* 2005;101:1192–1197.
28. Rodriguez J, Taboada M, Carceller J, et al. Stimulating popliteal catheters for postoperative analgesia after hallux valgus repair. *Anesth Analg* 2006;102:258–262.
29. Stevens MF, Werdehausen R, Golla E, et al. Does interscalene catheter placement with stimulating catheters improve postoperative pain or functional outcome after shoulder surgery? A prospective, randomized and double-blinded trial. *Anesth Analg* 2007;104:442–447.
30. Hayek SM, Ritchey RM, Sessler D, et al. Continuous femoral nerve analgesia after unilateral total knee arthroplasty: stimulating versus nonstimulating catheters. *Anesth Analg* 2006;103:1565–1570.
31. Morin AM, Eberhart LH, Behnke HK, et al. Does femoral nerve catheter placement with stimulating catheters improve effective placement? A randomized, controlled, and observer-blinded trial. *Anesth Analg* 2005;100:1503–1510.
32. Barrington MJ, Olive DJ, McCutcheon CA, et al. Stimulating catheters for continuous femoral nerve blockade after total knee arthroplasty: a randomized, controlled, double-blinded trial. *Anesth Analg* 2008;106:1316–1321.

33. Mariano ER, Loland VJ, Sandhu NS, et al. Ultrasound guidance versus electrical stimulation for femoral perineural catheter insertion. *J Ultrasound Med* 2009;28:1453–1460.

34. Mariano ER, Cheng GS, Choy LP, et al. Electrical stimulation versus ultrasound guidance for popliteal-sciatic perineural catheter insertion: a randomized controlled trial. *Reg Anesth Pain Med* 2009;34:480–485.

35. Mariano ER, Loland VJ, Bellars RH, et al. Ultrasound guidance versus electrical stimulation for infraclavicular brachial plexus perineural catheter insertion. *J Ultrasound Med* 2009;28:1211–1218.

36. Mariano ER, Loland VJ, Sandhu NS, et al. A trainee-based randomized comparison of stimulating interscalene perineural catheters with a new technique using ultrasound guidance alone. *J Ultrasound Med* 2010;29:329–336.

37. Chelly JE, Williams BA. Continuous perineural infusions at home: narrowing the focus. *Reg Anesth Pain Med* 2004;29:1–3.

38. Borgeat A, Ekatodramis G, Kalberer F, et al. Acute and nonacute complications associated with interscalene block and shoulder surgery: a prospective study. *Anesthesiology* 2001;95:875–880.

39. Boezaart AP, de Beer JF, Nell ML. Early experience with continuous cervical paravertebral block using a stimulating catheter. *Reg Anesth Pain Med* 2003;28:406–413.

40. Ilfeld BM, Morey TE, Enneking FK. Continuous infraclavicular brachial plexus block for postoperative pain control at home: a randomized, double-blinded, placebo-controlled study. *Anesthesiology* 2002;96:1297–1304.

41. Ilfeld BM, Morey TE, Enneking FK. Continuous infraclavicular perineural infusion with clonidine and ropivacaine compared with ropivacaine alone: a randomized, double-blinded, controlled study. *Anesth Analg* 2003;97:706–712.

42. Mariano ER, Afra R, Loland VJ, et al. Continuous interscalene brachial plexus block via an ultrasound-guided posterior approach: a randomized, triple-masked, placebo-controlled study. *Anesth Analg* 2009;108:1688–1694.

43. Mariano ER, Loland VJ, Ilfeld BM. Interscalene perineural catheter placement using an ultrasound-guided posterior approach. *Reg Anesth Pain Med* 2009;34:60–63.

44. Neal JM. Ultrasound-guided regional anesthesia and patient safety: an evidence-based analysis. *Reg Anesth Pain Med* 2010;35:S59–S67.

45. Ekatodramis G, Macaire P, Borgeat A. Prolonged Horner syndrome due to neck hematoma after continuous interscalene block. *Anesthesiology* 2001;95:801–803.

46. Weller RS, Gerancher JC, Crews JC, et al. Extensive retroperitoneal hematoma without neurologic deficit in two patients who underwent lumbar plexus block and were later anticoagulated. *Anesthesiology* 2003;98:581–585.

47. Klein SM, D'Ercole F, Greengrass RA, et al. Enoxaparin associated with psoas hematoma and lumbar plexopathy after lumbar plexus block. *Anesthesiology* 1997;87:1576–1579.

48. Clendenen SR, Robards CB, Wang RD, et al. Case report: continuous interscalene block associated with neck hematoma and postoperative sepsis. *Anesth Analg* 2010;110:1236–1238.

49. Chelly JE, Greger JR, Casati A, et al. What has happened to evidence-based medicine? *Anesthesiology* 2003;99:1028–1029.

50. Horlocker TT, Wedel DJ, Rowlingson JC, et al. Regional anesthesia in the patient receiving antithrombotic or thrombolytic therapy: American Society of Regional Anesthesia and Pain Medicine Evidence-Based Guidelines (Third Edition). *Reg Anesth Pain Med* 2010;35:64–101.

51. Tuominen MK, Pere P, Rosenberg PH. Unintentional arterial catheterization and bupivacaine toxicity associated with continuous interscalene brachial plexus block. *Anesthesiology* 1991;75:356–358.

52. Mulroy MF. Systemic toxicity and cardiotoxicity from local anesthetics: incidence and preventive measures. *Reg Anesth Pain Med* 2002;27:556–561.

53. Loubert C, Williams SR, Helie F, et al. Complication during ultrasound-guided regional block: accidental intravascular injection of local anesthetic. *Anesthesiology* 2008;108:759–760.

54. Klein SM. Beyond the hospital: continuous peripheral nerve blocks at home. *Anesthesiology* 2002;96:1283–1285.

55. Klein SM, Benveniste H. Anxiety, vocalization, and agitation following peripheral nerve block with ropivacaine. *Reg Anesth Pain Med* 1999;24:175–178.

56. Weinberg GL. Current concepts in resuscitation of patients with local anesthetic cardiac toxicity. *Reg Anesth Pain Med* 2002;27:568–575.

57. Cook LB. Unsuspected extradural catheterization in an interscalene block. *Br J Anaesth* 1991;67:473–475.

58. Mahoudeau G, Gaertner E, Launoy A, et al. Interscalenic block: accidental catheterization of the epidural space. *Ann Fr Anesth Reanim* 1995;14:438–441.

59. De Biasi P, Lupescu R, Burgun G, et al. Continuous lumbar plexus block: use of radiography to determine catheter tip location. *Reg Anesth Pain Med* 2003;28:135–139.

60. Frohm RM, Raw RM, Haider N, et al. Epidural spread after continuous cervical paravertebral block: a case report. *Reg Anesth Pain Med* 2006;31:279–281.

61. Rotzinger M, Neuburger M, Kaiser H. Inadvertant epidural placement of a psoas compartment catheter. Case report of a rare complication. *Anaesthesist* 2004;53:1069–1072.

62. Litz RJ, Vicent O, Wiessner D, et al. Misplacement of a psoas compartment catheter in the subarachnoid space. *Reg Anesth Pain Med* 2004;29:60–64.

63. Pousman RM, Mansoor Z, Sciard D. Total spinal anesthetic after continuous posterior lumbar plexus block. *Anesthesiology* 2003;98:1281–1282.

64. Souron V, Reiland Y, De Traverse A, et al. Interpleural migration of an interscalene catheter. *Anesth Analg* 2003;97:1200–1201.

65. Moore DC, Batra MS. The components of an effective test dose prior to epidural block. *Anesthesiology* 1981;55:693–696.

66. Ilfeld BM, Morey TE, Wang RD, et al. Continuous popliteal sciatic nerve block for postoperative pain control at home: a randomized, double-blinded, placebo-controlled study. *Anesthesiology* 2002;97:959–965.

67. Capdevila X, Macaire P, Dadure C, et al. Continuous psoas compartment block for postoperative analgesia after total hip arthroplasty: new landmarks, technical guidelines, and clinical evaluation. *Anesth Analg* 2002;94:1606–1613.

68. Singelyn FJ, Contreras V, Gouverneur JM. Epidural anesthesia complicating continuous 3-in-1 lumbar plexus blockade. *Anesthesiology* 1995;83:217–220.

69. Faust A, Fournier R, Hagon O, et al. Partial sensory and motor deficit of ipsilateral lower limb after continuous interscalene brachial plexus block. *Anesth Analg* 2006;102:288–290.

70. Al Nasser B, Palacios JL. Femoral nerve injury complicating continuous psoas compartment block. *Reg Anesth Pain Med* 2004;29:361–363.

71. Hebl JR. Ultrasound-guided regional anesthesia and the prevention of neurologic injury: fact or fiction? *Anesthesiology* 2008;108:186–188.

72. Neal JM, Wedel DJ. Ultrasound guidance and peripheral nerve injury: is our vision as sharp as we think it is? *Reg Anesth Pain Med* 2010;35:335–337.

73. Reiss W, Kurapati S, Shariat A, et al. Nerve injury complicating ultrasound/electrostimulation-guided supraclavicular brachial plexus block. *Reg Anesth Pain Med* 2010;35:400–401.

74. Cohen JM, Gray AT. Functional deficits after intraneural injection during interscalene block. *Reg Anesth Pain Med* 2010;35:397–399.

75. West GA, Haynor DR, Goodkin R, et al. Magnetic resonance imaging signal changes in denervated muscles after peripheral nerve injury. *Neurosurgery* 1994;35:1077–1085.

76. Singelyn FJ, Aye F, Gouverneur JM. Continuous popliteal sciatic nerve block: an original technique to provide postoperative analgesia after foot surgery. *Anesth Analg* 1997;84:383–386.

77. Tuominen M, Haasio J, Hekali R, et al. Continuous interscalene brachial plexus block: clinical efficacy, technical problems and bupivacaine plasma concentrations. *Acta Anaesthesiol Scand* 1989;33:84–88.

78. Borgeat A, Kalberer F, Jacob H, et al. Patient-controlled interscalene analgesia with ropivacaine 0.2% versus bupivacaine 0.15% after major open shoulder surgery: the effects on hand motor function. *Anesth Analg* 2001;92:218–223.

79. Lehtipalo S, Koskinen LO, Johansson G, et al. Continuous interscalene brachial plexus block for postoperative analgesia following shoulder surgery. *Acta Anaesthesiol Scand* 1999;43:258–264.

80. Ekatodramis G, Borgeat A. Subcutaneous tunneling of the interscalene catheter. *Can J Anaesth* 2000;47:716–717.

81. Klein SM, Nielsen KC, Buckenmaier III CC, et al. 2-Octyl cyanoacrylate glue for the fixation of continuous peripheral nerve catheters. *Anesthesiology* 2003;98:590–591.

82. Ilfeld BM, Enneking FK. Continuous peripheral nerve blocks at home: a review. *Anesth Analg* 2005;100:1822–1833.

83. Ilfeld BM, Wright TW, Enneking FK, et al. Total shoulder arthroplasty as an outpatient procedure using ambulatory perineural local anesthetic infusion: a pilot feasibility study. *Anesth Analg* 2005;101:1319–1322.

84. Bleckner LL, Bina S, Kwon KH, et al. Serum ropivacaine concentrations and systemic local anesthetic toxicity in trauma patients receiving long-term continuous peripheral nerve block catheters. *Anesth Analg* 2010;110:630–634.

85. Cuvillon P, Ripart J, Lalourcey L, et al. The continuous femoral nerve block catheter for postoperative analgesia: bacterial colonization, infectious rate and adverse effects. *Anesth Analg* 2001;93:1045–1049.

86. Gaumann DM, Lennon RL, Wedel DJ. Continuous axillary block for postoperative pain management. *Reg Anesth Pain Med* 1988;13:77–82.

87. Stojadinovic A, Auton A, Peoples GE, et al. Responding to challenges in modern combat casualty care: innovative use of advanced regional anesthesia. *Pain Med* 2006;7:330–338.

88. Capdevila X, Bringuier S, Borgeat A. Infectious risk of continuous peripheral nerve blocks. *Anesthesiology* 2009;110:182–188.

89. Bergman BD, Hebl JR, Kent J, et al. Neurologic complications of 405 consecutive continuous axillary catheters. *Anesth Analg* 2003;96:247–252.

90. Neuburger M, Buttner J, Blumenthal S, et al. Inflammation and infection complications of 2285 perineural catheters: a prospective study. *Acta Anaesthesiol Scand* 2007;51:108–114.

91. Adam F, Jaziri S, Chauvin M. Psoas abscess complicating femoral nerve block catheter. *Anesthesiology* 2003;99:230–231.

92. Neuburger M, Lang D, Buttner J. Abscess of the psoas muscle caused by a psoas compartment catheter. Case report of a rare complication of peripheral catheter regional anaesthesia. *Anaesthesist* 2005;54:341–345.

93. Tucker CJ, Kirk KL, Ficke JR. Posterior thigh abscess as a complication of continuous popliteal nerve catheter. *Am J Orthop* (Belle Mead NJ) 2010;39:E25–E27.

94. Capdevila X, Jaber S, Pesonen P, et al. Acute neck cellulitis and mediastinitis complicating a continuous interscalene block. *Anesth Analg* 2008;107:1419–1421.

95. Capdevila X, Pirat P, Bringuier S, et al. Continuous peripheral nerve blocks in hospital wards after orthopedic surgery: a multicenter prospective analysis of the quality of postoperative analgesia and complications in 1,416 patients. *Anesthesiology* 2005;103:1035–1045.

96. Head S, Enneking FK. Infusate contamination in regional anesthesia: what every anesthesiologist should know. *Anesth Analg* 2008;107:1412–1418.

97. Hebl JR. The importance and implications of aseptic techniques during regional anesthesia. *Reg Anesth Pain Med* 2006;31:311–323.

98. Grant SA, Neilsen KC. Continuous peripheral nerve catheters for ambulatory anesthesia. *Curr Anesthesiol Rep* 2000;2:304–307.

99. Hogan Q, Dotson R, Erickson S, et al. Local anesthetic myotoxicity: a case and review. *Anesthesiology* 1994;80:942–947.

100. Mulroy MF, Norris MC, Liu SS. Safety steps for epidural injection of local anesthetics: review of the literature and recommendations. *Anesth Analg* 1997;85:1346–1356.

101. Sadeh M, Czywewski K, Stern LZ. Chronic myopathy induced by repeated bupivacaine injections. *J Neurol Sci* 1985;67:229–238.

102. Kytta J, Heinonen E, Rosenberg PH, et al. Effects of repeated bupivacaine administration on sciatic nerve and surrounding muscle tissue in rats. *Acta Anaesthesiol Scand* 1986;30:625–629.

103. Parris WC, Dettbarn WD. Muscle atrophy following nerve block therapy. *Anesthesiology* 1988;69:289.

104. Zink W, Graf BM. Local anesthetic myotoxicity. *Reg Anesth Pain Med* 2004;29:333–340.

105. Zink W, Seif C, Bohl JR, et al. The acute myotoxic effects of bupivacaine and ropivacaine after continuous peripheral nerve blockades. *Anesth Analg* 2003;97:1173–1179.

106. Zink W, Bohl JR, Hacke N, et al. The long term myotoxic effects of bupivacaine and ropivacaine after continuous peripheral nerve blocks. *Anesth Analg* 2005;101:548–554.

107. Nouette-Gaulain K, Dadure C, Morau D, et al. Age-dependent bupivacaine-induced muscle toxicity during continuous peripheral nerve block in rats. *Anesthesiology* 2009;111:1120–1127.

108. Pandin PC, Vandesteene A, d'Hollander AA. Lumbar plexus posterior approach: a catheter placement description using electrical nerve stimulation. *Anesth Analg* 2002;95:1428–1431.

109. Tuominen M, Pitkanen M, Rosenberg PH. Postoperative pain relief and bupivacaine plasma levels during continuous interscalene brachial plexus block. *Acta Anaesthesiol Scand* 1987;31:276–278.

110. Denson DD, Raj PP, Saldahna F, et al. Continuous perineural infusion of bupivacaine for prolonged analgesia: pharmacokinetic considerations. *Int J Clin Pharmacol Ther Toxicol* 1983;21:591–597.

111. Ekatodramis G, Borgeat A, Huledal G, et al. Continuous interscalene analgesia with ropivacaine 2 mg/ml after major shoulder surgery. *Anesthesiology* 2003;98:143–150.

112. Kaloul I, Guay J, Cote C, et al. Ropivacaine plasma concentrations are similar during continuous lumbar plexus blockade using the anterior three-in-one and the posterior psoas compartment techniques: [Les concentrations plasmatiques de ropivacaine sont similaires pendant le bloc continu du plexus lombaire realise par voie anterieure trois-en-un et par voie posterieure de la loge du psoas]. *Can J Anaesth* 2004;51:52–56.

113. Anker-Moller E, Spangsberg N, Dahl JB, et al. Continuous blockade of the lumbar plexus after knee surgery: a comparison of the plasma concentrations and analgesic effect of bupivacaine 0.250% and 0.125%. *Acta Anaesthesiol Scand* 1990;34:468–472.

114. Rosenberg PH, Pere P, Hekali R, et al. Plasma concentrations of bupivacaine and two of its metabolites during continuous interscalene brachial plexus block. *Br J Anaesth* 1991;66:25–30.

115. Pere P, Tuominen M, Rosenberg PH. Cumulation of bupivacaine, desbutylbupivacaine and 4-hydroxybupivacaine during and after continuous interscalene brachial plexus block. *Acta Anaesthesiol Scand* 1991;35:647–650.

116. Dahl JB, Christiansen CL, Daugaard JJ, et al. Continuous blockade of the lumbar plexus after knee surgery– postoperative analgesia and bupivacaine plasma concentrations. A controlled clinical trial. *Anaesthesia* 1988;43:1015–1018.

117. Tuominen M, Rosenberg PH, Kalso E. Blood levels of bupivacaine after single dose, supplementary dose and during continuous infusion in axillary plexus block. *Acta Anaesthesiol Scand* 1983;27:303–306.

118. Buckenmaier CC III, Rupprecht C, McKnight G, et al. Pain following battlefield injury and evacuation: a survey of 110 casualties from the wars in Iraq and Afghanistan. *Pain Med* 2009;10:1487–1496.

119. Chelly JE, Greger J, Gebhard R. Ambulatory continuous perineural infusion: are we ready? [letter; comment]. *Anesthesiology* 2000;93:581–582.

120. Ilfeld BM, Enneking FK. A portable mechanical pump providing over four days of patient-controlled analgesia by perineural infusion at home. *Reg Anesth Pain Med* 2002;27:100–104.

121. Singelyn FJ, Gouverneur JM. Extended "three-in-one" block after total knee arthroplasty: continuous versus patient-controlled techniques. *Anesth Analg* 2000;91:176–180.

122. Singelyn FJ, Seguy S, Gouverneur JM. Interscalene brachial plexus analgesia after open shoulder surgery: continuous versus patient-controlled infusion. *Anesth Analg* 1999;89:1216–1220.

123. Singelyn FJ, Vanderelst PE, Gouverneur JM. Extended femoral nerve sheath block after total hip arthroplasty: continuous versus patient-controlled techniques. *Anesth Analg* 2001;92:455–459.

124. Iskandar H, Rakotondriamihary S, Dixmerias F, et al. Analgesia using continuous axillary block after surgery of severe hand injuries: self-administration versus continuous injection. *Ann Fr Anesth Reanim* 1998;17:1099–1103.

125. di Benedetto P, Casati A, Bertini L. Continuous subgluteus sciatic nerve block after orthopedic foot and ankle surgery: comparison of two infusion techniques. *Reg Anesth Pain Med* 2002;27:168–172.

126. Eledjam JJ, Cuvillon P, Capdevila X, et al. Postoperative analgesia by femoral nerve block with ropivacaine 0.2% after major knee surgery: continuous versus patient-controlled techniques. *Reg Anesth Pain Med* 2002;27:604–611.

127. Rawal N, Axelsson K, Hylander J, et al. Postoperative patient-controlled local anesthetic administration at home. *Anesth Analg* 1998;86:86–89.

128. Rawal N, Allvin R, Axelsson K, et al. Patient-controlled regional analgesia (PCRA) at home: controlled comparison between bupivacaine and ropivacaine brachial plexus analgesia. *Anesthiology* 2002;96:1290–1296.

129. Ganapathy S, Amendola A, Lichfield R, et al. Elastomeric pumps for ambulatory patient controlled regional analgesia. *Can J Anaesth* 2000;47:897–902.

130. Ilfeld BM, Morey TE, Enneking FK. The delivery rate accuracy of portable infusion pumps used for continuous regional analgesia. *Anesth Analg* 2002;95:1331–1336.

131. Ilfeld BM, Morey TE, Enneking FK. Delivery rate accuracy of portable, bolus-capable infusion pumps used for patient-controlled continuous regional analgesia. *Reg Anesth Pain Med* 2003;28:17–23.

132. Ilfeld BM, Morey TE, Enneking FK. Portable infusion pumps used for continuous regional analgesia: delivery rate accuracy and consistency. *Reg Anesth Pain Med* 2003;28:424–432.

133. Ilfeld BM, Morey TE, Enneking FK. New portable infusion pumps: real advantages or just more of the same in a different package? *Reg Anesth Pain Med* 2004;29:371–376.

134. Kalichman MW, Moorhouse DF, Powell HC, et al. Relative neural toxicity of local anesthetics. *J Neuropathol Exp Neurol* 1993;52:234–240.

135. Ribeiro FC, Georgousis H, Bertram R, et al. Plexus irritation caused by interscalene brachial plexus catheter for shoulder surgery. *Anesth Analg* 1996;82:870–872.

136. Blumenthal S, Borgeat A, Maurer K, et al. Preexisting subclinical neuropathy as a risk factor for nerve injury after continuous ropivacaine administration through a femoral nerve catheter. *Anesthiology* 2006;105:1053–1056.

137. Horlocker TT, O'Driscoll SW, Dinapoli RP. Recurring brachial plexus neuropathy in a diabetic patient after shoulder surgery and continuous interscalene block. *Anesth Analg* 2000;91:688–690.

138. Williams BA, Murinson BB. Diabetes mellitus and subclinical neuropathy: a call for new paths in peripheral nerve block research. *Anesthiology* 2008;109:361–362.

139. Borgeat A, Aguirre J, Curt A. Case scenario: neurologic complication after continuous interscalene block. *Anesthiology* 2010;112:742–745.

140. Ilfeld BM, Yaksh TL. The end of postoperative pain–a fast-approaching possibility? And, if so, will we be ready? *Reg Anesth Pain Med* 2009;34:85–87.

141. Borgeat A, Kalberer F, Jacob H, et al. Patient-controlled interscalene analgesia with ropivacaine 0.2% versus bupivacaine 0.15% after major open shoulder surgery: the effects on hand motor function. *Anesth Analg* 2001;92:218–223.

142. Ilfeld BM, Duke KB, Donohue MC. The association between lower extremity continuous peripheral nerve blocks and patient falls after knee and hip arthroplasty. *Anesth Analg* 2010;111:1552–1554.

143. Kandasami M, Kinninmonth AW, Sarungi M, et al. Femoral nerve block for total knee replacement - a word of caution. *Knee* 2009;16:98–100.

144. Feibel RJ, Dervin GF, Kim PR, et al. Major complications associated with femoral nerve catheters for knee arthroplasty: a word of caution. *J Arthroplasty* 2009;24:132–137.

145. Brodner G, Buerkle H, Van Aken H, et al. Postoperative analgesia after knee surgery: a comparison of three different concentrations of ropivacaine for continuous femoral nerve blockade. *Anesth Analg* 2007;105:256–262.

146. Ilfeld BM, Moeller LK, Mariano ER, et al. Continuous peripheral nerve blocks: is local anesthetic dose the only factor, or do concentration and volume influence infusion effects as well? *Anesthiology* 2010;112:347–354.

147. Capdevila X, Dadure C, Bringuier S, et al. Effect of patient-controlled perineural analgesia on rehabilitation and pain after ambulatory orthopedic surgery: a multicenter randomized trial. *Anesthiology* 2006;105:566–573.

148. Muraskin SI, Conrad B, Zheng N, et al. Falls associated with lower-extremity-nerve blocks: a pilot investigation of mechanisms. *Reg Anesth Pain Med* 2007;32:67–72.

149. Offerdahl MR, Lennon RL, Horlocker TT. Successful removal of a knotted fascia iliaca catheter: principles of patient positioning for peripheral nerve catheter extraction. *Anesth Analg* 2004;99:1550–1552.

150. Motamed C, Bouaziz H, Mercier FJ, et al. Knotting of a femoral catheter. *Reg Anesth* 1997;22:486–487.

151. MacLeod DB, Grant SA, Martin G, et al. Identification of coracoid process for infraclavicular blocks. *Reg Anesth Pain Med* 2003;28:485.

152. David M. Knotted peripheral nerve catheter. *Reg Anesth Pain Med* 2003;28:487–488.

153. Burgher AH, Hebl JR. Minimally invasive retrieval of knotted nonstimulating peripheral nerve catheters. *Reg Anesth Pain Med* 2007;32:162–166.

154. Capdevila X, Biboulet P, Morau D, et al. Continuous three-in-one block for postoperative pain after lower limb orthopedic surgery: where do the catheters go? *Anesth Analg* 2002;94:1001–1006.

155. Spansberg NL, Anker-Moller E, Dahl JB, et al. The value of continuous blockade of the lumbar plexus as an adjunct to acetylsalicyclic acid for pain relief after surgery for femoral neck fractures. *Eur J Anaesthesiol* 1996;13:410–412.

156. Singelyn FJ, Ferrant T, Malisse MF, et al. Effects of intravenous patient-controlled analgesia with morphine, continuous epidural analgesia, and continuous femoral nerve sheath block on rehabilitation after unilateral total-hip arthroplasty. *Reg Anesth Pain Med* 2005;30:452–457.

157. Singelyn FJ, Deyaert M, Joris D, et al. Effects of intravenous patient-controlled analgesia with morphine, continuous epidural analgesia, and continuous three-in-one block on postoperative pain and knee rehabilitation after unilateral total knee arthroplasty. *Anesth Analg* 1998;87:88–92.

158. Singelyn FJ, Gouverneur JM. Postoperative analgesia after total hip arthroplasty: i.v. PCA with morphine, patient-controlled epidural analgesia, or continuous "3-in-1'" block?: a prospective evaluation by our acute pain service in more than 1,300 patients. *J Clin Anesth* 1999;11:550–554.

159. Ilfeld BM, Morey TE, Thannikary LJ, et al. Clonidine added to a continuous interscalene ropivacaine perineural infusion to improve postoperative analgesia: a randomized, double-blind, controlled study. *Anesth Analg* 2005;100:1172–1178.

160. Stierwaldt R, Ulsamer B. Complications during the use of a catheter for continuous lumbar plexus block during implantation of a total hip endoprosthesis. *Reg Anaesth* 1991;14:38–39.

161. Chin KJ, Chee V. Perforation of a Pajunk stimulating catheter after traction-induced damage. *Reg Anesth Pain Med* 2006;31:389–390.

162. Lee BH, Goucke CR. Shearing of a peripheral nerve catheter. *Anesth Analg* 2002;95:760–761.

163. Klein SM, Steele SM, Nielsen KC, et al. The difficulties of ambulatory interscalene and intra-articular infusions for rotator cuff surgery: a preliminary report. [Difficultes des perfusions interscalenes et intra-articulaires ambulatoires pour la reparation de la coiffe des rotateurs: un rapport preliminaire]. *Can J Anaesth* 2003;50:265–269.

164. Pere P. The effect of continuous interscalene brachial plexus block with 0.125% bupivacaine plus fentanyl on diaphragmatic motility and ventilatory function. *Reg Anesth* 1993;18:93–97.

165. Borgeat A, Perschak H, Bird P, et al. Patient-controlled interscalene analgesia with ropivacaine 0.2% versus patient-controlled intravenous analgesia after major shoulder surgery: effects on diaphragmatic and respiratory function. *Anesthesiology* 2000;92:102–108.

166. Sardesai AM, Chakrabarti AJ, Denny NM. Lower lobe collapse during continuous interscalene brachial plexus local anesthesia at home. *Reg Anesth Pain Med* 2004;29:65–68.

167. Smith MP, Tetzlaff JE, Brems JJ. Asymptomatic profound oxyhemoglobin desaturation following interscalene block in a geriatric patient. *Reg Anesth Pain Med* 1998;23:210–213.

168. Capdevila X, Macaire P, Aknin P, et al. Patient-controlled perineural analgesia after ambulatory orthopedic surgery: a comparison of electronic versus elastomeric pumps. *Anesth Analg* 2003;96:414–417.

169. Macaire P, Gaertner E, Capdevila X. Continuous post-operative regional analgesia at home. *Minerva Anestesiol* 2001;67:109–116.

170. Johnson T, Monk T, Rasmussen LS, et al. Postoperative cognitive dysfunction in middle-aged patients. *Anesthesiology* 2002;96:1351–1357.

171. Ilfeld BM, Esener DE, Morey TE, et al. Ambulatory perineural infusion: the patients' perspective. *Reg Anesth Pain Med* 2003;28:418–423.

172. Swenson JD, Bay N, Loose E, et al. Outpatient management of continuous peripheral nerve catheters placed using ultrasound guidance: an experience in 620 patients. *Anesth Analg* 2006;103:1436–1443.

173. Davis JJ, Swenson JD, Greis PE, et al. Interscalene block for postoperative analgesia using only ultrasound guidance: the outcome in 200 patients. *J Clin Anesth* 2009;21:272–277.

174. Klein SM, Nielsen KC, Greengrass RA, et al. Ambulatory discharge after long-acting peripheral nerve blockade: 2382 blocks with ropivacaine. *Anesth Analg* 2002;94:65–70.

175. Corda DM, Enneking FK. A unique approach to postoperative analgesia for ambulatory surgery. *J Clin.Anesth* 2000;12:595–599.

176. Ilfeld BM. Ambulatory perineural local anesthetic infusion: portable pump and dosing regimen selection. *Tech Reg Anesth Pain Manag* 2004;8:90–98.

177. Sawaki Y, Parker RK, White PF. Patient and nurse evaluation of patient-controlled analgesia delivery systems for postoperative pain management. *J Pain Symptom Manage* 1992;7:443–453.

178. Remerand F, Vuitton AS, Palud M, et al. Elastomeric pump reliability in postoperative regional anesthesia: a survey of 430 consecutive devices. *Anesth Analg* 2008;107:2079–2084.

179. Ilfeld BM, Morey TE. Use of term "patient-controlled" may be confusing in study of elastometric pump. *Anesth Analg* 2003;97:916–917.

180. Zahnd D, Aebi S, Rusterholz S, et al. A randomized crossover trial assessing patient preference for two different types of portable infusion-pump devices. *Ann Oncol* 1999;10:727–729.

COMPLICATIONS OF SYMPATHETIC BLOCK

22

Complications Associated with Stellate Ganglion and Lumbar Sympathetic Blocks

Richard L. Rauck and James P. Rathmell

To the regional anesthesiologist and pain specialist, the sympathetic nervous system is important because it supplies efferent impulses responsible for vascular tone and because the sympathetic chain carries afferent nociceptive impulses toward the spinal cord. A number of acute posttraumatic and chronic neuropathic pain conditions are maintained through nociceptive impulses that travel through the sympathetic nervous system. These conditions often improve with sympathetic blockade.

Pain arising from the viscera and sympathetically maintained pain that arises after injury in the periphery can be effectively relieved in many instances by using local anesthetic or neurolytic blockade of the sympathetic nervous system at one of three main levels: the cervicothoracic ganglia (including the stellate ganglion), the celiac plexus, or the lumbar ganglia. Pain that is relieved by sympathetic blockade is termed sympathetically maintained pain (Box 22-1).

A recent critical review of the literature used an evidence-based analysis of outcome studies to provide recommendations for appropriate applications of sympathetic blocks (Box 22-2).[1] The primary uses supported by available evidence include diagnosis of pain that is responsive to sympathetic blockade (e.g., complex regional pain syndrome [CRPS]) and the treatment of ischemic pain. The usefulness of repeated sympathetic blocks in the treatment of either CRPS or postherpetic neuralgia (PHN) is unclear from the available evidence. The most comprehensive and recent reviews, one published in 2002 and the more recent in 2010, both question the efficacy of local anesthetic sympathetic blockade as a long-term treatment for CRPS.[2,3] Efficacy of sympathetic blockade is based almost entirely

BOX 22-2 Uses for Sympathetic Blockade in Pain Therapy

1. Pain Diagnosis: Sympathetic blocks can establish whether pains are nonresponsive or responsive to such blocks. However, response to sympathetic blockade should not be the basis for establishing or excluding a diagnosis of CRPS.
2. Neuropathic Pain Therapy:
   (a) PHN. A critical review of the literature regarding the use of sympathetic blocks in the treatment of acute herpes zoster pain and in the treatment of PHN found little support for the widely held view that sympathetic blocks reduced the incidence of long-term reduction of pain in these disorders. Attempts to reduce PHN by combining such blocks with aggressive drug therapies during acute herpes infection warrant further study.
   (b) CRPS (RSD) treatments are seen as evolutionary at present, with the role of sympathetic blocks being only part of a balanced pain-treatment strategy.
3. Ischemic Pain: Permanent sympathetic block with neurolytic or thermocoagulation techniques provides up to 50% long-term improved blood flow and reduction of pain and ulceration for patients with advanced peripheral vascular disease. This is particularly appropriate at lumbar levels in which percutaneous techniques are safe when conducted with real-time imaging control.

BOX 22-1 Sympathetically Maintained Pain and Complex Regional Pain Syndrome

Patients with complex regional pain syndrome (CRPS) often experience persistent pain and vasomotor changes (swelling, edema, and temperature and color changes in the affected area) that suggest altered function of the sympathetic nervous system. Blockade of the sympathetic ganglia that serve the affected region often leads to significant pain relief in those with CRPS. The term *sympathetically maintained* pain was coined by neuroscientists to explain the pain relief that ensues after blockade of the sympathetic ganglia. Pain that persists despite sympathetic blockade is termed *sympathetically independent pain.*

CRPS is divided into type 1 (reflex sympathetic dystrophy) and type 2 (causalgia). CRPS types 1 and 2 both occur after traumatic injury. CRPS type 1 follows injuries such as strains, sprains, and fractures, in which there is not injury to a major nerve or nerve plexus. CRPS type 2 shares the same clinical features as CRPS type 1 (persistent pain and signs of sympathetic dysfunction), but follows a major nerve trunk injury such as a gunshot wound involving the brachial plexus.

on case series. Less than one-third of patients obtain full pain relief, and transient pain relief is common. The absence of control groups in case series may lead to overestimation of the treatment response, which can explain the usual findings, suggesting that sympathetic blocks are effective. Likewise, systematic review of the use of sympathetic blockade for treating herpes zoster or PHN suggests that this area also remains in need of further study.[4] Despite the limited available data to support their usefulness, the use of sympathetic blocks is a well-established part of treating many of these painful disorders, and this approach to the treatment is likely to remain in common use for the foreseeable future.

Most techniques for the blockade of the sympathetic nerves have been described for decades. Sympathetic blocks (including stellate ganglion, celiac plexus, and lumbar sympathetic blocks [LSBs]) have been used for more than half a century. Practitioners have developed a relatively good understanding of the risks and complications of performing these procedures. Some newer techniques (such as hypogastric plexus block and newer approaches to the sympathetic nerves such as transdiscal approaches) have been described, but little is known about the risks of these approaches. This chapter focuses on known and potential complications of the various approaches to blockade of the stellate ganglion and lumbar sympathetic chain. The risks associated with celiac plexus, hypogastric plexus, and ganglion impar block are described in Chapters 23 and 24.

► STELLATE GANGLION BLOCK

Definition and Scope

Complications from stellate ganglion block can arise from inadvertent vascular, epidural, or intrathecal injection (Box 22-3). Needle trauma can result in injuries to vessels or nervous tissue in the neck. Pneumothorax can also occur following a stellate ganglion block. Infections are uncommon. There are no published reports available that offer an estimate of the frequency of complications associated with stellate ganglion block. In a recent survey of members of the Canadian Anesthesiologists' Society, approximately one-third of the anesthesiologists surveyed reported that they incorporate chronic pain as part of their practices and that the most commonly practiced interventions included stellate ganglion block (61%) and lumbar sympathetic block (50%), suggesting that these techniques remain in common use.[5] Most complications described, however, appear only in the form of sporadic case reports.

Mechanism of Causation

Intravascular Injection

Several arteries and veins lie in close proximity to the intended injection site, the anterior tubercle of C6 or C7 (Fig. 22-1). Injections into the vein do not commonly result in sequelae because the volume and concentration of local anesthetic should not produce a toxic effect. The risk of local anesthetic toxicity can further be reduced by the use of dilute local anesthetic concentrations such as 0.25% bupivacaine.

Arterial injections do not offer the same measure of safety. As little as 2.5 mg of bupivacaine or a mixture of 1.25 mg of bupivacaine and 5 mg of lidocaine injected into the vertebral or internal carotid artery has been reported to produce almost immediate generalized seizure.[6] Vertebral injections occur when the needle is inserted too medially

---

BOX 22-3 Complications Associated with Stellate Ganglion Block

Common

- Recurrent laryngeal and phrenic nerve block
- Brachial plexus block

Uncommon

- Pneumothorax
- Generalized seizure
- Total spinal anesthesia
- Severe hypertension

Rare

- Transient locked-in syndrome
- Paratracheal hematoma
- Soft tissue infection/osteomyelitis

---

and posteriorly. The practitioner often contacts the bone but mistakes the posterior tubercle for the anterior tubercle. Slight withdrawal of the needle from the posterior tubercle, particularly if in a medial position, can produce a vertebral artery injection.

The carotid artery also lies near the site of entry for a stellate ganglion block. It is advisable to feel for the carotid pulse and then retract the vessel laterally prior to inserting the needle. This should prevent insertion into the carotid artery in most cases. Injection into the carotid artery can be expected to produce effects similar to those of vertebral artery injection.

Rarely is this procedure performed secondary to direct inflammation of the ganglion. Sympathetic blocks (e.g., stellate ganglion block) are performed diagnostically and therapeutically to produce sympathetic denervation. Local anesthetics effectively block these nerves temporarily. Long-term benefits have been reported following local anesthetic blocks. The addition of corticosteroids has not been demonstrated to enhance the effect of the local anesthetic. If there has been trauma at the site of the ganglion (e.g., a gunshot wound), injection of corticosteroid with local anesthetic would seem reasonable. Routine administration of corticosteroid in these injections might be questioned because of the risk of intra-arterial injection into the vertebral, carotid, or spinal radicular artery. Specifically, particulate corticosteroids (suspensions such as methylprednisolone acetate) can cause an embolic stroke if unintentionally injected into any of these arteries.

Epidural or Intrathecal Injection

The cervical spinal nerves traverse the intervertebral foramen near the location for a stellate ganglion block (Fig. 22-1). If the needle is positioned posterior to the anterior tubercle, it can be placed into either the epidural compartment or into a dural sleeve that accompanies the spinal nerve. Whereas cerebrospinal fluid would be expected upon aspiration if the needle were inside the subarachnoid space, this may be overlooked as the practitioner focuses on the more likely risk of vascular aspiration and injection. Paresthesias in the distribution of the brachial plexus may or may not occur. If present, one should consider repositioning the needle more anteriorly.

Epidural injection of 10 mL of local anesthetic at the C6 or C7 level produces variable effects and is dependent on the concentration of local anesthetic and on whether the entire volume of drug is injected. In our experience, epidural injection (with high concentration of local anesthetic) can produce a profound sensory and motor block but often spares the phrenic nerve. Subjective respiratory distress is common secondary to the block of the intercostal nerves. It is important to understand the delayed onset of epidural blockade, particularly with bupivacaine or ropivacaine, where 15 to 20 minutes are required until the most profound effects of the local anesthetic are apparent. Thus, assuring that patients are monitored closely for this interval is essential.

Intrathecal injection of local anesthetic at this site commonly produces a total spinal block. Loss of airway reflexes and phrenic nerve function often occurs. Patients often describe as initial symptoms difficulty breathing or an inability to move their arms. Contralateral motor block develops as further confirmation of intrathecal injection along with the block of the lower extremities.

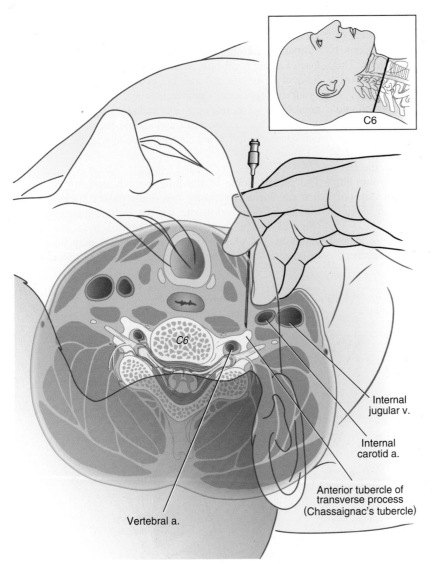

FIGURE 22-1. Axial diagram of stellate ganglion block. The great vessels of the neck are gently retracted laterally and the needle is seated on the anterior tubercle of the transverse process of C6 (Chassaignac's tubercle). Note the position of the vertebral artery within the foramen transversarium, the spinal nerve and dural cuff, and the carotid artery and jugular vein.

Labels in figure:
- Internal jugular v.
- Internal carotid a.
- Anterior tubercle of transverse process (Chassaignac's tubercle)
- Vertebral a.
- C6

Recurrent Laryngeal and Phrenic Nerve Blocks

Recurrent laryngeal and phrenic nerve blocks are frequent side effects of a stellate ganglion block. They occur from local anesthetic injection that spills from the area of the ganglion. Because diffusion of drug is required to obtain a satisfactory block, it can be expected that these nerves will often be temporarily blocked. Symptoms of a recurrent laryngeal nerve block include hoarseness and, occasionally, respiratory stridor. Patients often complain of difficulty in getting their breath and the sensation of a lump in the throat. Phrenic nerve block rarely presents as a problem for patients unless they have preexisting and severe respiratory compromise. The potential for producing phrenic nerve block is one reason bilateral stellate ganglion blocks are rarely performed at the same time. Most practitioners wait several days to a week between injections.

Horner's Syndrome

Horner's syndrome is often observed following a stellate ganglion block. In fact, many practitioners look for Horner's syndrome as evidence of sympathetic denervation following the injection of local anesthetic onto the stellate ganglion. Thus, Horner's syndrome is best characterized as an expected side effect in that effective block of the stellate ganglion cannot be achieved without the appearance of these signs and symptoms. Horner's syndrome consists of miosis (pupillary constriction, ptosis [drooping of the upper eyelid] and enophthalmos [recession of the globe within the orbit]). Signs of successful stellate ganglion block are listed in Box 22-4. The presence of Horner's syndrome does not necessarily equate to sympathetic denervation of the upper extremity. A study by Malmqvist et al.[7]

BOX 22-4 Signs of Successful Stellate Ganglion Block

- Horner's syndrome
  - Miosis (pupillary constriction)
  - Ptosis (drooping of the upper eyelid)
  - Enophthalmos (recession of the globe within the orbit)
- Anhidrosis (lack of sweating)
- Nasal congestion
- Venodilation in the hand and forearm
- Increase in temperature of the blocked limb by at least 1°C

used five measures of sympathetic denervation (including the presence of Horner's syndrome, increased temperature of the blocked extremity, and sympathogalvanic skin response) to evaluate the effectiveness of a stellate ganglion block. The authors found that only 15 of 54 blocks had four or five positive measures following stellate ganglion block.

A study by Hogan et al.[8] examined the distribution and spread of contrast following stellate ganglion block using magnetic resonance imaging. They found that injectate was not delivered to the stellate ganglion but rather passed anterior to it (with or without caudad extension to the stellate ganglion). This could produce Horner's syndrome but not sympathetic denervation to the extremity. Other sites of spread included the brachial plexus, the subclavian plexus, and the epidural or subarachnoid spaces.

Horner's syndrome following stellate ganglion injection with local anesthetic resolves when the local anesthetic

effect ends. Ideally, the analgesic effect outlives the Horner's syndrome. Use of neurolytic solutions can produce permanent Horner's syndrome when injected near the stellate ganglion. Use of dilute neurolytic solutions (3%) has been reported by Racz et al. as safe and may not produce permanent Horner's syndrome (personal communication). However, the use of neurolytic solutions near the stellate ganglion cannot be advocated for routine cases and should be used only in special situations following clear discussion with the patient.

Pneumothorax

The pleural dome of the lung extends variably above the first rib. Most commonly, this dome passes laterally to the intended C6 injection site for the stellate ganglion block (Fig. 22-2). In the anterior C7 approach to the stellate ganglion, the pleural dome is closer and may be entered in unusual cases. This can be accentuated in patients with

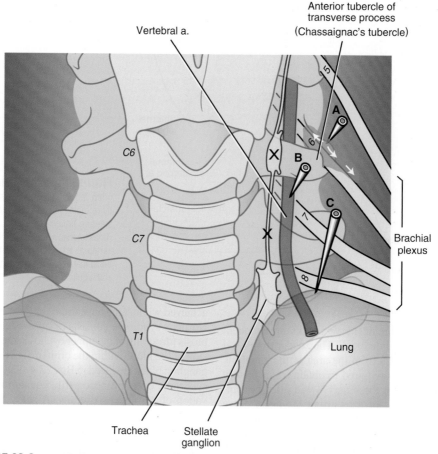

FIGURE 22-2. Complications of stellate ganglion block. The stellate ganglion conveys sympathetic fibers to and from the upper extremities and the head and neck. The ganglion is comprised of the fused superior thoracic ganglion and the inferior cervical ganglion and is named for its fusiform shape (in many individuals, the two ganglia remain separate). The stellate ganglia lie over the head of the first rib at the junction of the transverse process and uncinate process of T1. The ganglion is just posteromedial to the cupola of the lung and medial to the vertebral artery, and these are the two structures most vulnerable. Stellate ganglion block is typically carried out at the C6 or C7 level to avoid pneumothorax, and a volume of solution that will spread along the prevertebral fascia inferiorly to the stellate ganglion is employed (usually 10 mL). When radiographic guidance is not used, the operator palpates the anterior tubercle of the transverse process of C6 (Chassaignac's tubercle), and a needle is seated in the location. With radiographic guidance, it is simpler and safer to place a needle over the vertebral body just inferior the uncinate process of C6 or C7. Incorrect needle placement can lead to **(A)** spread of the injectate adjacent to the spinal nerves where they join to form the brachial plexus, **(B)** damage to the vertebral artery or intraarterial injection, or **(C)** pneumothorax. Local anesthetic can also course proximally along the spinal nerves to the epidural space. (Modified from Rathmell JP. *Atlas of Image-guided Intervention in Regional Anesthesia and Pain Medicine.* 2nd ed. Philadelphia, PA: Lippincott Williams & Wilkins, 2012, with permission.)

pulmonary disease and hyperinflated lungs, such as patients with chronic obstructive pulmonary disease.

The posterior approach to the upper thoracic sympathetic chain is extremely close to the parietal pleura. Anyone using this approach should be cautious and guided by fluoroscopy or computed tomographic techniques. Pneumothorax can result despite careful attention to detail, and patients should be warned of this potential complication prior to a posterior approach of the sympathetic chain or stellate ganglion.

Brachial Plexus Block

Brachial plexus block can occur following a stellate ganglion injection. The majority of sympathetic nerves that travel to the upper extremity leave the sympathetic chain to accompany the somatic nerves of the brachial plexus. A few sympathetic nerves of the upper extremity, often referred to as the anomalous Kuntz nerves, may not pass through the stellate ganglion but later join the brachial plexus.[9] These upper extremity sympathetic fibers can only be blocked by either a brachial plexus block or a posterior approach to the upper thoracic sympathetic chain.

In a standard anterior (C6) approach to the stellate ganglion, the brachial plexus will not be blocked. However, partial block of the nerve roots that form the brachial plexus is commonly seen after a stellate ganglion block. This occurs most commonly when the needle has been inserted too deeply, bypasses the anterior tubercle, and rests on the posterior tubercle. After retraction from the posterior tubercle, the injection of local anesthetic is likely to block one or more of the roots of the brachial plexus.

Other Complications

A hematoma following a stellate ganglion block is always possible. Indeed, paratracheal hematoma causing airway obstruction and death has been reported after stellate ganglion block.[10] This occurs most commonly if the vertebral artery or carotid artery has been entered. A more serious, although very rare, situation develops if a plaque is dislodged following unintentional arterial puncture of either the carotid or the vertebral artery. Presentation would be expected to mimic an evolving stroke. This should be viewed as a medical emergency, with life support and direct transport to an emergency facility.

Similarly, unintentional puncture can also produce an arterial wall dissection. This is more likely in the rare situation in which the needle rests in the wall of the artery, negative aspiration is noted, and subsequent injection of the local anesthetic produces the dissection. Symptomatic patients should be stabilized or resuscitated and taken directly to an emergency facility.

Infections are very uncommon following stellate ganglion injections, but there are case reports of cervical vertebral osteomyelitis.[11,12] In our practice, alcohol preparation of the site and the use of good technique with sterile surgical gloves have prevented any infectious complication in 20 years' experience. More formal surgical preparation with a betadine (or similar) solution and sterile drape is reasonable and warranted. Many examiners believe it is important, however, to watch the patient during the injection for immediate feedback if an intravascular injection occurs. Thus, draping the patient's face should be avoided or performed carefully. If an infection occurs, the most likely organism would be a strain of *Staphylococcus* unless the esophagus was inadvertently entered. Because the needle can contact the bone during the procedure, any infection should be treated with antibiotics and followed closely. An infectious disease consultation should be considered in patients who do not respond to a course of oral antibiotics.

Two separate case reports have reported a transient locked-in syndrome following stellate ganglion block.[13,14] In both cases, the patient remained conscious but was unable to breathe or move, with sparing of eye movement. The authors of both reports believed these cases were the result of intra-arterial injections of the vertebral artery. In our practice, we have seen two cases of a similar presentation in 20 years. However, we attributed both cases to acquiring a total spinal injection. Whether these cases represent a different phenomenon or a misdiagnosis is unclear. Fortunately, in all four cases (ours and the published cases), the patients recovered uneventfully. Care should be taken to provide sedation and frequent reassurance to these patients, as they are conscious but unable to move or breathe.

Wallace and Milholland[15] have reported a case of contralateral and bilateral Horner's syndrome following stellate ganglion injection. They also reported a bilateral recurrent laryngeal nerve block, which can potentially produce lifethreatening airway compromise.

Kimura et al.[16] have reported severe hypertension following stellate ganglion block. They reported seven patients who developed systolic blood pressures over 200 mm Hg after a stellate ganglion block. They postulated that local anesthetic diffused along the carotid sheath, resulting in block of the vagus nerve, attenuation of the baroreceptor reflex, and subsequent unopposed sympathetic activity.

Prevention and Treatment

Intravascular Injection

Careful aspiration prior to injection helps to prevent intravascular injection but is not 100% effective. Slight movement of the needle can change the position from extravascular to intravascular. Attaching tubing to the needle and having a second person perform the aspirations and injections may further decrease the chance of intravascular injections, although no studies have been performed to confirm this. Incremental injections of local anesthetic injection are also advocated by many to minimize the chance of a large intravascular injection.

In recent years, the use of ultrasound as an alternative to blind or fluoroscopy-guided techniques for performing stellate ganglion block has been described.[17] The stellate ganglion is a superficial structure and the use of ultrasound allows ready identification of the adjacent soft tissue and vascular structures that cannot be seen with fluoroscopy (Fig. 22-3). Ultrasound can be reliably used to avoid these vascular structures[18] and the use of ultrasound is likely to supplant other techniques for performing stellate ganglion block.

If an intravascular (arterial) injection occurs, a grand mal seizure often results. Fortunately, these are transient and usually resolve prior to initiation of any therapy. Therapy is directed at maintaining an airway and preventing oral (teeth or tongue) trauma. Oxygen should be administered as soon as possible, although the seizure often ends before therapy can be initiated. The most serious risk from a grand mal seizure is aspiration of vomitus. For this reason, it is

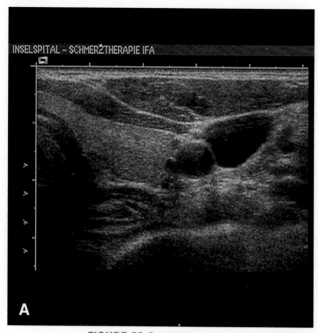
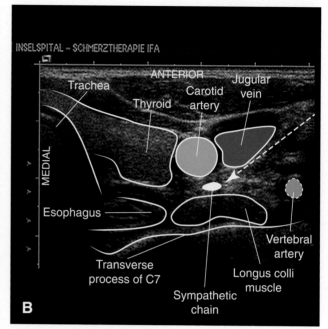

FIGURE 22-3. Anatomy relevant to stellate ganglion block as seen on ultrasound. A: Transverse (short-axis) ultrasound view at the level of the transverse process of C7. **B:** Labeled image. Note that the vertebral artery can be seen anterior to the echogenic transverse process at the level of C7. The vertebral artery cannot be seen clearly at the C6 level on ultrasound, as it lies posterior to the echogenic transverse process within the foramen transversarium. At the level of C7, the superior margin of the thyroid is seen just lateral to the trachea. The *dashed arrow* indicates the optimal trajectory for placing a needle using an in-plane approach, for example placing the needle in a lateral to medial direction with the shaft in the transverse plane of the ultrasound image. (Ultrasound image courtesy of Urs Eichenberger MD, PhD, University Department of Anesthesiology and Pain Therapy, University Hospital of Bern, Bern, Switzerland, 2011. Reproduced from Rathmell JP. *Atlas of Image-guided Intervention in Regional Anesthesia and Pain Medicine.* 2nd ed. Philadelphia, PA: Lippincott Williams & Wilkins, 2012, with permission.)

advisable to have a patient adhere to an "npo" status prior to the procedure. An intravenous line should be considered, particularly in patients with potentially difficult airways or larger than average necks.

Epidural or Intrathecal Injection

Epidural injection (with high concentration of local anesthetic) can produce a profound sensory and motor block but often spares the phrenic nerve. Subjective respiratory distress is common secondary to block of the intercostal nerves. If airway reflexes are intact, continuous oxygen saturation monitoring and cardiac monitoring will allow the patient to be cared for with supportive care (oxygen and IV fluids) and not require intubation. Small doses of benzodiazepines can be administered to allay the patient's fears while the block subsides.

Intrathecal injection of local anesthetic at this site commonly produces a total spinal block. Loss of airway reflexes and phrenic nerve function often occurs. Patients often describe as initial symptoms difficulty breathing or an inability to move their arms. Contralateral motor block develops as further confirmation, along with block of the lower extremities. Intubation and assisted ventilation are required until the block abates. Blood pressure, cardiac, and oxygen saturation monitoring should be performed until the block resolves. The duration of the block depends on the drug and the total dose injected. The patient will commonly remain awake during the event. Once the airway is protected and

vital signs stabilized, some sedation to keep the patient comfortable is advised. Verbal reassurance of the patient can further calm fears and assure them that the effects they are experiencing are temporary.

Recurrent Laryngeal and Phrenic Nerve Block

Symptoms of a recurrent laryngeal nerve block include hoarseness and, occasionally, respiratory stridor. Patients often complain of difficulty in getting their breath and the sensation of a lump in their throats. Symptomatic treatment is sufficient along with the reassurance that these sensations will resolve as the local anesthetic dissipates. Patients should be cautioned to drink clear liquids initially after a stellate ganglion block to make sure that their upper airway anatomy is not compromised. Once they feel comfortable swallowing liquids, they can progress to regular food. Phrenic nerve block rarely presents as a problem for patients unless they have preexisting severe respiratory compromise. The potential for producing phrenic nerve block is one reason bilateral stellate ganglion blocks are rarely performed at the same time. Most practitioners wait several days to a week between injections.

Pneumothorax

If air is aspirated during the placement of the needle, the examiner should decide if the trachea or pulmonary parenchyma has been entered. Breath sounds should be examined following the procedure if one suspects a pulmonary problem. Any abnormalities should be followed up with a chest x-ray. Inspiration and expiration films should be considered. With the common availability of bedside ultrasound, the diagnosis of even small pneumothoraces can now be made rapidly at the bedside[19]; use of time-motion mode (M-mode) ultrasound simplifies the diagnosis dramatically.

Delayed presentation of a pneumothorax is always possible. If a pneumothorax is suspected but unconfirmed, patients should be warned to call or go to an emergency facility if they become symptomatic. Patients who develop a pneumothorax should be hospitalized and watched closely, with appropriate consultation with a pulmonologist or a cardiothoracic surgeon if this is indicated.

Brachial Plexus Block

In a standard anterior (C6) approach to the stellate ganglion, the brachial plexus will not be blocked. However, partial block of the nerve roots that form the brachial plexus is commonly seen after a stellate ganglion block. This occurs most commonly when the needle has been inserted too deeply, bypasses the anterior tubercle, and rests on the posterior tubercle. After retraction from the posterior tubercle, the injection of local anesthetic is likely to block one or more of the roots of the brachial plexus.

There are no long-term sequelae of a block of the brachial plexus with local anesthetic. An intraneural injection is almost impossible, but extreme radiating pain during injection should be avoided in the unlikely event that the needle has pierced the epineurial layer of the nerve. Outpatients who develop a partial brachial plexus motor block should be warned about being insensate for possibly 24 hours or more (depending on the volume and concentration of local anesthetic used) and should avoid putting the extremity in an unsafe position, such as one where a burn could occur. Use of a sling may help diminish any risk associated with a motor block.

Partial brachial plexus block may make interpretation of the stellate ganglion block difficult. Complete sympathetic denervation may not coexist if the stellate ganglion is not equally blocked or the entire brachial plexus denervated. Patients can also be distracted by the motor block and experience dysesthesias, anesthesia dolorosa, and so on. Although complete brachial plexus denervation can be an excellent therapeutic modality for patients with severe dystonia and CRPS, partial block following stellate ganglion block should be viewed as an undesired (although most frequently harmless) side effect.

Other Complications

Hematoma. A hematoma following a stellate ganglion block occurs most commonly if the vertebral artery or carotid artery has been entered. In the event of a hematoma, direct pressure should be held by the examiner or nurse following known puncture of an artery. Communication with the patient should continue to make sure that there is no arterial compromise to the cerebral cortex while pressure is maintained.

Plaque Dislodgement. Presentation following dislodgement of a plaque after unintentional arterial puncture of either the carotid or the vertebral artery or following arterial wall dissection would be expected to mimic an evolving stroke. This should be viewed as a medical emergency, with life support and direct transport to an emergency facility indicated.

Infection. Risk of infection is minimized by the use of alcohol preparation of the site and good technique with sterile surgical gloves. More formal surgical preparation with betadine or a similar solution and sterile drapes can also be recommended. Many examiners believe it is important, however, to watch the patient during the injection for immediate feedback if an intravascular injection occurs and therefore recommend avoiding the use of drapes over the patient's face or positioning them carefully.

If an infection occurs, the most likely organism would be a strain of *Staphylococcus* unless the esophagus was inadvertently entered. Any infection should be treated with antibiotics and followed closely. An infectious disease consultation should be considered in patients who do not respond to a course of oral antibiotics.

Locked-in Syndrome. In the event of suspected locked-in syndrome (where the patient remains conscious but unable to breathe or move, with sparing of eye movement), supportive care should be instituted immediately—with respiratory support, sedation, and frequent reassurance (in that the patient will be conscious but unable to move or breathe).

Bilateral Recurrent Laryngeal Nerve Block. Bilateral recurrent laryngeal nerve block can produce life-threatening airway compromise and must be monitored closely. Intubation may be required if patients cannot sustain acceptable oxygen saturation.

▶ LUMBAR SYMPATHETIC BLOCK

Scope, Frequency, and Mechanism

LSB is commonly performed for either diagnostic or therapeutic purposes in patients with suspected sympathetically mediated pain in the lower extremities. It is also performed in patients with compromised vascular supply to the lower extremity. It may also be done occasionally in patients with other neuropathic lower extremity pain, such as diabetic neuropathy and PHN (although often with limited success). A recent prospective study of 216 LSBs performed with radiographic guidance demonstrated a 21.3% (46/216) incidence of injection into the psoas and 12.5% (27/216) incidence of intravascular injection of contrast.[20] There are no published data that present any estimate of the frequency of other complications associated with this block, and the complications described in the following discussion are derived from case reports. Complications that have been reported with LSB include intravascular injection, intraspinal injection, infection (including discitis), postdural puncture headache (PDPH), and hematoma formation (Box 22-5).

BOX 22-5 Complications of LSB

- Intravascular injection (generalized seizure, cardiovascular collapse)
- Intraspinal injection (spinal or epidural block)
- Infection (retroperitoneal abscess, discitis)
- PDPH
- Hematoma (superficial, retroperitoneal)

Mechanism of Causation

Intravascular Injection

On the left side of the spine, the aorta lies close to the needle-placement site for an LSB and the inferior vena cava is near the placement site for needles placed on the right side (Fig. 22-4). Large volumes of local anesthetic, particularly bupivacaine, injected into either vessel can cause seizures and/or cardiovascular collapse if injected into either vessel. Resuscitation can be prolonged and difficult if bupivacaine is injected.

Intraspinal Injection

It is possible for the needle to enter the intervertebral foramen and penetrate the dural sleeve of a spinal nerve with final placement in either the epidural or the intrathecal space, although this occurs less frequently now that fluoroscopy is commonly used during these procedures. Entry into the spinal canal when using the "blind" technique (i.e., using surface landmarks alone to guide needle placement) occurs when the angle of needle placement is too shallow and aims directly toward the intervertebral foramen rather than the anterolateral surface of the vertebral body.

Complications of Neurolytic Lumbar Sympathetic Block

Fluoroscopic use should decrease the incidence of complications from LSB injections. A comparison of alcohol and phenol demonstrated that alcohol blocks were more likely to produce an L2 neuralgia than was phenol. However, either agent can produce an L2 neuralgia, and this complication can occur with good spread of contrast. For this reason, some practitioners advocate the use of radiofrequency (RF) denervation. Multiple lesions are required with RF to achieve adequate denervation.[21] There is insufficient published information on the RF technique to understand if it will reduce the incidence of neuralgia. However, neuralgia has been reported in several cases following neurolytic LSB using RF.[21]

Discitis

The intervertebral disc lies near the path of an LSB needle (Fig. 22-4). It is not uncommon for the needle to unintentionally pass through part of the disc. Normally, this does not result in a complication, but discitis can occur.

Postprocedural Bleeding

Many patients who are taking a blood thinner or anticoagulant visit pain clinics for interventional procedures. All of the procedures discussed in this chapter have significant blood vessels in the vicinity of the needles used for the procedure. Maier et al.[22] have reported severe bleeding in two patients following LSB: a large subcutaneous hematoma in one case and a massive retroperitoneal hematoma in the second. Both patients were receiving irreversible platelet aggregation inhibitors (toclopidine or clopidogrel).

Other Complications

Postdural Puncture Headache. PDPH after LSB has been reported in two cases.[23] The cases most likely occurred as a result of the needle passing near a nerve root sleeve

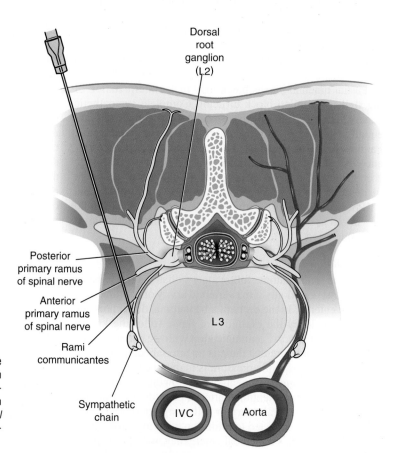

FIGURE 22-4. Axial diagram of LSB. A single needle passes over the transverse process, and the tip is in position adjacent to the lumbar sympathetic ganglia over the antero-medial surface of the L3 vertebral body. (Reproduced from Rathmell JP. *Atlas of Image-guided Intervention in Regional Anesthesia and Pain Medicine.* 2nd ed. Philadelphia, PA: Lippincott Williams & Wilkins, 2012, with permission.)

Dorsal root ganglion (L2)

Posterior primary ramus of spinal nerve

Anterior primary ramus of spinal nerve

Rami communicantes

Sympathetic chain

IVC

Aorta

L3

that contained spinal fluid. One patient underwent an unsuccessful attempt at an epidural blood patch.

Unintended Motor Block. Needles that are placed too laterally and posteriorly will come to rest in the psoas sheath or muscle. A striated appearance on fluoroscopy is indicative of needle placement into the muscle. If local anesthetic is injected, patients will develop a motor block of the lumbar plexus with resultant lower extremity weakness.

Renal Trauma/Ureter Puncture. Renal trauma or puncture of a ureter can occur with needles that begin too far laterally. Most practitioners avoid inserting the needle any more than 7 to 8 cm from the midline. Fortunately, sequelae are minimal unless a neurolytic is injected, resulting in possible ureteral stricture or extravasation of urine.

Prevention and Treatment

Intravascular Injection

Intravascular injection of large volumes of local anesthetic, particularly bupivacaine, can cause seizures and/or cardiovascular collapse. Resuscitation can be prolonged and difficult if bupivacaine is injected. Careful, frequent aspiration and intermittent injection is recommended. In a recent evaluation of 216 LSBs, the authors found that injection at the L2 level had a lower incidence of intravascular injection than injection at the L3 or L4 levels[20]; this same group found that the use of a live fluoroscopy technique was necessary to detect intravascular needle placement in most cases. If the solution contains epinephrine, changes in heart rate may serve as a signal of intravascular injection. A detailed description of local anesthetic toxicity can be found in Chapter 7.

Intraspinal Injection

Intraspinal injection should occur rarely, if ever, with the proper use of radiographic guidance during LSB. If a local anesthetic is the only drug used, side effects should resolve over time. Supportive care and vasopressors may be required. Neurolytic LSBs should only be performed using an imaging technique to ensure that the needle is sufficiently anterior and that no drug will track back into the intraspinal space.

Discitis

Historically, complete surgical drape, gown, and so on are not used for an LSB (as one might for a discogram). Whether this increases the risk of discitis is unclear. However, it would seem prudent to avoid the intervertebral disc whenever possible, given the potentially serious consequences of discitis. Our practice has seen one serious discitis from a "blind" LSB done before fluoroscopy was in common use. The patient ultimately required surgery and partial vertebrectomy to resolve the infection.

Postprocedural Bleeding

Stopping the use of anticoagulants or other drugs used to inhibit platelet aggregation carries its own set of risks. Patients have suffered embolic strokes when appropriately stopped from their anticoagulant medications prior to interventional procedures. The risk/benefit ratio of stopping or continuing any of these drugs should be carefully considered.

Alternative therapies may be appropriate. Consulting the patient's primary care physician or the specialist that is prescribing the anticoagulant may be indicated. (See Chapter 4 for a detailed discussion of the risks and recommendations for conduct of neural blockade in patients receiving anticoagulation.)

Other Complications

Postdural Puncture Headache. The diagnosis and management of PDPH is discussed in Chapter 9. Although epidural blood patch is not an unreasonable treatment, the location of the dural puncture is likely to be far lateral, near the intervertebral foramen, and this approach may well fail. We have seen PDPH develop following LSB, more commonly when performed without fluoroscopy. Our experience was similar to the previously referenced author in that epidural blood patch was not effective in treating the headache symptoms. However, all cases appear to be transient and resolve over a matter of days.

Unintended Motor Block. If femoral plexus block with resultant lower extremity weakness appears, patients should be observed and cautioned about what to expect. If bupivacaine is injected, the lower extremity weakness can last for hours and patients should be cautioned to move about carefully to avoid falling. Close monitoring may be indicated, depending on the patient.

Renal Trauma and Ureter Puncture. Renal trauma or puncture of a ureter can occur when needles begin far laterally. Most practitioners avoid inserting the needle any more than 7 to 8 cm from the midline. Fortunately, sequelae are minimal unless a neurolytic solution is injected. This may result in ureteral stricture or extravasation of urine.

▶ SUMMARY

Complications from sympathetic nerve blocks are typically self-limiting. Vascular structures lie in close proximity to the most commonly blocked plexi and sympathetic chain. Care should be used to avoid large intravascular injections of local anesthetics, particularly bupivacaine. Phenol can also cause problems when injected intravascularly in large amounts. Corticosteroids injected in the neck (e.g., stellate ganglion block) pose specific risks.

Intervertebral discs lie close to the path taken by many of the needles used for these nerve blocks. Whereas "transdiscal" approaches have been described for many of these procedures,[24] the practitioner should always consider the risk/benefit ratio before deciding on any given approach. Infections have been readily treated, although deep fascial infections can develop into abscesses and ultimately seed the epidural space if left untreated.

Finally, somatic nerve roots also lie near the sympathetic nerves in most areas of the body. The use of fluoroscopy aids the practitioner in minimizing the risk of damaging a nerve root, but does not eliminate this risk entirely. If the patient can be kept awake enough to communicate, permanent damage should be unlikely even if a needle contacts a neural structure during the procedure. Transient paresthesias or neuritis is commonly self-limiting and resolves over several weeks without specific treatment.

References

1. Boas RA. Sympathetic nerve blocks: in search of a role. *Reg Anesth Pain Med* 1998;23:292–305.

2. Cepeda MS, Lau J, Carr DB. Defining the therapeutic role of local anesthetic sympathetic blockade in complex regional pain syndrome: a narrative and systematic review. *Clin J Pain* 2002;18:216–233.

3. Tran de QH, Duong S, Bertini P, et al. Treatment of complex regional pain syndrome: a review of the evidence. *Can J Anaesth* 2010;57:149–166.

4. Wu CL, Marsh A, Dworkin RH. The role of sympathetic nerve blocks in herpes zoster and postherpetic neuralgia. *Pain* 2000;87: 121–129.

5. Peng PW, Castano ED. Survey of chronic pain practice by anesthesiologists in Canada. *Can J Anaesth* 2005;52:383–389.

6. Kozody R, Ready LB, Barsa JE, et al. Dose requirement of local anaesthetic to produce grand mal seizure during stellate ganglion block. *Can Anaesth Soc J* 1982;29:489–491.

7. Malmqvist EL, Bengtsson M, Sorensen J. Efficacy of stellate ganglion block: a clinical study with bupivacaine. *Reg Anesth* 1992;17:340–347.

8. Hogan QH, Erickson SJ, Haddox JD, et al. The spread of solutions during stellate ganglion block. *Reg Anesth* 1992;17:78–83.

9. Cho HM, Lee DY, Sung SW. Anatomical variations of rami communicantes in the upper thoracic sympathetic trunk. *Eur J Cardiothorac Surg* 2005;27:320–324.

10. Kashiwagi M, Ikeda N, Tsuji A, et al. Sudden unexpected death following stellate ganglion block. *Leg Med* (Tokyo) 1999;1:262–265.

11. Shimada Y, Marumo H, Kinoshita T, et al. A case of cervical spondylitis during stellate ganglion block. *J Nippon Med Sch* 2005;72:295–299.

12. Maeda S, Murakawa K, Fu K, et al. A case of pyogenic osteomyelitis of the cervical spine following stellate ganglion block. *Masui* 2004;53:664–667.

13. Dukes RR, Alexander LA. Transient locked-in syndrome after vascular injection during stellate ganglion block. *Reg Anesth* 1993;18:378–380.

14. Tuz M, Erodlu F, Dodru H, et al. Transient locked-in syndrome resulting from stellate ganglion block in the treatment of patients with sudden hearing loss. *Acta Anaesthesiol Scand* 2003;47:485–487.

15. Wallace MS, Milholland AV. Contralateral spread of local anesthetic with stellate ganglion block. *Reg Anesth* 1993;18:55–59.

16. Kimura T, Nishiwaki K, Yokota S, et al. Severe hypertension after stellate ganglion block. *Br J Anaesth* 2005;94:840–842.

17. Gofeld M, Bhatia A, Abbas S, et al. Development and validation of a new technique for ultrasound-guided stellate ganglion block. *Reg Anesth Pain Med* 2009;34:475–479.

18. Nix CM, Harmon DC. Avoiding intravascular injection during ultrasound-guided stellate ganglion block. *Anaesthesia* 2011;66: 134–135.

19. Ueda K, Ahmed W, Ross AF. Intraoperative pneumothorax identified with transthoracic ultrasound. *Anesthesiology* 2011;115:653–655.

20. Hong JH, Kim AR, Lee MY, et al. A prospective evaluation of psoas muscle and intravascular injection in lumbar sympathetic ganglion block. *Anesth Analg* 2010;111:802–807.

21. Rocco AG. Radiofrequency lumbar sympatholysis. The evolution of a technique for managing sympathetically maintained pain. *Reg Anesth* 1995;20:3–12.

22. Maier C, Gleim M, Weiss T, et al. Severe bleeding following lumbar sympathetic blockade in two patients under medication with irreversible platelet aggregation inhibitors. *Anesthesiology* 2002;97:740–743.

23. Artuso JD, Stevens RA, Lineberry PJ. Post dural puncture headache after lumbar sympathetic block: a report of two cases. *Reg Anesth* 1991;16:288–291.

24. Ohno K, Oshita S. Transdiscal lumbar sympathetic block: a new technique for a chemical sympathectomy. *Anesth Analg* 1997;85: 1312–1316.

23

Complications Associated with Neurolytic Celiac Plexus Block

Indy M. Wilkinson, Steven P. Cohen, and Michael A. Erdek

▶ DEFINITION AND SCOPE

Neurolytic celiac plexus block (NCPB) is a therapeutic analgesic technique predominantly employed in the management of patients suffering from visceral pain due to intra-abdominal malignancies. The block is achieved by the injection of neurolytic solutions (e.g., alcohol or phenol) around the celiac plexus or splanchnic nerves. In view of the inherent risks involved with neurolysis, most practitioners proceed with NCPB only after a positive response to a "prognostic" block performed with local anesthetic. Indications for NCPB primarily include intra-abdominal malignancies, but there is anecdotal evidence to suggest that this procedure may be effective in treating noncancer pain such as that caused by chronic pancreatitis as well.[1,2] Pain related to esophageal cancer, gastric cancer, colorectal cancer, gallbladder cancer, cholangiocarcinoma, and liver metastases has been treated effectively with a celiac plexus block.[3] It has also been shown to be helpful in the treatment of pediatric patients with hepatoblastoma and neuroblastoma.[4,5]

The National Cancer Institute estimates that there are over 43,000 new cases of pancreatic cancer each year in the United States alone. Combined with the NCI estimates for the yearly incidence of colorectal cancer (140,000), gastric cancer (21,000), esophageal cancer (16,000), gallbladder cancer (10,000), and cancer of the small intestine (7,000), there are over 200,000 new cases of malignancies amenable to NCBP diagnosed each year in the United States.[6] Most frequently though, NCPB is employed in the treatment of pain caused by pancreatic cancer, with some patients experiencing relief for half a year or longer. Anatomical location of the tumor seems to affect the efficacy of the block, with cancer confined to the head of the pancreas showing a more favorable response compared with that involving the body or tail, or spread to other structures.[7] This may be because metastatic or direct spread indicates a more advanced tumor. In a randomized controlled trial by Wong et al. involving patients with pancreatic cancer, NCPB was shown to provide superior analgesia to pharmacological therapy, as well as a reduction in systemic opioid use with a concomitant reduction in untoward, medication-related side effects.[8] Because NCPB targets the visceral component of pain, celiac plexus block with local anesthetic solutions can also be used as a "diagnostic" test used to differentiate visceral from somatic pain. However, up to 28% of patients who obtain a successful diagnostic celiac plexus block with local anesthetic fail to achieve a positive outcome with neurolytic blockade.[9] There is some evidence to suggest that lower baseline opioid doses and not using sedation during the diagnostic block may be associated with positive outcome from NCPB.[10]

Anatomy

The celiac plexus and splanchnic nerves are responsible for relaying the majority of visceral pain from the abdomen (Fig. 23-1). The celiac plexus is comprised of a complex network of presynaptic sympathetic nerves and ganglia overlying the anterolateral surface of the abdominal aorta surrounding the origin of the celiac artery at roughly the T12/L1 vertebral levels. The largest of all anatomical plexuses, it is made up of nerve fibers branching mainly from the greater (T5-T9), lesser (T10-T11), and least (T12) splanchnic nerves. Postsympathetic fibers leaving the ganglia synapse directly on the upper abdominal organs, excluding the descending colon, sigmoid colon, rectum, and pelvic viscera. Celiac plexus block is often carried out using computed tomography (CT), and this allows direct visualization of the structures that are adjacent to the celiac plexus as well as the structures that lie directly along the path of the advancing needle (Fig. 23-2).

Block Techniques

Celiac plexus blocks can be performed via multiple techniques including posterior and anterior approaches. The posterior approaches can be further classified into transcrural (aka anterocrural), retrocrural (through or adjacent to the vertebral disc), and its variant bilateral splanchnic nerve block (Fig. 23-1). The less frequently employed anterior approach can be further categorized into percutane-

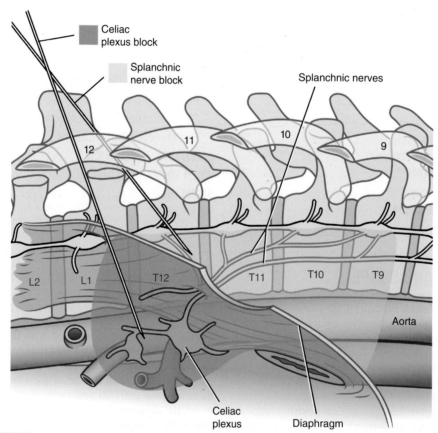

FIGURE 23-1. Anatomy of the celiac plexus and splanchnic nerves. The celiac plexus is comprised of a diffuse network of nerve fibers and individual ganglia located in close proximity to the anterolateral surface of the aorta at the T12/L1 vertebral level. Presynaptic sympathetic fibers travel from the thoracic sympathetic chain toward the celiac ganglia, traversing over the anterolateral aspect of the inferior thoracic vertebrae as the greater (T5-T9), lesser (T10-T11), and least (T12) splanchnic nerves. Celiac plexus block using a transcrural approach places the local anesthetic or neurolytic solution in direct contact with the celiac ganglion anterolateral to the aorta. The needles pass through the crura of the diaphragm en route to the celiac plexus. In contrast, for splanchnic nerve block, the needles remain posterior to the diaphragmatic crura in close apposition to the T12 vertebral body. Shading indicates the pattern of solution spread for each technique. (Reproduced from Rathmell JP. *Atlas of Image-Guided Intervention in Regional Anesthesia and Pain Medicine.* 2nd ed. Philadelphia, PA: Lippincott Williams & Wilkins, 2012, with permission.)

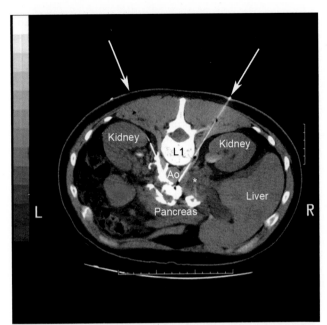

FIGURE 23-2. CT after the placement of two transcrural needles for NCPB. Neurolytic solution (10% phenol in iohexol 100 mg/mL) has been injected through both needles (10 mL on each side). The arrows indicate the approximate needle trajectory on each side. Contrast extends over the left anterolateral surface of the aorta and anteriorly along the posterior surface of the pancreas. There is a large soft tissue mass adjacent to the right-sided needle (asterisk) consistent with lymphadenopathy or metastatic tumor. (Reproduced from Rathmell JP, Gallant JM, Brown DL. Computed tomography and the anatomy of celiac plexus block. *Reg Anesth Pain Med* 2000;25:411–416, with permission.)

ous and laparoscopic techniques. In addition, celiac plexus neurolysis can be accomplished intraoperatively by the surgeon under direct visualization. Ideally, the technique utilized should be dictated by the patient's anatomy, tumor burden, and the likelihood of complications, which can vary based on technique.

Most of the techniques employed for celiac plexus block are described in terms of their relationship to the diaphragmatic crura. The crura of the diaphragm are tendinous structures that extend posteroinferiorly from the diaphragm and attach to the vertebral column. In the transcrural approach, the needles are inserted posteriorly and are advanced such that they traverse the crura and continue to the vicinity of the celiac plexus. This technique places the block solution anterolateral to the aorta in direct contact with the celiac plexus proper. In this approach, the diaphragm can act as a barrier to posterior spread of neurolytic solution, possibly decreasing the likelihood of it contacting and inadvertently damaging a spinal segmental artery or radicular tissue. In the transaortic variation of the transcrural block, generally done from the left side, the abdominal aorta is intentionally pierced in a posteroanterior direction in order to reach the celiac plexus on its anterolateral surface. Tissues traversed by the advancing needle during the transcrural technique include skin, subcutaneous adipose tissue, lumbar paraspinal muscles, the posterior abdominal wall, and the crura of the diaphragm. Structures in close proximity to the passage of the needle are the epidural and intrathecal spaces, the kidneys, and the pancreas.

In the retrocrural approach, the needles begin posteriorly, usually at the cephalad portion of L1, and are advanced superiorly and anteriorly, stopping proximal to the crura. In this technique, the advancement of the needle stops before it reaches the aorta and might therefore reduce the risk of aortic trauma. In addition, smaller volumes of solution are needed for this technique, and the diaphragm works as a barrier to reduce the influence of extensive tumor burden on the spread of the neurolytic solution.

Variations of the classic two-needle retrocrural technique utilize a single-needle approach. In one adaptation, a long needle is inserted under fluoroscopy guidance until the tip is positioned cephalad to the celiac artery to achieve a wider, bilateral spread of neurolytic solution.[11] In a second variant, a small-gauge needle is inserted transdiscally through one of the lower thoracic levels, until the tip is situated in the midline just anterior to the annulus fibrosus. A single-needle approach has been shown to decrease fluoroscopy time when compared with the classic technique[12] and is probably less painful owing to reduced tissue trauma.[13] Traversing an intervertebral disc carries the risk of discitis,[14] a higher incidence of nerve root injury, and possibly increased disc degeneration at long-term follow-up.[15] Risk mitigation strategies include using a smaller gauge needle to minimize the likelihood of disc degeneration; the judicious use of sedation to diminish the risk of nerve injury; and employing a double-needle technique, which has been postulated to reduce the risk of discitis during lumbar discograms.[16] Whereas some experts have advocated prophylactic antibiotics to reduce the risk of discitis, systematic reviews have failed to support this.[15,17,18]

Splanchnic nerve block is a variant of the retrocrural technique, with the main difference being that it warrants the needles being placed more cephalad at the mid- to anterior border of the T12 vertebral body. Both the splanchnic and classic retrocrural approaches block the splanchnic nerves via the cephalad spread of solution and are essentially the same technique. Whereas arguments have been made advocating the use of one approach over the other, no evidence exists that supports the superiority of either.

In the percutaneous anterior approach, the patient lies in the supine position. The origin of the celiac trunk is identified using ultrasound or CT. After superficial injection of local anesthesia, a 15 cm needle is ultrasonographically guided into the preaortic area near the origin of the celiac trunk where local anesthetic and/or neurolytic solution is injected.[19] Pain relief with this technique is comparable to that associated with posterior approaches.[20] Advantages of the anterior approach include the fact that it is done with the patient in the supine position, which is significantly more comfortable for many patients with terminal intra-abdominal malignancies. In addition, the needle trajectory does not traverse any major neural structures other than the celiac plexus itself and therefore may be associated with a lower theoretical risk of neurologic complications. Disadvantages of the anterior approach include the possibility of piercing the bowel, and there is a case report of a patient developing a retroperitoneal abscess with the formation of a vascular-enteric fistula following this technique.[21] The laparoscopic anterior approach may decrease some of these risks owing to its performance under direct visualization but carries with it the inherent risks associated with general anesthesia.

Neurolytic Solutions

Neurodestructive agents such as ethanol and phenol are typically employed during the neurolytic procedure. The most commonly used neurolytic agent is ethanol. Typical concentrations range between 50% and 100%, with volumes ranging between 20 and 50 mL, though somewhat smaller volumes are needed for retrocrural techniques.[22] The mechanism of action of ethanol is thought to be via the extraction of cholesterol and phospholipids from neural cell membranes, causing precipitation of lipoproteins and mucoproteins.[9] Ethanol can produce severe pain when injected by itself. Therefore, some experts advocate injecting 5 to 10 mL of local anesthetic 5 minutes prior to the administration of ethanol to minimize discomfort. Another approach is to dilute 100% ethanol by 50% with a local anesthetic.

Some authors have advocated the use of phenol in a concentration >6% because phenol (often mixed with glycerin) induces necrosis when applied directly to the neural tissue.[9,23] At lower concentrations, it has reversible local anesthetic effects, rendering it less effective for long-term analgesia. Phenol produces nonselective tissue destruction by denaturing proteins in axons and adjacent blood vessels. The degree of damage after peripheral nerve block is concentration-dependent, and the changes range from segmental demyelination to complete Wallerian degeneration.[24] One advantage of phenol is the fact that it is painless on injection. Disadvantages of phenol include its slower and shorter duration of action. Axonal regeneration occurs more rapidly than after ethanol. In addition, its increased viscosity limits its usefulness in clinical practice.

▶ FREQUENCY AND MECHANISM OF SPECIFIC COMPLICATIONS

Although NCPB is a relatively safe procedure, it may be associated with a variety of complications. These complications range from minor, often expected untoward effects of successful celiac plexus/splanchnic nerve blockade, to those that are major and life-threatening. The potential for complications must be considered carefully while being cognizant of the fact that in many patients with limited life expectancies associated with intra-abdominal malignancies, the analgesic benefit of the procedure outweighs these risks. Nonetheless, all potential complications should be discussed with patients and/or their legal power of attorney prior to the procedure.

In a randomized controlled study by Wong et al.[8] involving 104 NCPBs, the most common complications were weakness or numbness in the T10-L2 distribution (8%), lower chest pain (3%), postural hypotension (2%), failure of ejaculation (2%), difficult urination (1%), and warmth and fullness of the leg (1%). In a review of 2,730 patients conducted between 1986 and 1990, the overall incidence of major complications from NCPB, such as paraplegia and bladder and bowel dysfunction, was 1 in 683 procedures.[25]

Ischia et al.[26] compared three percutaneous NCPB techniques—transaortic approach, classic retrocrural approach, and bilateral splanchnic blocks—in a prospective study involving 61 patients with pancreatic cancer. Although there were no differences in analgesic efficacy or major complications among the various approaches, orthostatic hypotension occurred more frequently with the retrocrural or splanchnic nerve blocks, and bowel hypermotility (e.g., diarrhea) was more common with the transaortic, transcrural technique.

Systemic Complications

When neurolysis is performed with ethanol, acetaldehyde toxicity may occur in individuals who lack the enzyme aldehyde dehydrogenase. This mutation occurs when a lysine residue replaces a glutamate in the active site at position 487 of ALDH-2 and is more common in East Asians. The accumulation of aldehyde in the blood results in palpitations, facial flushing, and hypotension. Alcohol neurolysis can also induce toxic reactions in patients treated with drugs that inhibit acetaldehyde dehydrogenase. In two separate case reports,[27,28] patients taking the drugs moxalactam and carmofur that inhibit this enzyme experienced disulfiram-like reactions characterized by temporary flushing, sweating, dizziness, vomiting, and hypotension following alcohol celiac plexus neurolysis. Other agents that possess this property include metronidazole, chloramphenicol, tolbutamide, chlorpropamide, and other β-lactam–type antibiotics.

Some patients who undergo blocks with alcohol may experience systemic effects similar to those observed after ethanol ingestion. Thompson and colleagues found that blood alcohol levels in five patients rose acutely over the first 20 minutes to a peak level of 0.021 g/dL following celiac plexus neurolysis with 50 mL of 50% alcohol.[29] Although this is only 25% of the common legal limit for alcohol intoxication, it is possible that cognitive effects may occur when higher concentrations are injected in elderly patients, or those with low body weights. Treatment of systemic complications is supportive in nature, as most are self-limited.

The intravascular injection, or rapid vascular uptake, of phenol may also result in systemic toxicity. In addition to sensory and motor deficits, the intravascular injection of phenol may result in convulsions resulting from an increase in acetylcholine in the central nervous system. Systemic doses of phenol in excess of typical clinical doses (more than 8 g) cause effects similar to those seen with local anesthetic overdose, such as generalized seizures and cardiovascular collapse. This effect may be at least partially due to an increase in acetylcholine in the central nervous system.[30] Clinical doses up to 1 g are unlikely to cause serious toxicity in the absence of intravenous injection.[31]

Neurologic Complications

Neurologic complications from NCPB primarily manifest as sensory and/or motor deficits distal to the celiac plexus in the trunk and lower extremities. Although the incidence is low (1 in 683 procedures resulted in paraplegia),[25] major neurologic deficits can cause dramatic reductions in the quality of life. There are multiple proposed mechanisms for these complications. The most widely accepted is the inadvertent injection of neurolytic solution into the vicinity of the neural tissue other than the celiac plexus or splanchnic nerves. Neural structures in close proximity to the needle trajectory that may be accidentally damaged include the spinal cord via the epidural and intrathecal space, thoracic and lumbar nerve roots exiting the vertebral foramen, and the lumbar

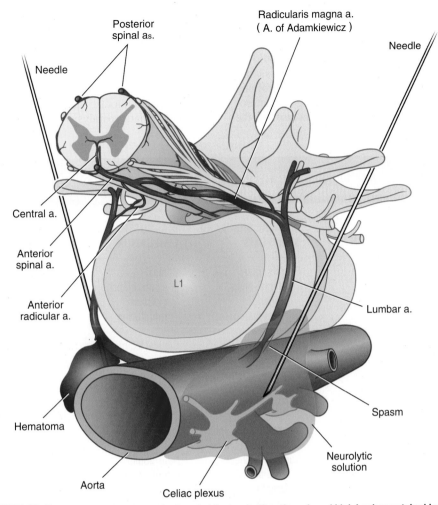

FIGURE 23-3. **Arterial supply of the spinal cord at the level of low thoracic and high lumbar vertebral levels.** The largest feeding artery to the spinal cord is the artery of Adamkiewicz (anterior radicular artery), which branches from the lumbar artery (in this figure).

plexus. Even in the absence of direct contact of these neural structures, interruption of their blood supply can cause necrosis and permanent deficits. Ethanol has been shown to induce vasospasm of the segmental lumbar arteries in dogs, and accidental injection into a radicular artery supplying the spinal cord may be a potential ischemic cause of paraplegia after celiac plexus block (Fig. 23-3).[22,32] If arterial vasospasm is suspected, immediate radiological consultation is needed, as previous studies have shown that the timely administration of intra-arterial vasodilators may reverse neurological sequelae.[33] It is important to emphasize that the use of radiographic guidance does not provide certain protection from neurologic complications. In a large series of 2,730 patients receiving NCPB, four cases of permanent paraplegia occurred.[25] In all four cases, radiographic guidance was used, including the use of radiographic contrast to confirm final needle placement.

Cardiovascular Complications

Cardiovascular complications range from mild transient orthostatic hypotension to the more serious major vascular complications of aortic dissection and pseudoaneurysm. Other vascular complications include phlebitis, vessel thrombosis, vasospasm, tissue ischemia, and damage to the microcirculation around small nerves. Orthostatic hypotension may occur for up to 5 days after NCPB in approximately 3% of patients.[8] Because the celiac plexus and splanchnic nerves are sympathetic networks, their blockade results in a relative increase in parasympathetic tone. The resulting vasodilation of the splanchnic vasculature can result in blood pooling and orthostatic hypotension. Ensuring adequate intravascular volume prior to the procedure may minimize this complication. Treatment includes hydration, supine bed rest, and avoiding sudden changes in position. Wrapping the lower extremities with elastic bandages has been successfully used in treating patients who developed orthostatic hypotension and needed to walk during the first week following the block. In refractory cases, alpha-1 agonists can be considered.

Aortic dissection and aortic pseudoaneurysm have been observed following NCPB.[34] Aortic injury can occur as a result of direct damage from the needle during the procedure, or injection of fluid into the vessel wall.[30] The latter scenario can usually be detected by contrast injection under fluoroscopy. Ethanol has been shown to have contractile effects in human aortic muscle cells by increasing the intracellular concentration of ionized calcium,[35] but whether this can clinically alter the complication rate is unknown. In addition, needle puncture of the aorta or the inferior vena cava may rarely result in retroperitoneal hemorrhage. Patients presenting with orthostatic hypotension and backache should be monitored with serial hematocrit testing to assure this complication does not go undetected. Complications involving the aorta are seen more frequently when using the anterocrural approach. If severe atherosclerotic disease of the abdominal aorta is present, or a graft is in place, clinicians should strongly consider using a retrocrural technique.

Pulmonary Complications

Pulmonary complications of NCPB include pulmonary trauma, pneumothorax, pleural effusion, chylothorax, and diaphragmatic paralysis.[36,37] These complications are

TABLE 23-1 Summary of Complications Associated with NCPB. Clinical Signs and Symptoms, Diagnostic Evaluation and Management

ORGAN SYSTEM	COMPLICATION	CLINICAL SIGNS AND SYMPTOMS	DIAGNOSTIC EVALUATION	MANAGEMENT
Systemic	Allergic reaction	Pruritis, rash, edema, hives, urticaria, hypotension, dyspnea	Clinical exam, blood pressure monitoring	Varies by severity of the reaction ranging from self-limited to antihistamine, corticosteroid, epinephrine, and airway management
	Alcohol intoxication	Euphoria, dysarthria, ataxia, loss of consciousness	Clinical exam, blood alcohol concentration	Supportive
Nervous	Seizure	Confusion, convulsions, urinary incontinence, loss of consciousness	Clinical exam, EEG	Airway management, benzodiazepines/barbiturates
	Sensory/motor deficits of the trunk/lower extremities	Numbness, weakness, paresis, paresthesia, paraplegia	Neurologic examination, radiologic imaging, EMG	Emergent neurology evaluation
Cardiovascular	Orthostatic hypotension	Positional hypotension, lightheadedness, syncope	Orthostatic blood pressure readings	Self-limited to hydration, leg wraps, alpha-1 agonists
	Hemorrhage	Pain, hypotension	Radiologic imaging	Self-limited to necessitating surgical or interventional radiological intervention
	Aortic dissection	Pain, hypotension	Radiologic imaging	Emergent surgery or interventional radiology
Pulmonary	Lung trauma, pneumothorax, chylothorax, pleural effusion	Dyspnea, hypotension, tachycardia, diminished or absent unilateral breath sounds	Radiographic imaging	Self-limited to needle decompression/chest tube
Gastrointestinal	Bowel hypermotility	Diarrhea, incontinence	Clinical exam	Loperamide, hydration, supportive
Genitourinary	Renal trauma	Hematuria, hypotension	Radiologic imaging	Urology consult
	Incontinence	Incontinence	Neurology consult	Limited treatment available
	Ejaculatory dysfunction	Sexual dysfunction	Neurologic and urologic evaluation	Limited treatment available

Radiographic refers to x-ray; radiologic to other forms.

exceedingly rare but can occur when higher vertebral levels are targeted. Pneumothorax results from needle puncture of the pleura. Pleural effusion may result from diaphragmatic irritation by a neurolytic agent injected into or proximal to the diaphragm.[38]

Gastrointestinal Complications

Gastrointestinal complications range from mild bowel hypermotility to direct trauma to gastrointestinal viscera. Bowel hypermotility is an expected side effect, but can be life-threatening in a debilitated, dehydrated patient.[39] As with orthostatic hypotension, NCPB causes bowel hypermotility as a result of an imbalance in the sympathetic/parasympathetic tone (favoring parasympathetic). Although bowel hypermotility is typically self-limited, treatment with loperamide or another antimotility agent can resolve symptoms in the short run. Bowel and pancreatic injury can occur as a result of direct needle trauma. If pancreatic injury occurs, only minimal elevations of amylase may be noted.[40]

Genitourinary Complications

Genitourinary complications include ejaculatory dysfunction, hematuria caused by renal trauma, and renal infarction after accidental neurolytic injection.[14] Injury to the kidney is more likely when needle insertion is more than 7.5 cm from the midline, a higher vertebral level is targeted (T11-12), or needle position is lateral to the vertebral body.[41]

▶ DIAGNOSTIC EVALUATION

Diagnosis and treatment of complications following NCPB is contingent upon the specific complication that is present and the organ system affected, as summarized in Table 23-1.

▶ WHEN TO SEEK FURTHER CONSULTATION

Minor complications like orthostatic hypotension and bowel hypermotility can be expected as the result of a successful NCPB, but any patient demonstrating hemodynamic instability should be monitored closely while a cause is being sought. If a major complication is suspected, the practitioner should seek immediate consultation by specialized services. Some of the major complications associated with NCPB such as aortic dissection and vasospasm can result in permanent sequelae if immediate action is not taken, and care must be taken to address them urgently.

▶ SUMMARY

Neurolytic celiac plexus blockade provides analgesia that is superior to pharmacologic therapy without the associated medication-related side effects in the setting of visceral pain due to intra-abdominal malignancies and pancreatitis. It is a relatively safe procedure, with the most frequently observed complications being minor and self-limited. Major complications, while rare, can be significant or even life-threatening if not dealt with immediately. The risk/benefit analysis of this procedure must therefore be carefully considered in the setting of each individual patient and explicitly discussed between patients and caregivers.

References

1. Whiteman M, Rosenberg H, Haskin P et al. Celiac plexus block for interventional radiology. *Radiology* 1986;161:836–838

2. Rykowski JJ, Hilgier M. Continuous celiac plexus block in acute pancreatitis. *Reg Anesth* 1995;20:528–532.

3. Eisenberg E, Carr DB, Chalmers TC. Neurolytic celiac plexus block for treatment of cancer pain: a meta-analysis. *Anesth Analg* 1995;80(2):290–295.

4. Berde C, Sethna N, Fisher D et al. Celiac plexus blockade for a 3-year-old boy with hepatoblastoma and refractory pain. *Pediatrics* 1990;5:779–781

5. Staats P, Kost-Byerly S. Celiac plexus blockade in a 7-year-old child with neuroblastoma. *J Pain Symptom Manage* 1995;10:321–324

6. Cancer Trends Progress Report—2009/2010 Update, National Cancer Institute, NIH, DHHS, Bethesda, MD, April 2010, http://progressreport.cancer.gov

7. Rykowski JJ, Hilgier M. Efficacy of neurolytic celiac plexus block in varying locations of pancreatic cancer: influence on pain relief. *Anesthesiology* 2000;92(2):347–354.

8. Wong GY, Schroeder DR, Carns PE, et al. Effect of neurolytic celiac plexus block on pain relief, quality of life, and survival in patients with unresectable pancreatic cancer: a randomized controlled trial. *JAMA* 2004;291(9):1092–1099.

9. Fugere F, Lewis G. Celiac plexus block for chronic pain syndromes. *Can J Anaesth* 1993;40:954–963

10. Erdek M, Halpert D, Fernandez M, et al. Assessment of celiac plexus block and neurolysis outcomes and technique in the management of refractory visceral cancer pain. *Pain Med* 2010;11(1):92–100.

11. De Cicco, M. Single-needle celiac plexus block: is needle tip position critical in patients with no regional anatomic distortions? *Anesthesiology* 1997;87(6):1301–1308.

12. Ugur F, Gulcu N, Boyaci A. Celiac plexus block with the long stylet needle technique. *Adv Ther* 2007;24(2):296–301.

13. Stojanovic MP, Dey D, Hord ES, et al. A prospective crossover comparison study of the single-needle and multiple-needle techniques for facet-joint medial branch block. *Reg Anesth Pain Med* 2005;30:484–490.

14. Kapoor SG, Huff J, Cohen SP. Systematic review of the incidence of discitis after cervical discography. *Spine J* 2010;10(8):739–745.

15. Carragee EJ, Don AS, Hurwitz EC, et al. Does discography cause accelerated progression of degeneration changes in the lumbar disc: a ten-year matched cohort study. *Spine* 2009;34(21):2338–2345.

16. Fraser RD, Osti OL, Vernon-Roberts B. Discitis after discography. *J Bone Joint Surg Br* 1987;69:26–35

17. Willems PC, Jacobs W, Duinkerke ES, et al. Lumbar discography: should we use prophylactic antibiotics? A study of 435 consecutive discograms and a systematic review of the literature. *J Spinal Disord Tech* 2004;17:243–247.

18. Sharma SK, Jones JO, Zeballos PP, et al. The prevention of discitis during discography. *Spine J* 2009;9:936–943

19. Zenz M, Kurs-Muller K, Strumpf M, et al. The anterior sonographic-guided celiac plexus blockade. Review and personal observations. *Anaesthesist* 1993;42(4):246–255.

20. Romanelli D, Beckmann C, Heiss F. Celiac plexus block: efficacy and safety of the anterior approach. *Am J Roentgenol* 1993;160:497–500.

21. Navarro-Martinez J, Montes A, Comps O, et al. Retroperitoneal abscess after neurolytic celiac plexus block from the anterior approach. *Reg Anesth Pain Med* 2003;28(6):528–530.

22. De Leon-Casasola OA, Ditonio E. Drugs commonly used for nerve blocking: neurolytic agents. In: Raj PP, ed. *Practical Management of Pain*. 3rd ed. St. Louis: Mosby, 2000:575–578.

23. Akhan O, Altinok D, Özmen MN, et al. Correlation between the grade of tumoral invasion and pain relief in patients with celiac ganglia block. *AJR* 1997;168:1565–1567.

24. Gregg RV, Constantini CH, Ford DJ, et al. Electrophysiologic and histopathologic investigation of phenol in renografin as a neurolytic agent. *Anesthesiology* 1985;63:239.

25. Davis DD. Incidence of major complications of neurolytic coeliac plexus block. *J R Soc Med* 1993;86:264–266.

26. Ischia S, Ischia A, Polati E, et al. Three posterior percutaneous celiac plexus block techniques: a prospective randomized study in 61 patients with pancreatic cancer pain. *Anesthesiology* 1992;76:534–540.

27. Noda J, Umeda S, Mori K, et al. Acetaldehyde syndrome after celiac plexus alcohol block. *Anesth Analg* 1986;65(12):1300–1302.

28. Noda J, Umeda S, Mori K, et al. Disulfiram-like reaction associated with carmofur after celiac plexus alcohol block. *Anesthesiology* 1987;67(5):809–810.

29. Thompson GE, Moore DC, Bridenbaugh DL, et al. Abdominal pain and alcohol celiac plexus nerve block. *Anesth Analg* 1977;56:1–5.

30. Sett SS, Taylor DC. Aortic pseudoaneurysm secondary to celiac plexus block. *Ann Vasc Surg* 1991;5:88–91.

31. Benzon HT. Convulsions secondary to intravascular phenol: a hazard of celiac plexus block. *Anesth Analg* 1979;58:150–151.

32. Brown DL, Rorie DK. Altered reactivity of isolated segmental lumbar arteries of dogs following exposure to ethanol and phenol. *Pain* 1994;56:139–143.

33. Vijayvergiya R, Otal PS, Bagga S, et al. Symptomatic carotid vasospasm caused by a distal-protection device during stent angioplasty of the right internal carotid artery. *Tex Heart Inst J* 2010;37(2):226–229.

34. Kaplan R, Schiff-Keren B, Alt E. Aortic dissection as a complication of celiac plexus block. *Anesthesiology*. 1995;83:632–635.

35. Johnson ME, Sill JC, Brown DL, et al. The effect of the neurolytic agent ethanol on cytoplasmic calcium in arterial smooth muscle and endothelium. *Reg Anesth* 1996;21:6–13.

36. Rosenthal J. Diaphragmatic paralysis complicating alcohol splanchnic nerve block. *Anesth Analg* 1998;86:845–846.

37. Fine PG, Bubela C. Chylothorax following celiac plexus block. *Anesthesiology* 1985;63:454–456.

38. Fujita Y, Takori M. Pleural effusion after CT-guided alcohol celiac plexus block. *Anesth Analg* 1987;66:911–912.

39. Matson JA, Ghia JN, Levy JH. A case report of a potentially fatal complications associated with Ischia's transaortic method of celiac plexus block. *Reg Anesth* 1985;10:193–196.

40. Lubenow TR, Ivankovich AD. Serum alcohol, CPK, and amylase levels following celiac plexus block with alcohol. *Reg Anesth* 1988;13(Suppl):64.

41. Moore DC. Celiac (splanchnic) plexus block with alcohol for cancer pain of the upper intra-abdominal viscera. In: Bonica JJ, Ventafridda V, eds. *Advances in Pain Research and Therapy.* Vol 2. New York, NY: Raven Press, 1979:357–371.

24

Complications Associated with Superior Hypogastric and Ganglion Impar Blocks

James M. Hitt and Oscar A. de Leon-Casasola

▶ DEFINITION AND SCOPE

The relevant anatomy and technique for superior hypogastric and ganglion impar blocks have been well described, but only limited observational data point to the usefulness of these techniques for treating pain arising from the pelvic viscera. Few complications have been reported as resulting from these techniques. Therefore, much of the following discussion focuses on *potential* complications.

Stretch, compression, invasion by tumor, or distension of visceral structures can result in a poorly localized noxious type of pain known as visceral pain. Patients experiencing visceral pain often describe the pain as vague, deep, squeezing, crampy, or colicky. Other signs and symptoms include referred pain (e.g., shoulder pain that appears when the liver's capsule of Gleason is distended due to tumor growth) and nausea/vomiting due to vagal irritation.

Visceral pain associated with cancer may be relieved with oral pharmacologic therapy that includes combinations of nonsteroidal anti-inflammatory drugs, opioids, and other adjuvant therapy. In addition to pharmacologic therapy, neurolytic blocks of the superior hypogastric plexus are also effective in controlling pelvic visceral pain due to cancer and should be considered as important adjuncts to pharmacologic therapy for the relief of severe pain experienced by cancer patients. These blocks rarely eliminate cancer pain, because patients frequently experience coexisting somatic and neuropathic pain. Therefore, oral pharmacologic therapy must be continued in the majority of these cases, albeit at lower doses. The goals of performing a neurolytic block of this nature are to maximize the analgesic effects of opioid or nonopioid analgesics while reducing the total daily dose of these agents to alleviate or reduce both the incidence and the severity of side effects.

▶ SUPERIOR HYPOGASTRIC PLEXUS BLOCK

Cancer patients with tumors within the organs of the pelvis may experience severe pain that is unresponsive to oral or parenteral opioids. Moreover, excessive sedation or other side effects may limit the acceptability and usefulness of oral opioid therapy and/or adjuvants. Therefore, an invasive approach that effectively controls pain would improve the quality of life of these patients.

Clinical Uses

Visceral pelvic pain associated with cancer and chronic nonmalignant conditions may be alleviated by blocking the superior hypogastric plexus.[1,2] Analgesia is possible because the afferent fibers innervating the organs in the pelvis travel in the sympathetic nerves, trunks, ganglia, and rami. Thus, a sympathectomy for visceral pain is analogous to a peripheral neurectomy or dorsal rhizotomy for somatic pain. A recent study[1] suggests that visceral pain is an important component of the cancer pain syndrome experienced by patients with cancer of the pelvis, even in advanced stages. Thus, percutaneous neurolytic blocks of the superior hypogastric plexus should be considered more often for patients with advanced stages of pelvic cancer.

Anatomy

The superior hypogastric plexus is situated in the retroperitoneum, bilaterally extending from the lower third of the fifth lumbar vertebral body to the upper third of the first sacral vertebral body (Fig. 24-1). It receives fibers from the inferior hypogastric plexus, which in turn receives all afferent fibers from the pelvic organs. Because the inferior hypogastric plexus is not a distinct structure, but rather a group of branched fibers, it would be difficult to perform a

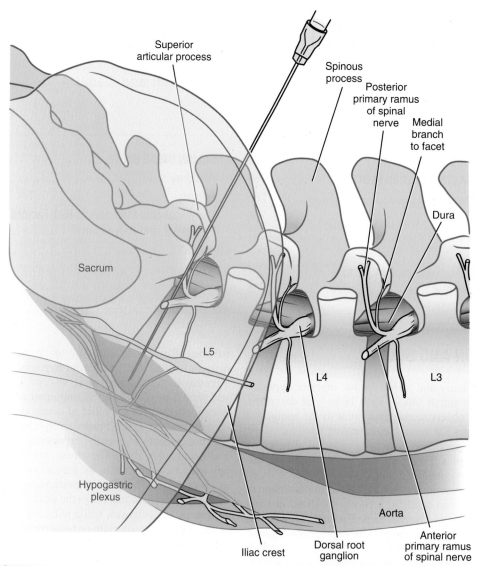

FIGURE 24-1. Anatomy of the superior hypogastric plexus. The superior hypogastric plexus is comprised of a loose web-like group of interlacing nerve fibers that lie over the anterolateral surface of the L5 vertebral body and extend inferiorly over the sacrum. Needles are positioned over the anterolateral surface of the L5/S1 intervertebral disc of the inferior aspect of the L5 vertebral bodies to block the superior hypogastric plexus. (Reproduced with permission from Rathmell JP. *Atlas of Image-guided Intervention in Regional Anesthesia and Pain Medicine.* 2nd ed. Philadelphia, PA: Lippincott Williams & Wilkins, 2012.)

neurolytic procedure at this level. Conversely, the superior hypogastric plexus has two well-defined ganglia, making it feasible to block.

Technique

Patients are placed in the prone position with a pillow under the pelvis to flatten the lumbar lordosis. Two 7-cm needles are inserted with the bevel directed medially 45 degrees and 30 degrees caudad so that the tips lie anterolateral to the L5-S1 intervertebral disc space. Aspiration is important to avoid injection into the iliac vessels. If blood is aspirated, a transvascular approach can be used. The accurate placement of the needle is verified via biplanar fluoroscopy. Anterior-posterior (AP) views should reveal the tip of the needle at the level of the junction of the L5 and S1 vertebral bodies. This is an important safety step to avoid potential spread of the neurolytic agent toward the L5. Lateral views will confirm the placement of the needle's tip just beyond the vertebral body's anterolateral margin. The injection of 3 to 5 mL of water-soluble contrast medium is used to verify the accurate needle placement and to rule out intravascular injection. In the AP view, the spread of contrast should be confined to the midline region. In the lateral view, a smooth posterior contour corresponding to the anterior psoas fascia indicates that the needle is at the appropriate depth. Figures 24-2 and 24-3 show adequate needle placement and contrast medium spread prior to neurolysis of the superior hypogastric plexus.

For a prognostic hypogastric plexus blockade or for patients with non–cancer-related pain, local anesthetic alone is used. For therapeutic purposes in patients with cancer-related pain, phenol is typically used as the neurolytic solution.

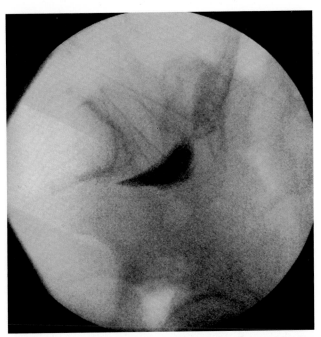

FIGURE 24-3. Superior hypogastric plexus block. Cross-lateral view of the lumbosacral region with two 22-gauge Chiba needles placed at the correct site and one placed in the upper third of the fifth lumbar vertebra. This last needle represents inappropriate needle placement.

The transdiscal approach has gained interest as an alternative to the classic approach for some patients. Barriers to the classic approach to the superior hypogastric plexus block (SHPB) include atherosclerotic disease of the iliac vessels, the L5 transverse process, the L5 nerve root, and the iliac crest. Two transdiscal approaches have been described—a traditional lateral approach that is performed similar to discography at the L5-S1 level[3] and a posteromedian approach that involves crossing the subarachnoid space.[4] Figures 24-4 and 24-5 illustrate needle placement for the transdiscal approach of the SHPB in the oblique and lateral views, respectively. Figure 24-5 demonstrates the spread of contrast in the retroperitoneal space where the superior hypogastric plexus lies.

Gamal et al.[3] compared the classic and transdiscal approach to the SHPB in 30 patients and reported that the transdiscal approach was associated with decreased procedure time, similar efficacy, and no complications. Despite lack of complications reported, the limited data available combined with recent data concerning long-term complications of discography raise some concerns for routine use of this approach.

The anterior approach to the SHPB has also been described using either CT guidance or ultrasound.[5,6] Prior to attempting an anterior approach to the SHPB, patients need to have preprocedure bowel and bladder preparation to limit the risk of visceral injury and possible intraabdominal or retroperitoneal infection. A case series of 10 patients reported that a CT-guided anterior approach is a safe and effective alternative approach for performing an SHPB.[5] This technique allows for detailed visualization of the aorta, iliac veins, and lumbar nerve roots, but it does involve inserting a needle through intestinal loops, which can result in transmitting intestinal flora to the retroperitoneum.

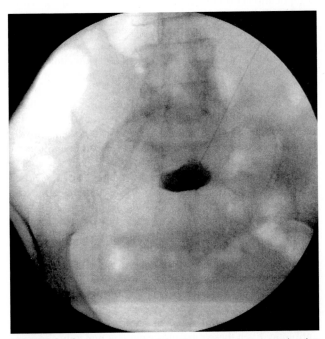

FIGURE 24-2. Superior hypogastric plexus block. Anteroposterior view of the lumbosacral area with a 22-gauge Chiba needle placed at the junction of the lumbosacral vertebrae. Notice that the injection of 3 mL of radiographic contrast was performed with a single needle to demonstrate the spread to the midline.

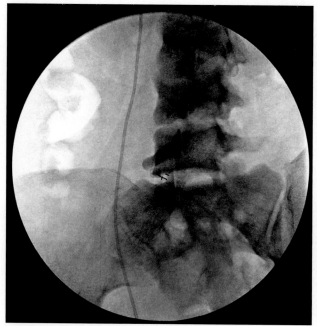

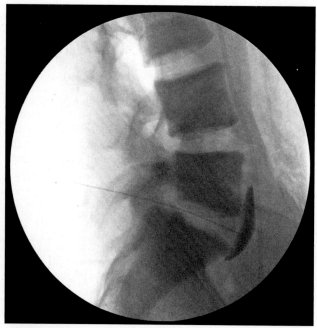

FIGURE 24-4. **Superior hypogastric plexus block, transdiscal approach.** Oblique view of the lumbosacral spine with localizing marks indicating the insertion site and path for a transdiscal approach to the superior hypogastric plexus.

FIGURE 24-5. **Superior hypogastric plexus block, transdiscal approach.** Lateral view of the lumbosacral area with a 22-gauge needle penetrating the L5/S1 disc. Note that the injection of 3 mL of contrast demonstrated spread in the retroperitoneum from the caudal half of the L5 vertebral body to the cephalad one-third of the S1 vertebral body.

Efficacy

The effectiveness of the block was originally demonstrated by documenting a significant decrease in pain via visual analog pain score (VAPS). In this study, Plancarte et al.[2] showed that the block was effective in reducing VAPSs in 70% of patients with pelvic pain associated with cancer. The majority of the enrolled patients had cervical cancer. In a subsequent study, 69% of patients experienced a decrease in VAPSs. Moreover, a mean daily opioid (morphine) reduction of 67% was seen in the success group (736 ± 633 reduced to 251 ± 191 mg/d) and 45% in the failure group (1,443 ± 703 reduced to 800 ± 345 mg/d).[1] In a more recent multicenter study, 159 patients with pelvic pain associated with cancer were evaluated. Overall, 115 patients (72%) had satisfactory pain relief after one or two neurolytic procedures. Mean opioid use decreased by 40% from 58 ± 43 reduced to 35 ± 18 equianalgesic mg/d of morphine 3 weeks after treatment in all the studied patients. This decrease in opioid consumption was significant for both the success group (56 ± 32 reduced to 32 ± 16 mg/d) and the failure group (65 ± 28 reduced to 48 ± 21 mg/d).[7] Success was defined in these two studies as the ability to reduce opioid consumption by at least 50% in the 3 weeks following the block and a decrease to <4/10 in the VAPSs.[1,7]

In a recent case report, Rosenberg et al.[8] reported on the efficacy of this block in a patient with severe chronic nonmalignant penile pain after transurethral resection of the prostate. Although the patient did not receive a neurolytic agent, a diagnostic block performed with 0.25% bupivacaine and 20 mg of methylprednisolone acetate was effective in relieving the pain for >6 months. The usefulness of this block in chronic benign pain conditions has not been adequately documented in a large cohort of patients.

Complications: Mechanism, Risk Factors, Treatment, and Prevention

The combined experience of more than 200 cases from the Mexican Institute of Cancer, Roswell Park Cancer Institute, and M.D. Anderson Cancer Center indicates that neurologic complications do not occur as a result of this block.[7] However, inadequate needle placement may lead to catastrophic results, as suggested by the fluoroscopy images shown in Figures 24-6 and 24-7. In this case, one of the needles was placed in the superior third of L5 and after injection of contrast medium, posterior extension with delineation of the L5 nerve root was noted. The tip of needle needs to be placed in the inferior third of L5 to avoid this potential problem. Moreover, careful evaluation of the postcontrast medium injection images must be done to rule out abnormal spread.

There are only a limited number of reports detailing the use of superior hypogastric plexus block, and none have reported complications with this procedure. Due to the close proximity of the iliac vessels, intravascular injection can easily occur. However, this should not present a problem unless there is evidence of atherosclerotic disease. If this is the case, there is the risk of dislodging a plaque and producing a distal embolism.

There are limited reports of experience with the transdiscal approach to the superior hypogastric plexus, but there are no reports of discitis, disc herniation, or disc rupture.[3,4] The risk of discitis can be reduced by employing strict sterile precautions and through the use of preprocedural prophylactic antibiotic. Even these measures cannot completely eliminate the risk of infectious complications in the form of discitis, which, when they occur, are painful and require long-term intravenous antibiotics. While the published data do not report disc-related complications, a recent study examined the long-term effects of discography on degenerative

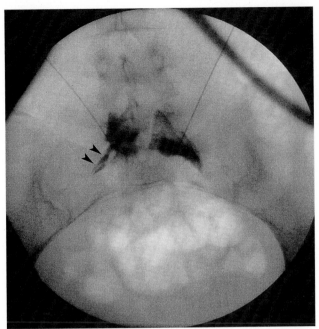

FIGURE 24-6. Superior hypogastric plexus block. Anteroposterior view of the lumbosacral area with a 22-gauge Chiba needle placed at the upper third of the fifth lumbar vertebra. Note that the injection of 3 mL of radiographic contrast resulted in posterior spread to the L5 spinal nerve (*arrowheads*). Injection of neurolytic solution in the position is likely to lead to direct neural injury to the L5 spinal nerve, with partial sensory and motor loss in the lower extremity.

changes of the lumbar discs.[9] This study was a retrospective, matched cohort study that used magnetic resonance imaging to measure the progression of disc degeneration at a 7- to 10-year follow-up after three-level provocative discography in asymptomatic or minimally symptomatic patients. The

cohort of subjects who underwent discography showed a statistically significant increase in disc degeneration, including progression of disc degeneration and new disc herniations, which were found disproportionately on the side of anular puncture.[9] These results suggest that there may be long-term effects of any annular puncture, and a transdiscal SHPB should be performed with these risks in mind.

The anterior approach for the SHPB also carries a risk of bowel or bladder perforation, retroperitoneal infection and abscess formation. The use of preprocedural bowel and bladder preparation can reduce this risk, but it is difficult to avoid the bowel completely. CT guidance can be used to visualize important vascular and neural structures, but the accuracy of the localization depends on patient immobility. Because this approach introduces unique infectious risks, its use must be weighed against the risk of using posterior approaches or the use of an intrathecal drug delivery system as alternative methods for controlling pain. Specific recommendations for minimizing the risk of complications during superior hypogastric plexus block are shown in Box 24-1.

▶ GANGLION IMPAR BLOCK

The ganglion impar is a solitary retroperitoneal structure located at the level of the sacrococcygeal junction. This unpaired ganglion marks the end of the two sympathetic chains. Visceral pain in the perineal area associated with malignancies may be effectively treated with neurolysis of the ganglion impar (Walther's).[10] It has been argued that patients who will benefit from this block frequently present with a vague, poorly localized pain that is frequently accompanied by sensations of urinary urgency and burning in the perineal region. However, the clinical value of this block is not clear because the published experience is limited.

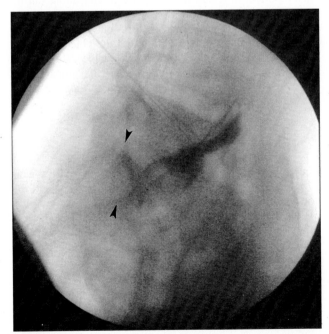

FIGURE 24-7. Superior hypogastric plexus block. A cross-lateral view of the image shown in Figure 24-6. Note the posterior spread of radiographic contrast (*arrowheads*) despite needle tip's positioning in the anterior aspect of the vertebral body.

> **BOX 24-1** Recommendations for Preventing Complications During Superior Hypogastric Plexus Block
>
> - Pay strict attention to needle placement. The tip of the needle needs to be at the junction of L5-S1.
> - Avoid the use of the traditional approach in patients with evidence of atherosclerotic disease of the iliac vessels. Under these circumstances, the transdiscal approach at the L5-S1 may be a better choice, but must be weighed against the increased risk of accelerated disc degeneration and development of new disc herniation or rupture.
> - The anterior approach is an alternative approach for blocking the superior hypogastric plexus, but the risk of retroperitoneal infection and bowel or bladder injury are significant and must be weighed against the benefits of the procedure. Alternative therapies, such as intrathecal drug delivery systems, may be better choices for controlling chronic pelvic pain.

Anatomy

The ganglion impar is a solitary retroperitoneal structure located anterior to the sacrococcygeal junction. This ganglion marks the end of the two sympathetic chains and is the only unpaired autonomic ganglion in the body. Gray communicating nerve fibers pass from the ganglion impar to the spinal nerves. Unlike the thoracic and upper lumbar levels, at the level of the ganglion impar, there are no white communicating nerve fibers passing from the spinal nerves to this sympathetic ganglion.[11] Visceral afferents innervating the perineum, distal rectum, anus, distal urethra, vulva, and distal third of the vagina converge at the ganglion impar. The original technique was described by Plancarte et al.[12] This technique calls for the patient to be positioned in the lateral decubitus position with the hips fully flexed. A standard 22-gauge 3.5-inch spinal needle is bent 1 inch from its hub to form a 30-degree angle. Then the needle is introduced under local anesthesia through the anococcygeal ligament with its concavity oriented posteriorly, and under fluoroscopic guidance it is directed along the midline at or near the sacrococcygeal junction while placing a finger in the rectum to avoid puncturing this structure. Retroperitoneal location is verified by the observation of the spread of 2 mL of water-soluble contrast medium. An alternative needle geometry, bending the needle to the shape of an arc, has been proposed by Nebab and Florence.[13]

Two alternative approaches for this block have been described. The first alternative is to place the patient in the lithotomy position.[14] This position straightens the path from the anococcygeal ligament to the ganglion impar and eliminates the need to bend the needle. In the second approach, the transsacrococcygeal approach,[15] the tip of the needle is directly placed in the retroperitoneal space by inserting a 20-gauge 1.5-inch needle through the sacrococcygeal ligament under fluoroscopy so that the tip of the needle is just anterior to the bone. This technique avoids the invasion of more caudal structures with the needle and the need to insert a finger in the rectal lumen.

For diagnostic blocks, local anesthetic alone is used. For neurolytic blocks, phenol is used. Cryoablation of the ganglion impar has been also described for repeated procedures via a transsacrococcygeal approach in a patient with chronic benign pain postabdominoperineal resection.[16]

Efficacy

There are three prospective observational studies that evaluated the efficacy of ganglion impar block. Plancarte et al.[12] evaluated 16 patients (13 women and 3 men) ranging in age from 24 to 87, with advanced cancer (cervix, 9; colon, 2; bladder, 2; rectum, 1; endometrium, 2) and persistent pain despite treatment (pharmacologic management resulted in a 30% global reduction in pain). Localized perineal pain was present in all cases and was characterized as burning and urgent in eight patients and of mixed character in eight patients. Pain was referred to the rectum (seven patients), perineum (six patients), or vagina (three patients). After a neurolytic block with a transanococcygeal approach, eight patients reported complete pain relief, with the remainder experiencing significant pain reduction (60%–90%). Blocks were repeated in two patients. Follow-up was carried out for 14 to 120 days and depended on survival.

Swofford and Ratzman[17] reported on the efficacy of the transsacrococcygeal approach. Twenty patients, with ages ranging from 35 to 70, with perineal pain unresponsive to previous intervention were studied (18 with a bupivacaine/steroid block and 2 with a neurolytic block). In the bupivacaine/steroid group, five patients reported complete (100%) pain relief, 10 patients reported >75% pain reduction, and three patients reported >50% pain reduction. Both neurolytic blocks resulted in complete pain relief. Duration of the pain relief varied from 4 weeks to long term.

Vranken et al.[18] studied the effect of the ganglion impar block in long-lasting treatment-resistant coccygodynia. Twenty patients (17 women and 3 men) with a diagnosis of coccygodynia (spontaneous, 7; fracture, 3; injury, 10) received a 5-mL injection of 0.25% bupivacaine. There was no pain reduction or increase of quality of life associated with the procedure. Thus, based on this study, it would appear that this block is not effective for the treatment of coccygodynia.

Complications: Mechanism, Risk Factors, Treatment, and Prevention

Although there is always the risk of damaging the adjacent structures to the ganglion impar, there are no complications reported from this technique. Plancarte et al.[19] has reported one case in which epidural spread of contrast within the caudal canal was observed. In this case, needle repositioning resolved the problem. Although published experience is limited and criteria to predict success or failure is not available, patients with perineal pain poorly localized with a burning character are considered candidates for the block. The procedure is considered safe, as no complications have been reported. In regard to preventing complications during ganglion impar block, the use of the transsacrococcygeal approach is not only easier to perform but should decrease the risk of rectal wall perforation and the potential development of an abscess. The limited available data and the uncontrolled nature of this data on ganglion impar block limit any conclusions that can be drawn regarding the safety or efficacy of this treatment.

▶ SUMMARY

Neurolysis of the superior hypogastric plexus and the ganglion impar may be used in patients with visceral pain of the pelvis and the perineal region, respectively. There are only limited available data of low quality on which to judge the safety and efficacy of these two unusual treatments. Nonetheless, there are few complications reported with either block. Strict adherence to technique is important to prevent potential complications. Moreover, the use of this technique for patients who do not have a significant visceral pain component is not warranted. The incidence of complications reported in the literature is very low, but complications do occur.

References

1. de Leon-Casasola OA, Kent E, Lema MJ. Neurolytic superior hypogastric plexus block for chronic pelvic pain associated with cancer. *Pain* 1993;54(2):145–151.

2. Plancarte R, Amescua C, Patt RB, et al. Superior hypogastric plexus block for pelvic cancer pain. *Anesthesiology* 1990;73(2):236–239.

3. Gamal G, Helaly M, Labib YM. Superior hypogastric block: transdiscal versus classic posterior approach in pelvic cancer pain. *Clin J Pain* 2006;22(6):544–547.

4. Nabil D, Eissa AA. Evaluation of posteromedial transdiscal superior hypogastric block after failure of the classic approach. *Clin J Pain* 2010;26(8):694–697.

5. Cariati M, De Martini G, Pretolesi F, et al. CT-guided superior hypogastric plexus block. *J Comput Assist Tomogr* 2002;26(3):428–431.

6. Mishra S, Bhatnagar S, Gupta D, et al. Anterior ultrasound-guided superior hypogastric plexus neurolysis in pelvic cancer pain. *Anaesth Intensive Care* 2008;36(5):732–735.

7. Plancarte R, de Leon-Casasola OA, El-Helaly M, et al. Neurolytic superior hypogastric plexus block for chronic pelvic pain associated with cancer. *Reg Anesth* 1997;22(6):562–568.

8. Rosenberg SK, Tewari R, Boswell MV, et al. Superior hypogastric plexus block successfully treats severe penile pain after transurethral resection of the prostate. *Reg Anesth Pain Med* 1998;23(6):618–620.

9. Carragee EJ, Don AS, Hurwitz EL, et al. 2009 ISSLS prize winner: does discography cause accelerated progression of degeneration changes in the lumbar disc: a ten-year matched cohort study. *Spine (Phila Pa 1976)* 2009;34(21):2338–2345.

10. de Leon-Casasola OA. Superior hypogastric plexus block and ganglion impar neurolysis for pain associated with cancer. *Tech Reg Anesth Pain Manag* 1997;1:27–31.

11. Gray H. *Gray's Anatomy*, Revised American, from the Fifteenth English Edition. New York, NY: Bounty Books, 1997.

12. Plancarte R, Amescua C, Patt RB. Presacral blockade of the ganglion impar (ganglion of Walther). *Anesthesiology* 1990;73:A751.

13. Nebab EG, Florence IM. An alternative needle geometry for interruption of the ganglion impar. *Anesthesiology* 1997;86(5):1213–1214.

14. Xue B, Lema MJ, de Leon-Casasola OA. Ganglion impar block. In: Benzon N, Raja S, Borook D, et al. eds. *Essentials of Pain Medicine and Regional Anesthesia*. Philadelphia, PA: Churchill Livingstone, 1999:329–331.

15. Wemm K Jr, Saberski L. Modified approach to block the ganglion impar (ganglion of Walther). *Reg Anesth* 1995;20(6):544–545.

16. Loev MA, Varklet VL, Wilsey BL, et al. Cryoablation: a novel approach to neurolysis of the ganglion impar. *Anesthesiology* 1998;88(5):1391–1393.

17. Swofford JB, Ratzman DM. A transarticular approach to blockade of the ganglion impar (ganglion of Walther). *Reg Anesth Pain Med* 1998;23:3S–103S.

18. Vranken J, Bannink I, Zuurmond WWA. Invasive procedures in patients with coccygodynia: caudal epidural infiltration, pudendal nerve block and blockade of the ganglion impar. *Anesth Pain Med* 2000;25:2S–25S.

19. Plancarte R, Velazquez R, Patt RB. Neurolytic blocks of the sympathetic axis. In: Patt R, ed. *Cancer Pain*. Philadelphia, PA: Lippincott-Raven, 1993:419.

COMPLICATIONS OF DEVICE PLACEMENT

25

Complications Associated with Intrathecal Drug Delivery Systems

F. Michael Ferrante and James P. Rathmell

In order to appreciate the significance of the development of intrathecal drug delivery systems as a therapeutic modality, it is important to understand their evolution. The presence of opioid receptors within the central nervous system was first discovered simultaneously by several investigators in 1973.[1] The presence of endogenous opioid peptides in the brain (enkephalins) that were ligands to these receptors was discovered in 1975,[2] lending credence to the hypothesis that exogenous opioid analgesia was the result of mimicry of endogenous opioid peptides at opioid receptors. Shortly thereafter, opioid receptors were discovered in primate spinal cord tissue,[3] and Yaksh and Rudy[4] demonstrated that opioids applied to rat spinal cord produced profound analgesia. Intraspinal analgesia was first achieved in humans in 1979 with subarachnoid administration of morphine,[5] and the first epidural administration of morphine followed shortly thereafter.[6] Thus, in a period of 6 years following the discovery of opioid receptors, intraspinal opioid analgesia had seen its birth.

Initially, intraspinal analgesia was administered via percutaneously placed or tunneled percutaneous catheters using intermittent bolus techniques. Subsequently, the Shiley-Infusaid Model 400 pump (Norwood, PA) had originally been developed for regional infusion of drugs (chemotherapy, heparin) to specific organs and was adapted to intrathecal delivery.

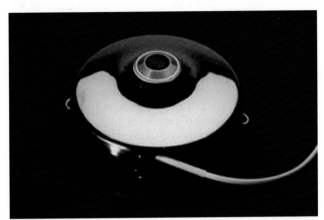

FIGURE 25-1. The Codman 3000 nonprogrammable, implantable intrathecal drug delivery pump. With the Codman system, intermittent injections can be given through a closed tip needle with a needle shaft aperture that directs fluid away from the drug reservoir chamber and directly into the catheter. Pump refills utilize an open tip needle without a needle shaft aperture, directing fluid into the inner drug reservoir chamber. Thus, the Codman system has required reliance upon proper needle type for refill or bolus in order to minimize the risk of overdose. (Image courtesy of DePuy Spine Inc., Raynham, MA.)

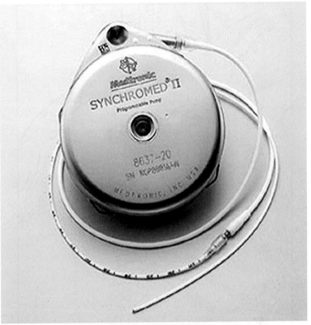

FIGURE 25-2. The Medtronic Synchromed II programmable, implantable intrathecal drug delivery pump. The design utilizes the technology of pacemakers to allow programmability. The pump consists of a lithium battery, a reservoir system, microprocessor, and antenna. An external programmer can communicate with the pump to change settings, allowing programmability. Access to the side port is limited by a wire mesh over the entry port that restricts needle access to 25-gauge or smaller needle. The side port connects directly to the intrathecal catheter, and access can allow sampling of CSF as well as direct administration of drug boluses. Limiting needle access to the sideport to smaller gauge needles reduces the chances of inadvertent administration of the reservoir refill directly in to the intrathecal space. (Image courtesy of Medtronic Inc., Minneapolis, MN.)

Both the Shiley-Infusaid pump and its present iteration, the Codman 3000 implantable constant flow infusion drug delivery system (Fig. 25-1, DePuy Spine, Inc., Raynham, MA), are battery-free systems without internal electronics. The design has an inner and outer chamber separated by an accordion-like bellows. The outer chamber has a propellant that is warmed by body temperature, producing a constant pressure on the bellows. This constant pressure causes the drug to flow out of the inner chamber, through a filter and flow restrictor, and then into the catheter. The Codman 3000 constant flow pump has three available reservoir sizes (16, 30, and 50 mL) with four factory-set flow rates. Because it is a constant flow pump, the only way to adjust dosage is to change the drug concentration manually during a pump refill.[7,8]

The Shiley-Infusaid pump had two potential sources of access, an inlet septum for access to the inner drug reservoir chamber during refill and a side port for intermittent injection. Unfortunately, there was no inherent fail-safe system to distinguish between the two ports, with potentially dire consequences. With the present Codman system (Fig. 25-1), intermittent injections can be given through a closed tip needle with a needle shaft aperture that directs fluid away from the drug reservoir chamber and directly into the catheter. Pump refills utilize an open tip needle without a needle shaft aperture, directing fluid into the inner drug reservoir chamber. Thus, the Codman system has required reliance upon proper needle type for refill or bolus in order to minimize the risk of overdose.

While Medtronic Inc. (Minneapolis, MN) manufactures a constant flow pump (Isomed System), it is best known for its production of programmable intrathecal drug delivery systems, specifically the Synchromed, Synchromed-EL, and now the Synchromed 2 (Fig. 25-2). The original Synchromed device entered the marketplace in 1991. The design utilizes the technology of pacemakers to allow programmability. The pump consists of a lithium battery, a reservoir system, microprocessor, and antenna. An external programmer can communicate with the pump to change settings, allowing programmability.

Implanted catheters with subcutaneous injection sites have been developed as intrathecal drug delivery systems such as the Port-a-Cath system (Fig. 25-3, Smiths Medical, St. Paul, MN). Such a design is not useful for long-term delivery (years) given it is implicitly an "open" system with the need for repetitive site instrumentation, potentially leading to infectious complications. Implanted catheters with subcutaneous injections sites do have utility for epidural administration of short to intermediate duration. The remainder of this chapter is limited to a discussion of complications associated with implanted intrathecal drug delivery pumps, which are now in common use for the treatment of a wide range of pain disorders (Box 25-1).

▶ SCOPE

Complications associated with intrathecal drug delivery systems can be categorized as surgical, infectious, device related (catheter and/or pump), and drug related. Intrathecal drug delivery systems have been in widespread use for more than two decades, and as a result there is significant experience with the complications associated with use of these devices. The reported incidence of adverse events ranges from 3% to 24%, most of which are minor and related to the infused drug.[9] Most device-related complications occur at the time of or within the first few months after implantation,

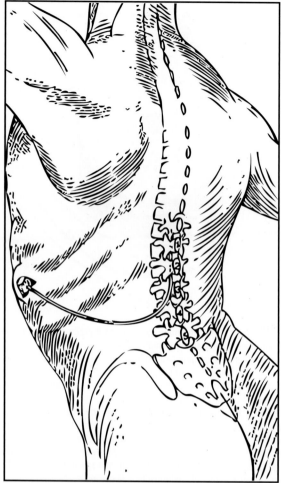

FIGURE 25-3. **The Port-a-Cath implanted catheter with subcutaneous injections port.** These percutaneously accessed systems have been used to provide long-term intrathecal infusions using an external reservoir and drug delivery pump. Such a design is not useful for long-term delivery (years) given it is implicitly an "open" system with the need for repetitive site instrumentation, invariably leading to infectious complications. Implanted catheters with subcutaneous injections sites do have utility for epidural administration of short to intermediate duration. (Illustration redrawn to illustrate the Port-a-Cath system, Smiths Medical, St. Paul, MN.)

BOX 25-1 Established Indications for Intrathecal Drug Delivery

Controlled trials support the use of intrathecal drug delivery for the following indications:
- Spasticity associated with cerebral palsy and spinal cord injury unresponsive to oral agents
- Chronic cancer-related pain poorly responsive to more conservative treatment

Limited observational data support the use of intrathecal drug delivery for the following indications:
- Chronic low back pain
- Complex regional pain syndrome (CRPS)
- Other forms of chronic neuropathic pain

---

and many of these surgical complications can be avoided with careful surgical technique and recent improvements in technology. In the largest available series, complications related to the device or catheter occurred in 21.1% of patients during the first 9 months after implantation.[10] Drug-related complications are common and typically evolve over several months following implantation.[9] In recent years, it has been recognized that long-term intrathecal drug delivery can lead to formation of inflammatory masses at the tip of the intrathecal catheter, within the thecal sac. Since the first reports of inflammatory mass formation, there has been increased reporting of this complication, and these reports have led to greater concern about the risk of significant neurologic injury.[11] Recent postmarketing surveillance reports alerted the manufacturer of the Synchromed device to a series of deaths that occurred early after pump implantation; this led to a large-scale epidemiologic study, which concluded that intrathecal drug therapy is associated with a significant increase in mortality rate.[12] The reasons for this increase are unclear, but possible mechanisms will be discussed below.

▶ DEFINITION, INCIDENCE, AND DIAGNOSIS

Surgical Complications

Intrathecal drug delivery involves the placement of an indwelling catheter within the thecal sac, and injury to the neuraxis can occur in several ways. During initial implantation, direct trauma to the spinal cord or spinal nerves can result from needle or catheter placement. Because the spinal nerves of the cauda equina float freely within the cerebrospinal fluid (CSF) below the L1-L2 level, this problem is unlikely if needle entry is below this level. Catheter complications can result from threading the catheter into the conus medullaris or other portions of the spinal cord, resulting in catastrophic neurologic injury, typically with paraparesis or complete paraplegia ensuing.[13,14] During direct placement of the catheter into the spinal cord parenchyma at the time of implantation, the awake patient is likely to report pain or paraesthesia, particularly reports of pain involving both sides of the trunk or both lower extremities. This complication may be more likely when the patient undergoes implantation while under general anesthesia, and some authors have concluded that pumps should be implanted under sedation only whenever possible, with a level of sedation that allows for verbal communication with the patient throughout catheter placement.[13] Other complications that may occur at or soon after the initial surgical period include CSF leak, hygroma formation, and chronic postdural puncture headache. The incidence of common complications occurring within the first months after implantation is shown in Table 25-1.

The tissue dissection required to place an intrathecal drug delivery system is minimal and limited to the subcutaneous tissues. Nonetheless, significant bleeding can occur and lead to the need for wound reexploration and evacuation of hematoma in the immediate postoperative period. Bleeding within the pocket can lead to the formation of a significant hematoma and, if left untreated, may lead to wound dehiscence. The diagnosis is typically obvious: the patient reports pain immediately postoperatively that is accompanied by progressive swelling at the surgical site. Bleeding within the spinal canal

TABLE 25-1 Frequency of Complications Associated with Implantation of Intrathecal Drug Delivery Systems

	N	%
Total number of patients	209	100
Number of patients with one complication (procedure or catheter related)	37	18.6
Number of patients with two or more complications (procedure or catheter related)	9	5.7

ADVERSE EVENT	NUMBER OF EVENTS	NUMBER OF EVENTS PER PATIENT YEAR
Catheter-related complication		
Leakage, cuts, or breaks in catheter	3	0.02
Catheter dislodgement/migration	2	0.01
Accessories (catheter-to-pump connector)	1	0.01
Catheter of pump disconnection	1	0.01
Total	7	0.05
Procedure-related complication		
Infection	15	0.10
Catheter dislodgement/migration	10	0.07
Occlusion or angulation (kink)	5	0.03
CSF leak/hygroma or spinal headache	4	0.03
Accessories (catheter-to-pump connector)	3	0.02
Leakage, cuts, or breaks in catheter	2	0.01
Catheter of pump disconnection	1	0.01
Loss of drug effect	1	0.01
Other (catheter in epidural space/no drug effect)	1	0.01
Total	42	0.29

Reproduced from Follett KA, Naumann CP. A prospective study of catheter-related complications of intrathecal drug delivery systems. *J Pain Symptom Manage* 2000;19:209–215, with permission.

can also occur after intrathecal catheter placement, resulting in epidural hematoma formation. Close attention should be paid to evaluation of the patient who presents with worsening back pain in the immediate postoperative period; the appearance of neurologic deficits warrants emergent imaging (magnetic resonance imaging [MRI] or computed tomography [CT]) and evacuation of the epidural hematoma, if present.

Leakage of CSF can result in immediate postprocedural headache and has the typical characteristics of a post dural-puncture headache: lack of any alternate cause and the onset of worsening of headache related to sitting upright or standing. While this headache is typically self-limited and responds to conservative treatment, the CSF leak can be persistent and lead to chronic positional headache. Ongoing CSF leakage can also flow along the course of the tunneled catheter from the thecal sac all the way to the subcutaneous pocket in the paraspinous region where the catheter is typically fastened to the paraspinous fascia. These subcutaneous

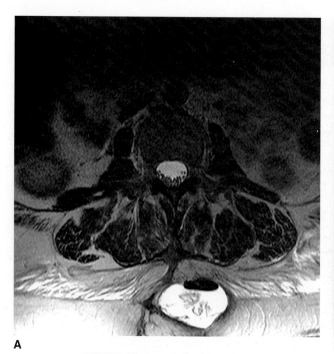

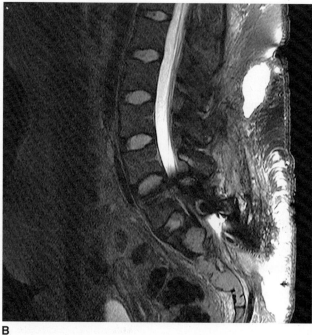

A   **B**

FIGURE 25-4. **Subcutaneous CSF hygroma associated with an implanted intrathecal drug delivery system as seen on MRI. A:** Axial T2-weighted MRI of the lumbosacral spine. **B:** Sagittal T2-weighted MRI of the lumbosacral spine. This patient presented with a large, fluctuant area just beneath the lumbar paraspinous incision. There was no pain, tenderness or erythema in the region. MRI demonstrates a large, high-signal fluid collection with an air-fluid level within located in the right paraspinous subcutaneous region where the intrathecal catheter was anchored to the subcutaneous tissue during implantation. Surgical exploration revealed clear fluid without evidence for infection. The catheter was removed and the pump was left *in situ*; several months later the catheter was replaced and connected with the existing pump and intrathecal therapy was resumed without incident.

CSF collections (termed a "hygroma"; Fig. 25-4) can become quite large and may even lead to breakdown of the overlying incision. The diagnosis of a CSF hygroma is suspected in the patient who presents with a painless, fluctuant swelling in the area underlying the paraspinous incision made at the time of catheter placement and is best confirmed using MRI.

Catheter kinks, breaks, leakage, dislodgement from the CSF, and disconnection from the pump all occur with some regularity. Catheter-related complications occurred immediately at the time of implant in 3.3% of cases in one large series; catheter dislodgement also occurred weeks or months after device placement in 9.7% of cases. The diagnosis of catheter-related complications can be quite difficult. The most common feature is unexplained, inadequate pain control. This leads to a search for the cause, and this search usually ensues after several dose escalations fail to provide pain relief. The diagnosis is best made by careful examination of the entire length of the catheter from the point where it attaches to the subcutaneous pump all the way along the subcutaneous course to the intrathecal tip of the catheter. When the catheter is completely dislodged from the intrathecal space, disconnected, or severed, this is obvious on simple radiographic inspection using fluoroscopy, x-ray, or CT (Fig. 25-5). Catheter kinks or leaks caused by small holes or breaks in the catheter are more difficult to diagnose. The best means is to access the intrathecal pump through the side port (Fig. 25-6), aspirate enough CSF to clear the catheter of drug, and inject nonionic radiographic contrast medium that is safe for myelography. Leaks along the course can be seen

as the radiographic contrast leaks in to the subcutaneous tissue. Correct intrathecal placement will be apparent when a normal myelogram appears; subtle misplacement, for example, subdural or epidural catheter location, can also be readily detected in this manner.

Infectious Complications

Infectious complications are uncommon and can occur within the neuraxis, along the course of the catheter or within the subcutaneous pump pocket. Infections within the neuraxis directly related to intrathecal dug delivery include meningitis and direct infection of the spinal cord near the catheter tip resulting in transverse myelitis.[15] Infection involving the implanted pump or catheter can result in the need to remove the device. The incidence of wound infection ranges from 0% to 4.5%, although higher rates of infection have been reported.[16] In early superficial infections, the diagnosis can be confused with seroma or hygroma. This is sometimes difficult because each of these complications can involve some redness, edema, and fluctuance of the pocket. The presence of a fever, elevated white blood count, elevated C-reactive protein, and elevated erythrocyte sedimentation rate raises the level of suspicion for an infectious process. In immunocompromised patients, these laboratory values may not change. In cases where purulent discharge with or without wound dehiscence develop, the diagnosis presents no dilemma. In all cases where infection is suspected, culture and Gram stain are helpful to verify the presence of infection

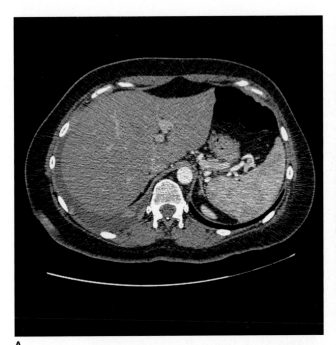
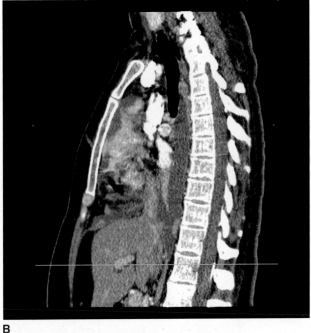

A   B

FIGURE 25-5. Sagittal (A) and axial (B) CT of the thorax in a patient with an intrathecal drug delivery system placed and providing pain relief for a patient with chest wall pain associated with metastatic lung cancer. The catheter tip can be seen in the midline in the posterior aspect of the thecal sac at the T9/T10 level. Reference line on the sagittal images corresponds with the level of the axial image shown.

and identify the causative organism. In cases where fever and malaise are present but no obvious device infection is found, other causes of infection should be sought.

Device-related Complications

Device-related complications typically occur distant from the original time of implantation and arise from problems with the catheter or the implanted pump. The most common complications are those associated with the intrathecal catheter, but problems with the pump and the subcutaneous pocket and course of the catheter may also arise. Follet and Naumann[10] reported a 9.7% rate of catheter-related complications in the first nine months after implantation. The most common complication was that of catheter dislodgement from the intrathecal space, and this study found that more than half of these dislodgements occurred in those where the catheter had not been anchored to the paraspinous fascia. The appearance of new kinks or breaks in the catheter occured with less frequency. A single case where the catheter had been perforated by the needle at the time of a pump refill was reported in the same series.

Migration of the catheter completely out of the spinal canal and into the subcutaneous tissues in the paraspinous region is most common. Migration to the subdural compartment[12] or the epidural space has also been described. In all three locations, a loss of the effectiveness of analgesia is likely to be the presenting symptom. It has been hypothesized that subdural catheter migration can also create a loculated region containing high concentrations of the infused drug between the dura mater and the arachnoid mater. This pocket is contained only by the fragile arachnoid membrane, and sudden rupture and release of the loculated drug into the intrathecal space could cause a sudden overdose. Migration can occur

into the foramen or toward the nerve root, causing radicular pain or sciatica.[17] Reports of catheter migration in to the spinal cord have also appeared[18]; however, it remains unclear in these cases if the catheter migrated or was actually placed into the cord at the time of implantation, only for symptoms to appear later.[14,18] Catheter placement or migration into the spinal cord can go undiagnosed until significant neurologic deficits appear; as with any suspected intrinsic injury to the spinal cord, imaging with MRI is the best means to establish a definitive diagnosis. When catheter migration is suspected, simple radiographic inspection using fluoroscopy, x-ray, or CT as described previously (see Device-related Complications) is the best means to establish the diagnosis.

In patients with indwelling pumps, a refill is required at intervals ranging from 14 to 120 days. During each refill, the pump reservoir must be accessed percutaneously, and there is a risk of inadvertent subcutaneous placement of the drug as well as device or intrathecal infection. Because high concentrations of drug are used and a large dose of the drug will be quickly absorbed if placed subcutaneously, this problem typically becomes life threatening within minutes. The risk of inadvertent subcutaneous placement can be minimized by ensuring that only those with adequate training and familiarity with the pump perform refills. Nonetheless, accessing the pump can be difficult, particularly in those who are obese and when the pump has been placed within a deeper plane. Use of radiographic guidance can simplify identifying the reservoir port (Fig. 25-6). The risk of infection is minimized by appropriate sterile technique, use of a bacteriostatic filter, and the antibacterial effects of any local anesthetics included in the infused agent. Despite the need to frequently perform this procedure, the infection rates appear to be low and should occur in <1% of all refills.[19] Drug overdose and device infection have also been reported

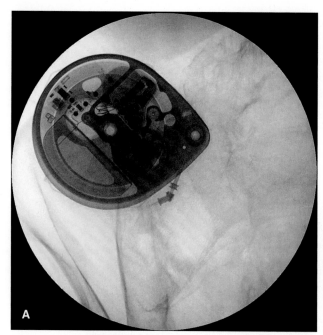
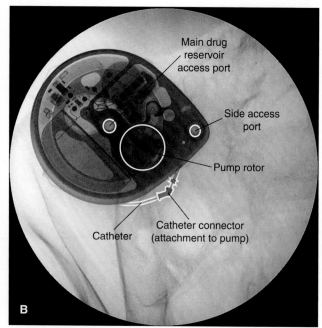

FIGURE 25-6. **A: Appearance of the Medtronic Synchromed II (Minneapolis, MN) 40 mL intrathecal drug delivery pump as seen *in situ* using fluoroscopy in the anterior-posterior plane. B:** Labeled image. Fluoroscopy can be used to readily identify the drug reservoir access port during routine periodic refilling of the pump using the 22-gauge Huber-type (non-coring) needle supplied by the manufacturer. By taking two sequential radiographs separated by several minutes, fluoroscopy can also be used to assess proper rotation of the rollers around the rotor in the peristaltic pump, as their position will change if the rotor is moving. Finally, fluoroscopy is essential when assessing the integrity of the catheter and its position within the CSF using the side access port. The side access port can be accessed with a 25-gauge needle; the side access port is specifically designed to prevent entry with the larger needle used for drug refills. Once the needle is in position, at least 0.3 mL of fluid must be withdrawn to clear the catheter of highly concentrated drug and prevent administration of an intrathecal bolus. Once the catheter has been cleared, radiographic contrast can be injected and the couse of the catheter examined along its entire length to detect any dislodgement or leaks. When the catheter is in proper position within the thecal sac, contrast will accumulate along the inner borders of the thecal sac producing a typical lumbar myelogram. Following the side port study, the pump must be carefully programmed to deliver a precise bolus in order to refill the catheter with drug and prevent a period during which no drug is being delivered.

after attempts to access the port and remove the drug by unauthorized persons. In one case, the patient was trying to gain access to and sell the drug in the pump and intravenous injection of the drug resulted in overdose.[20]

In most patients, the implanted device causes an inflammatory reaction, and the body creates a fibrous capsule around the device. This fibrous capsule holds the device firmly in position. In malnourished patients, the device can erode through the subcutaneous tissue and other structures. Tissue breakdown can also lead to disastrous erosion into an artery or vein.[21]

The noninfectious buildup of serosanguineous fluid in the pocket can lead to a seroma that may impede the ability of the wound to heal (see Chapter 26). This can lead to pain, wound breakdown, and dehiscence. Seroma is usually diagnosed by the appearance of a painful erythematous fluctuant mass surrounding the implanted device accompanied by normal laboratory values, lack of fever, and lack of night sweats. Diagnosis is confirmed by aspiration of straw-colored fluid that does not show bacteria on microscopic analysis or subsequent culture. Long-term skin breakdown can occur because of fat necrosis of the subcutaneous tissue. This often accompanies a significant change in weight, most commonly a drop in body mass index.

Intrathecal catheters can develop fibrosis around the catheter tip that results in difficulty aspirating or injecting

through the catheter side port. The extent of fibrosis is variable. Minor fibrosis at the catheter tip can go unnoticed, causing problems only when trying to aspirate CSF through the side port. More extensive fibrosis can lead to dangerous inflammatory masses. The occurrence of inflammatory masses surrounding the tip of intrathecal catheters during long-term intrathecal infusion of morphine was first reported in 1999, and, in more recent years, the number of reports and agents associated with inflammatory masses has grown. The inflammatory mass appears to be a chronic fibrotic, noninfectious mass that develops at the tip of the intrathecal catheter over the course of months or years. As the inflammatory mass grows larger, patients often present with neurologic signs and symptoms that reflect direct compression of the spinal cord or other neural elements by the expanding mass.[11] Theories regarding the process that leads to inflammatory mass formation include mast cell degranulation creating inflammation of the surrounding tissue. The mast cell theory is well supported by work in animal models, including dogs and sheep.[22] Other theories include a nitric oxide response, allergic response, or a reaction to the foreign body of the catheter material, but have little support in the literature. These reactions are a result of the local response to high concentrations of opioid at the catheter tip. Reported cases have been most directly linked to high concentrations of morphine and hydromorphone, although similar granulomas have now been reported with baclofen alone[23] as well as combination therapy that included clonidine.[24] A consensus statement by a panel of experts recommended that the concentration of morphine be limited to 30 mg/mL and that the concentration of hydromorphone be limited to 20 mg/mL. Because of the reported cases with these two drugs, new interest has arisen in using smaller and more lipid-soluble molecules such as fentanyl or sufentanil. The current literature is limited regarding complications arising from these drugs. The normal course of presentation of an inflammatory mass is an initial loss of pain relief, followed by progressive neurologic loss. The described neurologic symptoms include loss of proprioception, referred pain at the level of the catheter tip, change in sensation, motor loss, and eventually bladder and bowel symptoms. If not diagnosed and treated, this process can progress to paraplegia.[11,25] Diagnosis is based on physician suspicion of this complication (Box 25-2). The gold standard for diagnosis is a T1-weighted MRI with and without gadolinium (Fig. 25-7). If the patient cannot undergo an MRI, the second choice for diagnosis is a CT myelogram. The radiologist may require education if not familiar with the appearance of these lesions.

Currently available programmable pumps are driven by a rotor that requires a motor with gears. Mechanical failure, including jamming of the gears or rotor failure, can occur and result in a stalled pump. Examination of the pump under fluoroscopy at timed intervals will reveal that there is no movement of the pump's rotor (Fig. 25-6).

Drug-related Complications

The reported frequency of complications associated with long-term infusion of opioids is shown in Table 25-2. Paice et al.[26] demonstrated in a multicenter review that complications can be common and can affect several body systems. Complications resulting directly from the use of intrathecal opioids include nausea and vomiting (25.2%), pruritis (13.3%), edema (11.7%), diaphoresis (7.2%), weakness (7.2%), weight gain (5.4%), and diminished libido (4.9%). Winkelmuller and Winkelmuller[27] showed a similarly high rate of adverse effects with intrathecal opioids. They reported complications, including constipation (50%),

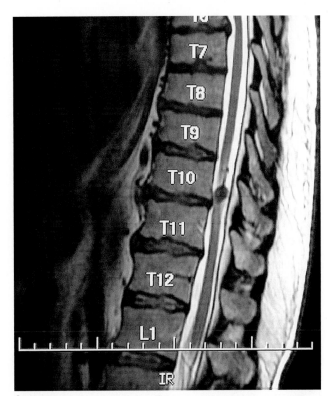

A

B

FIGURE 25-7. MRI study of a patient with an inflammatory mass surrounding the tip of an implanted intrathecal drug delivery catheter. **A:** Midline sagittal T2-weighted image. The inflammatory mass involves the dorsal aspect of the spinal cord at the level of the inferior end plate of T10. **B:** Axial T2-weighted image through the inflammatory mass. The mass displaces the spinal cord toward the left.

BOX 25-2 Diagnosis of Inflammatory Mass Formation During Long-term Intrathecal Drug Delivery

- Maintain a high index of suspicion.
- Suspect when pain control has been adequate but is suddenly lost.
- Suspect when any new neurologic signs or symptoms appear, including new onset of pain, loss of sensation, or weakness in the trunk or lower extremities, as well as new onset of urinary retention or bowel or bladder incontinence.
- The diagnostic study of choice is MRI with gadolinium enhancement.

---

difficulty urinating (42.7%), nausea (36.6), impotence (26.8%), vomiting (24.4%), nightmares (23.2%), pruritis (14.6%), sweating (8.5%), edema (6.1%), and decreased libido (4. 9%).

Other common side effects occur with intrathecal infusion. Peripheral edema of the lower extremities has been reported with opioids, most commonly morphine. The incidence of this complication appears to vary from

TABLE 25-2 Complications Reported with Long-term Intrathecal Infusion of Opioids

COMPLICATION	REPORTED FREQUENCY (%)
Constipation	50
Difficulty urinating	42.7
Nausea and vomiting	24.4–36.6
Impotence	26.8
Nightmares	23.2
Pruritus	13.3–14.6
Edema	6.1–11.7
Diaphoresis	7.2–8.5
Weakness	7.2
Weight gain	5.4
Diminished libido	4.9

Data derived from Paice JA, Penn RD, Shott S. Intraspinal morphine for chronic pain: a retrospective, multicenter study. *J Pain Symptom Manage* 1996;11:71–80; Winkelmuller M, Winkelmuller W. Long-term effects of continuous intrathecal opioid treatment in chronic pain of nonmalignant etiology. *J Neurosurg* 1996;85:458–467.

1% to 20%, depending on the vascular status of patients prior to implantation. The mechanism appears to be related to a direct effect on the pituitary from intrathecal opioids.[28] Inflammatory mass of the catheter tip appears to be a direct result of a reaction to the infused drug, most commonly morphine. This complication was discussed in the previous section.

Several other drugs are commonly delivered as chronic intrathecal infusions. Clonidine is active at the alpha receptors and can cause hypotension and somnolence. It is also associated with severe rebound hypertension with the sudden withdrawal or reduction.[29] Ziconotide (SNX-111) is a synthetic analogue of an N-type voltage-dependent calcium channel blocker that was first isolated from the marine snail Conus magnus. Ziconotide was approved for intrathecal use by the United States Food and Drug Administration (FDA) in late 2004 and has shown some promise in treating refractory pain associated with cancer and acquired immunodeficiency syndrome (AIDS).[20] In this double-blind, placebo-controlled trial, 111 patients aged 24 to 85 with cancer or AIDS with pain more than 50 mm on a visual analog pain scale were randomized to receive either ziconotide or placebo intrathecally. Intrathecal ziconotide or placebo was administered over 5 to 6 days followed by a 5-day maintenance period. There was significantly better pain reduction in those receiving ziconotide than those receiving placebo, but side effects occurred almost universally in those receiving ziconotide

(Table 25-3). Indeed, the high frequency of side effects mandates slow dose escalation over a prolonged time period and has led to limited use of this new agent.

Placement of the incorrect drug or concentration within the pump can prove disastrous. If a sudden change in analgesia, increased somnolence, or other effects appear soon after the reservoir has been refilled, a drug error should be suspected. In these circumstances, the drug must be sent for analysis. Possible causes include giving the wrong patient the intended drug, mislabeling by the pharmacist, or improper calculation when preparing or ordering the drug.[31] The first sign of the placement of an inaccurate drug may be patient distress or respiratory depression. Because of this troubling diagnostic dilemma, it is critical to double check each refill solution at the pharmacy and in the pain center to ensure accuracy. Additional testing is needed to determine accuracy of concentration, stability, and lack of bacterial contaminates.[32]

▶ PREVENTION AND TREATMENT

Prevention and Treatment of Surgical Complications

Prevention of most immediate surgical complications relies on careful surgical technique. Wound hematoma is best prevented by meticulous hemostasis during intraoperative dissection and wound closure. The incidence of surgical site infection can be reduced significantly by the use of preoperative antibiotics.[33] There is no consensus on the best means to provide anesthesia for the implantation of an indwelling intrathecal drug-delivery system. Some practitioners advocate for use of sedation, keeping patients awake enough to respond during the initial catheter placement, so that they can report any contact with neural structures. Other practitioners use general anesthesia for these procedures. In either circumstance, the use of radiographic guidance to guide initial intrathecal needle and catheter placement is advisable, as this allows precise needle direction to the midline below the level of the conus medullaris (below L2), where the risk of encountering neural structures is minimized.

The risk of shearing of the intrathecal catheter can be minimized by avoiding withdrawing the catheter through the needle once it has been advanced. With this said, the catheter can often be easily withdrawn and readvanced through the needle without damage to the catheter. This is more likely when the angle of entry into the thecal sac is shallow, close to the plane of the dura mater (<45 degrees from the plane of the back). This shallow angle ensures that the catheter does not have to make an abrupt turn at the needle tip and reduces the chances that the catheter will shear or be otherwise damaged on the bevel of the needle. In the event of catheter fracture within the subarachnoid space, a new catheter is required. There is no consensus regarding the need to remove the retained catheter fragment. Removal requires laminectomy and durotomy. Experience with fractured ventriculoperitoneal shunts offers good evidence that the presence of a retained catheter in the intrathecal space presents little risk over time and that the risk of surgical exploration and removal may well be greater than leaving the catheter fragment in place.

TABLE 25-3 Complications Reported with Short-term Intrathecal Infusion of Ziconotide (SNX-111)

	NO. OF PATIENTS (%)	
	ZICONOTIDE ($n = 72$)	PLACEBO COMPLICATION ($n = 40$)
Patients with any	70 (97.2)	29 (72.5) adverse event
Patients with any	22 (30.6)	4 (10.0) serious adverse event
Cardiovascular system	24 (33.3)	4 (10.0)
Postural hypotension	17 (23.6)	2 (5.0)
Hypotension	6 (8.3)	2 (5.0)
Nervous system	60 (83.3)	14 (35.0)
Dizziness	36 (50.0)	4 (10.0)
Nystagmus	33 (45.8)	4 (10.0)
Somnolence	17 (23.6)	3 (7.5)
Confusion	15 (20.8)	2 (5.0)
Abnormal gait	9 (12.5)	0
Urogenital system	23 (31.9)	0
Urinary retention	13 (18.1)	0
Urinary tract infection	7 (9.7)	0

Adapted from Staats PS, Yearwood T, Charapata SG, et al. Intrathecal ziconotide in the treatment of refractory pain in patients with cancer and AIDS. *JAMA* 2003;291:62–70. Ref. [30].

Direct trauma to the cord or nerve roots can result in paralysis, pain, and traumatic radiculitis. Treatment is initiated as soon as the diagnosis is confirmed by MRI: intrinsic injury to the spinal cord may result in an increase in T2-weighted signal within the substance of the spinal cord; MRI is unlikely to show any abnormalities immediately following spinal nerve injury. Neurosurgical consultation and initiation of high-dose intravenous steroids should be considered. If the injury involves a catheter, removal of the catheter should be urgently performed. CSF leak is treated conservatively by fluid intake, bed rest, and caffeine. If that should fail, some would consider an epidural blood patch. If the clinician chooses to perform a blood patch, two important risks should be considered. Care must be taken to avoid shearing the catheter with the needle, and the introduction of a foreign body should be considered. The foreign body, blood, may serve as a culture medium if an infection develops.

Postoperative bleeding is treated with a pressure dressing and observation. If the hematoma is rapidly expanding, immediate surgical reexploration is needed. Treatment is evacuation of the hematoma, irrigation of the wound, identification the bleeding source, and hemostasis. Recurrent bleeding may suggest a bleeding disorder, and consultation with a hematologist may be needed. The considerations regarding management of anticoagulant agents prior to surgery are similar to the considerations surrounding neuraxial blockade (see Chapter 4). The risk of discontinuing antiplatelet agents prior to surgery should be discussed with each patient's primary care physician so that an appropriate analysis of the risk of recurrent thromboembolic event can be weighed against the risk of perioperative bleeding.

Excessive tension on the margins of the wound created during implantation can lead to skin breakdown and/or cellulitis, mandating device removal. This is normally apparent in the immediate postoperative period, but may develop much later in the course of treatment. During implantation, it is important to ensure that the pocket created is large enough to allow for good apposition of the wound margins without tension on the suture line. If excessive tension on the skin overlying the implanted device appears chronically, the surgeon should consider pocket revision. If properly monitored, a pump should be suitable in patients with low body mass index. This group includes cancer patients who have poor nutritional status and small children. Literature in spasticity shows that toddlers are able to tolerate pump placement if vigilance is paid to wound care and pocket monitoring.[34]

The pump can flip within the pocket after implantation so that the access port is facing toward the abdominal wall. This can occur due to a change in body habitus that leads to laxity in the tissue of the abdominal wall. The pump can also flip if the patient repeatedly attempts to move it within the pocket. In these instances, the pump may be repositioned, and an abdominal binder can be used to hold it in position. Eventually, surgical correction may be required. This process involves removing some of the surrounding adipose tissue to anchor the pump to the fascia. In the morbidly obese, this may be impossible because it may lead to the pump being so far from the surface that it can no longer communicate with the telemetry device used in programming. In these cases, a Dacron pouch may be used to anchor to the surrounding tissue in the hope that fibrosis will develop to avoid further movement of the pump.

Prevention and Treatment of Infectious Complications

Prevention of infection is best accomplished through meticulous use of sterile technique, gentle tissue dissection, and sound wound closure. Because implanted devices used for chronic pain therapy extend to the neuraxis and infection can prove catastrophic, routine antimicrobial prophylaxis is warranted in all patients (Table 25-4). The Centers for Disease Control and Prevention published an extensive *Guideline for Prevention of Surgical Site Infection* in 1999[35] that discusses all aspects of prevention in detail, and a recent review of infectious complications associated with chronic pain therapies[33] has also recently appeared. Infection of a pump is a much more serious issue, and treatment options vary with the severity of tissue involvement. In superficial infections, treatment options include oral antibiotics and observation or open incision and drainage. In either treatment scenario, the goal is to preserve the system. Once infection has spread

to the deeper tissues, treatment is removal of the pump and catheter and initiation of antibiotics by either an oral or intravenous route. Consultation with an infectious disease specialist can be helpful when determining the proper antibiotic regimen. Culture results can be used to guide therapy. If the device is replaced in the future, the infectious disease specialist may be helpful in identifying preoperative precautions to reduce the risk of recurrent infection.

In the event of neuraxial infection, rapid intervention is required. Meningitis is seen in <0.1% of all cases of infection associated with implanted intrathecal drug delivery devices[36] and is treated in a manner consistent with other patients with meningitis. There is no consensus in the literature on the need to remove the device in the setting of meningitis. Epidural abscess is a much more serious event in most situations and can result in paralysis if rapid action is delayed. This problem is identified by pain in the back outside the character of typical postoperative pain, fever, and malaise. Diagnosis is confirmed by MRI or CT, and treatment often requires surgical drainage of the abscess and removal of the catheter. Transverse myelitis, in which neurologic symptoms appear on both sides of midline and are thought to arise from inflammatory changes within the spinal cord, is a rare complication and is likely closely associated with inflammatory granuloma formation or infection. Treatment consists of a high-dose intravenous steroid administration and consultation with an infectious disease specialist to rule out and treat any identifiable viral or bacterial causes of this disorder.[15]

After removing an implanted device because of tissue infection, wound dehiscence, or seroma, the clinician must be vigilant to avoid withdrawal symptoms caused by abrupt cessation of opioid, clonidine, and/or baclofen.[9] The most common reason to revise or remove a pump is because the battery reached the end of its useful life. Battery exhaustion is expected, and available devices will need replacement every 2 to 5 years, on average. Significant overdosing can occur at the time of pump replacement, and vigilance must be maintained to correctly identify the drug dose, catheter length, and bridge bolus. This can usually be accomplished in the outpatient setting with minimal risk, but when uncertainties about the bridge dosing arise during pump replacement, the patient should be admitted for careful observation until the entire bridge bolus has been completed, and significant time at the new baseline infusion has elapsed.

Prevention and Treatment of Device-related Complications

Catheter malfunction is the most common problem seen with implanted pumps. This problem can lead to withdrawal, increased pain, and the need for surgical correction. Prevention of catheter migration is accomplished by careful anchoring of the catheter to the paraspinous fascia. Indeed, the incidence of catheter migration is doubled when this simple anchoring step is omitted.[10] Careful attention to the course that the intrathecal catheter takes at the time of implantation can minimize the risk of kinking; the catheter should be coiled without abrupt angles. Diagnosis of catheter malfunction is often made by plain x-ray, a side port study using radiographic contrast (as described previously), or MRI. Treatment includes correction of the identified problem. If the catheter has migrated out of

TABLE 25-4 Recommended Antibiotic Prophylaxis Prior to Implantation of an Implanted Intrathecal Drug Delivery

ANTIBIOTIC	DOSE AND ADMINISTRATION
Cefazolin	1–2 g IV 30 min prior to incision
Clindamycin (β-lactam allergic patients)	600 mg IV 30 min prior to incision
Vancomycin prior (methicillin-resistant *Staphylococcus aureus* carriers)	1 g IV over 60 min to incision

Adapted from Rathmell JP, Lake T, Ramundo MB. Infectious risks of chronic pain treatments: injection therapy, surgical implants, and intradiscal techniques. *Reg Anesth Pain Med* 2006;31:346–352.

the subarachnoid space, the entire catheter must be replaced. If catheter migration has occurred into a foramen or to a different level, the catheter position may be corrected by pulling it back to the midline. Catheter migration into the spinal cord is rare and requires consultation with a neurosurgeon and removal of the system. Catheter kinking or fracture can necessitate replacing the entire catheter. If the lesion is at the level of the anchor or near the midline incision, a splicing kit can be used so that only the posterior wound needs to be explored. If the catheter fractures at a more proximal location, the entire catheter should be replaced.

Catheter fibrosis (minor fibrosis without a large inflammatory mass) can lead to decreased drug effect and is apparent when there is pain on injection through the side port. This complication can be treated by either pulling the catheter back or revising the distal portion of the catheter. Some experts suggest a revision of the intrathecal portion of the catheter and a change to a different vertebral level in this situation.

Although one cannot totally avoid seroma, its incidence can be reduced by careful attention to surgical technique. By avoiding excessive tissue trauma and paying close attention to homeostasis, the occurrence of tissue leakage of serosanguineous fluid can be reduced and subsequently the occurrence of seroma will be reduced. Once a seroma is diagnosed, treatment involves sterile aspiration of the seroma fluid with analysis of the fluid to rule out infection. A straw-colored fluid without other signs or symptoms of infection suggests a noninfectious seroma. If aspiration is performed repeatedly without resolution of the symptoms, surgical incision and drainage may be needed. A drain may be used to avoid repeat collection of fluid, but is somewhat controversial because of the perceived risk of increased infection. Recurrent seroma can lead to the need to revise the pocket, moving the pump to a new location.

Skin breakdown over the long term can occur and lead to cellulitis and exposure of the device, mandating removal. If pain develops around the pump, a careful exam should be performed to rule out the need for surgical revision, before skin breakdown occurs.

Mechanical failure, including a stalled rotor or a jammed gear in a programmable pump, requires replacement of the entire device. Pump replacement is also required if the side port develops a leak or if the access port develops a loss of integrity.

A catheter tip granuloma, an inflammatory mass at the catheter tip, varies in its presentation. Deer[37] showed in a series of consecutive patients examined by MRI that patients can have these lesions but show no symptoms. Coffey and Burchiel[11] presented a series of patients with much more troubling outcomes, including paraplegia. In asymptomatic patients, treatment may consist of repeat MRI and observation or of catheter revision. Animal studies have shown that persistent exposure to the inciting drug leads to persistent advancement of the lesion. The infusion of saline may lead to lesion regression, but results in cessation of the therapy. As a result, many clinicians opt for removing the catheter. Any time catheter revision is planned, the patient should be kept responsive. The incision is made and the catheter is exposed. Once the catheter is located, it should be gently removed. If resistance develops or unexpected pain occurs, the catheter should be left in place. Options at this point include occluding the catheter at the ligament with suture or surgical clips and leaving it in place or surgical resection

to remove the mass. In cases where there is no obvious neurologic compromise, the need for surgical resection is not usually warranted. After the initial diagnosis of the lesion, the clinician should immediately discontinue the offending agent and switch drugs or initiate saline. Options include removal of the catheter, revision of the catheter one to two levels below the current level, or replacement of the catheter. The nuances of surgical management of catheter tip granulomas have been the subject of a recent review.[38] Once the catheter has been corrected, the offending agent should be avoided in the future, and alternative drugs should be used.

Prevention and Treatment of Drug-related Complications

The most successful means of minimizing drug-related complications during intrathecal delivery is to be thoroughly familiar with each agent and to avoid drugs that are not well supported in published reports. In extreme cases, such as those of patients with terminal cancer, the use of novel agents may be an acceptable alternative. Recent studies have shown that ketamine and meperidine are possible alternatives in these cases.[39,40]

Complications from opioids (such as nausea and vomiting, pruritis, dysuria, constipation, edema, diaphoresis, weakness, weight gain, and diminished libido) generally dissipate over time with no specific treatment. Of these problems, edema can be persistent and troubling. Treatment consists of conservative measures, including diuretics and support stockings. Maximizing control of edema prior to implant in those with long-standing problems may also help in reducing the subsequent incidence of this problem. If these options are not successful, a change of drug is required.

Constipation can be problematic, although it is less common than with other routes of opioid administration. Similar to those receiving long-term oral opioid analgesics, treatment is to place the patient on a good bowel regimen and increase activity and fiber in the diet. Reduction of testosterone has been described in relation to oral and intrathecal opioids (see Chapter 34). Once this problem has been confirmed by laboratory studies, treatment includes testosterone replacement by an oral or transdermal route. Because there are data suggesting supplemental testosterone can lead to a worsening of prostate cancer, it is important to receive a normal prostate specific serum level prior to prescribing replacement therapy.

Some drugs have complications specific to their receptor-mediated actions. Clonidine is active at alpha receptors. To prevent somnolence or hypotension, the dose of this drug should be elevated with caution. Side effects are more likely to occur if the catheter is in the high thoracic or cervical region. Bupivacaine has also been shown to cause specific problems with loss of sensation. This can be avoided by starting at a low dose of 1 to 2 mg/d and increasing the dose with caution.

Ziconotide has specific problems related to its infusion (Table 25-3). These problems include dizziness, confusion, hallucination, somnolence, and nausea. Recent work in follow-up studies[41,42] shows that a slow titration can reduce the incidence of these problems and improve the ability of patients to tolerate the drug.

Complications of drug mislabeling or the presence of contaminants must be corrected at the pharmacy level. The physician should have discussions with the pharmacy they use to provide the pump drugs and ensure they are using international standards to make compounds and create admixtures. The pharmacist should also be well versed in the concentrations of drugs that are safe to administer in the device.

Finally, recent large-scale population studies suggest that there is an increase in mortality in those patients who receive intrathecal drug delivery for the treatment of chronic noncancer pain when compared to controls that are matched for overall level of disease severity.[12] The reasons for this increase in mortality are unclear, but in a small series of fatalities reported through the FDA's MedWatch system, several of these cases point to deaths occurring within the first 24 to 48 hours after initial implantation or revision of an implanted drug delivery system. Extensive analysis suggests that some of these deaths may be related to errors in programming or sudden reinstitution of intrathecal therapy after long intervals when no drug was being delivered due to malfunction of the system. Close attention must be paid to programming of the device and calculation of the initial drug infusion rate when a new system is being placed or an existing system revised. Specific steps to minimize the risk of drug overdose during initial implantation of system revision have been proposed (Box 25-3).[43]

▶ WHEN TO SEEK CONSULTATION

It is important to remember the value of consultants in cases where complications arise. In cases where a potential risk is permanent neurologic damage, it is imperative to ask for the advice of a neurosurgeon or orthopedic spine surgeon. Likewise, infectious disease consultants can prove invaluable in selecting and guiding therapy whenever device or wound infection is suspected. In those patients with coexisting disease, judicious use of appropriate specialist consultants will improve patient care.

▶ SUMMARY

Intrathecal drug delivery is a viable alternative treatment to long-term pharmacologic management with oral agents. Like spinal cord stimulation, intrathecal drug delivery has proven efficacious, cost effective, and satisfying to many patients with chronic and cancer-related pain. The prevention, recognition, and treatment of complications are a vital part of the successful use of these devices.

References

1. Brownstein MJ. A brief history of opiates, opioid peptides, and opioid receptors. *Proc Natl Acad Sci U S A* 1993;90(12):5391–5393.
2. Hughes J, Smith TW, Kosterlitz HW, et al. Identification of two related pentapeptides from the brain with potent opiate agonist activity. *Nature (London)* 1975;258:577–580.
3. LaMotte C, Pert CB, Snyder SH. Opiate receptor binding in primate spinal cord: distribution and changes after dorsal horn resection. *Brain Res* 1976;112:407–412.
4. Yaksh TL, Rudy TA. Analgesia mediated by a direct spinal action of narcotics. *Science* 1976;192:1357–1358.
5. Wang JK, Nauss LA, Thomas JE. Pain relief by intrathecally applied morphine in man. *Anesthesiology* 1979;50:149–151.
6. Behar M, Magora F, Olschwang D, et al. Epidural morphine in treatment of pain. *Lancet* 1979;1:527–528.
7. Ferrante FM. Neuroaxial infusion in the management of cancer pain. *Oncology* 1999;13:30–36.
8. Faaber J, Koulousakis A, Staats P. Clinical protocols for titrating constant flow implantable pumps in patients with pain or spasticity. *Neuromodulation* 2005;8:121–130.
9. Thimineur MA, Kravitz E, Vodapally MS. Intrathecal opioid treatment for chronic non-malignant pain: a 3-year prospective study. *Pain* 2004;109:242–249.
10. Follett KA, Naumann CP. A prospective study of catheter-related complications of intrathecal drug delivery systems. *J Pain Symptom Manage* 2000;19:209–215.
11. Coffey RJ, Burchiel KJ. Inflammatory mass lesions associated with intrathecal drug infusion catheters: report and observations on 41 patients. *Neurosurgery* 2002;50:78–86.
12. Coffey RJ, Owens ML, Broste SK, et al. Mortality associated with implantation and management of intrathecal opioid drug infusion systems to treat noncancer pain. *Anesthesiology* 2009;111:881–891.
13. Harney D, Victor R. Traumatic syrinx after implantation of an intrathecal catheter. *Reg Anesth Pain Med* 2004;29:606–609.
14. Huntoon MA, Hurdle MF, Marsh RW, et al. Intrinsic spinal cord catheter placement: implications of new intractable pain in a patient with a spinal cord injury. *Anesth Analg* 2004;99:1763–1765.
15. Ubogu EE, Lindenberg JR, Werz MA, et al. Transverse myelitis associated with *Acinetobacter baumannii* intrathecal pump catheter-related infection. *Reg Anesth Pain Med* 2003;28:470–474.
16. Torrens JK, Stanley PJ, Ragunathan PL, et al. Risk of infection with electrical spinal-cord stimulation. *Lancet* 1997;349:729.
17. Milbouw G. An unusual sign of catheter migration: sciatica. *Neuromodulation* 2005;8:233.
18. Albrecht E, Durrer A, Chedel D, et al. Intraparenchymal migration of an intrathecal catheter three years after implantation. *Pain* 2005;118:274–278.
19. Dario A, Scamoni C, Picano M. The infection risk of intrathecal drug infusion pumps after multiple refill procedures. *Neuromodulation* 2005;8:36.

BOX 25-3 Specific Steps to Minimize the Risk of Drug Overdose During the Initial Implantation or Revision of an Existing Intrathecal Drug Delivery System

1. Initiating intrathecal therapy with the lowest dose that can be reasonably predicted to provide efficacy.
2. Avoid use of concomitant central nervous system depressants in the immediate postimplantation period.
3. Gain an expert understanding of the intrathecal drug pump, its construction, and proper programming.
4. Personally oversee all aspects of the initial programming.
5. Avoid use of excessively concentrated solutions during initiation of therapy to minimize the delay in onset of drug effects associated with slow infusion rates.
6. Routinely calculate when new drug will first enter the intrathecal space and warn the patient and their caregivers to be most vigilant during this interval of time.

Adapted from Rathmell JP, Miller MJ. Death after initiation of intrathecal drug therapy for chronic pain: assessing risk and designing prevention. *Anesthesiology* 2009;111:706–708.

20. Burton AW, Conroy B, Garcia E, et al. Illicit substance abuse via an implanted intrathecal pump. *Anesthesiology* 2005;89:1264–1267.

21. Narouze S, Yonan S, Malak O. *Inferior Epigastric Artery Erosion: A Rare Complication of Intrathecal Drug Delivery System. Abstract.* San Francisco, CA: American Society of Regional Anesthesia and Pain Medicine, 2003.

22. Yaksh TL, Horais KA, Tozier NA, et al. Chronically infused intrathecal morphine in dogs. *Anesthesiology* 2003;99:174–187.

23. Deer TR, Raso LJ, Garten TG. Inflammatory mass of an intrathecal catheter in patients receiving baclofen as a sole agent: a report of two cases and a review of the identification and treatment of the complication. *Pain Med* 2007;8:259–262.

24. Toombs JD, Follett KA, Rosenquist RW, et al. Intrathecal catheter tip inflammatory mass: a failure of clonidine to protect. *Anesthesiology* 2005;102:687–690.

25. Follett KA. Intrathecal analgesia and catheter-tip inflammatory masses. *Anesthesiology* 2003;99:5–6.

26. Paice JA, Penn RD, Shott S. Intraspinal morphine for chronic pain: a retrospective, multicenter study. *J Pain Symptom Manage* 1996;11:71–80.

27. Winkelmuller M, Winkelmuller W. Long-term effects of continuous intrathecal opioid treatment in chronic pain of nonmalignant etiology. *J Neurosurg* 1996;85:458–467.

28. Aldrete JA, Couto da Silva JM. Leg edema from intrathecal opiate infusions. *Eur J Pain* 2000;4:361–365.

29. Hassenbusch SJ, Gunes S, Wachsman S, et al. Intrathecal clonidine in the treatment of intractable pain: a phase I/II study. *Pain Med* 2002;3:85–91.

30. Staats PS, Yearwood T, Charapata SG, et al. Intrathecal ziconotide in the treatment of refractory pain in patients with cancer and AIDS. *JAMA* 2003;291:62–70.

31. Miele VJ, Price KO, Bloomfield S, et al. A review of intrathecal morphine therapy related granulomas. *Eur J Pain* 2006;10:251–261.

32. Coyne PJ, Hansen LA, Laird J, et al. Massive hydromorphone dose delivered subcutaneously instead of intrathecally: guidelines for prevention and management of opioid, local anesthetic, and clonidine overdose. *J Pain Symptom Manage* 2004;28:273–276.

33. Rathmell JP, Lake T, Ramundo MB. Infectious risks of chronic pain treatments: injection therapy, surgical implants, and intradiscal techniques. *Reg Anesth Pain Med* 2006;31:346–352.

34. Albright AL, Awaad Y, Muhonen M, et al. Performance and complications associated with the synchromed 10-ml infusion pump for intrathecal baclofen administration in children. *Neurosurgery* 2004;101(1 suppl):64–68.

35. The Centers for Disease Control and Prevention. Guideline for prevention of surgical site infection. *Infect Control Epidemiol* 1999;20:217–278.

36. Follett KA, Boortz-Marx RL, Drake JM, et al. Prevention and management of intrathecal drug delivery and spinal cord stimulation system infections. *Anesthesiology* 2004;100:1582–1594.

37. Deer T. A prospective analysis of intrathecal granuloma in chronic pain patients: a review of the literature and report of a surveillance study. *Pain Physician* 2004;7:225–228.

38. Zacest AC, Carlson JD, Nemecek A, et al. Surgical management of spinal catheter granulomas: operative nuances and review of the surgical literature. *Neurosurgery* 2009;65:1161–1164.

39. Benrath J, Scharbert G, Gustorff B, et al. Long-term intrathecal S(+)-ketamine in a patient with cancer-related neuropathic pain. *Br J Anaesth* 2005;95:247–249.

40. Souter KJ, Davies JM, Loeser JD, et al. Continuous intrathecal meperidine for severe refractory cancer pain: a case report. *Clin J Pain* 2005;21:193–196.

41. Wallace MS, Rauck R, Fisher R, et al. Intrathecal ziconotide for severe chronic pain: safety and tolerability results of an open-label, long-term trial. *Anesth Analg* 2008;106:628–637.

42. Webster LR, Fisher R, Charapata S, et al. Long-term intrathecal ziconotide for chronic pain: an open-label study. *J Pain Symptom Manage* 2009;37:363–372.

43. Rathmell JP, Miller MJ. Death after initiation of intrathecal drug therapy for chronic pain: assessing risk and designing prevention. *Anesthesiology* 2009;111:706–708.

Complications Associated with Spinal Cord Stimulation

Timothy R. Deer and Jason E. Pope

Spinal cord stimulation (SCS) is an important part of modern pain algorithms. Although it is considered an advanced therapy, it is an established treatment that has been utilized for both neuropathic and mixed pain for many years. SCS was first introduced into clinical practice in the late 1960s by Dr. Norman Shealy at the University Hospitals of Cleveland.[1] The concept at that time was to interrupt or change pain signals traveling to the brain in order to reduce suffering. This idea was based on the gate control theory that had been published in 1965 as an explanation for the observation that nonpainful stimuli like light touch or massage can reduce the perception of pain; Wall and Melzack hypothesized that pain perception resulted from a balance between inhibitory and excitatory fibers in the tracts controlling pain (Fig. 26-1).[2] The gate control theory was important as the initial theory behind the use of SCS, but to date there has been no scientific confirmation that this theory is accurate.

Over the past five decades, the implantation of SCS systems has evolved in many areas, including patient selection and technology as well as a focus on improved outcomes and improved health care utilization. The increase in physician implantation has been driven by a sharpened focus on pain treatment by the medical community and society, a desire to reduce the need for chronic opioid medications, and the goal of improving function. With the increase in the number of patients being offered SCS therapy, there has been a focus on improving technology by both physician innovators and medical device manufacturers.

The initial systems used for SCS had a single lead with one anode and one cathode. These rudimentary devices also had limited ability to be programmed and consisted of nothing more than an on/off mechanism triggered by a handheld magnet. Evolution of newer devices and implant techniques has improved effectiveness by using multiple electrode arrays with a variety of cathode and anode combinations, multiple leads to increase paraesthesia coverage, and smaller generators to improve comfort and acceptance. In recent years, rechargeable batteries, percutaneously placed paddle leads, and new patient pain mapping software have been introduced and show promise for improving the usefulness of SCS even further. Because of variances in approval criteria, some products, such as those used to introduce percutaneous paddle leads and new paddle constructs, are available outside the United States prior to being available in the United States. It is important for physicians to be up-to-date on evolving technologies since

Gate-Control Theory of Melzack and Wall

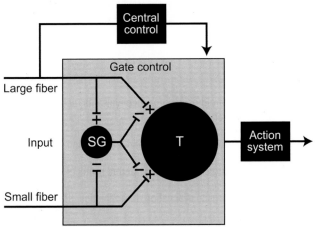

FIGURE 26-1. Schematic diagram of the gate control theory as proposed by Melzack and Wall in 1965. The theory suggests that sensory input from the periphery converges on a group of secondary neurons (T) in the spinal cord, which, in turn, convey sensory input to higher centers in the brain. This transmission of sensory input from first-order to second-order neuron within the spinal cord serves as the "Gate" for sensory input and is modified by interneurons located within the substantia gelatinosa. If nonnociceptive sensory input traveling via large nerve fibers converges on the same secondary neurons, this nonpainful input closes the "Gate" preventing transmission of painful nociceptive input. SCS was developed based on the gate control theory with the idea that stimulating nonnociceptive fibers electrically might close the gate and reduce pain perception. While the gate control theory has proven overly simplistic, the concept that nonnociceptive nerve traffic can modify pain perception has proven true.

BOX 26-1 Established Indications for Spinal Cord Stimulation

- Chronic lumbar radiculopathy
- Chronic cervical radiculopathy
- Neuropathic limb pain secondary to spinal disease prior to initial surgery
- Failed cervical surgery syndrome with radicular component
- Failed back surgery syndrome (including persistent pain in the back and/or the extremities)
- Primary axial back pain prior to intrathecal drug administration
- Spinal stenosis
- Postherpetic neuralgia
- Peripheral nerve injury
- Brachial plexopathy
- Radiation neuritis
- Complex Regional Pain Syndrome (Types I and II)
- Raynaud's syndrome
- Ischemic pain of the extremity
- Visceral pain syndromes including abdominal pain from pancreatitis
- Visceral pain syndromes including pelvic pain from interstitial cystitis
- Angina pectoris
- Diabetic peripheral neuropathy and other neuropathies of the upper and lower extremities

many of these new technologies will impact practice by improving the success of stimulation and reducing the rate of complications.

Early retrospective case series[3] and prospective, observational trials[4] established the usefulness of SCS for treating chronic pain after prior lumbar surgery, particularly chronic radicular pain. Recently, SCS proved to provide superior pain relief, based on visual analog scales and global patient satisfaction, when compared to repeat operation in those patients having recurrent or persistent pain following prior lumbar fusion.[5] Critically important in this era of cost-based medicine, the available evidence suggests that SCS results in a net savings to the health care system when compared with conservative pain treatment techniques.[6] SCS in conjunction with a structured physical therapy program also leads to better functional improvement in patients with complex regional pain syndrome than physical therapy alone.[7] SCS is now established as an effective technique for treating many types of chronic pain (Box 26-1). Like any surgical technique, particularly those requiring placement of an indwelling device, complications will arise in a small number of patients. It is important to understand the potential complications when offering this therapy to patients. Complications can be broken down into those relating to the neuraxis, those involving the device and its components, and those occurring in the tissues outside the spine. In order to have success in managing these complications, the physician must understand the complications that can occur, how to recognize them, and the best corrective measures for each (Table 26-1).

▶ SCOPE OF THE PROBLEM

The incidence of complications associated with spinal cord stimulator placement has been reported in frequencies ranging from 0% to 81%, depending on the author and significance of the adverse event reported. In a systematic analysis focusing on higher quality studies, the mean complication rate was 34% when reviewing multiple data pools. In this same analysis, the need to do a surgical revision was 23%, while those requiring explant was 11%. Life-threatening or serious complications occurred <1% of the time.[8] Cameron performed an extensive review of literature encompassing 3,679 patients and reported a complication rate of 36%. In another long-term analysis of 102 implanted patients, the surgical revision rate was 32% over a 10-year follow-up period.[9] Burchiel and colleagues found a 17% revision rate with patients implanted for 1 year or more.[10] Kumar[11] found lead complication rates to be 5.3%, epidural fibrosis rates of 19%, and infection rates of 2.7%. Furthermore, Kumar et al.,[12] in a later study, reported a frequency of stimulators requiring revision of approximately 25% to 33%, and of those requiring revision, 85% remained satisfied with the results.

The most serious complications involve the spine and associated structures. Device complications are much more common and require more frequent surgical attention. The complications surrounding programming and device computer malfunction are a frustration to the patient and clinician, but are minor when compared to the potentially life-threatening problems that involve spinal structures.

TABLE 26-1 Complications Associated with SCS, Their Diagnosis, and Treatment

COMPLICATION	DIAGNOSIS	TREATMENT
Complications involving the neuraxis		
Nerve injury	CT or MRI, EMG/NCS/physical exam	Steroid protocol, anticonvulsants, neurosurgery consult
Epidural fibrosis	Increased stimulation amplitude	Lead programming and lead revision
Epidural hematoma	Physical exam, CT or MRI	Surgical evacuation, steroid protocol
Epidural abscess	Physical exam, CT or MRI, CBC, blood work	Surgical evacuation, IV antibiotics, ID consult
PDPH	Positional headache, blurred vision, nausea	IV fluids, rest, blood patch
Complications outside the neuraxis		
Seroma	Serosanguineous fluid in pocket	Aspiration, if no response surgical drainage
Hematoma	Blood in pocket	Pressure and aspiration, surgical revision
Pain at generator	Pain on palpation	Topical lidocaine patches, injection, revision
Wound infection	Fever, rubor, drainage	Antibiotics, incision and drainage, removal
Device-related complications		
Unacceptable programming	Lack of stimulation in area of pain	Reprogramming of device, revision of leads
Lead migration	Inability to program, x-rays	Reprogramming, surgical revision
Current leak	High impedance, pain at leak site	Revision of connectors, generator, or leads
Generator failure	Inability to read device	Replacement of generator

Complications of structures outside the neuraxis vary in severity and can be as simple as pain at an incision or generator or as complicated as serious wound infections leading to sepsis.[13–16] Kemler[17] reported that biologic complications from SCS typically occur within 3 months of implant, while device complications occur later, but typically still within the first 2 years after implantation.

▶ DEFINITION, INCIDENCE, AND DIAGNOSIS OF COMPLICATIONS ASSOCIATED WITH SPINAL CORD STIMULATION

Complications Involving the Neuraxis

Among the most serious and urgent complication of SCS is the development of an epidural hematoma. The incidence of this complication is low, and no reliable estimate of the incidence can be made from the existing literature, although it is thought to be <1%. While unproven, because SCS involves placing a large introducer needle into the epidural space and then threading an electrode many levels cephalad within the spinal canal, it seems likely that the incidence of epidural hematoma formation would be somewhat higher than that during single shot or continuous epidural analgesia. Exact numbers are not available. The development of an epidural hematoma can lead to paralysis if not treated in a timely fashion.[18] The patient may complain of numbness developing in the immediate postoperative period. This numbness may be accompanied by severe back or leg pain. Weakness in the postoperative period should be seen as a red flag for suspicion of an epidural hematoma. Risk factors for developing this complication include use of anticoagulants, aspirin, nonsteroidal anti-inflammatory drugs, or other drugs affecting platelet function. Readers are directed to the American Society of Regional Anesthesia guidelines for regional anesthesia in the patient receiving anticoagulation therapy.[19] Other risks include difficult lead placement with multiple lead passes, the need to place a surgical lead requiring laminectomy, and reoperation in an area previously implanted. This complication is more common with surgical instrumentation requiring extensive bone removal.[8]

Diagnosis of an epidural hematoma in this setting requires computed tomography (CT). Magnetic resonance imaging (MRI) can be obtained if the device has been removed. While MRI has been done in patients with implants in place without difficulty, MRI has not been approved by the Food and Drug Administration for use in patients with indwelling SCS leads[20–22] over concerns that the strong magnetic field may induce inductive heating within the epidural lead and resultant tissue injury.

Another serious and potentially life-threatening complication is infection of the spinal structures. Possible infections include epidural abscess, discitis, and meningitis. The incidence of such infections is small, and no data exist on the exact percentage, but most authors have quoted an incidence of <1 in a 1,000.[23] Epidural abscess is the most common of these complications, and considerations are similar to those discussed for epidural analgesia (see chapter on infectious complications). Meglio et al.[24] described a case of an intradural and epidural abscess with associated paraplegia in a patient with a recently explanted spinal cord stimulator. Discitis and meningitis often result as a progression of the epidural abscess into surrounding tissues. The patient with a developing epidural abscess often complains of severe pain in the area of the lead implant. An elevated temperature above 101 degrees Fahrenheit may also be suggestive of abscess formation and bacteremia. The development of radiating pain in a dermatomal or nondermatomal fashion may indicate progression of the abscess. Risk factors for abscess formation include an immunocompromised state, uncontrolled diabetes mellitus, chronic dialysis, a history of organ transplant with ongoing immunosuppressive medications, history of chronic skin infections, history of methicillin-resistant staphylococcal aureus infection, and localized skin infection or breakdown at the surgery site. Diagnosis of an epidural abscess or discitis can be confirmed by CT or using MRI, once the device has been removed. The diagnosis of bacterial meningitis diagnosis is best confirmed by prompt cerebral spinal fluid (CSF) analysis.[23]

Neurologic injury of the spinal cord or nerve roots is a potential risk of SCS. Direct trauma to neural structures caused by the epidural needle used to introduce the electrode is the most common reported mechanism for this complication, and other mechanisms include injury by lead placement, lead removal, and traction on nerves while placing a surgical laminectomy lead. In many reported cases of nerve injury, the patient was under general anesthesia or deep sedation at the time of injury and could not respond with complaints of a paraesthesia at the time of neural contact. Meyer et al.[25] described such a case where an intradural percutaneous lead was discovered at C2 on postoperative CT in a patient that was undergoing a planned IPG replacement (but unplanned lead replacement) under general anesthesia. The patient developed quadriparesis due to direct injury to the spinal cord.[25] Evaluation should be guided by the symptoms reported by the patient. Imaging studies are unlikely to reveal any abnormalities following isolated injury to a single nerve root, even in the patient reporting ongoing painful dysesthesiae. In contrast, any patient who develops signs or symptoms suggesting injury to the spinal cord should undergo immediate imaging with CT (in the event the epidural electrode remains in place) or MRI (if the lead was removed). MRI is far more sensitive in delineating subtle

injury to the substance of the spinal cord itself. In some cases, direct visualization of the cord or nerve tissue by open surgical examination is required to confirm an injury, remove a paddle lead, or repair a dural tear. Electromyograms and nerve conduction studies can also be helpful in defining the location and extent of nerve injury, but may not show an abnormality for several weeks following injury (see Chapter on Nerve Injury).[26]

A more frequent but less-worrisome neuraxial complication is that of inadvertent dural puncture. In a study involving patients with complex regional pain syndrome reported by Kemlar, 11% of 36 patients in the randomized clinical trial had evidence of postdural puncture headache (PDPH).[27] Other authors have noted similar rates of this complication. Factors that may predispose to this complication are previous surgery in the area of needle placement, calcified ligaments, obesity, and patient movement. Technique may also play a role with a higher rate of dural puncture occurring with the midline approach, steep angle of needle placement (above 45 degrees), and the use of a needle to introduce a retrograde lead. An extremely rare, but more severe complication is a dural tear with subsequent chronic CSF leak. This can lead to chronic positional headache, nausea, tinnitus, and malaise. The introduction of a foreign body into the epidural space can result in scarring of the epidural tissues. Lenarson et al.[28] reported a histologically confirmed foreign body reaction causing symptomatic compression of the cervical spinal cord secondary to a percutaneous epidural SCS lead. Epidural fibrosis is a predictable result of lead placement into the epidural space, although it has been described as a complication.[29] Scarring begins shortly after lead introduction and, as stimulation is dependent on tissue impedance, may adversely alter the therapeutic stimulation characteristics. Kumar et al.[30] describe "system tolerance" as loss of analgesic effect despite, continued concordant paraesthesia coverage, partly attributed to the epidural scarring.

Patients who require SCS often have significant pathologic changes of the bony spine, and these abnormalities can progress in the years following placement of an implanted system. In cases where a lead is successfully placed, the development of spinal stenosis may result in compression of the spinal structures, and the presence of an electrode in the epidural space may well contribute to the degree of central canal stenosis, resulting in new radicular symptoms or signs of myelopathy.[31] Diagnosis of spinal stenosis in the patient with an indwelling lead is made by history, physical exam, and eventually by CT myelography most often in consultation with a neurosurgeon.

Complications Involving Nonspinal Tissues

Infection involving the implanted pulse generator pocket or the paraspinous course of the electrode can result in the need to remove the device. The incidence of wound infection ranges from 0% to 4.5%, although some have reported higher rates of infection.[32] Diagnosis of infection is most often straightforward, with erythema, tenderness, and drainage of purulent material from the sites of surgical placement of the lead and/or IPG. In deep-seated infections or early in the course of infection, laboratory values may help define the presence and severity of infection: elevated white blood count, elevated C-reactive protein, and elevated erythrocyte sedimentation rate. These tests are nonspecific markers of inflammation and may indicate a postoperative atelectasis, blood clot, or urinary tract infection. An elevated white blood cell count, with a left shift in the differential cell count toward neutrophils along with abnormality in either of the other two studies should prompt increased vigilance by the implanting physician. Infections may occur in the pocket, lead placement incision, or tunneled subcutaneous tissue. Infections may involve only the superficial tissues or may be widespread, extending from the pocket to the epidural space.

The noninfectious buildup of serosanguineous fluid in the pocket can lead to a seroma that may impede the ability of the wound to heal, can cause pain, and can lead to poor patient satisfaction even if the device is providing effective pain relief. Seroma is diagnosed when normal laboratory values are present, wound Gram stain and culture are negative, fever is absent, yet an erythematous, swollen, fluctuant wound is present. Diagnosis is confirmed by aspiration of straw-colored fluid that does not show bacteria on microscopic analysis or subsequent culture. Adherence to meticulous surgical technique can reduce the risk of seroma, but cannot eliminate it entirely.[33]

The Centers for Disease Control and Prevention release guideline statements regarding surgical site infection perioperative prevention strategies, including commentary on surgeon, patient, and environmental factors.[34] Of the factors listed in Box 26-2, appropriate hand preparation by the surgeon, a sterile operating theater environment, type of skin preparatory solution (chlorhexidine is preferred to povidone iodine), use of preoperative antibiotics administered 30 minutes prior to incision, and wound irrigation are all supported by conclusive scientific study. Preoperative bathing, the use of antibiotic irrigation, occlusive drapes, dressing removal time, antibacterial ointments, or postoperative antibiotics have only anecdotal evidence and may contribute to microbial antibiotic resistance.[35] Bleeding can occur in the wound of the generator or lead placement area. The bleeding can range from superficial bruising to large volume hematoma requiring treatment.[36] Bedder et al.[37] commented on the use of bacterial ointment after closure, describing that routine antibiotic ointment may increase antibiotic resistance, increase allergy to the antimicrobial, and increase susceptibility to skin necrosis.

Postoperative pain can occur in patients with spinal cord stimulators and connectors. The incidence of this problem is low and is estimated to be between 0.8% and 5.6%,[8,12] but when present can lead to patient dissatisfaction and even the need for explantation or revision of the system. The differential diagnosis includes neuroma at the surgical site, subcutaneous skin irritation, and bony irritation caused by the device coming in to contact with the anterior superior iliac spine or costal margin; diagnosis is straightforward and based on clinical judgment and physical exam. If neuroma is suspected, diagnosis may be enhanced by transient relief after an injection of local anesthetic. In some patients, weight loss that occurs with increased activity after successful implantation leads to loss of superficial adipose and may result in pain at the site of superficial wires, connectors, and generators. In the event the device becomes too superficial it can result in skin breakdown and skin infection. Without proper treatment, this can lead to loss of the device.[8]

BOX 26-2 Avoiding Infection and Seroma Formation

- Screen the patient preoperatively for signs or symptoms of skin, dental, urinary, or pulmonary infection.
- If signs or symptoms suggestive of infection are present, obtain a preoperative white blood cell count with differential.
- Administer prophylactic antibiotics 30 min before start of device placement.
- Recommend that the patient bathe with chlorhexidine or similar agent the morning of surgery.
- If the patient has a history of MSRA infection or colonization, use intranasal mupirocin or similar antibiotic for 72 h prior to surgery (consider consultation with an infectious disease specialist for guidance regarding eradication of MRSA colonization).
- Review that the antibiotic covers common microbes detected in your facility.
- Prepare the skin using at least six successive applications of chlorhexidine that extend least 24 inches outside of your suspected surgical field.
- Use chlorhexidine gluconate surgical preparation solution.
- If hair removal is required to prepare the operative field, clipping is suggested over shaving. If shaving is required, it should be performed immediately before the surgical skin preparation.
- Drape at least 12 inches outside of your projected operative field.
- Avoid direct contact with the C-arm once it is moved into the lateral position.
- Adhere to meticulous sterile technique.
- Adhere to meticulous gentle surgical technique during tissue dissection, avoiding aggressive blunt dissection.
- Irrigate the wounds under low pressure with copious amounts of saline prior to closure.
- Ensure complete hemostasis within the pocket and paraspinous incisions.
- Ensure all dead space is closed and a layered closure is performed.
- Ensure that all skin edges are even and no tension is on the skin during closing.
- Consider the use antibiotic ointment on the incisions prior to placing the sterile dressing.

Complications Involving the Implanted Device

Device-related complications are often difficult to distinguish from overall adverse events in published reports. Taylor and colleagues[38] reported an overall 43% device complication rate. Many of these events were not felt to be significant. Others estimated complications requiring revision neared 25% to 33%, while complication requiring explant was approximately 11%.[8,12] Alo and colleagues[39] reported significant adverse events of the device requiring revision in 6% of patients and device removal in a similar number of patients. The most common complication of SCS is the loss of paraesthesia capture and the loss of perceived stimulation overlapping with the area of chronic pain. In many cases, this complication is the result of lead migration, dead zones in the epidural space, or changes in the patient's pain pattern. "Dead zones" are areas in the epidural space that do not result in perceived stimulation by the patient even at high amplitudes and pulse widths. Modern lead technology incorporates an array of 4 to 16 electrodes. When paraesthesia capture is lost, a change in programming using alternate electrodes within the array can often reproduce a satisfactory pattern of stimulation.[40,16] The cause for a change in stimulation pattern or loss of coverage is established using plain films with a comparison of lead placement in the postoperative period and after loss of stimulation, computer analysis for impedance and amplitude requirements, and reexamination of the patient to assess change in disease status or progression of disease (Box 26-3).

When reprogramming does not resolve the loss of stimulation, and x-rays do not show migration, the system must be analyzed for other problems. Computer analysis will be helpful in revealing a disruption in the circuit. In the setting of high impedance, the diagnosis of current leak can be confirmed. The most common problem in this setting is loss of current from the connector or generator site. Fluid in the connector is a common cause. Other differential diagnosis includes a break in the electrode or wiring. Surgical exploration with testing of the lead, connectors, and generator is often the only means to identify the problem.

In chronic lead implantation, the patient may experience a loss of stimulation that is not explained by reprogramming, x-ray analysis, or impedance abnormalities. In these cases, the patient must be evaluated for critical spinal stenosis. The difficulty of this diagnosis is that all other parameters may be normal, but stimulation is significantly different than the previous pattern. The gold standard of diagnosis is CT myelogram.[41] Lead migration is another device-related complication that may lead to failure of

stimulation. The incidence of lead migration has been reduced in recent years due to improved anchoring techniques. There are juxtaposed reports that surgical leads have a lower incidence of lead migration than percutaneously placed leads.[42,43] IPG placement has been suggested to influence lead migration, and placement of the IPG in the abdomen is better than the diagnostic workup for lead migration that includes an initial attempt to reprogram the leads. When reprogramming does not lead to a recapture of stimulation, a series of anterior-posterior and lateral films are obtained of the lead placement area of the spine. The films can be compared to the initial postoperative films to diagnose migration.[44] Painful stimulation occurs as a result of a current leakage in the system, change in programming, lead migration, or change in disease state. Current leak is diagnosed by computer analysis showing exceptionally high impedance. The device should be turned off until proper diagnostic workup is completed. Lead fracture may occur leading to device failure. This complication, most often seen with surgical paddle leads, results in initial increasing impedance followed by eventual loss of stimulation.[8,16]

Positional stimulation can occur due to the lead falling away from the neural structures with patient movement and was recently described by Abejon and Feler.[45] Other causes of this problem are the development of epidural fibrosis or the presence of an epidural fat pad or vessel under the lead. The diagnoses of these problems are often made by diagnostic exclusion of other causes, since there is no good way to image these structures. An analysis has shown that 6% of patients experience pain at the connector site or generator. Pain at the implant site can occur because of the hardness of the anchor, irritation by connection devices, or pain from the generator. This is more common in patients who experience weight gain.[8,16]

Other reported complications include skin burns caused by overcharging a rechargeable device. In these situations, the battery heats as it charges, and because of the superficial nature of the device, it can cause skin burns of varying significance. The IPG itself can flip within the implant pocket and result in the inability to program or charge a device. In these cases, the generator flips over and suddenly is no longer able to communicate with external telemetry. This can be caused by creating a pocket that is larger than the device, by an increase in patient weight resulting in a change in subcutaneous adipose, or by the patient having a nervous habit of manipulating the device.[46]

▶ TREATMENT OF COMPLICATIONS ASSOCIATED WITH SPINAL CORD STIMULATION

Treatment of Complications Involving the Neuraxis

The most common postoperative complication of the neuraxis is puncture of the dura. When an accidental puncture of the dura occurs, the initial treatment is commonly conservative and includes hydration, oral or parenteral caffeine, oral or parenteral analgesics, or methods to increase CSF pressure, like the use of abdominal binders. The use of

---

BOX 26-3 Diagnosing the Cause for Loss of Stimulation in the Patient with an Implanted Spinal Cord Stimulator

- Examine the patient and the device.
- Perform an analysis using the clinician computer programmer.
- Check to ensure that the implanted pulse generator is functional and battery life remains.
- Check lead impedance (excessive impedance or no impedance reading may indicate lead fracture).
- Reprogram the lead configuration in attempts to regain stimulation.
- Obtain a plain AP and lateral x-ray of the region where the epidural spinal cord stimulation lead was placed and compare to films obtained at the time of initial placement.
- Check lead-IPG interface under fluoroscopy to ensure appropriate contact.

prophylactic blood patch has not been shown to prevent the occurrence of PDPHs, yet they are commonly employed. The decision to perform a blood patch is complicated, because of the worry of introducing blood into a space with a foreign body. No data are available to suggest the best course if the symptoms do not abate with conservative measures. The authors would recommend blood patches be performed as the last resort in these cases. Commonly, PDPH occurs with a frequency estimated as high as 85% following a 16- to 18-gauge needle, so entry with a 14-gauge spinal cord stimulator needle is likely high.[47] Once the headache occurs, correct diagnosis is essential, as other headaches can mimic PDPH. Epidural blood patch success for PDPH is approximately 60% to 70%.

The development of postimplant epidural fibrosis results in no adverse event in most patients. In the event that stimulation changes because of epidural fibrosis, the treatment of choice is reprogramming. Reprogramming options include changing the electrode array to move the cathode to an area where fibrosis does not exist, by changing the amplitude or by changing the frequency. When stimulation cannot be recaptured to an acceptable level, surgical revision is required.[8]

In the event of potentially catastrophic complications, an emergent response is required. In cases of epidural hematoma, the diagnosis must be made quickly and treated within an 8-hour window.[48] Treatment usually involves surgical evacuation of the clot. In some instances when the hematoma is small, careful observation is used. When epidural abscess is diagnosed, treatment involves surgical decompression, infectious disease consultation, and proper antibiotic coverage. Nerve injury or spinal cord injury is sometimes difficult to delineate from nerve root irritation. When spinal cord injury is suspected, consideration should be given to administration of high-dose intravenous steroids in consultation with a neurosurgeon. Neurosurgical consultation is recommended, but in the absence of hematoma or abscess there is usually little that can be done surgically to correct the problem.[18,23]

Treatment of Complications Involving the Nonspinal Tissues

Because implanted devices used for chronic pain therapy extend to the neuraxis and infection can prove catastrophic, routine antimicrobial prophylaxis is warranted in all patients (Table 26-2). The Centers for Disease Control and Prevention published an extensive guideline for prevention of surgical site Infection in 1999 that discusses all aspects of prevention in detail[49] and again in a review of infectious complications associated with chronic pain therapies.[50] Infection of the superficial tissues can be treated conservatively with oral and topical antibiotics (Fig. 26-2). If a conservative approach is chosen, the patient should be carefully monitored. If signs of spread of the infection to deeper structures or to surrounding tissues are suspected, surgical incision and drainage is the treatment of choice (Fig. 26-3). Irrigation with a high volume irrigator containing antibiotic solution may be helpful in reducing the risk of the organism spreading in the tissues. Debridement of any tissue that appears unhealthy may also be of help in resolving the problem.[32]

TABLE 26-2 Recommended Antibiotic Prophylaxis Prior to Implantation of a Spinal Cord Stimulation System[49]	
ANTIBIOTIC	**DOSE AND ADMINISTRATION**
Cefazolin	1–2 g iv 30 min prior to incision
Clindamycin (β-lactam allergic patients)	600 mg iv 30 min prior to incision
Vancomycin (methicillin-resistant *Staphylococcus aureus* (MRSA) carriers)	1 g iv over 60 min prior to incision

Infection of the tissue containing the leads or generator requires surgical debridement, removal of the device, and, in many cases, hospitalization for intravenous antibiotics. In some instances, the device can be salvaged, but the likelihood of salvaging the device is small, and there should be a low threshold for explant. In all instances of infection, cultures should be taken, and sensitivity to the chosen antibiotic regimen should be assessed. If the patient appears systemically ill, blood cultures should also be obtained. Initially, the patient should be started on broad spectrum coverage

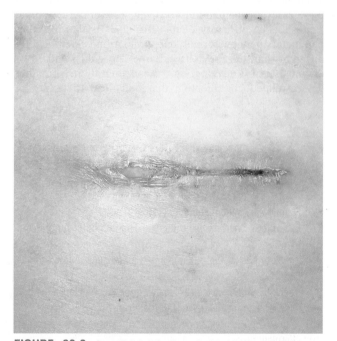

FIGURE 26-2. Superficial infection of the incision overlying an implanted pulse generator. There is scant purulent discharge draining from the medial extent of the incision. Infection of the superficial tissues can be treated conservatively with oral and topical antibiotics. If a conservative approach is chosen, the patient should be carefully monitored. If signs of spread of the infection to deeper structures or to surrounding tissues are suspected, surgical incision and drainage is the treatment of choice.

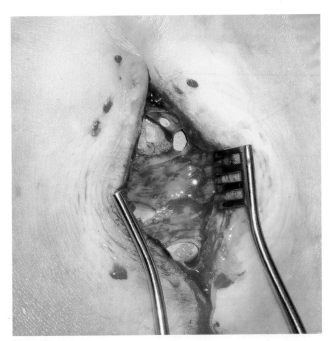

FIGURE 26-3. Deep tissue infection with pus tracking along the implanted spinal cord stimulator leads within the paraspinous region. Surgical incision and drainage with removal of all components of the implanted device is the treatment of choice. Irrigation with a high volume irrigator containing antibiotic solution may be helpful in reducing the risk of the organism spreading in the tissues. Debridement of any tissue that appears unhealthy may also be of help in resolving the problem.

such as vancomycin and gentamycin. When culture results are available, the antibiotic can be adjusted in consultation with an infectious disease expert. In serious infections, the antibiotics should be used intravenously until fever has been absent for 72 hours and then converted to oral agents if cultures show sensitivity.

Seroma can lead to wound dehiscence and loss of the device. The initial treatment of seroma is compression of the tissue and observation. In the event of increasing seroma volume despite conservative treatment, sterile aspiration is recommended. If the seroma recurs on a frequent basis, surgical exploration of the wound is recommended. Attention should be given to good hemostasis, irrigation, and debridement with cautery of any tissue that appears inflamed. The best treatment of a seroma is avoidance. The incidence of seroma can be reduced by gentle manipulation of tissue at the initial time of implant, careful attention to homeostasis, and careful sizing of the pocket to ensure the size of the pocket closely approximates the size of the device.[33] Bleeding in the pocket or lead implant site can lead to discomfort and, in some cases, the need for surgical evacuation. Initial treatment includes compression of the wound and discontinuation of any drug that may increase the risk of bleeding. If these conservative measures fail, treatment is surgical exploration and evacuation of clot and hematoma may be necessary. If surgical evacuation does not occur in a timely fashion, it can lead to wound dehiscence.

Treatment of neuroma should initially be conservative. Options include the use of topical local anesthetics, anticonvulsants, or nonsteroidal anti-inflammatory drugs. TENS

units, massage, and ultrasound have also been found to be helpful in some cases. If these conservative measures fail, treatment involves injections with local anesthetic and steroid or in severe cases surgical revision of the incision.[15]

Treatment of Complications Involving the Implanted Device

The most commonly seen complaint relating to the device in the studies analyzed in this chapter is the loss of appropriate capture of stimulation. The initial treatment involves reprogramming of the device. Changes in pulse width, electrode configuration, active lead selection, and frequency may be used as strategies to overcome this adverse outcome. Systems with 16 electrodes and high-frequency stimulation capabilities should be considered as the primary choice in the future. By using these more sophisticated devices, the need for surgical revision may be reduced.[8,14–16] In patients whom reprogramming creates an acceptable stimulation pattern, but pain relief is not achieved, there is some evidence that spinal infusion of baclofen may result in stimulation salvage and improved outcomes.[33]

When stimulation is lost due to migration (Fig. 26-4) of the lead that cannot be corrected by programming, surgical revision is required. Migration may be prevented by immobilization by bracing and movement restriction in the first 4 to 6 weeks after surgery. Migration may also be reduced by careful attention to surgical technique when anchoring the lead. Kumar et al.[12] describe placing the nose of the anchor in the tissue to avoid lead kinking (Fig. 26-5). Many physicians correct lead migration by revising the leads, again using a percutaneous technique to place the new leads. In the event that a percutaneous lead migrates on more than one occasion, the use of a surgical lead should be considered.

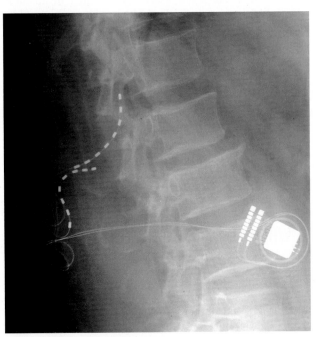

FIGURE 26-4. Lead migration. One of the two SCS leads has migrated out of the epidural space. This is easily detected using plain radiographs.

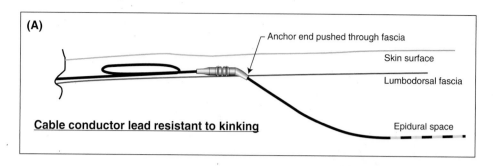

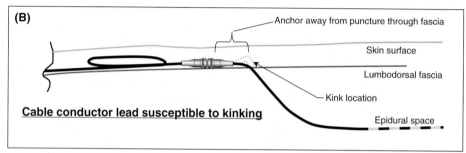

FIGURE 26-5. Appropriate anchor placement as described by Kumar et al.[12]

Positional stimulation is most commonly seen with percutaneous leads. Revision to a surgical lead may correct this issue; however, it is not always successful. Initial treatment should be 6 weeks of immobilization by bracing to see if the positional changes will resolve.

Painful stimulation may occur as a result of lead placement or migration near a nerve root or due to stimulation of the ligamentum flavum or other spinal structures. Nerve root stimulation requires surgical revision. Stimulation of tissues other than the spinal cord is more common with percutaneous leads because of the circumferential nature of the stimulation pattern. The initial treatment is reprogramming, but in cases where this does not resolve the definitive treatment is to replace the percutaneous lead with a unidirectional paddle lead. New technology will allow this to be done percutaneously without the need for partial laminectomy.

Spinal stenosis may be present prior to implant or develop while the leads are in place. In the event of critical stenosis that becomes symptomatic after lead placement, the treatment is surgical decompression and revision of the lead. In patients who have not been implanted, decompression of the stenotic area should be addressed prior to consideration of lead placement. In cases where there is some doubt about the long-term risks of stenosis, informed consent should be given, and the use of new low profile, low diameter leads should be considered.[37]

WHEN TO SEEK CONSULTATION

It is important to remember the value of consultants in cases where complications arise. In cases where there is potential risk for permanent neurologic injury, it is imperative to ask for the advice of a neurosurgeon or orthopedic spine surgeon. Likewise, infectious disease consultants can be invaluable, particularly in cases where a previous infection has been reported or in patients who are at high risk, for example, the immunocompromised. In cases where coexisting disease increases the risks to the patient, it may be helpful to have a specialist evaluate them and make perioperative recommendations. One good example would be consultation with an endocrinologist in a patient who has elevated blood glucose and hemoglobin A1C levels.

PATIENT EDUCATION, INFORMED CONSENT, AND LEGAL DOCUMENTATION

Physicians, nurses, and physician extenders are all critical in giving a team educational approach to SCS. Many device companies offer educational materials, models, videos, and Web site information to better inform the patient and their families. With any interventional pain procedure, good patient education in the preoperative period can serve to improve outcomes. In patients considering SCS, it is important to educate them on how the procedure is expected to affect their disease state, and what alternatives are available in their situation. Important areas of education include the techniques involved in the placement of a trial and permanent lead system, the need for postoperative care, the rehabilitation process after implant, and the specific activity limitations the patient will have after implant. Perhaps the most critical area of patient education is that of setting realistic expectations. The patient should understand the goals of pain reduction and functional restoration. If their expectations are unreasonable, the chance of a perceived complication is increased dramatically. In patients who are psychologically unstable, abnormal mental responses can be confused with actual physical complications. In the process of patient education, a psychological evaluation should be performed to both educate and evaluate psychological stability.[35]

When obtaining informed consent for SCS, the complications noted in this chapter should be discussed. Risks of epidural hematoma, epidural abscess, nerve injury, or paralysis are extremely rare and should be discussed in a reassuring manner as possible, but unlikely complications. Other risks to be discussed include wound infection, bleeding, PDPH, lead migration, and mechanical device failure. The failure to achieve pain relief is not a complication, but should be discussed in the education phase and properly documented.

Documentation is important for many reasons, including compliance, billing, and notation of medical necessity. When discussing these devices, it must be stressed that proper documentation of failure of conservative treatment, education of the patient, and a witnessed discussion of informed consent should be noted in the record. It is also important to document the patient's responsibilities and the postoperative requirements of the caregivers.

▶ SUMMARY

As with any surgical approach to disease management, the physician must consider the risks to benefit ratio in patients being considered for SCS. In this chapter, we have covered many outcomes that are undesirable for the patient and have discussed how to limit or avoid these adverse events. Based on the relatively low risk and the potential benefit in the properly selected patient, SCS should be considered in the pain treatment algorithm of appropriate patients who have failed to improve with more conservative approaches.

Close attention to surgical technique, patient selection, cost effectiveness, and overall outcome is essential to gaining optimal response to these implantable technologies. Prevention, recognition, and treatment of complications are vital parts of the use of these devices.

References

1. Shealy CN, Mortimer JT, Hagfors NR. Dorsal column electroanalgesia. *J Neurosurg* 1970;32(5):560–564.
2. Melzack R, Wall PD. The gate control theory of pain mechanisms. *Science* 1965:150:170–179.
3. Burchiel KJ, Anderson VC, Wilson BJ, et al. Prognostic factors of spinal cord stimulation for chronic back and leg pain. *Neurosurgery* 1995;36(6):1101–1110;discussion 1110–1111.
4. Burchiel KJ, Anderson VC, Brown FD, et al. Prospective, multicenter study of spinal cord stimulation for relief of chronic back and extremity pain. *Spine* 1996;21(23):2786–2794.
5. North RB, Kidd DH, Farrokhi F, et al. Spinal cord stimulation versus repeated lumbosacral spine surgery for chronic pain: a randomized, controlled trial. *Neurosurgery* 2005;56(1):98–106;discussion 106–107.
6. Mekhail NA, Aeschbach A, Stanton-Hicks M. Cost benefit analysis of neurostimulation for chronic pain. *Clin J Pain* 2004;20(6):462–468.
7. Kemler MA, Barendse GA, van Kleef M, et al. Spinal cord stimulation in patients with chronic reflex sympathetic dystrophy. *N Engl J Med* 2000;343(9):618–624.
8. Turner JA, Loeser JD, Deyo RA, et al. Spinal cord stimulation for patients with failed back surgery syndrome or complex regional pain syndrome: a systematic review of effectiveness and complications. *Pain* 2004;108(1–2):137–147.
9. Quigley DG, Arnold J, Eldridge PR, et al. Long-term outcome of spinal cord stimulation and hardware complications. *Stereotact Funct Neurosurg* 2003;81(1–4):50–56.
10. Burchiel KJ, Anderson VC, Brown FD, et al. Prospective, multicenter study of spinal cord stimulation for relief of chronic back and extremity pain. *Spine* 1996;21(23):2786–2794.
11. Kumar A, Felderhof C, Eljamel MS. Spinal cord stimulation for the treatment of refractory unilateral limb pain syndromes. *Stereotact Funct Neurosurg* 2003;81(1–4):70–74.
12. Kumar K, Buchser E, Linderoth B, et al. Avoiding complications from spinal cord stimulation: practical management recommendations an international panel of experts. *Neuromodulation.* 2007;10:24–33.
13. North RB, Ewend MG, Lawton MT, et al. Failed back surgery syndrome: 5-year follow-up after spinal cord stimulator implantation. *Neurosurgery* 1991;28:692–699.
14. Krames E. Spinal cord stimulation: indications, mechanism of action, and efficacy. *Cur Rev Pain* 1999;3:419–426.
15. North RB, Wetzel FT. Spinal cord stimulation for chronic pain of spinal origin: a valuable long-term solution. *Spine* 2002;27:2584–2591.
16. Heidecke V, Rainov NG, Burkert W. Hardware failures in spinal cord stimulation for failed back surgery syndrome. *Neuromodulation* 2000;3:27–30.
17. Kemler MA, et al. Avoiding complications from spinal cord stimulation: practical recommendations from an international panel of experts. *Neuromodulation* 2007;10:24–33.
18. Franzini A, Ferroli P, Marras C, et al. Huge epidural hematoma after surgery for spinal cord stimulation. *Acta Neurochir (Wien)* 2005;147(5):565–567;discussion 567.
19. Horlocker TT, Rowlingson JC, Enneking FK, et al. Regional anesthesia in the patient receiving antithrombotic or thrombolytic therapy: American Society of Regional Anesthesia and Pain Medicine Evidence–Based Guidelines (Third Edition). *Reg Anesth Pain Med* 2010;35(1):64–101.
20. Advanced Neuromodulation Systems FDA Labeling (Plano, TX).
21. Medtronic Neurological FDA Labeling (Minneapolis, MN).
22. Advanced Bionics FDA Labeling (Boston, MA).
23. Martin RJ, Yuan HA. Neurosurgical care of spinal epidural, subdural, and intramedullary abscesses and arachnoiditis. *Orthop Clin North Am* 1996;27(1):125–136.
24. Meglio M, Cioni B, Rossi GF. Spinal cord stimulation in management of chronic pain. A 9-year experience. *J Neurosurg* 1989;70:519–524.
25. Meyer SC, Swartz K, Johnson JP. Quadriparesis and spinal cord stimulation: case report. *Spine* 2007;32(19):E565–E568.
26. Mailis-Gagnon A, Furlan AD, Sandoval JA, et al. Spinal cord stimulation for chronic pain. *Cochrane Database Syst Rev* 2004;(3):CD003783.
27. Kemler MA, Barendse GA, van Kleef M, et al. Spinal cord stimulation in patients with chronic reflex sympathetic dystrophy. *N Engl J Med* 2000;343(9):618–624.
28. Lennarson PJ, Guillen T. Spinal cord compression from a foreign body reaction to spinal cord stimulation: a previously unreported complication. *Spine* 2010;35(25):E1516–E1519.
29. Deer TR, Stewart CD. Complications of spinal cord stimulation: identification, treatment and prevention. *Pain Med* 2008;9:S93–S101.
30. Kumar K, Wilson JR, Taylor RS, et al. Complications of spinal cord stimulation, suggestions to improve outcome, and financial impact. *J Neurosurg Spine* 2006;5:191–203.
31. Barolat G. Spinal cord stimulation for chronic pain management. *Arch Med Res* 2000;31(3):258–262.
32. Torrens JK, Stanley PJ, Ragunathan PL, et al. Risk of infection with electrical spinal-cord stimulation. *Lancet* 1997;349(9053):729.
33. Winkler PA, Herzog C, Weiler C, et al. Foreign-body reaction to silastic burr-hole covers with seroma formation: case report and review of the literature. *Pathol Res Pract* 2000;196(1):61–66.
34. Mangram AJ, Horan TC, Pearson ML, et al. The Hospital Infection Control Practices Advisory Committee. Guideline for Prevention of Surgical Infection, 1999. *Infect Cont Hosp Epidemiol* 1999;20(4):247–278.
35. Bedder MS, Bedder HF. Spinal cord stimulation surgical technique for the nonsurgically trained. *Neuromodulation* 2009;12(1):1–19.
36. Mortimer H. Tissue viability. Post-operative wounds: a nurse-led change in wound dressings. *Nurs Stand.* 1993;8(7):56–58.

37. Access lead data on file for FDA IDE. Advanced Neurological Systems. Plano, Texas.

38. Taylor RS, Van Buyten JP, Buchser E. Spinal cord stimulation for chronic back and leg pain and failed back surgery syndrome: a systematic review and analysis of prognostic factors. *Spine* 2005;30(1):152–160.

39. Alo KM, Holsheimer J. New trends in neuromodulation for the management of neuropathic pain. *Neurosurgery.* 2002;50(4):690–703; discussion 703–704.

40. Deer TR. Current and future trends in spinal cord stimulation for chronic pain. *Curr Pain Headache Rep* 2001;5:503–509.

41. Burton A. Spinal Cord Stimulation. American Society of Anesthesiologists. Course Text Book. Annual Meeting. 2004.

42. Cameron T. Safety and efficacy of spinal cord stimulation for the treatment of chronic pain: a 20-year literature review. *J Neurosurg* 2004;100:254–267.

43. Rosenow JM, Stanton-Hicks M, Rezai AR, et al. Failure modes of spinal cord stimulation hardware. *J Neurosurg Spine* 2006;5:183–190.

44. Deer T. An Overview of Implantable Devices. American Society of Anesthesiologists. Course Text Book. Annual Meeting. 1999.

45. Abejon D, Feler C. Is impedance a parameter to be taken into account in spinal cord stimulation? *Pain Physician* 2007;10(4): 533–540.

46. North RB, Calkins SK, Campbell DS, et al. Automated, patient-interactive, spinal cord stimulator adjustment: a randomized controlled trial. *Neurosurgery* 2003;52(3):572–580;discussion 579–580.

47. Pope JE, Stanton-Hicks M. Accidental subdural spinal cord stimulator lead placement and stimulation. *Neuromodulation:Technology at the Neural Interface* 2011;14(1):30–32;discussion 33.

48. Vandermeulen EP, Van Aken H, Vermylen J. Anticoagulants and spinal-epidural anesthesia. *Anesth Analg* 1994;79:1165–1177.

49. Infection Control and Hospital Epidemiology 1999;20:217–278.

50. Rathmell JP, Lake T, Ramundo MB. Infectious risks of chronic pain treatments: injection therapy, surgical implants, and intradiscal techniques. *Reg Anesth Pain Med* 2006;31:346–352.

COMPLICATIONS OF NEURAXIS APPROACHES

27

Complications Associated with Epidural, Facet Joint, and Sacroiliac Joint Injections

Stephen E. Abram

Injections of long-acting corticosteroid agents into and adjacent to the spinal canal are performed routinely for patients with back and neck pain. Epidural steroid injection has become an accepted and widely used treatment for sciatica and cervical radiculopathy, its primary indications. The technique is also used by some physicians for axial low back and neck pain and for neural claudication associated with spinal stenosis, despite lack of evidence of benefit for these indications.[1,2] Cervical and lumbar zygapophyseal (facet) joint injections are performed frequently for patients in whom pathology involving these joints is thought to be a source of pain. Many physicians believe that facet injections are purely diagnostic, whereas others indicate that some patients experience persistent relief (i.e., 6 months or more) when long-acting corticosteroids are injected along with the local anesthetic.[3] Similarly, local anesthetic injection of the sacroiliac joint is used to determine whether that structure is a source of pain, and some patients experience prolonged benefit from the addition of "depot" steroids (depot therapy refers to injection of a drug together with a substance that slows the release and prolongs the action of the drug).[4]

Despite warnings about the neurotoxic potential of neuraxial injection of corticosteroids,[5] there are few reports of serious complications associated with epidural, zygapophyseal, or sacroiliac joint injection of long-acting corticosteroids. Unfortunately, there is no mandatory reporting of complications in the United States, and thus the true incidence of serious side effects and complications cannot be determined. The American Society of Anesthesiologists Closed Claims Study provides some insight, reporting on 114 complications claimed to be caused by epidural steroid injections that resulted in malpractice litigation.[6] Unfortunately, only legal cases that have been completed can be reported, and thus cases brought to litigation in the past several years are unlikely to be included. A listing of the types of complications cited in that report is shown in Box 27-1. Complications that have been reported following epidural, facet joint, and sacroiliac corticosteroid injections include neurotoxicity, neurologic injury, pharmacologic effects of corticosteroids and coadministered agents, and other less frequent problems discussed in this chapter.

▶ NEUROTOXICITY

The intrathecal injection of neurotoxic substances can result in arachnoiditis or cauda equina syndrome. The dura and arachnoid provide considerable protection against chemical injury to intraspinal neural structures. However, arachnoiditis and neurologic injury can occur if there is sufficient chemical irritation or inflammation. The first reported cases of arachnoiditis were mainly postinfectious and often followed syphilis or tuberculosis infections. Iatrogenic cases became a concern when it was discovered that arachnoiditis could be induced by intrathecal injection of oily radiographic contrast materials. It is most commonly found among patients who have undergone multiple diagnostic and surgical procedures of the spine, and thus it is often difficult to determine the inciting cause. Spine surgery is a recognized etiology.

Arachnoiditis and Cauda Equina Syndrome

Definition

Arachnoiditis is an inflammatory condition involving the leptomeninges and underlying neural structures. The mildest form consists of arachnoid adhesions. Adhesive arachnoiditis is a severe and often progressive form that is associated with neuropathic pain and neurologic dysfunction. Some cases are associated with calcific deposits involving the inflamed meninges and are known as calcific arachnoiditis. The inflammatory response triggers fibrin exudates that cause nerve roots to adhere to each other and to the dural sac. The subsequent repair process produces dense collagen adhesions, hyalinization of the arachnoid membrane, and loss of cerebrospinal fluid (CSF).[7] Commonly encountered symptoms are listed in Box 27-2. Radiographic findings are characterized by three patterns, described in Box 27-3.[8]

BOX 27-1 Primary Outcome for Claims Related to Epidural Steroid Injections

Nerve injury	28
Infection	24
Death/brain damage	9
Headache	20
Increased pain, no relief	10

From Fitzgibbon DR, Posner KL, Caplan RA, et al. Chronic pain management: American Society of Anesthesiologists Closed Claims Project. Anesthesiology 2004;100:98–105.

BOX 27-2 Symptoms of Adhesive Arachnoiditis

- Constant, burning pain in lower back and legs
- Urinary frequency, incontinence
- Muscle spasm, back, and legs
- Variable sensory loss
- Variable motor dysfunction

Cauda equina syndrome is a complex and variable entity associated with compression or injury to the lumbar spinal nerve roots that comprise the cauda equina within the thecal sac. The syndrome is characterized by bilateral sciatica, saddle hypesthesia, lower extremity weakness, and bowel, bladder, and sexual dysfunction. Symptoms are confined to the lumbosacral nerve root distribution, but are otherwise indistinguishable from those of arachnoiditis. Cauda equina syndrome can be caused by adhesive arachnoiditis as well as other abnormalities affecting the cauda equina (e.g., external compression of the cauda equina by a large central intervertebral disc herniation, epidural hematoma, or abscess; Fig. 27-1).

Scope

Arachnoiditis and cauda equina syndrome are uncommon conditions and represent a distinct minority of cases among patients with severe back and leg pain. The true prevalence of these conditions among patients who have undergone multiple diagnostic and surgical procedures of the spine is not known.

Pathophysiology

Concern regarding the neurotoxic potential of epidural steroid injections relates almost entirely to the consequences of unintentional intrathecal placement of corticosteroid suspensions. Much of this concern arose from the practice of treating advanced cases of multiple sclerosis (MS) with intrathecal methylprednisolone acetate (MPA). The earliest report of arachnoiditis following intrathecal steroid injections[9] cited two cases of adhesive arachnoiditis among a series of 23 patients who received a total of 83 injections of MPA. The author of that report expressed concern that the drug vehicle, polyethylene glycol, initiated the inflammatory response. A third case of arachnoiditis, described by the author as "sclerosing pachymeningitis," was diagnosed in a patient with advanced MS.[10] Prior to steroid therapy, her symptoms included urinary dysfunction, sensory changes in the legs, and upper motor neuron signs. She received six intrathecal injections of MPA over the course of a year, with transient symptomatic improvement and no apparent complications. Her disease progressed dramatically over the following 2 years. She received an additional two injections shortly before her death with no apparent benefit. Postmortem examination revealed severe arachnoiditis with necrotizing and hemorrhagic changes. A fourth case of arachnoiditis that occurred in a patient who received intrathecal MPA treatment for MS occurred after multiple injections over a 2-year period.[11] Myelographic findings were compatible with the diagnosis, and thickening and calcification of the meninges were noted when a laminectomy was performed.

One case of myelographically documented arachnoiditis has been reported following intrathecal MPA treatment

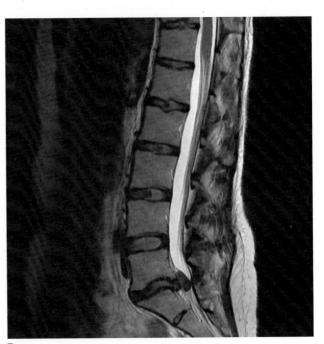

A   **B**

FIGURE 27-1. **MRI of the lumbosacral spine demonstrating compression of the cauda equina caused by a large lumbar intervertebral disc herniation.** A 31-year-old with a history of prior L5/S1 discectomy underwent an uncomplicated interlaminar epidural steroid injection for treatment of acute radicular pain in the left S1 distribution associated with a recurrent disc herniation. The day following the epidural steroid injection, she presented emergently with new onset of perineal numbness and inability to urinate, raising concern of epidural hematoma related to the injection. Repeat MRI of the lumbosacral spine revealed a large progression in the extent of her central and left-sided L5/S1 disc herniation causing compression of the cauda equina. **A:** Axial T2-weighted image at the level of L5/S1. **B:** Sagittal T2-weighted image near midline. (Images provided by J.P. Rathmell.)

for lumbar disc disease.[12] The patient had a "traumatic tap" during the injection. The arachnoiditis would probably be characterized as group 1 according to the Delamarter classification,[8] in that the patient's symptoms resolved following discectomy. A case of cauda equina syndrome was reported in a patient who received 14 intrathecal injections and 4 epidural injections of MPA over an 18-month period.[13] Her initial response to the injections was beneficial and uncomplicated except for the occurrence of transient urinary incontinence following one of the early procedures. After the last injection, she developed persistent sacral anesthesia and urinary retention.

Aseptic Meningitis

Definition

Aseptic meningitis is a generally benign condition that produces signs of neurologic irritation, including burning pain in the legs, headache, meningismus, and in severe cases seizures. Fever and nausea are often reported. CSF examination reveals pleocytosis, elevated protein, and decreased glucose. The introduction of virtually any substance, including normal saline or water, into the subarachnoid space can produce the syndrome.[14] Seghal et al.[15] documented the occurrence of aseptic meningitis following intrathecal injections of 40 to 200 mg MPA. They found a dose-related polymorphonuclear pleocytosis beginning within 24 hours and lasting about 6 days. At doses over 80 mg, they documented elevation of CSF proteins and clinical signs of meningeal irritation. On the other hand, Goldstein et al.[16] were unable to show any CSF changes or symptoms of meningeal irritation in patients with MS treated with 40 mg MPA.

Scope

Several cases of aseptic meningitis have been reported following intrathecal corticosteroid injections.[1,17–19] One of these cases was severe, producing headache, fever, nausea, bilateral leg pain, and seizures.[1] CSF culture was negative. There was elevation of CSF protein, leukocytes, and red blood cells. Symptoms were prolonged, resolving after 3 weeks. One case of aseptic meningitis was reported following an epidural injection of MPA.[20] No local anesthetic was injected with the steroid, and, thus, a dural puncture with intrathecal migration of the drug cannot be ruled out.

Mechanism of Neurotoxicity

It is difficult to determine which component of the steroid preparation, if any, is neurotoxic. Nelson et al.[9] suggested that polyethylene glycol is the offending agent. This speculation was based on studies demonstrating that 78% to 80% propylene glycol, an ingredient in a long-acting local anesthetic preparation of the drug efocaine, causes nerve injury.[21,22] It has a molecular weight of 78. The polyethylene glycol preparation used in steroid suspensions has a molecular weight of 3,350 and is present in concentrations of 2.8% to 3%. Benzon et al.[23] studied the acute effects of polyethylene glycol on nerve conduction in both sheathed and unsheathed neurons in rabbits. They found no functional change with concentrations of 3% and 10% and slowing of conduction with 20% and 30%. A 40% concentration abolished conduction, but the effect was reversible following washout in both sheathed and unsheathed preparations. Benzyl alcohol 0.9% is pre-

sent in several steroid suspension preparations, including multidose vials of Depo-Medrol brand MPA (Pharmacia & Upjohn, Kalamazoo, MI) and Aristocort Intralesional brand triamcinolone diacetate (American Cyanamid, Madison, NJ). Two animal studies reported on histologic changes following neuraxial injection of the triamcinolone/benzyl alcohol preparation. Delaney et al.[24] performed light and electron microscopy studies of nerve roots, cord root entry zone, and meninges after epidural injections of triamcinolone diacetate plus lidocaine in cats. They found mild inflammatory changes 30 days after injection with complete resolution by 120 days. Abram[25] examined the spinal cord and meninges of rats injected intrathecally four times at 5-day intervals with triamcinolone diacetate. Animals demonstrated no neurologic dysfunction. There were no histologic differences between steroid- and saline-injected animals. There have been reports of aseptic meningitis following intracisternal injections of pyrogen-free serum albumen plus 0.9% benzyl alcohol.[26] Deland[27] therefore assessed the effects of intracisternal injections of benzyl alcohol 0.9% to 9% in dogs. The highest concentration (10 times the concentration used as a preservative in pharmaceutical agents) produced transient neurologic dysfunction related to local anesthetic effects, but there was no evidence of aseptic meningitis at any concentration. Few histologic abnormalities were noted, and these were seen as frequently in saline controls. Hahn et al.[28] reported a case of motor blockade following intrathecal cancer chemotherapy with cytosine arabinoside diluted in bacteriostatic water containing 1.5% benzyl alcohol. Function returned to normal after washout with saline. The authors subsequently showed that benzyl alcohol caused nerve root injury in animal studies.

In Australia, where there was substantial public controversy about the risk of arachnoiditis following epidural MPA injection during the 1990s, some physicians have begun to use Celestone Chronodose (Schering-Plough, Kenilworth, NJ) for steroid epidurals. This product contains betamethasone 5.7 mg, betamethasone sodium phosphate 3.9 mg (in solution), and betamethasone acetate 3 mg (in suspension) per milliliter in an aqueous vehicle-containing sodium phosphate, sodium phosphate monobasic, disodium edetate, benzalkonium chloride, and water. Despite the absence of both polyethylene glycol and benzyl alcohol, a study in sheep demonstrated the development of histopathologic changes of arachnoiditis following intrathecal injection of 2 mL or more of this preparation.[29] The product is available in the United States as Celestone Soluspan (Schering-Plough, Kenilworth, NJ). As is the case with all of the commercially available corticosteroid suspensions, it does not have a product indication for epidural injection for the treatment of sciatica.

Prevention of Neurotoxicity

It is not clear whether a single intrathecal injection is likely to cause serious harm. As noted previously, the reported cases of arachnoiditis were associated with multiple intrathecal injections, and in most cases there was preexisting neurologic disease. A recent study of intrathecal MPA for postherpetic neuralgia failed to find any evidence of either aseptic meningitis or arachnoiditis among 89 patients treated with four 60-mg injections.[30] Patients were followed for 2 years and underwent diagnostic lumbar punctures and

MRIs. On the other hand, arachnoiditis, cauda equina syndrome, and aseptic meningitis are complications of intrathecal, not epidural, steroid injections. The surest way to prevent their occurrence is to see that the injected drugs are not administered intrathecally. The use of a test dose of local anesthetic will help prevent intrathecal administration. Likewise, fluoroscopic guidance and injection of contrast can be helpful, as the pattern of intrathecal dye spread can be distinguished from that of epidural spread. If accidental dural puncture occurs, epidural injection at another level can still result in intrathecal spread of the injected drug. There is yet another reason to temporarily abandon the procedure if accidental dural puncture occurs. It is likely that flow of CSF into the epidural space will dilute the injected steroid or will carry it away from the targeted neural structures.

Treatment of Neurotoxicity

There is no definitive treatment for arachnoiditis. Symptomatic treatment is the same as for other forms of neuropathic pain. For aseptic meningitis, symptomatic treatment and reassurance are all that is required.

▶ NEUROLOGIC INJURY

Scope and Mechanism of Injury

In the Closed Claims Study, nerve injury occurred in 14 patients following epidural steroid injection.[6] Six of these resulted in paraplegia and one in quadriplegia. Spinal cord damage can occur from needle entry into the cord. Such injuries are generally mild unless there is bleeding into the cord. More severe injury will occur if material is injected into the substance of the spinal cord. Another mechanism of injury is injection of steroid suspension into a radicular artery with embolization of end arteries in the spinal cord. This type of injury was implicated in a fatal case of massive cerebellar injury following a transforaminal injection of triamcinolone acetonide.[31] The authors of this case report demonstrated that all of the corticosteroid suspensions they tested contained particles large enough to occlude capillaries and arterioles. Embolization has not been implicated as a mechanism for injury following caudal or interlaminar epidural steroid injections. However, there are arteries in the posterior epidural and subarachnoid spaces that communicate with those supplying the cord, and embolization with suspended corticosteroid material is theoretically possible. While intravascular dye spread has been documented during interlaminar cervical epidural steroid injection,[32] all of the reported cases were documented as venous injections, which would not be expected to produce any neurologic injury.

Embolization of a radicular artery is theoretically possible during cervical facet injection with particulate steroid preparations. Heckman et al.[33] reported a case of transient quadriplegia following a C5-6 facet injection using 1% lidocaine. They postulated radicular artery injection as the cause. The procedure was done without fluoroscopy, so the final needle position could not be determined. Undoubtedly, the outcome would have been disastrous had particulate steroid been included in the injectate.

Direct Spinal Cord Trauma

Needle injury or injection into the cord is a significant risk for cervical, thoracic, and upper lumbar epidural injections. Two cases of spinal cord injury following cervical epidural steroid injections were reported by Hodges et al.[34] Both cases used fluoroscopic guidance, both cases were performed at C5-6, and in both cases the patient was sedated with a combination of midazolam and propofol. It was postulated that the patients failed to respond to needle contact with the cord because of the sedation. Both patients experienced persistent upper extremity pain and lower extremity paresthesias. Four unreported cases of spinal cord injury resulted in litigation in which the author served as an expert witness (all of these claims are now closed). The first resulted from a cervical epidural steroid injection performed in an anesthetized patient that resulted in a fatal injury to the upper cervical cord and medulla. Two additional cervical epidural steroid injections resulted in significant and permanent pain and neurologic injury. All of these cervical procedures were performed at C5-6 or above, and all involved the use of moderate to deep sedation. The fourth case was a lumbar epidural steroid injection performed without fluoroscopic guidance. The patient received general anesthesia because of allergy to local anesthetic. Complete and permanent motor and sensory block of one leg became evident immediately after the procedure. MRI showed a new lesion in the conus. Field et al.[35] reported three cases of transient neurologic injury that followed otherwise uneventful cervical epidural steroid injections in awake patients. All three patients had large disc herniations that caused effacement of the epidural fat and spinal fluid surrounding the spinal cord at the level of injection (Fig. 27-2). The authors hypothesized that direct injury to the spinal cord or dorsal nerve root could occur even without dural puncture when narrowing or obliteration of the epidural space caused by a large disc herniation displaces the spinal cord posteriorly.

Prevention of Direct Spinal Cord Trauma

There is enough evidence from case reports of direct trauma to the spinal cord following epidural steroid injections to suggest the following guidelines:

1. Examine MRI images before the procedure. Avoid injection at cervical or thoracic levels where the spinal cord has been displaced posteriorly. Consider advancing a catheter from below in such situations.

2. Avoid entry into the epidural space above C6-7. MRI scans and cryomicrotome anatomic studies indicate that there is no space between the ligamentum flavum and the dura at C5-6 and above.

3. Obtain a lateral fluoroscopic view before injecting anything. Ensure that the needle is in the most dorsal aspect of the epidural space. In the low-cervical spine, the shoulders may obscure the lateral view. The use of the "swimmer's view" (one arm raised 180 degrees overhead and the other arm at the side) may allow visualization of the needle and the spine.[36]

4. Avoid deep sedation or general anesthesia during the procedure. The patient should be alert enough to respond to paresthesias induced by needle contact with neural structures, though this precaution does not guarantee safety.

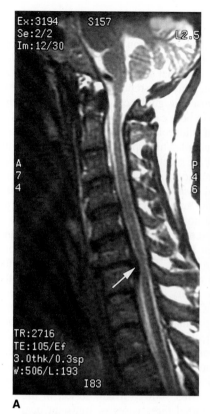
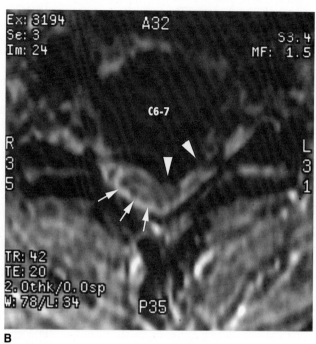

FIGURE 27-2. Field et al.[35] reported three cases of transient neurologic injury that followed otherwise uneventful cervical epidural steroid injections in awake patients. All three patients had large disc herniations causing effacement of the epidural fat and spinal fluid surrounding the spinal cord at the level of injection. **A:** Midline sagittal T2-weighted MRI showing large disc herniation at the C6/7 level (*arrow*) that effaces the epidural fat and CSF signal both anterior and posterior to the spinal cord. **B:** Axial T1-weighted MRI showing a large central and left-sided disc herniation (*arrowheads*) displacing the spinal cord (*arrows*) to the right posterolateral limits of the spinal canal. (Reproduced from Field J, Rathmell JP, Stephenson JH, et al. Neuropathic pain following cervical epidural steroid injection. *Anesthesiology* 2000;93:885–888, with permission.)

Simon et al.[37] reported a case of intramedullary injection of contrast during a C1-2 myelogram. A total of 15 mL iohexol was injected, resulting in unilateral arm weakness and diffuse hyperreflexia. Presumably, the patient was awake (there was no mention of sedation) and reported no sensation during needle placement but experienced paresthesias in the face, neck, and arm during injection of the dye. Similarly, Tripathi et al.[38] reported a case of cord injury following a T11-12 epidural steroid injection in a nonsedated patient who experienced no paresthesias during needle placement or during injection.

Treatment of Direct Spinal Cord Trauma

In most cases, there is probably little that can be done to minimize the extent of neurologic dysfunction after the traumatic event has occurred. High-dose intravenous corticosteroid may be of benefit. High-dose intravenous steroids administered in the hours immediately following traumatic spinal cord injury have been shown to result in a significant reduction in neuronal injury.[39] The patient who experienced intramedullary iohexol was treated promptly with an intravenous bolus of 30 mg/kg methylprednisolone followed by 5.4 mg/kg/h for 48 hours. Her symptoms reportedly began to improve within 4 hours of steroid treatment.[39]

▶ PHARMACOLOGIC EFFECT OF CORTICOSTEROIDS

Hypercorticism and Adrenal Suppression

Scope and Pathophysiology

Cushing syndrome, a characteristic pattern of obesity with associated hypertension, is the result of abnormally high blood levels of cortisol resulting from hyperfunction of the adrenal cortex. Prolonged exogenous administration of glucocorticoids results in a clinical pattern identical to the spontaneous disorder and is frequently called cushingoid syndrome. The active corticosteroid in MPA and other depot steroid preparations is slowly released over a period of days to 1 to 2 weeks. It is common for patients to report side effects, mostly during the first 3 posttreatment days. Fluid retention and weight gain[40] as well as increased blood pressure[36] and congestive heart failure[41] have been reported after epidural steroid injections. Cushingoid side effects, usually beginning 1 to several weeks after epidural steroid injections, have been reported by several authors.[42–44] These include facial swelling, buffalo hump, skin bruising, and scaly skin lesions. The most dramatic case occurred in a patient who had received a single cervical epidural injection of 60 mg MPA. Over the following month, he developed a 20-lb weight gain, moon facies, buffalo hump, and neck thickening. These symptoms persisted for 1 year. Laboratory investigation showed markedly reduced serum cortisol levels and no response to adrenocorticotropic hormone (ACTH). Cortisol levels rose slowly, but were still low (normal at 6 months). Jacobs et al.[45] documented marked suppression of plasma cortisol levels in 12 patients who each received a single epidural injection of 80 mg MPA. Plasma cortisol and ACTH levels were significantly depressed at 1, 7, 14, and 21 days after treatment. The ability of exogenous ACTH to increase plasma cortisol levels was also reduced over a 3-week period. Kay et al.[46] assessed the adrenal response to a series of three weekly epidural injections of 80 mg triamcinolone diacetate. Suppression of serum cortisol and ACTH began within 45 minutes of the initial injection and remained low 7 days after each of the first two injections. Levels were nearly normal 30 days after the last injection. Patients sedated with midazolam during the procedures had greater and more prolonged suppression. Another symptom of hypercorticism is steroid-induced myopathy, which is characterized by progressive proximal muscle weakness, increased serum creatinine kinase levels, and a myopathic electromyogram (EMG) and muscle biopsy specimen. This has been reported following a single epidural dose of triamcinolone.[47] All patients who have been taking steroids for long periods develop reversible myofiber atrophy, but this is not steroid myopathy unless it progresses to become a necrotizing myopathy.

Prevention of Hypercorticism and Adrenal Suppression

Because the most severe reported case of Cushing syndrome and adrenal suppression occurred after a single, relatively small steroid dose, it is unlikely that this complication can be avoided in susceptible patients. Repeat procedures should not be done for patients who have persistent improvement following a single injection.

Treatment of Hypercorticism and Adrenal Suppression

Patients undergoing surgery within a few weeks of receiving depot steroids should be evaluated for adrenal suppression or should receive steroid coverage during the perioperative period. Otherwise, no specific treatment is indicated.

Epidural Lipomatosis

Definition and Scope

An increase in the amount of fat in the epidural space can be seen in some patients who have been treated with systemic corticosteroids (see Chapter 10). There is concern that epidural steroid administration can produce similar increases in the amount of epidural fat. Although this is probably a rare phenomenon, there is some evidence that epidural lipomatosis can be caused or aggravated by epidural steroid injection. Sandberg and Lavyne[48] published a case report of a 68-year-old man who presented with right sciatica and MRI documentation of spinal stenosis but normal volume of epidural fat. He was treated with two epidural injections, 1 month apart, of MPA 120 mg. Three years later, he presented with bilateral sciatica and neural claudication. MRI demonstrated persistent spinal stenosis and mild epidural lipomatosis. He underwent three injections, a month apart, of triamcinolone

diacetate 80 mg. He experienced transient improvement after each injection and then persistent worsening of symptoms. MRI 3 months after the last injection showed a substantial increase in epidural fat from L2 to L5, with compression of the thecal sac. He underwent multilevel laminectomy and removal of epidural fat with subsequent improvement in symptoms. Another case report discussed a patient who had been on chronic steroid treatment for asthma and who was treated with epidural steroids without prior spine imaging. A subsequent MRI demonstrated severe epidural lipomatosis.[49] It was not known if the condition was exacerbated by the epidural injection.

Diagnosis, Prevention, and Treatment

Epidural lipomatosis is an unlikely complication of epidural steroid injections. However, it should be ruled out by MRI in patients with a history of chronic steroid use before proceeding.

Allergy to Corticosteroids

Although rare, allergic reaction to steroid suspension has been documented. Simon et al.[50] reported a delayed allergic reaction to triamcinolone diacetate that began a week after an epidural steroid injection. Following the patient's recovery, skin testing resulted in recurrence of symptoms after 12 hours.

Altered Glucose Tolerance

Definition and Scope

Glucocorticoid administration reduces the hypoglycemic effect of insulin[51] and interferes with blood glucose control in diabetic patients. Following injection of depot steroids, diabetic patients generally report increased blood glucose levels and insulin requirements for 48 to 72 hours. Surprisingly, there is almost no medical literature on the effect of long-acting steroid administration on blood sugar control in diabetics. There is some information available on the effect of exogenous corticosteroids on glucose metabolism in normal patients.

Pellacani et al.[52] studied the effect of two doses of 40 mg soluble methylprednisolone administered intravenously 12 hours apart. They documented a significant reduction in glucose tolerance 2 hours after the second injection with return to normal by 24 hours. Injection of MPA or other steroid suspensions would be expected to have a less profound but more prolonged effect. Ward et al.[53] studied the metabolic effect of a single caudal injection of triamcinolone acetonide. They found that fasting glucose levels and serum glucose response to insulin were significantly depressed, and serum insulin levels were significantly increased 24 hours after injection. All three values had returned to normal after 1 week.

Treatment of Altered Glucose Tolerance

Glucose levels in diabetic patients should be monitored closely during the week following any type of depot steroid injection. Patients need to be informed that adjustment of insulin dose may be required. Brittle diabetics should consult their internist or endocrinologist prior to initiating steroid treatment.

BOX 27-4 Adverse Systemic Effects of Corticosteroids

- Glucose intolerance
- Hypokalemia
- Hypertension
- Myopathy
- Cutaneous changes
- Truncal obesity
- Pancreatitis
- Psychotic reactions
- Dementia
- Benign intracranial hypertension
- Seizures
- Osteoporosis
- Aseptic necrosis, femoral, or humeral head
- Adrenal insufficiency
- Increased intraocular pressure
- Cataract
- Hyperlipidemia

Other Side Effects and Complications of Corticosteroid Therapy

Both short- and long-term corticosteroid therapies are associated with a substantial number of adverse effects. Although many of these side effects and complications have not been reported following injections of steroid suspensions, most are possible, particularly if injections are repeated over prolonged intervals. Box 27-4 provides a list of many of these adverse effects.

▶ PHARMACOLOGIC EFFECT OF COADMINISTERED AGENTS

Definition, Scope, and Pathophysiology

Local anesthetics are often administered in conjunction with epidural corticosteroids. The primary reason is to determine whether the steroid has reached the affected nerve root. The assumption is that if the patient experiences temporary relief from the anesthetic, the steroid is in the right place. This goal can be accomplished with a very small amount of local anesthetic (e.g., 20–30 mg lidocaine). Nevertheless, much larger quantities are sometimes used, and intrathecal or intravascular injection can produce systemic toxicity or high spinal anesthesia (see Chapter 7). Even low doses of local anesthetic accidentally injected intrathecally in the cervical region can have profound effects on blood pressure, cardiac output, and respiration. Five cases of death or brain damage following accidental intrathecal injection of local anesthetic plus steroid were cited in the Closed Claims Study.[6] Most of those patients were not given a local anesthetic test dose. Another case report cited apnea and cardiovascular collapse following accidental intrathecal injection of 6 mL 1.5% lidocaine plus 80 mg triamcinolone acetonide in a 70-year-old woman.[54] No test dose was administered. The patient was resuscitated but remained unconscious for 10 hours. She subsequently recovered without permanent injury. Opioids are rarely coadministered with epidural corticosteroids. The Closed Claims Study[6] reported three cases of brain damage or death related to delayed respiratory depression from morphine coadministered epidurally with steroids.

Prevention of Complications from Pharmacologic Effects of Coadministered Agents

The amount of local anesthetic that is coadministered with epidural steroids should be limited to a dose that would not produce a serious systemic reaction if injected into a blood vessel or produce a high spinal if injected intrathecally. It is probably wise to omit local anesthetic from cervical epidural injections. Opioids should not be coadministered with epidural steroids in outpatients, and the practice is best avoided altogether.

▶ DURAL PUNCTURE COMPLICATIONS

Scope

Accidental dural puncture during attempted epidural injection is associated with a headache incidence of over 50%.[55] The headache incidence among patients undergoing attempted epidural steroid injection has not been reported. Postdural puncture headache and associated symptoms are discussed in Chapter 9.

Introduction of air into the subdural or subarachnoid space during attempted epidural needle placement can produce pneumocephalus and an immediate headache that can last up to several days. The most likely cause is dural puncture arising from using a loss of resistance technique with air.[56,57] However, headache following the introduction of air into the subarachnoid space was documented after a cervical epidural steroid injection performed by a hanging drop technique.[58]

Prevention of Dural Puncture Complications

Use of a needle with a smaller gauge than the usual 17- to 18-gauge epidural needle will most likely result in a lower incidence of headache should a dural puncture occur. On the other hand, it is not known whether accidental dural puncture would occur more often using a smaller needle. There is evidence that the use of a smaller-gauge needle increases the incidence of incorrect needle placement.[59] Once accidental dural puncture has been confirmed, it may be possible to reduce the risk of developing postdural puncture headache by injecting 10-mL preservative-free normal saline before removing the needle.[55]

▶ BLEEDING COMPLICATIONS

Scope of the Problem

Intraspinal bleeding is a potentially devastating complication that can result in paraplegia or quadriplegia. This complication is discussed in detail in Chapter 4. Back pain and headache may be the presenting complaints. Both epidural[60] and subdural[61] hematomas have been reported following epidural steroid injections. The epidural hematoma was treated successfully with surgical decompression. The subdural hematoma initially produced quadriplegia. The patient recovered after surgery but developed meningitis 8 days later and subsequently died. Neither patient had a coagulopathy. The epidural hematoma patient had undergone six previous cervical epidural steroid injections and had been taking indomethacin at the time of the procedure. Benzon et al.[62] reported a case of quadriplegia following a cervical epidural steroid injection in a patient who had been taking clopidogrel and diclofenac. Following surgical decompression, the patient regained upper extremity function, but his lower extremities remained paralyzed. The Closed Claims Study cites two cases of spinal cord injury resulting from epidural hematomas following epidural steroid injections.[6] Both patients had been receiving anticoagulants. The report did not indicate whether these were done at the lumbar, thoracic, or cervical level.

Prevention of Bleeding Complications

The most important risk factor is, of course, coagulopathy—either primary or pharmacologic. Anticoagulants and antiplatelet drugs such as clopidogrel and ticlopidine are contraindications to epidural injections of any sort. On the other hand, nonsteroid anti-inflammatory drugs (NSAIDs), including aspirin, do not appear to appreciably increase the risk of epidural bleeding. Horlocker et al.[63] reported no major hemorrhagic complications among 1,035 patients who received a total of 1,214 epidural steroid injections. One-third of patients had been taking NSAIDs at the time of treatment (134 on aspirin, 249 on other NSAIDs, and 34 on multiple drugs).

The only published reports of epidural hematomas resulting in neurologic complications occurred following cervical injections. Given the rarity of reports of this complication, no conclusion regarding relative risk of cervical versus lumbar epidural injections can be drawn.

▶ INFECTIOUS COMPLICATIONS: INFECTIONS OF THE SPINE

Scope and Pathophysiology

Infectious complications following epidural or intraarticular injections are rare (see Chapter 5), but the risk is undoubtedly higher in diabetic patients. Epidural abscess is a condition that can occur spontaneously, in the absence of injection or instrumentation of the spinal canal. Tang et al.[64] reviewed 46 cases of spontaneous epidural abscess and found that 46% occurred in diabetic patients. Common presenting symptoms included paralysis (80%), localized spinal pain (89%), radicular pain (57%), and chills and fever (67%). The erythrocyte sedimentation rate was always elevated. *Staphylococcus aureus* was the organism isolated in about half the cases. Hooten et al.[65] recently reviewed the cases of epidural abscess following epidural steroid injections in the medical literature. They found

14 cases, 2 of which also presented with meningitis. A synopsis of the patient characteristics and outcomes for those cases as well as another case[66] not included in that review is shown in Box 27-5. Infection was listed in the Closed Claims Study[6] as a cause for litigation in 24 cases involving epidural steroid injections. There were 12 cases of meningitis and 3 cases of osteomyelitis. There were seven cases of epidural abscess, six requiring surgical decompression, and one resulting in permanent lower extremity motor dysfunction. In one claim, there was both meningitis and epidural abscess and in one a combination of meningitis, abscess, and osteomyelitis. A single case of bacterial discitis was reported following caudal steroid injection.[67] This occurred following injection of 120 mg triamcinolone in a 73-year-old woman with mild diabetes mellitus. One month after injection, she returned with increased back pain. MRI revealed L4-5 discitis and adjacent osteomyelitis. Biopsy culture grew *Pseudomonas aeruginosa*. She was successfully treated with intravenous ciprofloxacin and gentamycin. There are a number of reports of septic arthritis of the facet and sacroiliac joints that occurred in the absence of injection or instrumentation. Systematic reviews have reported 27 cases of facet joint infection[68] and 166 cases of bacterial sacroiliitis.[69] Facet joint sepsis may be complicated by psoas and epidural abscess, meningitis, endocarditis, and widespread sepsis.

There have been several reports of septic complications of facet joint injections of steroids.[70–77] These include septic arthritis,[71,72] paraspinal abscess,[70,71] epidural abscess,[73] meningitis,[74] bacterial endocarditis,[76] and fatal generalized sepsis.[77] In only one case was the patient identified as a diabetic.[75] One of the cases in which an epidural abscess occurred resulted in permanent motor and sensory loss in

---

BOX 27-5 Data Regarding Cases of Epidural Abscess Following Epidural Steroid Injections

Total number of cases	15
Onset within 1 week	9
Onset beyond 1 week	6
Patients with diabetes	5
Caudal epidural injection	1
Lumbar epidural injection	10
Thoracic epidural injection	1
Cervical epidural injection	3
Required laminectomy	11
Deaths	2
Residual motor dysfunction	5

From Hooten WM, Kinney MO, Huntoon MA. Epidural abscess and meningitis after epidural corticosteroid injection. *Mayo Clin Proc* 2004;79:682–686 and Huang RC, Shapiro GS, Lim M, et al. Cervical epidural abscess after epidural steroid injection. *Spine* 2004;29:E7–E9.

the lower extremities. One of the patients with a paraspinous abscess was treated successfully with needle aspiration followed by antibiotics. Most cases required surgical incision and drainage.

There is one reported case of bacterial sacroiliitis after sacroiliac joint injection with steroid.[78] No details of the case were available.

Fungal infection following epidural steroid injection is an extremely rare complication. A case of "torula meningitis" was reported by Shealy[79] following an intrathecal MPA injection (torula refers to yeast-like fungi that are nonpathogenic but may be allergenic; this report probably, though incorrectly, refers to *Cryptococcus*). No details of the case, such as the time course after injection or the outcome, were presented. Another case involved the formation of an *Aspergillus abscess* in the spinal canal 6 weeks following the last of three epidural steroid injections in a healthy 31-year-old woman.[80] There was no history of immune system compromise. She presented with lower extremity weakness, perianal numbness, and loss of rectal sphincter tone. MRI revealed intrathecal masses at T10-11 and T12-L1. A thick-walled intradural abscess was found at the initial laminectomy. She was treated with surgical drainage and intravenous amphotericin. Because of continued back pain, a repeat MRI was performed, showing an epidural abscess extending from L3, through S-1, L4-5 discitis and osteomyelitis, plus persistence of the T10-11 intradural lesion. More extensive laminectomy and drainage was carried out with improvement in neurologic symptoms but persistence of back pain.

Prevention of Spine Infections

Meticulous sterile technique with attention to skin preparation should prevent the large majority of infectious complications. Steroid injections should be avoided if there is any potential source of bacteria, such as a urinary tract infection or sinusitis. The use of antibiotic prophylaxis is controversial. The incidence of infection following epidural or intraarticular steroid injection is too low to justify routine prophylactic antibiotic use, and there is no data on the benefit of prophylaxis in immunocompromised patients. Antibiotic prophylaxis has been recommended for certain radiologic interventions, but no randomized controlled trials have been performed in that subspecialty either.[81,82] An added concern regarding routine preprocedure antibiotic administration is the development of resistant strains of pathogens. Vancomycin has been widely used as an alternate antibiotic to prevent and treat gram-positive infections, which are the most likely type to occur after steroid injections. There is now increasingly widespread vancomycin resistance among strains of enterococci and *S. aureus*.[81]

Treatment of Spine Infections

Most cases of epidural or paravertebral abscess require surgical drainage. Surgical decompression is urgently indicated if there is any neurologic compromise. While waiting for cultures, treatment with antibiotics that cover *S. aureus* is appropriate, as this is the most commonly isolated organism.

► OTHER SIDE EFFECTS AND COMPLICATIONS

Retinal hemorrhage resulting in visual defects has been reported after epidural injections.[83] These have occurred following administration of relatively high volumes (40–120 mL) of saline or local anesthetic. One case of retinal hemorrhage occurred following epidural injection of 80 mg MPA plus 20 mL 0.125% bupivacaine. The patient experienced decreased vision in one eye several hours after the procedure. Ophthalmologic examination revealed bilateral retinal hemorrhages. Some visual acuity returned, but the patient was left with some loss of acuity and a central scotoma in one eye. The cause of this lesion is thought to be a rapid increase in CSF pressure producing a rise in retinal vein pressure and subsequent hemorrhage. This complication is preventable by limiting the volume of epidural injection to a few milliliters. If larger volumes are used, injection should be carried out very slowly.

A 42-year-old man was diagnosed with bilateral subcapsular cataract formation following repeated treatment with epidural steroids.[84] The patient received 10 epidural injections of 80 mg MPA over a 6-year period. The interval between injections was never <3 months. Symptoms began 6 weeks after his last injection. This type of cataract is a known complication of chronic systemic corticosteroid therapy. Persistent hiccup, lasting 4 days, was reported after a thoracic epidural injection of betamethasone and lidocaine.[85] Hiccups subsided after repeated treatment with metoclopramide. Hiccups recurred after a second epidural steroid injection and again responded to metoclopramide. DeSio et al.[86] reported 12 cases of facial flushing and/or generalized erythema after epidural injection of triamcinolone diacetate 80 to 120 mg. Ten cases involved lumbar injections (two were cervical). Symptoms began 24 to 48 hours after the procedure and lasted about 72 hours. Cicala et al.[87] reported facial flushing in 13 cases of cervical epidural MPA injection. The phenomenon has also been reported following steroid injection of the shoulder capsule.[88] The cause of this side effect is unknown.

Vasovagal reactions, resulting in bradycardia and hypotension, and often accompanied by nausea and altered consciousness, are fairly common among patients undergoing procedures within or near the spinal canal. The incidence of vasovagal reactions during epidural steroid injections was shown to be significantly higher for patients undergoing cervical epidural injections (8%) than for those undergoing lumbar epidurals (1%).[89] The difference remained significant after correction for confounding variables such as sitting position.

► SUMMARY

There is a very low incidence of serious complications from injection of corticosteroid suspensions into the epidural space, facet joints, or sacroiliac joint. Nevertheless, some complications can be devastating. There is a greater likelihood of serious complications such as cord injury and high spinal from cervical epidural injections than from lumbar or caudal injections. Diabetic and immunocompromised patients are at greater risk of infectious complications. Careful history and physical examination will help identify risk factors such as diabetes, immunosuppression, coagulopathy, and occult infection. Patients should be informed of the most serious complications as well as common minor complications such as accidental dural puncture and post-dural puncture headache. They should be instructed to promptly report neurologic changes, new or increasing pain, headache, and fever. A system of night and weekend coverage should be available, and patients should know how to contact the on-call physician.

There is some controversy regarding injection into the epidural space following accidental dural puncture. In that circumstance, subarachnoid spread of injectate is likely. Although the risk of serious consequences such as meningitis and arachnoiditis is low, they are possible. In addition, there is a possibility that if the patient later develops arachnoiditis as a result of ongoing disease or surgery, it might be attributed to the injection. At this time, there is no evidence that epidural injection of steroids, without dural puncture, will produce either aseptic meningitis or arachnoiditis.

References

1. Abram SE. The use of epidural steroid injections for the treatment of lumbar radiculopathy. *Anesthesiology* 1999;91:1937–1941.
2. Delport EG, Cucuzzella AR, Marley JK, et al. Treatment of lumbar spinal stenosis with epidural steroid injections: a retrospective outcome study. *Arch Phys Med Rehabil* 2004;85:479–484.
3. Carrera GF. Lumbar facet joint injection in low back pain and sciatica: preliminary results. *Radiology* 1980;137:665–667.
4. Slipman CW, Lipetz JS, Plastaras CT, et al. Fluoroscopically guided therapeutic sacroiliac joint injections for sacroiliac joint syndrome. *Am J Phys Med Rehabil* 2001;80:425–432.
5. Nelson DA. Dangers from methylprednisolone acetate therapy by intraspinal injection. *Arch Neurol* 1988;45:804–806.
6. Fitzgibbon DR, Posner KL, Caplan RA, et al. Chronic pain management: American Society of Anesthesiologists Closed Claims Project. *Anesthesiology* 2004;100:98–105.
7. Wright MN, Denney LC. A comprehensive review of spinal arachnoiditis. *Orthop Nurs* 2003;22:215–219.
8. Delamarter R, Ross J, Masaryk T, et al. Diagnosis of lumbar arachnoiditis by magnetic resonance imaging. *Spine* 1990;15:4304–4310.
9. Nelson DA, Vates TS, Thompson RB. Complications from intrathecal steroid therapy in patients with multiple sclerosis. *Acta Neurol Scand* 1973;49:176–188.
10. Bernat JL, Sadowski CH, Vincent FM, et al. Sclerosing spinal pachymeningitis. *J Neurol Neurosurg Psychiatry* 1976;39:1124–1128.
11. Carta F, Canu C, Datti R, et al. Calcification and ossification of the spinal arachnoid after intrathecal injection of Depo Medrol. *Zentralbl Neurochir* 1987;48:256–261.
12. Ryan MD, Taylor TKF. Management of lumbar nerve root pain by intrathecal and epidural injection of depot methylprednisolone acetate. *Med J Aust* 1981;2:532–534.
13. Cohen FL. Conus medullaris syndrome following multiple intrathecal corticosteroid injections. *Arch Neurol* 1979;36:228–230.
14. Bedford THB. The effect of injected solutions on the cell count of the cerebrospinal fluid. *Br J Pharmacol* 1948;3:80–83.
15. Seghal AD, Tweed DC, Gardner WH, et al. Laboratory studies after intrathecal corticosteroids. *Arch Neurol* 1963;9:74–78.
16. Goldstein NP, McKenzie BE, McGuckin WF. Changes in cerebrospinal fluid of patients with multiple sclerosis after treatment with intrathecal methylprednisolone acetate: a preliminary report. *Mayo Clin Proc* 1962;37:657–668.
17. Gutknecht DR. Chemical meningitis following epidural injections of corticosteroids. *Am J Med* 1987;82:570.
18. Plumb VJ, Dismukes WE. Chemical meningitis related to intrathecal corticosteroid therapy. *South Med J* 1977;70:1241.
19. Abram SE. Subarachnoid corticosteroid injection following inadequate response to epidural steroids for sciatica. *Anesth Analg* 1978;57:313–315.
20. Morris JT, Konkol KA, Longfield RN. Chemical meningitis following epidural methylprednisolone injection. *Infect Med* 1994;11:439–440.
21. Margolis G, Hall HE, Nowill WK. An investigation of efocaine, a long acting local anesthetic agent. *Arch Surg* 1953;61:715–730.
22. Chino N, Awad EA, Kottke FJ. Pathology of propylene glycol administered by perineural and intramuscular injection in rats. *Arch Phys Med Rehabil* 1974;55:33–38.
23. Benzon HT, Gissen AJ, Strichartz GR, et al. The effect of polyethylene glycol on mammalian nerve impulses. *Anesth Analg* 1987;66:553–559.
24. Delaney TJ, Rowlingson JC, Carron H, et al. Epidural steroid effects on nerves and meninges. *Anesth Analg* 1980;59:610–614.
25. Abram SE. Subarachnoid corticosteroid injection following inadequate response to epidural steroids for sciatica. *Anesth Analg* 1978;57:313–316.
26. Barnes B, Fish M. Chemical meningitis as a complication of isotope cisternography. *Neurology* 1972;22:83–91.
27. Deland FH. Intrathecal toxicity studies with benzyl alcohol. *Toxicol Appl Pharmacol* 1973;25:153–156.
28. Hahn AF, Feasby TE, Gilbert JJ. Paraparesis following intrathecal chemotherapy. *Neurology* 1983;33:1032–1038.
29. Latham JM, Fraser RD, Moore RJ, et al. The pathologic effects of intrathecal betamethasone. *Spine* 1997;22:1558–1562.
30. Kotani N, Kushikata T, Hashimoto H, et al. Intrathecal methylprednisolone for intractable postherpetic neuralgia. *N Engl J Med* 2000;343:1514–1519.
31. Tiso RL, Cutler T, Catania JA, et al. Adverse central nervous system sequelae after selective transforaminal block: the role of corticosteroids. *Spine J* 2004;4:468–474.
32. Kaplan MS, Cooke J, Collins JG. Intravascular uptake during fluoroscopically guided cervical interlaminar steroid injection at C6-7: a case report. *Arch Phys Med Rehabil* 2008;89:553–558.
33. Heckmann JG, Maihofner C, Lanz S, et al. Transient tetraplegia after cervical facet joint injection for chronic neck pain administered without imaging guidance. *Clin Neurol Neurosurg* 2006;108:709–711.
34. Hodges SD, Castleberg RL, Miller T, et al. Cervical epidural steroid injection with intrinsic spinal cord damage: two case reports. *Spine* 1998;23:2137–2140.
35. Field J, Rathmell JP, Stephenson JH, et al. Neuropathic pain following cervical epidural steroid injection. *Anesthesiology* 2000;93:885–888.
36. Abbasi A, Malhotra G. The "swimmer's view" as alternative when lateral view is inadequate during interlaminar cervical epidural steroid injections. *Pain Med* 2010;11:709–712.
37. Simon SL, Abrahams JM, Sean GM, et al. Intramedullary injection of contrast into the cervical spinal cord during cervical myelography: a case report. *Spine* 2002;27:E274–E277.
38. Tripathi M, Nath SS, Gupta RK. Paraplegia after intracord injection during attempted epidural steroid injection in an awake-patient. *Anesth Analg* 2005;101:1209–1211.
39. Forrest JB. The response to epidural steroid injections in chronic dorsal root pain. *Can J Anaesth* 1980;27:40–46.
40. Hall ED, Springer JE. Neuroprotection and acute spinal cord injury: a reappraisal. *NeuroRx* 2004;1:80–100.
41. Goebert HW, Jallo SJ, Gardner SJ, et al. Painful radiculopathy treated with epidural injection of procaine and hydrocortisone acetate: results in 113 patients. *Anesth Analg* 1961;40:130–134.
42. Knight CL, Burnell JC. Systemic side effects of extradural steroids. *Anaesthesia* 1980;35:593–594.

43. Stambough JL, Booth RE, Rothman RH. Transient hypercorticism after epidural steroid injection. *J Bone Joint Surg* 1984;66A:1115–1116.

44. Tuel SM, Meythaler JM, Cross LL. Cushing's syndrome from methylprednisolone. *Pain* 1990;40:81–84.

45. Jacobs S, Pullan PT, Potter JM, et al. Adrenal suppression following extradural steroids. *Anaesthesia* 1983;38:953–956.

46. Kay J, Findling JW, Raff H. Epidural triamcinolone suppresses the pituitary-adrenal axis in human subjects. *Anesth Analg* 1994;79:501–505.

47. Boonen S, Van Distel G, Westhovens R, et al. Steroid myopathy induced by epidural triamcinolone injection. *Br J Rheumatol* 1995;34:385–386.

48. Sandberg DI, Lavyne MH. Symptomatic spinal epidural lipomatosis after local epidural corticosteroid injections: case report. *Neurosurgery* 1999;45:162–165.

49. Mchaourab AS, Hamill-Ruth RJ. Should imaging studies be routinely performed prior to epidural steroid injections? *Anesthesiology* 2001;95:1539–1540.

50. Simon DL, Kunz RD, German JD, et al. Allergic or pseudoallergic reaction following epidural steroid deposition and skin testing. *Reg Anesth* 1989;14:253–255.

51. Munck A. Glucocorticoid inhibition of glucose uptake by peripheral tissues: old and new evidence, molecular mechanisms and physiological significance. *Perspect Biol Med* 1971;14:265–269.

52. Pellacani A, Fornengo P, Bruno A, et al. Acute methylprednisolone administration induces a transient alteration of glucose tolerance and pyruvate dehydrogenase in humans. *Eur J Clin Invest* 1999;29:861–867.

53. Ward A, Watson J, Wood P, et al. Glucocorticoid epidural for sciatica: metabolic and endocrine sequelae. *Rheumatology* 2002;41:68–71.

54. Lee PKW, Kim JM. Lumbar epidural blocks: a case report of a life-threatening complication. *Arch Phys Med Rehabil* 2000;81:1587–1590.

55. Charsley MM, Abram SE. The injection of intrathecal normal saline reduces the severity of postdural puncture headache. *Reg Anesth Pain Med* 2001;26:301–305.

56. Abram SE, Cherwenka RW. Transient headache immediately following epidural steroid injection. *Anesthesiology* 1979;50:461–462.

57. Katz JA, Lukin R, Bridenbaugh PO, et al. Subdural intracranial air: an unusual cause of headache after epidural steroid injection. *Anesthesiology* 1991;74:615–618.

58. Simopoulos T, Peeters-Asdourian C. Pneumocephalus after cervical epidural steroid injection. *Anesth Analg* 2001;9:1576–1577.

59. Liu SS, Melmed AP, Klos JW, et al. Prospective experience with a 20-gauge Tuohy needle for lumbar epidural steroid injections: is confirmation with fluoroscopy necessary? *Reg Anesth Pain Med* 2001;26:143–146.

60. Williams KN, Jackowski A, Evans PJD. Epidural hematoma requiring surgical decompression following repeated epidural steroid injections for chronic pain. *Pain* 1990;42:197–199.

61. Reitman CA, Watters W. Subdural hematoma after cervical epidural steroid injection. *Spine* 2002;27:E174–E176.

62. Benzon HT, Wong HY, Siddiqui T, et al. Caution in performing epidural injections in patients on several antiplatelet drugs. *Anesthesiology* 1999;91:1558.

63. Horlocker T, Bajwa ZH, Zubaira A, et al. Risk assessment of hemorrhagic complications associated with nonsteroidal anti-inflammatory medications in ambulatory pain clinic patients undergoing epidural steroid injection. *Anesth Analg* 2002;95:1691–1697.

64. Tang HJ, Lin HJ, Liu YC, et al. Spinal epidural abscess-experience with 46 patients and evaluation of prognostic factors. *J Infect* 2002;45:76–81.

65. Hooten WM, Kinney MO, Huntoon MA. Epidural abscess and meningitis after epidural corticosteroid injection. *Mayo Clin Proc* 2004;79:682–686.

66. Huang RC, Shapiro GS, Lim M, et al. Cervical epidural abscess after epidural steroid injection. *Spine* 2004;29:E7–E9.

67. Yue WM, Tan SB. Distant skip level discitis and vertebral osteomyelitis after caudal epidural injection: a case report of a rare complication of epidural injections. *Spine* 2003;28:E209–E211.

68. Muffoletto AJ, Ketonen LM, Mader JT, et al. Hematogenous pyogenic facet joint infection. *Spine* 2001;26:1570–1576.

69. Vyskocil JJ, McIlroy MA, Brennan TA, et al. Pyogenic infection of the sacroiliac joint: case reports and review of the literature. *Medicine* 1991;70:188–197.

70. Cook NJ, Hanrahan P, Song S. Paraspinal abscess following facet joint injection. *Clin Rheumatol* 1999;18:52–53.

71. Orpen NM, Birch NC. Delayed presentation of septic arthritis of a lumbar facet joint after diagnostic facet joint injection. *J Spinal Disord Tech* 2003;16:285–287.

72. Alcock E, Regaard A, Browne J. Facet joint injection: a rare cause of epidural abscess formation. *Pain* 2003;103:209–210.

73. Magee M, Kannangara, S, Dennien B, et al. Paraspinal abscess complicating facet joint injection. *Clin Nucl Med* 2000;25:71.

74. Gaul C, Neundorfer B, Winterholler M. Iatrogenic (para-) spinal abscesses and meningitis following injection therapy for low back pain. *Pain* 2005;116:407–410.

75. Park MS, Moon SH, Hahn SB, et al. Paraspinal abscess communicated with epidural abscess after extra-articular facet joint injection. *Yonsei Med J* 2007;48:711–714.

76. Hoelzer BC, Weingarten TN, Hooten WM, et al. Paraspinal abscess complicated by endocarditis following a facet joint injection. *Eur J Pain* 2008;12:261–265.

77. Kim SY, Han SH, Jung MW, et al. Generalized infection following facet joint injection: a case report. *Korean J Anesthesiol* 2010;58(4):401–404.

78. Svendsen RN. Purulent arthritis after blockade treatment. *Ugeskr Laeger* 1993;155:2414–2415.

79. Shealy CN. Dangers of spinal injections without proper diagnosis. *JAMA* 1966;197:156–158.

80. Saigal G, DonavanPost MJ, Kozic D. Thoracic intradural *Aspergillus abscess* formation following epidural steroid injection. *Am J Neuroradiol* 2004;25:642–644.

81. Ryan JM, Ryan BM, Smith TP. Antibiotic prophylaxis in interventional radiology. *J Vasc Interv Radiol* 2004;15:547–556.

82. Spies JB, Rosen RJ, Lebovitz AS. Antibiotic prophylaxis in vascular and interventional radiology: a rational approach. *Radiology* 1988;166:381–387.

83. Purdy EP, Ajimal GS. Vision loss after epidural steroid injection. *Anesth Analg* 1998;86:119–122.

84. Chen YC, Garaj N, Clavo A, et al. Posterior subcapsular cataract formation associated with multiple lumbar epidural corticosteroid injections. *Anesth Analg* 1998;86:1054–1055.

85. Slipman CW, Shin CH, Patel RK, et al. Persistent hiccup associated with thoracic epidural injection. *Am J Phys Med Rehabil* 2001;80:618–621.

86. DeSio JM, Kahn CH, Warfield CA. Facial flushing and/or generalized erythema after epidural steroid injection. *Anesth Analg* 1995;80:617–619.

87. Cicala RS, Westbrook L, Anjel JJ. Side effects and complications of cervical epidural steroid injections. *J Pain Symptom Manage* 1989;4:64–66.

88. Jacobs LG, Barton MA, Wallace AW, et al. Intraarticular distension and steroids in the management of capsulitis of the shoulder. *BMJ* 1991;302:1498–1501.

89. Trentman TL, Rosenfeld DM, Seamans DP, et al. Vasovagal reactions and other complications of cervical vs. lumbar translaminar epidural steroid injections. *Pain Pract* 2009;9:59–64.

28

Complications Associated with Transforaminal Injections

Nikolai Bogduk

▶ DEFINITION

Transforaminal injections are injections delivered into an intervertebral foramen of the vertebral column. The target is typically the spinal that lies in the foramen. When used for diagnostic purposes, the drug injected is a local anesthetic agent. When used as a therapeutic intervention, a combination of a local anesthetic and a corticosteroid preparation is injected. Most operators use lidocaine (in concentrations of 0.5%, 1%, or 2%), although some use small volumes of bupivacaine (0.5%). The steroid preparation depends on operator preference and the availability of the preferred preparation. Choices include betamethasone, dexamethasone, triamcinolone, and methylprednisolone. In different jurisdictions around the world, some steroid preparations are proscribed for spinal use by the manufacturer.

Diagnostic transforaminal blocks are used to pinpoint the particular spinal nerve responsible for radicular pain when imaging studies are ambiguous. Some operators use them to confirm a diagnosis of discogenic pain. For diagnostic transforaminal injections, there are no published reports of complications, either because the procedure is not commonly practiced or because the agent injected is innocuous.

The situation is different for therapeutic transforaminal injections of corticosteroids. The procedure is widely practiced, and an abundance of literature on its complications has arisen.

▶ SCOPE OF THE PROBLEM AND PROPOSED MECHANISM OF CAUSATION

Cervical Transforaminal Injections

The hazards of cervical transforaminal injections are predicated by where the injection is performed and what is injected (Fig. 28-1). The needle is placed next to the spinal nerve and close to the dural sac and spinal cord. As well, the vertebral artery lies immediately outside the intervertebral foramen, and radicular arteries lie within the foramen. Each of these various anatomic relations has, to greater or lesser extents, been associated with complications.

Complications have been described in case reports,[1–9] in what amount to practice audits[10–13] and in a survey of 1,340 physicians.[14] The latter yielded 54 cases of complications, some of which included those described in the case reports. In broad terms, these complications can be categorized as miscellaneous and vascular (Table 28-1).

Some of the miscellaneous complications are enigmatic, for lack of sufficient information or because the cause of the complication was not pursued, such as death (cause not specified), transient amnesia, organic brain syndrome, seizure, headache, and dyspnea. Others are attributable to the needle and might apply to any paraspinal procedure, such as vasovagal episode, nausea, pain at the injection site, pain, and hematoma. Other complications are attributable

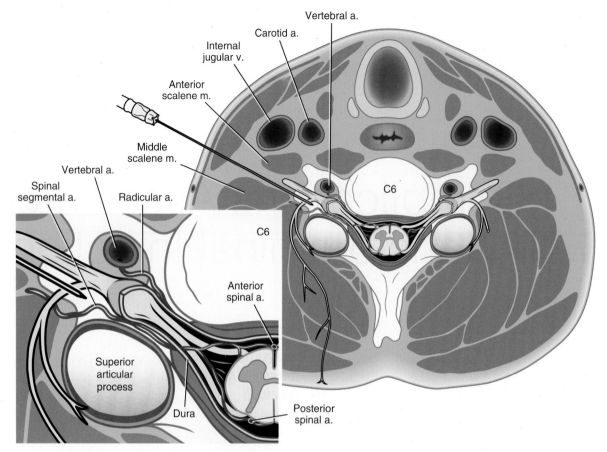

FIGURE 28-1. **Axial view of cervical transforaminal injection at the level of C6.** The needle has been inserted along the axis of the foramen, and is in final position against the posterior aspect of the intervertebral foramen. Insertion along this axis places the needle behind the spinal nerve, and behind the vertebral artery, which lies anterior to the foramen. **Inset:** A spinal artery arises from the vertebral artery. It supplies the vertebral column. Another spinal artery enters the intervertebral foramen from the ascending cervical artery or deep cervical artery. It furnishes radicular branches that accompany the nerve roots and ultimately reach the anterior and posterior spinal arteries of the spinal cord. (Modified from Rathmell JP. *Atlas of Image-guided Intervention in Regional Anesthesia and Pain Medicine.* 2nd ed. Philadelphia, PA: Lippincott Williams & Wilkins, 2012, with permission.)

to the agents injected, such as allergy to steroids or contrast medium. Some complications are idiosyncratic to the location of the injection in the cervical spine, such as dural puncture, sympathetic blockade, nerve root weakness, and nerve root injury. Direct spinal cord injury should not be a complication of cervical transforaminal injections, because guidelines for the procedure stipulate that the needle should be placed no further than midway across the intervertebral foramen and its position checked radiographically before any agent is injected.[15,16] In the case reported[3] (Table 28-1), the position of the needle was not checked before contrast medium was injected into the spinal cord. Similarly, high spinal anesthesia implies that the position of the needle was not checked before local anesthetic was injected intrathecally.

Some authors have identified complaints such as increased pain, light-headedness, and nausea as complications of cervical transforaminal injections.[11,12] However, these complaints were no more common than in a control group who did not undergo injections.[12] Therefore, they cannot be admitted as complications of transforaminal injections.

More often reported have been vascular complications. In addition to those listed in Table 28-1, several have been described in detail in case reports (Table 28-2). Vascular complications have involved the distribution of the vertebral artery or a radicular artery.

In the case of vertebrobasilar infarction, postulated causes include air embolism,[5] vasospasm,[14] aneurysm,[7,14] and steroid embolism.[6,14] Air embolism is certainly a risk if air is injected in an attempt to verify epidural placement of a needle; but doing so is neither a standard nor a common practice in the conduct of transforaminal injections. Vasospasm may sound attractive as a postulate, but is incompatible with past experience when radiologists were accustomed to directly puncturing vertebral arteries in the conduct of four-vessel angiography. Consequently, inducing a dissecting aneurysm, dislodging a mural plaque, and steroid embolism remain the likely causes of vertebrobasilar infarctions caused by cervical transforaminal injections. Passing a needle through the vertebral artery might dislodge a mural plaque. Injecting contrast medium or other material into the wall of the artery, instead of its lumen, could cause a dissecting aneurysm.

TABLE 28-1 Complications Associated with Cervical Transforaminal Injection of Steroids, as Reported by Various Authors

	SOURCE AND NUMBER OF CASES						
Miscellaneous	A	B	C	D	E	F	G
Death (cause not specified)	5						
Transient global amnesia							1
Organic brain syndrome			1				
Seizure	2				1		
Headache	2			45			5
Dyspnea						1	
Vasovagal episode	1					19	1
Increased pain at injection site				20			
Epidural hematoma	1						
Paraspinal hematoma	1					1	
Anaphylaxis to betamethasone					1		
Allergy to contrast medium						1	1
Dural puncture				1			
Transient sympathetic block						6	
Transient weakness upper limb							6
Nerve root injury	1	1					
Direct spinal cord injury			1				
High spinal anesthesia	3						
Vascular							
Vertebrobasilar infarction	16						
Spinal cord infarction	12						
Combined spinal and vertebrobasilar infarction	2						
Transient ischemic attack	3						
Spinal cord edema	2						
Brainstem edema	1						
Brain edema	1						
Cortical blindness	1						

A. In a survey of 1,340 physicians.[14]
B. Case report.[2]
C. Case report.[3]
D. Practice audit of 89 procedures on 37 patients.[12]
E. Practice audit of 4,612 procedures.[10]
F. Practice audit of 799 procedures.[11]
G. Practice audit of 1,036 procedures.[13]

TABLE 28-2 Key Features of Case Reports of Vascular Complications of Cervical Transforaminal Injections of Corticosteroids

SOURCE	SITE OF INJECTION	PATHOLOGY	ARTERY IMPLICATED	AGENT INJECTED
Brouwers et al.[1]	C6	Spinal cord infarction	Radicular	Triamcinolone
Windsor et al.[2]	C6	Spinal cord infarction	Radicular	Betamethasone
Ludwig and Burns[4]	C6	Spinal cord infarction	Radicular	triamcinolone
McMillan and Crumpton[5]	C5, C6	Occipital lobe infarction	Vertebral	Air
Tiso et al.[6]	C6	Cerebellar infarction Occipital infarction	Vertebral	Triamcinolone
Rozin et al.[7]	C6	Cerebral edema Brainstem hemorrhage Cerebellar hemorrhage	Vertebral	Methylprednisolone
Suresh et al.[8]	C5	Brainstem infarction	Vertebral	Triamcinolone
Wallace et al.[9]	C7 C5	Brainstem infarction Transient ischemia	Vertebral Vertebral	Not stated Not stated

Such a process has been verified at postmortem in two cases.[9] Steroid embolism could occur if the position of the needle is not checked, and if flow of contrast medium into the vertebral artery is not recognized.

Laboratory studies have shown that triamcinolone, betamethasone, and methylprednisolone preparations each form particles or aggregates that are larger than red blood cells.[6,17] Such particles or aggregates, therefore, could be capable of obstructing small vessels. Dexamethasone is the only commonly used corticosteroid that does not form particles or aggregates. It seems more than circumstantial that complications have been reported only in cases were particulate steroids have been used (Table 28-2). There have been no reports of complications when dexamethasone has been used.[14]

Two animal studies have demonstrated the ability of particulate steroids to cause infarctions. In one study, particular and nonparticular steroids were injected into the internal carotid artery of rats; lesions in the central nervous system occurred only in those animals into whom particular steroids were injected; no lesions, and no clinical deficits, were encountered in those animals injected with dexamethasone.[18] In the other study, either particulate or nonparticulate steroids were injected into the vertebral arteries of pigs.[19] All animals injected with particulate steroids failed to regain consciousness and showed clinical, magnetic resonance, and histopathologic features consistent with cerebrovascular insult. Animals who received nonparticulate steroids showed no evidence of neurologic injury, clinically, on imaging, or at postmortem.

In the case of spinal cord infarction, the leading contention is that the transforaminal injection compromises a radicular artery that happens to reinforce the anterior spinal artery (although in one case,[2] a posterior spinal artery was implicated). Reinforcing radicular arteries can occur at any cervical level, but appear to be more common at lower cervical levels.[20] Some authors have suggested that the needle used irritates the radicular artery in the intervertebral foramen and causes vasospasm.[1,4,21] While this proposition is conceptually entertainable, no direct evidence of it has been produced. In contrast, circumstantial evidence does support the contention that, if unintentionally injected into a radicular artery, particulate steroids can act as an embolus and cause infarction in the territory of the anterior spinal artery.

Two cases have been described in which digital subtraction angiography was used to capture images of a radicular artery during the injection of a test-dose of contrast medium in the course of a cervical transforaminal injection.[20,22] These cases showed that intra-arterial injection could occur even if the needle was correctly placed in the posterior quadrant of the intervertebral foramen (Fig. 28-2). An additional case report showed filling of a radicular artery during an injection of contrast medium high in the foramen.[23] In all three cases, filling of the radicular artery was recognized, the procedure was terminated, and the patient suffered no ill effects.

Another case report described a patient in whom digital substraction angiography showed no vascular uptake during injection of a test-dose of contrast medium, but after injection of local anesthetic the patient developed neurologic symptoms consistent with anesthetization of the anterior and anterolateral cervical spinal cord.[24] The patient recovered in 20 minutes and suffered no lasting ill effects.

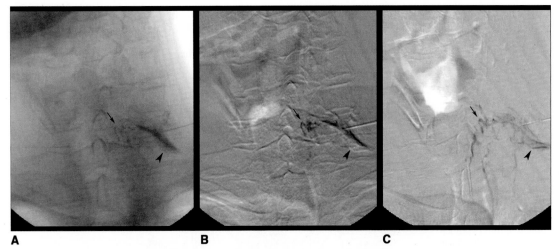

FIGURE 28-2. Anterior-posterior of the cervical spine during C7/T1 transforaminal injection (digital subtraction sequence after contrast injection). An anteroposterior view of an angiogram obtained after injection of contrast medium, prior to planned transforaminal injection of corticosteroids. **A**: Image as seen on fluoroscopy. The needle lies in the left C7-T1 intervertebral foramen no further medially than its mediolateral point. Contrast medium outlines the exiting nerve root (*arrowhead*). The radicular artery appears as a thin thread passing medially from the site of injection (*small arrow*). **B**: Digital subtraction angiogram reveals the radicular artery extending medially more clearly (*small arrow*). **C**: Digital subtraction angiogram after pixel-shift re-registration reveals that the radicular artery (*small arrow*) extends to the midline to join the anterior spinal artery. (Reproduced from Rathmell JP, Aprill C, Bogduk N. Cervical transforaminal injection of steroids. *Anesthesiology* 2004;100:1595–1600, with permission.)

Together, these case reports provided circumstantial evidence that spinal cord function could be compromised if a reinforcing radicular artery was occluded. Irreversible injury could occur if particulate steroids acted as an embolus in the radicular artery or the anterior (or posterior) spinal artery.

Lumbar Transforaminal Injections

The complications of lumbar transforaminal injections can be categorized as minor and major. An audit of 322 injections determined that minor complications occur in about 9% of cases.[25] In descending order of prevalence, minor complications include transient headaches (3%), increased back pain (2%), facial flushing (1%), increased leg pain (0.6%), and vasovagal reaction (0.3%). These complications are reminiscent of those associated with lumbar interlaminar and caudal injections. None was associated with any lasting morbidity.

Major complications involve the reinforcing radicular artery known as the artery of Adamkiewicz. Although this artery typically arises at thoracic levels, it can occur at any segmental level.[26] Estimates of its prevalence at lumbar and sacral levels differ. An artery of Adamkiewicz has been reported low as L1 or L2 in about 10%[27] or 1%[28] of people and more rarely at even lower levels. In those with a low-lying radicular artery, it is a hazard for lumbar transforaminal injections (Fig. 28-3).

Eight cases of paraplegia have been reported followed lumbar transforaminal injection of steroids.[26,29–32] All cases involved the injection of particulate steroids. The implication is that all patients suffered steroid embolism of an artery of Adamkiewicz, following unrecognized intra-arterial injection. The countervailing interpretation is that the needle induced vasospasm.

▶ PREVENTION

Guidelines for the conduct of cervical transforaminal injections[15,16] are designed to avoid the complications of this procedure. These guidelines stipulate that the target zone must be approached along a correctly obtained oblique view (and not, e.g., simply along a lateral view). The needle should be directed first of all onto the superior articular process behind the target foramen. These two measures guard against encountering the vertebral artery, which should lie anterior to the course of the needle. Thereafter, the needle should be readjusted to enter the intervertebral foramen tangential to its posterior wall, at about its middle (Fig. 28-4). The needle should not pass further medially than half-way across the width of the foramen. Once the needle has been placed, a test-dose of contrast medium should be injected and its flow carefully monitored during injection. That injection tests two things. First, under normal circumstances, it should show that the injectate correctly flows along the target nerve and into the lateral epidural space. Simultaneously, but more critically, it shows if intravascular injection occurs. Identification of small arteries is enhanced by using digital subtraction angiography.

Close attention is required to notice if the injection is intra-arterial. The rapid flow through arteries means that intra-arterial contrast medium will appear only fleetingly. This event is unlikely to be captured by postinjection spot films. The flow of contrast medium must be monitored by continuous fluoroscopic screening throughout the injection.

Intra-arterial injection must not only be recognized, but it must also be correctly interpreted. In some cases, flow of contrast medium along the vertebral artery has been misinterpreted as indicating correct flow in the epidural

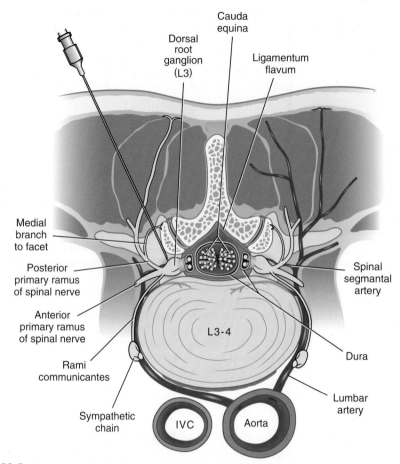

FIGURE 28-3. **Axial view of lumbar transforaminal selective nerve root injection.** On the right of the specimen, a needle has been placed in the intervertebral foramen, aiming at the nerve root complex. On the left, a radicular artery is accompanying the nerve roots. Such a vessel could be susceptible to penetration during a transforaminal injection. (Modified from Rathmell JP. *Atlas of Image-guided Intervention in Regional Anesthesia and Pain Medicine.* 2nd ed. Philadelphia, PA: Lippincott Williams & Wilkins, 2012, with permission.)

space.[22] It is also pertinent to realize that arterial flow to the spinal cord will not necessarily occur at the segmental level at which injection is being performed. It has been shown, in the thoracic spine, that retrograde filling of a radicular artery can occur, back to its parent vessel, from which the injectate can then flow to the spinal cord through a vessel at an adjacent segment.[33]

The guidelines for lumbar transforaminal injections[24] outline similar principles. A test-dose of contrast medium with real-time fluoroscopic monitoring is essential. Furthermore, during this test, a full view of the lumbar spine that includes several segments cephalad of the level of injection should be used. In one unpublished case, the operator missed cephalad intra-arterial flow of contrast medium because, although the entire lumbar spine was in view, the injection was at L1, and the contrast medium flowed to thoracic levels, which were not shown on-screen.

Some commentators have advocated conducting cervical transforaminal injections under computed tomography (CT) guidance, purportedly on the grounds that it is more accurate and safer.[7,9] However, CT is neither more accurate nor safer.

CT shows the location of the needle in a single view, but this does not render CT more accurate; it is only more convenient. In geometric terms, fluoroscopy is no less accurate. Its inconvenience is that it requires a second view to confirm depth of insertion.

It is true that CT allows the vertebral artery to be seen during insertion of the needle; but even so, CT is not fail-safe. Subintimal injection into the vertebral artery has occurred even though operators have used CT guidance.[9] The implication is that operators can fail to recognize penetration of the vertebral artery despite using CT.

More critically, CT displays only one plane of section; it does not display events cephalad or caudad of that plane. This is the paramount advantage of fluoroscopy. Anteroposterior fluoroscopy provides a full frontal view of the cervical spine. When test-doses of contrast medium are injected, this view will show intra-arterial flow, if it occurs, through ascending vessels such as the vertebral artery or a radicular artery. Such flow will not be seen on single-axial CT scans, and it is so fleetingly brief that it is unlikely to be captured on serial scans. Identifying such intra-arterial flow is crucial to avoiding steroid embolism. If it is seen, the procedure should be terminated, in order to avoid the consequences of steroid embolism.

With respect to arguments about accuracy and safety, it is frustrating that most of the case reports of central nervous system injury provide no illustrations of the technique used; for the few for which illustrations are available,

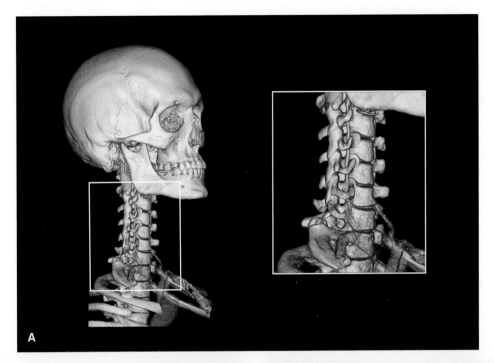

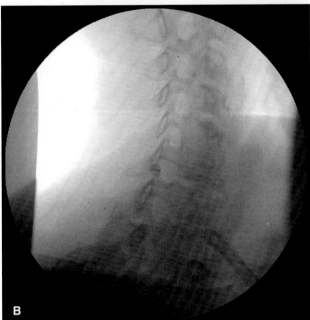

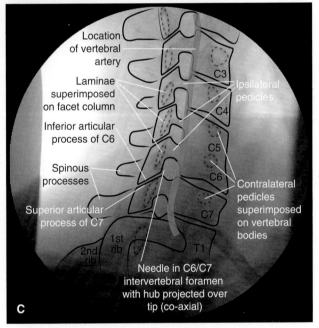

FIGURE 28-4. A: Bony anatomy relevant to cervical transforaminal injection. Three-dimensional reconstruction CT of the cervical spine as viewed from the anterior oblique approach used for cervical transforaminal injection. **Inset** matches the anatomic area in the radiographs shown in Figure 6-3B, C. **B**: Right oblique view of the cervical spine during right C6/C7 transforaminal injection. The needle is in proper position in the posterior aspect of the foramen for right C6/C7 transforaminal injection (C7 nerve root). Note that this patient has had a prior C5/C6 interbody fusion, and it is difficult to discern a disc space between these two vertebrae. **C**: The approximate position of the vertebral artery near the anterior aspect of the intervertebral foramina is shown in red. (Reproduced with permission from Rathmell JP. *Atlas of Image-guided Intervention in Regional Anesthesia and Pain Medicine.* 2nd ed. Philadelphia, PA: Lippincott Williams & Wilkins, 2012.)

those illustrations are incomplete or inadequate. Observers, therefore, cannot ascertain if the procedure was correctly performed. Material available to expert witnesses engaged in legal proceedings concerning unpublished cases suggests that correct technique has not always been used.

In some cases of cervical injections, failure to obtain a correct oblique view has been implicated. Under those conditions, the vertebral artery lies in line with the course of the needle into the intervertebral foramen. Yet even that factor alone does not explain why injections are so often made into the vertebral artery. Two additional failures must apply: failure to check the depth of insertion on anteroposterior views (or to interpret those views correctly) and failure to administer a test-dose of contrast medium (or to interpret its flow correctly).

▶ **DIAGNOSIS AND TREATMENT**

Neurologic complications of transforaminal injections are typically catastrophic. They are clinically obvious upon onset of spinal weakness and numbness. Their recognition requires no special investigations. Magnetic resonance imaging of the spinal cord and hindbrain serves only to identify the location and extent of the neurologic damage. In that regard, changes in the spinal cord or brainstem may not become evident until 2 days or more after injury.

There is no emergency management known to be able to reverse spinal cord or brainstem injury. Immediate treatment amounts to ventilatory and cardiovascular support as may be indicated and necessary. Subsequent management and rehabilitation follow standard protocols for spinal cord injury or hindbrain infarction.

▶ **SUMMARY**

In principle, transforaminal injections should be safe procedures if performed according to recommended guidelines.[15,16,34] To date, no evidence has been published to contradict this principle. The published evidence of complications is either incomplete or indicates that critical steps have been omitted or neglected.

References

1. Brouwers PJAM, Kottnik EJBL, Simon MAM, et al. A cervical anterior spinal artery syndrome after diagnostic blockade of the right C6-nerve root. *Pain* 2001;91:397–399.
2. Windsor RE, Strom S, Sugar R, et al. Cervical transforaminal injection: review of the literature, complications, and a suggested technique. *Pain Phys* 2003;6:457–465.
3. Lee JH, Lee JK, Seo BR, et al. Spinal cord injury produced by direct damage during cervical transforaminal epidural injection. *Reg Anesth Pain Med* 2008;33:377–379.
4. Ludwig MA, Burns SP. Spinal cord infarction following cervical transforaminal injection. A case report. *Spine* 2005;30:E266–E268.
5. McMillan MR, Crumpton C. Cortical blindness and neurologic injury complicating cervical transforaminal injection for cervical radiculopathy. *Anesthesiology* 2003;99:509–511.
6. Tiso RL, Cutler T, Catania JA, et al. Adverse central nervous system sequelae after selective transforaminal block: the role of corticosteroids. *Spine J* 2004;4:468–474.
7. Rozin L, Rozin R, Koehler SA, et al. Death during a transforaminal epidural steroid nerve root block (C7) due to perforation of the left vertebral artery. *Am J Forensic Med Pathol* 2003;24:351–355.
8. Suresh S, Berman J, Connell DA. Cerebellar and brainstem infarction as a complication of CT-guided transforaminal cervical nerve root block. *Skeletal Radiol* 2007;36:449–452.
9. Wallace MA, Fukui MB, Williams RL, et al. Complications of cervical selective nerve root blocks performed with fluoroscopic guidance. *AJR Am J Roentgenol* 2007;188:1218–1221.
10. Schellhas KP, Pollei SR, Johnson BA, et al. Selective cervical nerve root blockade: experience with a safe and reliable technique using an anterolateral approach for needle placement. *AJNR Am J Neuroradiol* 2007;28:1909–1914.
11. Pobiel RS, Schellhas KP, Eklund JA, et al. Selective cervical nerve root blockade: prospective study of immediate and longer term complications. *AJNR Am J Neuroradiol* 2009;30:507–511.
12. Huston CW, Slipman CW, Garvin C. Complications and side effects of cervical and lumbosacral selective nerve root injections. *Arch Phys Med Rehabil* 2005;86:277–283.
13. Ma DJ, Gilula LA, Riew KD. Complications of fluoroscopically guided extraforaminal cervical nerve blocks. An analysis of 1036 injections. *J Bone Joint Surg Am* 2005;87:1025–1030.
14. Scanlon GC, Moeller-Bertram T, Romanowsky SM, et al. Cervical transforaminal epidural steroid injections. More dangerous than we think? *Spine* 2007;32:1249–1256.
15. Standards Committee of the International Spine Intervention Society. Cervical transforaminal injection of corticosteroids. In: Bogduk N, ed. *Practice Guidelines for Spinal Diagnostic and Treatment Procedures*. San Francisco, CA: International Spine Intervention Society, 2004:237–248.
16. Rathmell JR, Aprill C, Bogduk N. Cervical transforaminal injection of steroids. *Anesthesiology* 2004;100:1595–1600.
17. Derby R, Date ES, Lee JH, et al. Size and aggregation of corticosteroids used for epidural injections. *Pain Med* 2008;9:227–234.
18. Dawley JD, Moeller-Bertram T, Wallace MS, et al. Intra-arterial injection in the rat brain. Evaluation of steroids used for transforaminal epidurals. *Spine* 2009;34:1638–1643.
19. Okubadejo G, Talcott M, Schmidt R, et al. Perils of intravascular methylprednisolone injection into the vertebral artery. An animal study. *J Bone Joint Surg* 2008;9:1932–1938.
20. Baker R, Dreyfuss P, Mercer S, et al. Cervical transforaminal injection of corticosteroids into a radicular artery: a possible mechanism for spinal cord injury. *Pain* 2002;103:211–215.
21. Nash T. Comment on 'a cervical anterior spinal artery syndrome after diagnostic blockade of the right C6-nerve root'. *Pain* 2002;96:217–218.
22. Bogduk N, Dreyfuss P, Baker R, et al. Complications of spinal diagnostic and treatment procedures. *Pain Med* 2008;6:S11–S34.
23. Verrils P, Nowesenitz G, Barnard A. Penetration of a cervical radicular artery during a transforaminal epidural injection. *Pain Med* 2010;11:229–231.
24. Karasek M, Bogduk N. Temporary neurologic deficit after cervical transforaminal injection of local anesthetic. *Pain Med* 2004;5:202–205.
25. Botwin KP, Gruber RD, Bouchlas CG, et al. Complications of fluoroscopically guided transforaminal lumbar epidural injections. *Arch Phys Med Rehabil* 2000;81:1045–1050.
26. Kennedy DJ, Dreyfuss P, Aprill CN, et al. Paraplegia following image-guided transforaminal lumbar spine epidural steroid injection: two case reports. *Pain Med* 2009;19:1389–1394.
27. Lazorthes G, Gouza A. Supply routes of arterial vascularization of the spinal cord. Applications to the study of vascular myelopathies. *Bull Acad Natl Med* 1970;154:34–41.
28. Lo D, Vallee JN, Spelle L, et al. Unusual origin of the artery of Adamkiewicz from the fourth lumbar artery. *Neuroradiology* 2002;44:153–157.
29. Houten JK, Errico TJ. Paraplegia after lumbosacral nerve root block: report of three cases. *Spine J* 2002;2:70–75.
30. Somyaji HS, Saifuddin A, Casey ATH, et al. Spinal cord infarction following therapeutic compute tomography-guided left L2 nerve root injection. *Spine* 2005;30:E106–E108.
31. Huntoon M, Martin D. Paralysis after transforaminal epidural injection and previous spinal surgery. *Reg Anesth Pain Med* 2004;29:494–495.
32. Glaser SE, Falco FM. Paraplegia following a thoracolumbar transforaminal epidural steroid injection: a case report. *Pain Phys* 2005;8:309–314.
33. Yin W, Bogduk N. Retrograde filling of a thoracic spinal artery during transforaminal injection. *Pain Med* 2009;10:689–692.
34. Standards Committee of the International Spine Intervention Society. Lumbar transforaminal injection of corticosteroids. k In: Bogduk N, ed. *Practice Guidelines for Spinal Diagnostic and Treatment Procedures*. San Francisco, CA: International Spine Intervention Society, 2004:163–187.

29

Complications Associated with Discography and Intradiscal Treatment Techniques

Leonardo Kapural, Karlo Houra, and Andrej Radic

Lumbar discogenic pain is caused by the pathophysiologic changes within the intervertebral disc as a primary nociceptive structure, but it can also be the result of reduced intradiscal mechanical load-bearing capacity and for that reason altered spinal biomechanics.[1] For this reason, more of the recent therapeutic strategies for discogenic pain are directed toward several general objectives: destruction of primary nociceptive fibers formed in the process of postinjury neovascularization and innervation of posterior annular tears; restoring previous cytokine immunochemistry within the nuclear and annular biochemical steady state; and reestablishing the intervertebral disc height and annular integrity.[2] Such minimally invasive therapeutic approaches vary and may involve radiofrequency technology, already in wide use clinically, or cytokine inhibition, gene modulation, or cellular replacement, all still considered experimental.[1-4] This chapter discusses complications related to presently available and emerging intradiscal therapies aimed at treating discogenic pain as well as complications associated with diagnostic provocative discography.

Unexpected anatomic variations of the structures that form the spine, including aberrant vascular and neural tissue of the spinal cord, may be the direct cause of procedural complications. However, more frequently, lack of experience and faulty or poorly designed equipment contribute to adverse outcomes. Depending on their pathologic mechanisms, the onset of clinical presentations of different complications is variable. Immediate complications are clearly associated with the procedure and include cauda equine syndrome, acute disc herniation, contrast dye-related anaphylaxis, bleeding, muscle spasm, or probe/electrode fracture[5] (Table 29-1). Other complications may present themselves days or weeks after the intervention; examples include discitis,

TABLE 29-1 Reported Complications of Intradiscal, Minimally Invasive Procedures Used in Diagnosis and Treatment of Discogenic Pain and for the Treatment of Disc Herniation

COMPLICATIONS ASSOCIATED WITH INTRADISCAL TREATMENTS

Infectious

Discitis

Epidural abscess

Vertebral osteomyelitis

Subdural empyema

Bacterial meningitis

Neural

Cauda equina syndrome

Spinal nerve damage with or without complex regional

Pain syndrome (causalgia)

Acute disc herniation

Allergic/immune hypersensitivity

Dye-induced anaphylaxis

Urticaria

Vascular

Retroperitoneal bleeding

Intramuscular hematoma

Others

Probe/electrode fracture with retained foreign body

Muscle spasm

Burns

Vertebral avascular necrosis

Acceleration of disc degeneration

vertebral osteomyelitis, epidural abscess, or early causalgia. Atypical presentations of some complications may occur, in part, due to other comorbidities. The following paragraphs describe complications related to discography, intradiscal injections and heating of the disc, and several percutaneous disc decompression (PDD) techniques.

COMPLICATIONS ASSOCIATED WITH PROVOCATIVE DISCOGRAPHY

Because of its nonspecific features, the diagnosis of discogenic pain is not easily made by clinical means alone. Useful tools in the search for the origin of back pain are provocative discography and magnetic resonance imaging (MRI) studies. Although of questioned diagnostic value,[6–8] provocative discography is the only test that may relate pathologic changes found on MRI to patient's pain.[8–11] Discography is performed in a procedure room under fluoroscopic guidance, which allows consistent visualization of the bony landmarks. The patient lies prone and the lumbar lordosis is corrected by placing a roll or soft wedge under the lower abdomen. Monitoring and light sedation are used and a fluoroscopy employing a lateral or extrapedicular approach using "tunnel vision" facilitates intradiscal needle placement.[12]

The overall rate of complications following provocative lumbar discography is low, with reports ranging from 0% to 2.5%. Discitis, epidural abscess, and bacterial meningitis have all been reported.[5–11]

More frequent procedural complications include acute paresthesias, muscle spasm, and minor bleeding. During provocative discography, excessive amounts of local anesthetic injected deep, closer to the disc/foramina just prior to intradiscal needle placement, may decrease the ability of the patient and proceduralist to detect spinal nerve contact during needle placement. To avoid potential neural injury, the needle should be directed into the region below the segmental spinal nerve, just lateral to the superior articular process, and above the superior vertebral endplate immediately below the targeted disc. The patient may experience a brief, sharp, painful sensation when the needle pierces the well-innervated outer annulus fibrosus. If the patient experiences any paresthesias during needle advancement, insertion of the needle must stop and needle redirected.

Provocative discography may lead to acute lumbar disc herniation. In five patients, postdiscography herniation was clinically manifest as an acute exacerbation of radicular leg pain and was accompanied by an acute foot drop in one of these patients. Acute disc pressurization caused either an increase in the size of preexisting herniation or formation of the new one, confirmed by the comparative lumbar MRI scans prior to and after completed discography. The authors concluded that annular weakness may be a predisposing factor to discography-related disc herniations.[13]

Chronic discitis is the most dreaded complication associated with discography, and its frequency is from 0% to 1.3% per disc injected,[14,15] or more precisely 0.15% per patient and 0.08% per disc injected.[14–17] It is believed to be due to inoculation of skin flora carried by the procedure needle into the intervertebral disc.[14,15] Commonest skin flora microorganisms are *Staphylococcus aureus* and *Staphylococcus epidermidis*, although gram-negative bacteria also have been reported as the cause of discitis.[15–19]

Preprocedural intravenous and/or intradiscal antibiotics are frequently used as a prophylactic measure. The occurrence of infectious discitis may be decreased with the use of intradiscal antibiotics mixed with the water-soluble contrast.

Iohexol lowers the MICs (minimal inhibitory concentrations) of the antibiotics if it is used together with cefazolin and gentamycin.[20]

Intravenous administration of some antibiotics may produce an unpredictable intradiscal concentrations. While clindamycin and vancomycin levels were detected in the rabbit discs after the intravenous administration, cephalothin and oxacillin were not.[21] In humans, gentamicin and cefazolin do penetrate the intervertebral disc to a greater degree than other cephalosporins or oxacillin, indicating selective intradiscal availability of different antibiotics.[22,23] The highest intradiscal concentration of cefazolins is achieved within the "golden period" of 15 to 81 minutes after 2 g are given intravenously.[24]

There were no cases of infectious discitis after the administration of antibiotics prior to discography in a 3-month follow-up study of 200 patients.[15] Another large study reported no complications of 1,477 performed provocative discographies in 523 patients.[25]

The antibiotics can be mixed with the contrast agent into a stable, nonprecipitating solution before injecting them into the disc. None of the 127 patients, according to Osti et al.,[26] developed clinical or radiological signs of chemical or bacterial discitis after discography, when 1 mg of cefazolin was added to 1 mL of contrast agent.[26]

It is difficult to determine if the incidence of discitis is more frequent following cervical, thoracic, or lumbar provocative discography. The incidence of discitis after cervical discography ranges from 0.16% to as high as 3%. One study reported cervical discitis in 7 out of 1,357 patients with the predominant presenting symptom being excessive neck pain soon after the discogram.[27] Two smaller series reported acute discitis in 1 out of 31 and 2 out of 269 disc injections.[28,29] There were no reported infectious complications after 89 thoracic discographies in 20 patients.[30]

In order to prevent discitis, both the North American Spine Society and the International Spinal Intervention Society guidelines recommend utilizing a two-needle approach, in which a larger needle is inserted through the skin first, and a smaller gauge needle is then passed through the larger needle to enter the disc.[17,31] The theory behind the two-needle technique is that the smaller needle that enters the disc never passes through the skin, thereby reducing the chances of bacterial contamination of the needle tip. Prior to routine use of prophylactic antibiotics, Fraser et al.[18] reported a rate of discitis with single nonstyletted versus double needles of 2.7% versus 0.7%.

The patient with discitis presents days or weeks after the procedure with severe, unremitting back or neck pain with or even without fever. It is needed to complete a physical exam, laboratory tests that include complete blood count with differential, C-reactive protein and blood cultures, and imaging. MRI is the preferred imaging modality[32,33] and, within 3 to 4 days of symptoms, shows increased T2 signal in the disc and endplate hyperemia. It is recommended to do targeted biopsy during acute phase, before the endplate breach when sterile environment is created by the activation of immune system.[34] Treatment of discitis is difficult and protracted, typically requiring long-term antibiotic. Discitis can lead to more complicated infections of the adjacent soft tissues, leading to abscess formation that may require surgical intervention.[35,36] Epidural abscess formation is a rare complication of provocative discography. Frequently, decompressive lumbar laminectomy is needed to evacuate the abscess.[37] There were reports of prevertebral abscess and a spinal subdural empyema as a unique complication of cervical discography.[27,36]

One case of urticaria was also reported in a study on 750 discographic injections performed in 250 patients.[38]

Prolonged pain after discography is often misinterpreted. The first study reporting prolonged low back pain after discography enrolled incarcerated subjects and an inappropriate contrast irritant, the ionic contrast media diatrizoate (Hypaque).[39] More recently, a study conducted on six patients with a diagnosis of somatization disorder, abnormal psychometric testing, or worker's compensation claims documented prolonged back pain after the discography.[40] It is difficult to generalize such phenomena to a normal patient population, as persistent somatic complaints including chronic pain are common in this group.[40,41]

Finally, recent controversy has arisen surrounding the likelihood that discography itself can lead to accelerated disc degeneration after the diagnostic test is performed. Carragee et al.[42] compared 52 control patient with 50 patients who underwent lumbar discography and analyzed their subsequent imaging studies 10 years later, looking for signs of progressive disc degeneration. They concluded that modern discography techniques using small gauge needles and limited pressurization resulted in accelerated disc degeneration, disc herniation, loss of disc height, and signal and the development of reactive endplate changes compared to match controls. The authors recommended that careful consideration of risk and benefit should be used in recommending procedures involving disc injection. This case-control study has significant limitations, but has raised significant controversy and concern about the role for discography in the diagnosis of discogenic pain.

It is important that lumbar discography be performed by a well-experienced physician, under sterile conditions using fluoroscopic imaging for proper needle placement, in order to minimize the risk of complications.[5,9]

▶ COMPLICATIONS ASSOCIATED WITH ANALGESIC DISCOGRAPHY

Analgesic discography is an alternative to traditional provocative discography and was designed in efforts to increase the diagnostic precision associated with tests aimed at identifying symptomatic disc degeneration. This test employs the intradiscal placement of small-bore infusion catheters, through which local anesthetic can be infused after placement. The catheters are placed, and then each disc is successively anesthetized in efforts to locate the symptomatic level. Little has appeared with regard to complications associated with this new procedure. Nonetheless, during analgesic discography, the diameter of the needle inserted is significantly larger than the needle size used during provocative discography (Fig. 29-1). This is necessary in order to thread the balloon catheter, used later on for postinsertion testing[43] (Fig. 29-1B). As we have already discussed, puncturing an intervertebral disc with a needle may lead to progressive disc disruption.[42] Greater progression of degenerative disc disease has been suggested in postdiscography discs, and it

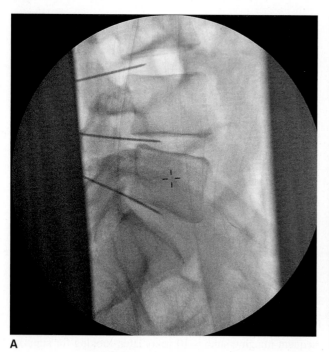 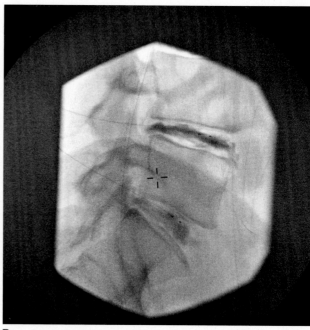

A   **B**

FIGURE 29-1. Intradiscal placement of the 18G introducers (A) used for the analgesic discography followed by insertion of intradiscal balloon (B) used during analgesic discography. Note a large diameter of the introducer that is required to be positioned within the intervertebral disc nucleus.

seems to be more rapid and severe in patients who had larger diameter size needles inserted into their intervertebral discs, suggesting that the large cannulae used during analgesic discography may be problematic.

▶ COMPLICATIONS ASSOCIATED WITH INTRADISCAL INJECTIONS

Chymopapain

Chymopapain has been used for years as a substance for intradiscal nuclear ablation (chemonucleolysis) in patients with contained disc herniations and ongoing back and leg pain. Chemonucleolysis uses chymopapain B, an injectable proteolytic enzyme. Chymopapain produces hydrolysis of noncollagenous protein that interconnects long-chain mucopolysaccharides; chymopapain also has a neurolytic effects on free nerve endings within the disc. This series of biochemical reactions leads to depolymerization of the nucleus pulposus, thereby lowering intradiscal pressure. Most patients who received such therapy were those suffering from contained disc protrusion and predominantly leg pain, but it has been used also for the treatment of discogenic lower back pain. An overall success rate of 72% was reported in one analysis of 17,000 patients treated with chymopapain for acute disc herniation and leg pain.[44,45]

There were 2.4% of patients with various side effects.[46] In 20% to 40% of cases, postinjection back pain and muscle spasm occurred as the most common side effects.[44–46] Chymopapain has not used in the United States since 1999 largely due to a series of patients with severe anaphylactic reactions after injection; nonetheless, this treatment is still common in other parts of the world.[44] The incidence of allergic reaction to chymopapain can be lowered from 1% to 0.3% by using IgE serum sensitivity testing prior to procedure.[47] It also appears that chemonucleolysis performed under local anesthesia lowers the risk of anaphylactic reaction.[48] Serious complications, like transverse myelitis, hemorrhage, and discitis, are rare. The overall morbidity rate related to this procedure is 0.399%, and the mortality rate is 0.02%.[46]

Intradiscal Steroids

It is questionable if there is any clinical benefit from repeated intradiscal steroid injections for the treatment of discogenic lower back pain; nonetheless, this treatment is still used by some practitioners. Observational studies suggest that patients with uncomplicated axial back pain presumed to be of discogenic origin had no long-term improvement in either functional capacity or pain scores.[49,50] However, when intradiscal steroid injections were used in patients with inflammatory end-plate changes, significant short-term improvements in pain scores and functional capacity have been reported.[38,39]

The most frequent and serious complication of such intradiscal steroid injections is formation of epidural calcifications, mainly when triamcinolone hexacetonide is used.[51] On occasion, this complication can first appear many years after an intradiscal injection of this agent.[52] Expanding calcifications become symptomatic in 14% to 68% of patients.[51,52] While this treatment is seldom used, it is important to keep in mind what previous study has revealed about the problems with this seemingly innocuous treatment.

► COMPLICATIONS ASSOCIATED WITH ANNULOPLASTY

The term annuloplasty is meant to refer to a group of minimally invasive procedures that are aimed at treating symptomatic degenerative disc disease. The dense innervation of the outer portion of the annulus fibrosus has been implicated as a cause of ongoing back pain associated with disruption of the outer annulus that appears with progressive disc degeneration. There are a number of different devices used to perform annuloplasty, but all employ some form of thermal energy in efforts to destroy free nerve endings. The incidence of complications during and after various annuloplasty procedures for discogenic pain range from 0% to as high as 10%[53,54] in different reports. These complications can be divided into early (appearing immediately after or within days of the procedure) and late (appearing weeks to months after the procedure) complications. Nerve injuries related to needle placement and/or thermal injuries together with infection, bleeding, and burns are early complications. Late complications include accelerated disc degeneration, vertebral avascular necrosis, and postprocedural disc herniation. Instrument malfunction or breakage during the procedure may also lead to significant injury of neural or vascular structures (Table 29-1). In the sections that follow, we will discuss the complications that have been associated with each specific method for performing percutaneous annuloplasty.

Intradiscal Electrothermal Therapy

Intradiscal electrothermal therapy (IDET) is a minimally invasive procedure in which controlled thermal energy is gradually delivered to the posterior the annulus fibrosus via an intradiscaly placed resistive coil.[55] IDET is performed under fluoroscopic guidance, while the patient is lightly sedated. A 17-gauge introducer needle is first inserted into the anterolateral part of the disc to be treated. The catheter is then threaded along the central aspect of the annulus. The distal part of the catheter is approximately 5 cm in length; once in position, the catheter is gradually heated to 90°C over 16 to 17 minutes. During this procedure, the intradiscal temperatures may range anywhere from 37°C to 65°C.[56] Inappropriate catheter placement and high temperatures delivered to the disc and the surrounding neural structures may cause nerve injury or osteonecrosis of endplate, which would manifest as a radicular pain, axial pain, or transient palsy. These complications, however, may also happen during other percutaneous invasive procedures and are not specific only to IDET. Catheter breakage[57](Figs.s 29-2 and 29-3), vertebral osteonecrosis,[58] and thermal injury to the cauda equina[59] have all been reported as serious complications of IDET. The proposed mechanism leading to catheter breakage and thermal injury to the cauda equine are shown in Figure 29-4. Some of the commonly listed risk factors for postsurgical spinal complications, such as obesity, history of leg pain, smoking, diabetes mellitus, and duration of the back pain, are unlikely to predict higher risk for complications after the IDET.[53] When compared to the nucleoplasty (see further discussion below) alone, frequency of complications was not higher in patients who received IDET combined with the nucleoplasty.[60] A

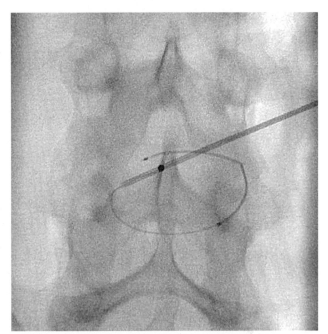

FIGURE 29-2. Repeated attempts to advance the IDET catheter can lead to kinking of the catheter and potential catheter breakage. Fluoroscopic anterior-posterior view combined with cranial tilt of the fluoroscope illustrates the extent of the IDET resistive coil kink.

study by Freeman et al.[54] reported no major complications in 38 patients with chronic discogenic back pain following the IDET. However, four patients had transient radiculopathy that resolved in a period of <6 weeks. In another study, temporary (<6 weeks) radicular signs and symptoms were reported by several patients, one patient complained of a new burning sensation in one leg and another patient had a foot drop. In two patients, nondermatomal paresthesias were present.[57] The paresthesias will occur in a small percentage of patients undergoing the IDET procedure, even when IDET is performed by the most skilled practitioners. Recently, Orr and Thomas published a case report in which an IDET catheter tip was broken off after an intradiscal kink, leaving a fragment of the catheter retained within the disc. The fragment subsequently migrated out of the disc and into the dural sac. The patient presented weeks later complaining of increased back pain, leg paresthesias, and dysesthesias, and the catheter fragment had to be surgically removed.[61] If the catheter is sheared, it should be left within the disc, as the current experience, aside from this one report, suggests a low likelihood for migration leading to need for surgical removal.

Discitis is another potential complication associated with IDET. Depending on the presence or absence of infection, it may be divided in septic or aseptic discitis. While intravenous antibiotics should be given 30 minutes before the procedure (please see discussion on discitis in discography section), intradiscal antibiotics should be administered after the IDET therapy. On withdrawal of the catheter, some authors do recommend an injection of cefazolin and local anesthetic to prevent discitis and ameliorate postprocedural pain.[57]

One of the published IDET studies reported a single case of discitis; this patient presented with increased low back pain, lethargy, night sweats, and spasm.[62] There are no other reports of discitis associated with IDET.

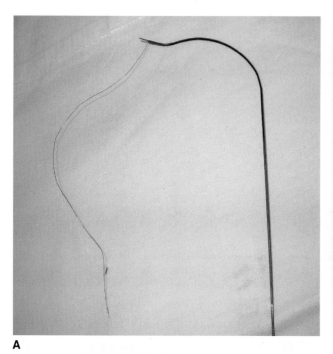

A

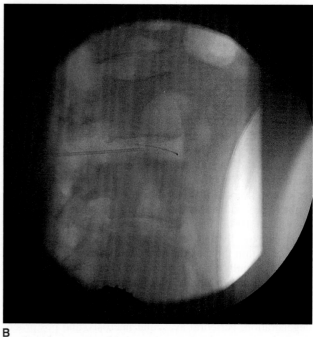

B

FIGURE 29-3. Uncoiled IDET catheter during the removal from the disc. The small uncoiled peace left retained within the posterior annulus. **A:** Uncoiled IDET catheter. **B:** Intradiscally retained uncoiled fragment of the same IDET catheter visible on the fluoroscopic lateral view (the IDET catheter introducer that has not been removed from the disc yet).

Cauda equina syndrome after IDET procedure was reported in one 56-year-old woman[63]; however, this complication may be underreported in the literature. This patient was deeply sedated, and the final IDET coil position was not confirmed in lateral radiographic plane.[63] The proposed mechanism of thermal injury to the cauda equine is extension of the thermal catheter in to the anterior epidural space (Fig. 29-4). The heating protocol that is used to perform IDET uses a slow, ramped increase in the temperature of the catheter. It is unlikely that significant injury can occur even when the catheter is placed too close to the cauda equina, unless the patient is deeply sedated. The awake or lightly sedated patient will report intolerable pain early in the course of treatment, leading to discontinuation or slowing of the IDET treatment.

Postprocedural disc herniation is a rare complication after IDET, with an incidence of 0.3%. This has been speculated to be due to thermally mediated loss of tensile strength of the collagen fibers.[56] Cohen et al.[53] published an episode of complicated disc herniation in a patient with worsening back pain after IDET, and with the MRI showed an increase in size of his disc protrusion at the IDET-treated disc level. However, one should take into consideration the natural progression of disc degeneration—expected changes of lumbar degenerative disc disease include increases in the size of disc protrusions as well as appearance of new disc herniations.

Radiofrequency Annuloplasty

Radiofrequency annuloplasty using the discTRODE (Covidien, Mansfield, MA) is another intradiscal technology used for treatment of discogenic pain that has proven to be ineffective.[64–67] This method employs a novel, flexible radiofrequency electrode that is directly placed within the posterolateral annulus. The electrode placement is guided by both, fluoroscopy and the electrical impedance values. A recent randomized prospective trial proved the discTRODE to be ineffective in improving back pain and function in patients with discogenic lower back pain.[67] There were no complications reported in any of the studies where discTRODE was used,[64–67] but similar considerations discussed for the other intradiscal techniques theoretically apply to this technique.

Intradiscal Biacuplasty

Intradiscal biacuplasty (Kimberly Clark, Atlanta GA) is a novel annuloplasty procedure intended to treat axial discogenic pain.[68–70] Two radiofrequency probes are placed into the disc, one on each side of the posterior annulus. A radiofrequency current is then passed in between the two probes, which allows denervation of the posterior annulus. The hollow lumen of the internally water-cooled probe permits an effective cooling of the electrode, allowing the delivery of greater energy to the annulus while preventing excessive spread of the heat distant from the site of treatment. Internally cooled electrodes can therefore produce much larger lesions compared to conventional electrodes. Up to now, no complications have been reported following annuloplasty using the biacuplasty technique.[68–70] Nonetheless, similar considerations discussed for the other intradiscal techniques theoretically apply to this technique.

▶ COMPLICATIONS ASSOCIATED WITH PERCUTANEOUS DISC DECOMPRESSION

Hijikata et al.[71] first reported the use of this minimally invasive, percutaneous surgical technique for the treatment of

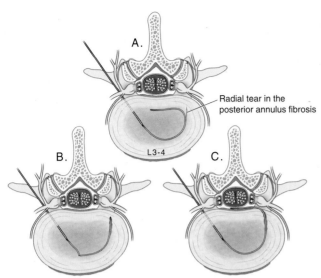

FIGURE 29-4. Mechanism that leads to catheter breakage and thermal injury to the cauda equina during IDET. A: Catheter in good position for IDET treatment with the thermally active portion of the catheter (*shaded*) along the inner aspect of the posterior annulus fibrosis. **B:** Radial tears that extend from the nucleus pulposus into the annulus fibrosis are common in patients with degenerative disc disease. The IDET catheter often extends into one or more of these radial tears during placement. Repeated attempts to forcibly advance the IDET catheter can lead to kinking of the catheter and catheter breakage. **C:** Radial tears can extend from the nucleus pulposus all the way to the outer limit of the annulus fibrosis. The IDET catheter can advance through a radial tear in the annulus and out into the anterior epidural space, where the catheter will lie in close proximity to the cauda equina. IDET treatment with the catheter in this position can cause direct thermal injury to the cauda equina.

disc herniation/protrusion in 1975. PDD collectively refers to any technique that can effectively remove a portion of the central nucleus pulposus, thereby reducing intradiscal pressure. Technically, chemonucleolysis (discussed above) is a form of PDD. In contrast to annuloplasty, which is designed to treat axial low back pain associated with disc degeneration, PDD is designed primarily to treat persistent radicular pain (leg pain) associated with small disc protrusions. Numerous procedures and several technologies have been described using either mechanical removal of the nuclear volume or delivery of heat to the nucleus in order to reduce intradiscal pressure, thereby allowing the disc protrusion to fall away from the adjacent spinal nerve and in this way eliminate radicular pain. Perioperative and postoperative complications related to those techniques are described below.

Automated Percutaneous Lumbar Decompression

Automated percutaneous disc decompression (APLD), using the Nucleotome (Clarus Medical, LLC, Minneapolis, MN) system, is performed in efforts to mechanically remove a portion of the central nucleus pulposus.[72–74] A side-shaving port with a blunt tip similar to devices used for meniscectomy during arthroscopic procedures is introduced through a cannula and placed within the nucleus in order to remove nuclear material. A small forceps is then placed through the same working cannula in order to remove residual fragments of disc material. Transient myofascial back pain is common in patients recovering from APLD at the site of cannula placement. Rarely, nerve damage, discitis, and bleeding can occur.

The incidence of discitis after APLD is 0.18%, and the incidence of paraspinous hematoma is about 0.09%.[75] The rate of overall complications is 1%. An initial controlled multicenter study reported only one case of discitis, one case of transient paresthesias, and one case of bleeding into the psoas muscle using this technique.[76] The frequency of discitis was even lower, occurring in nine out of 1,525 patients (0.06%) in another large study.[77] Finally, there were two cases of cauda equina syndrome reported following APLD in patients who were heavily sedated during the procedure.[78,79] The APLD technique was the earliest PDD technique developed and underwent extensive validation studies; from this early work, the limits of PDD were clearly established. Much of the early work on PDD enrolled patients with large disc herniations, including those with extruded disc fragments. These patients did not improve following APLD, rather only those with small, contained disc herniations or disc protrusions are likely to respond to APLD or any of the other PDD techniques. It is generally accepted that heavy sedation and general anesthesia should be not provided during interventional percutaneous spinal procedures because of possibly masking immediate clinical signs and symptoms.

Minimally Invasive Disc Removal

Minimally invasive disc removal with the Dekompressor (Stryker Medical, Kalamazoo, MI) device consists of battery-powered rotary cutting device that employs Archimedes principle to remove a portion of the central nucleus pulposus through a small-diameter cannula. The concept is identical to the APLD technique, but simply employs a different means to mechanically remove the nuclear material. The cannula serves as a channel for the tissue removal. The procedure is performed using the fluoroscopic guidance and under a mild sedation. Two clinical case series reported no complications when the Decompressor was used for treatment of small, contained disc protrusions. The procedure was either computed tomography or fluoroscopy guided and performed under local anesthesia.[80,81] More recently, Dekompressor probe breakage within the target disc has been described.[82]

Percutaneous Laser Disc Decompression

Laser technology has been used for over 20 years to decompress the nucleus pulposus of the lumbar discs in patients with small, contained disc herniations. The probe design used for percutaneous laser disc decompression (PLDD) was modified over the years, and the introducer diameter is smaller today than it was when the first such procedure was conducted in 1986. The mechanism of action is similar to other technologies, relying on vaporization of the nucleus pulposus rather than mechanical removal. The laser probe is placed within the disc by passing through the posterior annulus fibrosus. The probe is large and raises concern about progression of degenerative disc disease and possibly of worsening back pain following treatment.[43] Discitis and osteomyelitis are rarely seen complications of PLDD procedure.[83–85] Such complications may be subdivided into septic and aseptic, based on the presence of microorganisms.

Injuries to the nerve roots or vascular structures are even less common.[83] Two studies reported single case of discitis, one in 577 treated discs[83] and another one in the group of 200 patients during follow up over 4 years after the procedure.[84] A case of causalgia was also reported as a complication after the laser PLDD, presumably due to either mechanical or thermal injury to the spinal nerve adjacent to the treated disc.[86]

Nucleoplasty

Nucleoplasty utilizes Coblation technology (ArthroCare Corporation, Austin, Texas), providing ablation and coagulation of the nucleus pulposus to decompress the disc and decrease the size of the contained disc herniation.[87] It may be that the extent of such decompression is minimal as in markedly degenerated discs, and a therapeutic effect is more likely in those with nondegenerated discs.[88] During nucleoplasty, a coblation treatment catheter is advanced through an introducer cannula to the nuclear-annular interface. The catheter is then slowly advanced while a radiofrequency energy is delivered through a specially designed catheter.[89,90] A localized energy field is created at the tip of the treatment catheter, causing formation of a high-energy plasma that vaporizes a small volume of tissue within the nucleus, thereby decreasing intradiscal pressure.

The most comprehensive study on the incidence of various complications after nucleoplasty reported as short-term side effects soreness at the needle insertion site (76%) followed by the presence of mild numbness and tingling in the painful extremities of 26% of the patients. Others reported either increased intensity of preexisting back pain (15%) or new areas of back pain (15%), but side effects resolved within 2 weeks of the procedure in the majority of patients. Mild numbness and tingling persisted in 15% and increased back pain in 4% of treated patients.[91] In a recent prospective, randomized multicenter trial, nucleoplasty was compared with repeat transforaminal injections for treating 90 patients with persistent leg pain associated with small lumbar disc protrusions.[92] Those patients treated with nulceoplasty had significantly reduced pain and better quality of life scores than those treated using repeated transforaminal injections, with improvement persisting to 2-years of follow-up. Procedure-related adverse events, including injection site pain, increased leg or back pain, weakness, and lightheadedness, were observed in five patients in the nucleoplasty group (7 events) and seven in the transforaminal group (14 events). The collective experience with nucleoplasty suggests that adverse events are typically mild and self-limited. Nonetheless, all of the PDD techniques carry theoretical risks of complications that are similar to those discussed for other intradiscal techniques.

▶ SUMMARY

Serious complications following percutaneous intradiscal procedures for back or leg pain are well described, but infrequent. Discitis and other infections are the most serious complications seen after discography, IDET, and different forms of PDD. Heavy sedation and general anesthesia may expose patients to added risk of neurologic injury when these techniques are performed by removing their ability to report pain and discomfort when neural structures are being compromised. Hemorrhagic complications are rare and typically occur as a consequence of concomitant anticoagulant use or in those with previously unknown hemorrhagic disorders.

References

1. Hurri H, Karppinen J. Discogenic pain. *Pain* 2004;112(3): 225–228.
2. Kapural L. Indications for minimally invasive disk and vertebral procedures. *Pain Med* 2008;9(S1):S65–S72.
3. Cassinelli EH, Hall RA, Kang JD. Biochemistry of intervertebral disc degeneration and the potential for gene therapy applications. *Spine J* 2001;1(3):205–214.
4. Freemont AJ. The cellular pathobiology of the degenerate intervertebral disc and discogenic back pain. *Rheumatology* 2009;48:5–10.
5. Kapural L, Cata J. Complications of minimally invasive procedures for discogenic pain. *Tech Reg Anesth Pain Med* 2007;11(3):-157–163.
6. Carragee EJ, Alamin TF, Carragee JM. Low-pressure positive discography in subjects asymptomatic of significant low back pain illness. *Spine* 2006;31(5):505–509.
7. Carragee EJ, Lincoln T, Parmar VS, et al. A gold standard evaluation of the "discogenic pain" diagnosis as determined by provocative discography. *Spine* 2006;31(18):2115–2123.
8. Derby R, Howard MW, Grant JM, et al. The ability of pressure-controlled discography to predict surgical and nonsurgical outcomes. *Spine* 1999;24:364–371.
9. Guyer RD, Ohnmeiss DD. Lumbar discography. *Spine J* 2003; 3:11S–27S.
10. Derby R, Lee SH, Kim BJ, et al. Pressure-controlled lumbar discography in volunteers without low back pain symptoms. *Pain Med* 2005;6(3):213–221.
11. Derby R, Lee SH, Kim BJ, et al. Comparison of discogenic findings in asymptomatic subject discs and the negative discs of chronic low back pain patients: can discography distinguish asymptomatic discs among morphologically abnormal disc? *Spine J* 2005;5(4):389–394.
12. Kapural L, Goyle A. Imaging for provocative discography and minimally invasive percutaneous procedures for discogenic pain. *Tech Reg Anesth Pain Med* 2007;11(2):73–80.
13. Poynton AR, Hinman A, Lutz G. Discography-induced acute lumbar disc herniation: a report of five cases. *J Spinal Disord Tech* 2005;18:188–192.
14. Tehranzadeh J. Discography 2000. *Radiol Clin North Am* 1998;36:463–495.
15. Willems PC, Jacobs W, Duinkerke ES, et al. Lumbar discography: should we use prophylactic antibiotics? A study of 435 consecutive discograms and a systematic review of the literature. *J Spinal Disord Tech* 2004;17:243–247.
16. Hoelscher GL, Gruber HE, Coldham G, et al. Effects of very high antibiotic concentrations on human intervertebral disc cell proliferation, viability, and metabolism in vitro. *Spine* 2000;25:1871–1877.
17. Guyer RD, Ohnmeiss DD. Lumbar discography. Position statement from the North American Spine Society Diagnostic and Therapeutic Committee. *Spine* 1995;20:2048–2059.
18. Fraser RD, Osti OL, Vernon-Roberts B. Discitis after discography. *J Bone Joint Surg Br* 1987;69:26–35.
19. Guyer RD, Collier R, Stith WJ, et al. Discitis after discography. *Spine* 1988;13:1352–1354.
20. Klessig HT, Showsh SA, Sekorski A. The use of intradiscal antibiotics for discography: an in vitro study of gentamicin, cefazolin, and clindamycin. *Spine* 2003;28:1735–1738.
21. Esimont FJ, Wiesel SW, Brighton CT, et al. Antibiotic penetration into rabbit nucleus pulposus. *Spine* 1987;12:254–256.

22. Thomas RW, Batten JJ, Want S, et al. A new in-vitro model to investigate antibiotic penetration of the intervertebral disc. *J Bone Joint Surg Br* 1995;77:967–970.

23. Rhoten RL, Murphy MA, Kalfas IH, et al. Antibiotic penetration into cervical discs. *Spine* 1995;37:418–421.

24. Boscardin JB, Ringus JC, Feingold DJ, et al. Human intradiscal levels with cefazolin. *Spine* 1992;17:S145–S148.

25. Maezawa S, Muro T. Pain provocation at lumbar discography as analyzed by computed tomography/discography. *Spine* 1992;17(11):1309–1315.

26. Osti OL, Fraser RD, Vernon-Roberts B. Discitis after discography. The role of prophylactic antibiotics. *J Bone Joint Surg Br* 1990;72:271–274.

27. Zeidman SJ, Thompson K, Ducker TB. Complications of cervical discography: analysis of 4400 diagnostic disc injections. *Neurosurgery* 1995;37:414.

28. Connor PM, Darden BV II. Cervical discography complications and clinical efficacy. *Spine* 1993;18:2035–2038.

29. Guyer RD, Ohnmeiss DD, Mason SL, et al. Complications of cervical discography: findings in a large series. *J Spinal Disord* 1997;10:95–101.

30. Wood KB, Schellhas KP, Garvey TA, et al. Thoracic discography in healthy individuals. A controlled prospective study of magnetic resonance imaging and discography in asymptomatic and symptomatic individuals. *Spine* 1999;24:1548–1555.

31. Bogduk N. Lumbar disc stimulation. In: Bogduk, N, ed. *Practice Guidelines for Spinal Diagnostic and Treatment Procedures.* San Francisco, CA: International Spine Intervention Society, 2004.

32. Modic MT, et al. Vertebral osteomyelitis: assessment using MR. *Radiology* 1985;157(1):157–166.

33. Ledermann HP, et al. MR imaging findings in spinal infections: rules or myths? *Radiology* 2003;228(2):506–514.

34. Aprill C. Diagnostic disc injections. In: Aprill C, ed. *The Adult Spine: Principles and Practice.* Philadelphia, PA: Lippincott-Raven, 1997:523–538.

35. Ravicovitch MA, Spallone A. Spinal epidural abscesses. Surgical and parasurgical management. *Eur Neurol* 1982;21(5):347–357.

36. Lownie SP, Ferguson GG. Spinal subdural empyema complicating cervical discography. *Spine* 1989;14(12):1415–1417.

37. Junila J, Niinimaki T, Tervonen O. Epidural abscess after lumbar discography. A case report. *Spine* 1997;22:2191–2193.

38. Bernard TNJ. Lumbar discography followed by computed tomography. Refining the diagnosis of low-back pain. *Spine* 1990;15:690–707.

39. Holt EP. The question of lumbar discography. *J Bone Joint Surg Am* 1968;50(4):720–726.

40. Carragee EJ, et al. Provocative discography in patients after limited lumbar discectomy: a controlled, randomized study of pain response in symptomatic and asymptomatic subjects. *Spine* 2000;25(23):3065–3071.

41. Ketterer MW, Buckholtz CD. Somatization disorder. *J Am Osteopath Assoc* 1989;89(4):489–490, 495.

42. Carragee EJ, Don AS, Hurwitz EL, et al. Does discography cause accelerated progression of degeneration changes in the lumbar disc: a ten-year matched cohort study. *Spine (Phila Pa 1976)* 2009;34:2338–2345.

43. Alamin T, Arawal V, Carragee EJ. Fad versus provocative discography: comparative results and post-operative clinical outcomes. Proceedings of the NASS 22nd annual meeting. *Spine J* 2007;7:39S–40S.

44. Maroon JC. Current concepts in minimally invasive discectomy. *Neurosurgery* 2002;51(5 suppl):137–145.

45. Brown MD. Update on chemonucleolysis. *Spine* 1996;21(24 suppl):S62–S68.

46. Nordby EJ, Wright PH, Schofield SR. Safety of chemonucleolysis. Adverse effects reported in the United States, 1982–1991. *Clin Orthop* 1993;293:122–134.

47. Agre K, Wilson RR, Brim M, et al. Chymodiactin postmarketing surveillance. Demographic and adverse experience data in 29,075 patients. *Spine* 1984;9(5):479–485.

48. Hall BB, McCulloch JA. Anaphylactic reactions following the intradiscal injection of chymopapain under local anesthesia. *J Bone Joint Surg* 1983;65(9):1215–1219.

49. Simmons JW, McMillin JN, Emery SF, et al. Intradiscal steroids. A prospective double-blind clinical trial. *Spine* 1992;17:S172–S175.

50. Khot A, Bowditch M, Powell J, et al. The use of intradiscal steroid therapy for lumbar spinal discogenic pain: a randomized controlled trial. *Spine* 2004;29:833–836.

51. Duquesnoy B, Debiais F, Heuline A, et al. Unsatisfactory results of intradiscal injection of triamcinolone hexacetonide in the treatment of sciatica caused by intervertebral disk herniation. *Presse Med* 1992;21:1801–1804.

52. Darmoul M, Bouhaouala MH, Rezgui M. Calcification following intradiscal injection, a continuing problem? *Presse Med* 2005;34:859–860.

53. Cohen SP, Larkin T, Abdi S, et al. Risk factors for failure and complications of intradiscal electrothermal therapy: a pilot study. *Spine* 2003;28:1142–1147.

54. Freeman BJ, Fraser RD, Cain CM, et al. A randomized, double-blind, controlled trial: intradiscal electrothermal therapy versus placebo for the treatment of chronic discogenic low back pain. *Spine* 2005;30:2369–2377.

55. Saal JA, Saal JS. Intradiscal electrothermal treatment for chronic discogenic low back pain: a prospective outcome study with minimum 1-year follow-up. *Spine* 2000;25:2622–2627.

56. Kleinstueck FS, Diederich CJ, Nau WH, et al. Acute biomechanical and histological effects of intradiscal electrothermal therapy on human lumbar discs. *Spine* 2001;26:2198–2207.

57. Biyani A, Andersson GB, Chaudhary H, et al. Intradiscal electrothermal therapy: a treatment option in patients with internal disc disruption. *Spine* 2003;28:S8–S14.

58. Djurasovic M, Glassman SD, Dimar JR, et al. Vertebral osteonecrosis associated with the use of intradiscal electrothermal therapy: a case report. *Spine* 2002;27:E325–E328.

59. Wetzel FT. Cauda equina syndrome from intradiscal electrothermal therapy. *Neurology* 2001;56:1607.

60. Cohen SP, Williams S, Kurihara C, et al: Nucleoplasty with or without intradiscal electrothermal therapy (IDET) as a treatment for lumbar herniated disc. *J Spinal Disord Tech* 2005;18:S119–S124.

61. Orr RD, Thomas SA. Intradural migration of broken IDET catheter causing a radiculopathy. *J Spinal Disord Tech* 2005;18:185–187.

62. Davis TT, Delamarter RB, Sra P, et al. The IDET procedure for chronic discogenic low back pain. *Spine* 2004;29:752–756.

63. Hsia AW, Isaac K, Katz JS. Cauda equina syndrome from intradiscal electrothermal therapy. *Neurology* 2000;55:320.

64. Finch PM, Price LM, Drummond PD. Radiofrequency heating of painful annular disruptions: one-year outcomes. *J Spinal Disord Tech* 2005;18:6–13.

65. Erdine S, Yucel A, Celik M. Percutaneous annuloplasty in the treatment of discogenic pain: retrospective evaluation of one year follow-up. *Agri* 2004;16:41–47.

66. Kapural L, Hayek S, Malak O, et al. Intradiscal thermal annuloplasty ersus intradiscal radiofrequency ablation for the treatment of discogenic pain: a prospective matched control trial. *Pain Med* 2005;6:425–431.

67. Kvarstein G, Mawe L, Indahl A, et al. A randomized double-blind controlled trial of intra-annular radiofrequency thermal disc therapy-A 12-month follow-up. *Pain* 2009;145:279–286.

68. Kapural L, Mekhail N, Sloan S, et al. Histological and temperature distribution studies in the lumbar degenerated and non-degenerated human cadaver discs using novel transdiscal radiofrequency electrodes. *Pain Med* 2008;9(1):68–75.

69. Kapural L, De la Garza M, Ng A, et al. Novel transdiscal biacuplasty for the treatment of lumbar discogenic pain: a 6 months follow-up. *Pain Med* 2008;9(1):60–67.

70. Kapural L. Intervertebral disc cooled bipolar radiofrequency (intradiscal biacuplasty) for the treatment of lumbar discogenic pain: a 12 month follow-up of the pilot study. *Pain Med* 2008;9(4):464.

71. Hijikata S, Yamagishi M, Nakagama T, et al. Percutaneous discectomy: a new treatment method for lumbar disc herniation. *J Toden Hops* 1975;5:5–13.

72. Onik G, Helms CA, Ginsburg LH, et al. Percutaneous lumbar diskectomy using a new aspiration probe. *AJR Am J Roentgenol* 1985;144:1137–1140.

73. Onik G, Maroon J, Davis GW. Automated percutaneous discectomy at the L5-S1 level. Use of a curved cannula. *Clin Orthop Relat Res* 1989;238:71–76.

74. Sortland O, Kleppe H, Aandahl M, et al. Percutaneous lumbar discectomy. Techinque and clinical result. *Acta Radiol* 1996;37:85–90.

75. Maroon JC, Allen R. A retrospective study of 1054 APLD cases: a twenty month clinical follow-up. *J Neurol Orthop Med Surg* 1989;10:335–337.

76. Onik G, Mooney V, Maroon JC, et al. Automated percutaneous discectomy: a prospective multi-institutional study. *Neurosurgery* 1990;26:228–232.

77. Teng GJ, Jeffery RF, Guo JH, et al. Automated percutaneous lumbar discectomy: a prospective multi-institutional study. *J Vasc Interv Radiol* 1997;8:457–463.

78. Onik G, Maroon JC, Jackson R. Cauda equina syndrome secondary to an improperly placed nucleotome probe. *Neurosurgery* 1992;30:412–414.

79. Epstein NE. Surgically confirmed cauda equina and nerve root injury following percutaneous discectomy at an outside institution: a case report. *J Spinal Disord* 1990;3:380–382.

80. Amoretti N, Huchot F, Flory P, et al. Percutaneous nucleotomy: preliminary communication on a decompression probe (dekompressor) in percutaneous discectomy. Ten case reports. *Clin Imaging* 2005;29:98–101.

81. Alo KM, Wright RE, Sutcliffe J, et al. Percutaneous lumbar discectomy: clinical response in an initial cohort of fifty consecutive patients with chronic radicular pain. *Pain Pract* 2004;4:19–29.

82. Domsky R, Goldberg ME, Hirsh RA, et al. Critical failure of a percutaneous discectomy probe requiring surgical removal during disc decompression. *Reg Anesth Pain Med* 2006;31:177–179.

83. Quigley MR. Percutaneous laser discectomy. [review] [17 refs]. *Neurosurg Clin N Am* 1996;7:37–42.

84. Gronemeyer DH, Buschkamp H, Braun M, et al. Image-guided percutaneous laser disk decompression for herniated lumbar disks: a 4-year follow-up in 200 patients. *J Clin Laser Med Surg* 2003;21:131–138.

85. Farrar MJ, Walker A, Cowling P. Possible Salmonella osteomyelitis of spine following laser disc decompression. *Eur Spine J* 1998;7:509–511.

86. Plancarte R, Calvillo O. Complex regional pain syndrome type 2 (causalgia) after automated laser discectomy. A case report. *Spine* 1997;22:459–461.

87. Chen YC, Lee SH, Saenz Y, et al. Histologic findings of disc, end plate and neural elements after coblation of nucleus pulposus: an experimental nucleoplasty study. *Spine J* 2003;3:466–470.

88. Chen YC, Lee SH, Chen D. Intradiscal pressure study of percutaneous disc decompression with nucleoplasty in human cadavers. *Spine* 2003;28:661–665.

89. Sharps LS, Zacharia I. Percutaneous disc decompression using nucleoplasty. *Pain Phys* 2002;5:121–126.

90. Singh V, Piryani C, Liao K. Percutaneous disc decompression using coblation (nucleoplasty) in the treatment of chronic discogenic pain. *Pain Phys* 2002;5:250.

91. Bhagia SM, Slipman CW, Nirschl M, et al. Side effects and complications after percutaneous disc decompression using coblation technology. *Am J Phys Med Rehabil* 2006;85:6–11.

92. Gerszten PC, Smuck M, Rathmell JP, et al. Plasma disc decompression compared with fluoroscopy-guided transforaminal epidural steroid injections for symptomatic contained lumbar disc herniation: a prospective, randomized, controlled trial. *J Neurosurg Spine* 2010;12:357–371.

30

The Role of Image Guidance in Improving the Safety of Pain Treatment

James P. Rathmell and Smith C. Manion

Just over a decade ago, radiographic guidance was used infrequently in the pain clinic—it was reserved for major procedures like neurolytic celiac plexus block. In more recent years, at least two forces have been at work, which have led to the widespread use of imaging modalities in the field of pain medicine. First, pain practitioners are now being called on to serve as diagnosticians. Patients and referring practitioners expect pain physicians to have familiarity with imaging modalities and their usefulness in diagnosing pain conditions. At the same time, pain practitioners have come to realize the usefulness of radiographic guidance in achieving precise anatomic placement of needles and catheters. Although the evidence supporting the need for routine radiographic guidance is still evolving, the intuitive appeal of this more precise approach has caught firm hold—to the point where the majority of practitioners now perform most of their injections using fluoroscopic guidance. In some cases, such as patients with intractable pain associated with metastatic cancer, diagnostic imaging studies have proven invaluable in the planning and implementation of therapy directed toward pain relief. Despite the intuitive appeal of the precise anatomic information relayed by diagnostic imaging studies and the use of fluoroscopy, computed tomography (CT), and, most recently, the use of ultrasound in the pain clinic, there is scant evidence that this approach improves the safety or efficacy of pain treatment. In this chapter, we review the available evidence that examines the usefulness of diagnostic imaging and image guidance in planning and implementing pain treatment.

▶ DEFINITION AND SCOPE

Use of Diagnostic Imaging to Improve Safety

Diagnostic imaging is used broadly across all of medical practice to investigate the anatomic basis for new onset of many symptoms indicative of disease, and pain is one of the most common of those presenting symptoms. Indeed, diagnostic imaging is the cornerstone of establishing anatomic diagnoses responsible for pain, such as new onset of radicular pain associated with intervertebral disc herniation. A broad discussion of the use of diagnostic imaging is beyond the scope of this chapter, but several directed examples where diagnostic imaging can provide critical information in planning treatment will be reviewed.

There is moderate evidence from controlled trials that epidural injection of steroids can speed the resolution of radicular pain in the early months after acute lumbar disc herniations.[1-3] The technique is now in widespread use. By extension from the evidence for lumbar disc herniation, this technique has also been used to treat radicular pain associated with thoracic and cervical disc herniations as well as pain associated with spinal stenosis. Two decades ago, use of diagnostic imaging to establish the exact anatomic level of disc herniation was becoming more commonplace. However, most practitioners actually performing epidural injections were doing so without expertise in interpreting these imaging studies, and they were most commonly using the blind loss-of-resistance technique to identify the epidural space.[4] Based on little scientific evidence, conventional wisdom at that time held that the injection should be placed at the level of the disc herniation to produce the best benefit. Thus, many practitioners simply placed these epidural injections based on the radiologists report: if there was a disc herniation at the C6/7 level, then the injection was placed at that level. Reports of spinal cord injury occurring during these injections began to appear, and the connection between contact with the spinal

cord and high-grade spinal stenosis was established.[4] Indeed, in high-grade stenosis of the central spinal canal arising from any cause, there may be complete effacement of the CSF and epidural fat, with direct pressure on the spinal cord. This is precisely the case in a small proportion of patients with large disc herniations (Fig. 30-1). In these cases, it is critical to recognize the lack of adequate room in the posterior epidural space to allow for safe needle entry and placement of the epidural steroid. Thus the use of diagnostic imaging and review of the images prior to attempting epidural injection is now routine. When there is severe canal stenosis, injection at the stenotic levels can be readily avoided by using fluoroscopy to precisely guide needle placement at an anatomic level where prior diagnostic imaging has demonstrated adequate room for needle entry.

Neurolytic celiac plexus block is another technique that has moderate scientific evidence from controlled trials supporting the ability to reduce pain and the need for analgesic use in patients with pain associated with intra-abdominal malignancies, particularly pancreatic cancer. The complications associated with this technique have been detailed in Chapter 23 and include renal trauma, trauma to the large vessels of the abdomen, and pneumothorax. The use of diagnostic imaging for identification and staging of pancreatic

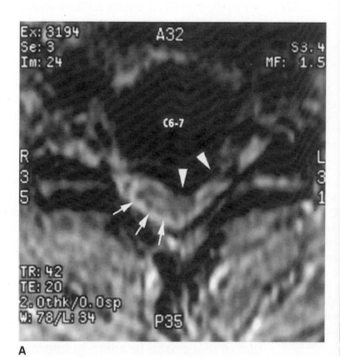

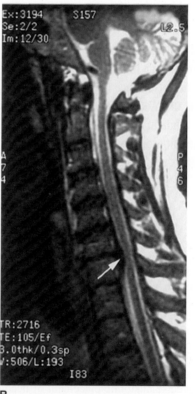

A   **B**

FIGURE 30-1. Cervical MRI in a patient with a large C6/7 disc herniation that causes significant stenosis of the central spinal canal. This patient developed neuropathic pain suggestive of minor spinal cord injury during epidural steroid injection conducted using a blind technique at the C6/7 level. Review of diagnostic imaging studies before injection would have identified this high-grade stenosis and use of fluoroscopy to select an intervertebral level where the stenosis was less severe may have prevented this injury. **A:** Axial T1-weighted magnetic resonance image at the C6/7 level. There is a large central herniated intervertebral disk that lateralizes to the left (*arrowheads*). The spinal cord is displaced toward the right posterior portion of the spinal canal (*arrows*). **B:** Sagittal T2-weighted image at the midline of the cervical spine. There is a large disk herniation at the C6/7 level, causing posterior displacement of the spinal cord (*arrow*) and effacement of the cerebrospinal fluid signal anterior to the spinal cord. (Reproduced from Field J, Rathmell JP, Stephenson JH, et al. Neuropathic pain following cervical epidural steroid injection. *Anesthesiology* 2000;93:885–888, with permission.)

cancer is standard practice worldwide; thus, these detailed anatomic studies are almost universally available at the time patients are referred for celiac plexus neurolysis. Close analysis of the diagnostic studies can assist in the planning stages to guide the spinal level of needle entry as well as the angle and depth of needle penetration. These planning measurements can be easily made on the diagnostic images and used to guide optimal needle placement during celiac plexus block done subsequently using either CT of fluoroscopy for guidance (Fig. 30-2). In this way, existing diagnostic studies can be used in the planning stages to avoid adjacent structures, thereby improving safety.

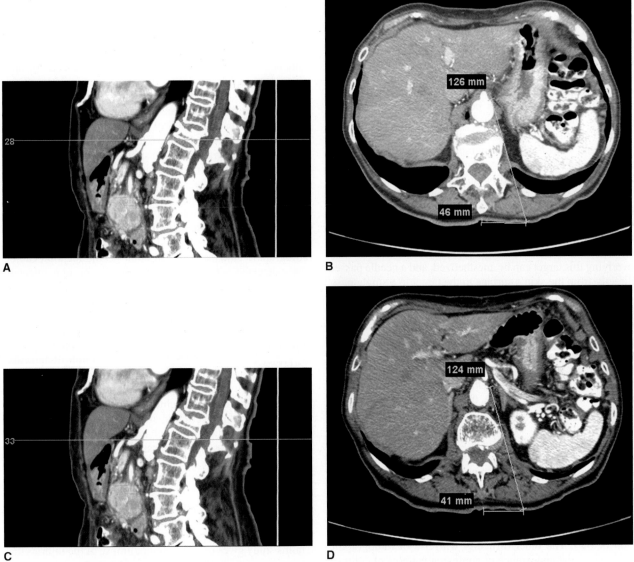

FIGURE 30-2. **Use of diagnostic CT angiography study of the abdomen in a patient referred for celiac plexus block to plan position and depth of needle placement.** The diagnostic CT angiogram can be used to determine the safest position to place needles and plan the final depth on needle insertion; these measurements can then be used to carry out the block with either fluoroscopy or CT guidance. **A:** Sagittal image through the celiac artery. The celiac artery arises from the aorta at the junction between the L1 and L2 vertebrae. This patient has a vertebral compression fracture of the L1 vertebral body. The line through this image corresponds with the axial image in Figure 30-2B. **B:** Axial image through the origin of the celiac artery from the anterior aorta, the typical site for celiac plexus block. Modern CT imaging software can be used to measure the distance from the anterolateral surface of the aorta to the skin surface (126 mm) and from the spinous process to the point of needle entry (46 mm). This patient has significant flattening of the diaphragms from chronic obstructive pulmonary disease. Performing the celiac plexus block at the level of L1 as shown will result in the needle traversing the pleura en route to the anterolateral surface of the aorta and is likely to result in a pneumothorax. **C:** Sagittal image 1 cm inferior to the origin of the celiac artery. The line through this image corresponds with the axial image in Figure 30-2D. **D:** Axial image 1 cm inferior to the origin of the celiac artery from the anterior aorta, below the inferior reflections of the pleura. The distance from the anterolateral surface of the aorta to the skin surface (124 mm) and from the spinous process to the point of needle entry (41 mm); similar measurements can be made for placement of the needle on the right side. Performing the celiac plexus block somewhat inferior to the celiac artery in this patient was carried out successfully: the needles were well below the pleura at this level.

Use of Image Guidance to Improve Safety

The earliest studies that point toward the superiority of image guidance in increasing the precision of epidural localization examine the success of the blind technique. One of the most quoted studies appeared in 1980 and demonstrated that using a blind technique correctly identified the epidural space when using the loss of resistance technique in only 30% of cases.[5] This study has been criticized, as the injectionists in the study were not frequent users of the loss of resistance technique. Indeed, when experienced physicians placed epidurals in the setting of labor and delivery, the success rose to 61.7% in comparison to a success rate of 47.7% in those who had performed <10 epidural injections previously.[6] In contrast, subsequent investigators reported a successful epidural injection in 97.5% of cases performed using fluoroscopic guidance and the caudal route.[7] Radiographic guidance can be used to display images in multiple planes at all spinal levels, and with use of radiographic contrast, the epidural space can be identified the vast majority of time (Figs. 30-3 and 30-4). The use of radiographic guidance using a coaxial technique can certainly improve the precision of needle placement, reducing or eliminating the need for redirection of the needle to reach the epidural space.[8] By aligning the axis of the x-ray beam with the final radiographic target—for example, the epidural space in the midline—the skin directly overlying this target can be anesthetized, and a needle passed directly from the skin's surface to the target in a single pass. Anteroposterior radiographs demonstrate the needle position from lateral to medial and cephalad to caudad; lateral radiographs demonstrate the needle's depth from the skin's surface (Figs. 30-3 and 30-4). However, only bony structures can be identified using fluoroscopy; thus, final needle advancement into the epidural space still requires use of the loss-of-resistance technique. Once the needle is in final position within the epidural space, the location can be confirmed by injecting a small volume of radiographic contrast. If the contrast spreads in a characteristic pattern without evidence of flow into a vascular structure, then the epidural location can be confirmed (Fig. 30-5). However, identification of intravascular needle location using fluoroscopy requires use of a live or real-time technique rather than single static images, as any contrast that flows into a blood vessel will be carried away within the blood stream and will no longer be seen on static images taken subsequently (see further discussion below). The other difficulty with use of radiographic guidance is the appearance of confusing patterns of contrast spread, particularly in patients who have had prior surgery and have fusion masses along the bony spine or scarring in the epidural space; we will discuss these problems in detail below. Thus, it is clear that the use of radiographic guidance does not *assure* the safety of image-guided injections, but the use of these techniques has strong intellectual appeal, indeed strong face validity as a means to improve safety: if you can directly visualize or more precisely infer the position of critical structures like blood vessels and the spinal cord, then it stands to reason that these structures can be avoided with the use of image guidance. Nonetheless, images can be confusing, practitioners have varying levels of skill, and despite the intuitive appeal of this approach, there is little evidence to support improved safety with image guidance. Indeed, in a recent study published by the American Society of Anesthesiologists (ASA) that examined closed malpractice claims, a subgroup of patients who sustained spinal cord injuries during the course of cervical spinal injections were examined in detail.[9] The use of radiographic guidance *was more common* in those who sustained spinal cord injuries than in those who had cervical procedures performed without radiographic guidance. It is tempting to jump to the conclusion that radiographic guidance made spinal cord injury more likely. However, it is equally plausible that the types of injections that led to spinal cord injury (in this case, cervical epidural steroid injection using an interlaminar technique) were simply done more often with radiographic guidance—thus the higher proportion of injuries associated with radiographic guidance. Without knowing how many total injections were done with and without radiographic guidance, we have no means to know the actual incidence of injury with each method of performing these injections. Nonetheless, the ASA Closed Claims report clearly demonstrates that direct trauma to the spinal cord can occur during the conduct of transforaminal injections, interlaminar epidural injections, and trigger point injections carried out at the level of the cervical spine even when image guidance is used.

Intravascular injection can lead to local anesthetic toxicity or catastrophic neural injuries to the brain or spinal cord, when particulate steroid is in use. With proper use of radiographic guidance, intravascular needle location can be easily detected *before* local anesthetic or steroid is injected; thus, use of radiographic guidance may well improve safety. The incidence of intravascular needle location exceeds 20% during cervical transforaminal injection,[10,11] and it is unclear what proportion of these injections are intravenous versus intra-arterial.[12] Use of digital subtraction technology appears to further increase the likelihood of detection of intravascular injection.[13] While intravascular injection is common during cervical transforaminal injection, the incidence during other pain treatment techniques is unclear. Nonetheless, the proximity of the vertebral artery during stellate ganglion block and the aorta during celiac plexus block make intra-arterial injection a distinct possibility, and means to detect intra-arterial needle location *before* injection of local anesthetic or steroid must be a routine part of performing these techniques.

It is impossible to gain any real estimate of the incidence of injuries occurring during the course of pain treatment, as there is no direct reporting mechanism. The ASA Closed Claims study gives us just a small glimpse of the injuries that can occur, with or without image guidance. Nonetheless, the incidence of these injuries appears to be exceedingly low, likely less than 1 in 10,000 injections and perhaps significantly lower; while it is difficult to estimate this risk with accuracy, in 2006, nearly 800,000 Medicare patients in the United States[14] received epidural injections and catastrophic neural injuries on record number <100 in total. What is quite clear from published studies is that the use of common injections for pain treatment has risen exponentially in the United States during the last decade[14] and that use of fluoroscopy to guide needle placement during these treatments is the rule rather than the exception. We are in desperate need of large-scale studies that examine the frequency of use of these treatments and their safety and effectiveness to guide practitioners in making rational decisions about using these techniques.

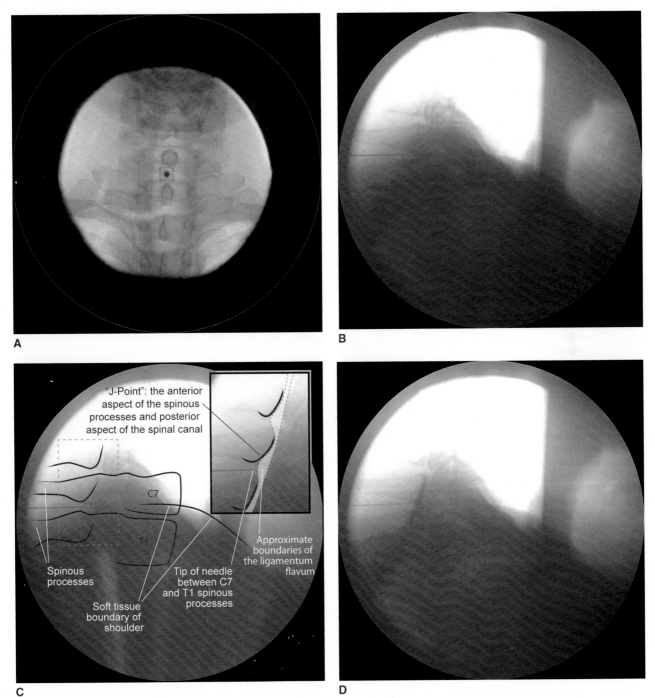

FIGURE 30-3. Radiographic identification of the cervical epdiural space. A: AP radiograph of the cervical spine during cervical interlaminar injection. A 20-gauge Tuohy needle is in position between the C7 and T1 laminae and spinous processes. The needle hub is projected directly over the needle tip and is positioned between the spinous processes. **B:** Lateral radiograph of the cervical spine near the cervicothoracic junction during interlaminar cervical epidural injection. A 22-gauge Tuohy needle is in place in the C7/T1 interspace extending toward the dorsal epidural space. **C:** Labeled image. The anterior most extent of the spinous process and the posterior most extent of the ligamentum flavum and spinal canal coincide with the "J-point" or the point where the inferior margin of the spinous process begins to arc in a cephalad direction, taking the appearance of the letter "J." The area outlined to the left of the image in the dashed box has been enlarged in the inset to the right, where the approximate borders of the ligamentum flavum have been outlined. **D:** The same lateral projection is shown with the needle in the epidural space after injection of 1 mL of radiographic contrast (iopamidol 200 mg/mL). The contrast extends in a linear stripe in a cephalad and caudad direction from the needle tip that outlines the dorsal (posterior) border of the dura mater.

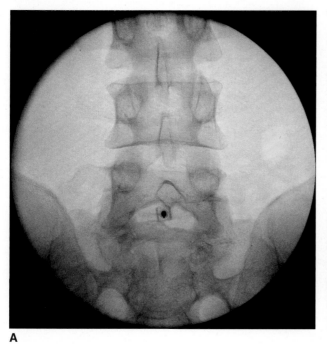

A

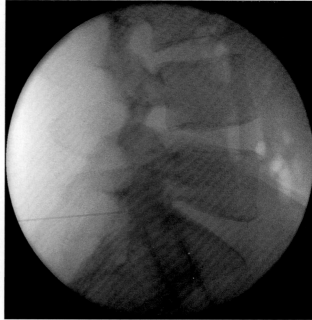

B

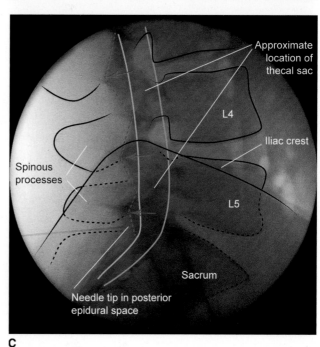

C

FIGURE 30-4. Radiographic identification of the lumbar epidural space. A: Anterior-posterior radiograph of the lumbar spine during interlaminar lumbar epidural injection. A 20-gauge Tuohy needle is in position between the L5 and S1 laminae with the hub projected directly over the needle tip. **B:** Lateral radiograph of the lumbar spine during interlaminar lumbar epidural injection. A Tuohy needle is in place in the L5/S1 interspace extending to the posterior epidural space. Clarity of lateral radiographs of the lumbar spine is often hindered by the overlying iliac crests. **C:** Labeled image. During lumbar interlaminar epidural injection, the needle can be safely advanced using the lateral radiograph to guide depth. The posterior-most extent of the ligamentum flavum lies just anterior to the junction of the spinous process with the laminae (*red arrows*). The needle can be safely advanced to this depth before starting the LOR technique during the last few millimeters of advancement through the ligamentum flavum to precisely identify the epidural space. The junction of the spinous process with the lamina can be easily identified in the lateral radiograph by following the inferior margin of the spinous processes anteriorly until the junction with the lamina is seen as a line that extends in an inferior and anterior direction (*dashed line*). The approximate location of the thecal sac is shown (*gray lines* indicate the approximate location of the anterior and posterior aspects of the dura mater).

▶ MECHANISM OF CAUSATION

Injuries associated with image-guided pain treatment fall into several broad categories. Bleeding and infectious complications are rare, but can be devastating, including epidural hematoma and epidural abscess—these complications have been discussed in detail in Chapters 4 and 5, respectively. Use of image guidance is unlikely to impact the incidence of either of these complications, but diagnostic imaging is integral to prompt diagnosis and treatment. In contrast, image guidance does play a critical role in avoiding direct trauma to neural structures as well as preventing unintended intravascular or intrathecal injection.

Direct Trauma to Neural Structures

Direct trauma to neural structures, including the spinal nerves at the level of the intervertebral foramina, the cauda equina, or the spinal cord itself, have all been associated with specific injections used in pain treatment. Specifically, direct needle contact with spinal nerves during transforaminal injection is not uncommon. This typically causes a transient paresthesia, which resolves promptly with redirection of the needle, but results in persistent pain in some individuals. Likewise, transforaminal injection is often carried out to treat radicular pain associated with foraminal stenosis and or nerve compression associated with disc herniation. In these

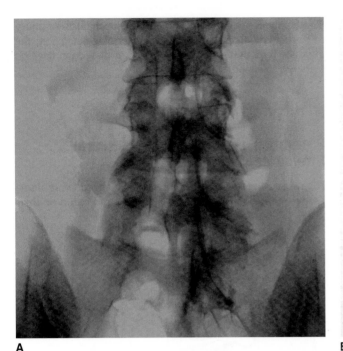
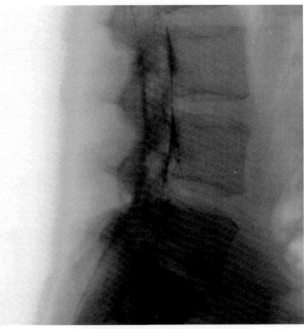

A   **B**

FIGURE 30-5. **Lumbar epidurography. A:** Anterior-posterior epidurogram of the lumbosacral spine. When larger volumes of injectate are used (in this image, 10 mL of contrast-containing solution), the injectate spreads extensively within the anterior and posterior epidural space and exits the intervertebral foramina, surrounding the exiting nerve roots. However, in the presence of significant obstruction to flow, as in this patient with a right L4/L5 disc herniation and compression of the exiting right L4 nerve root, the injectate often follows the path of least resistance, exiting the foramina on the side opposite from the disc herniation. **B:** Lateral epidurogram of the lumbosacral spine. When larger volumes of injectate are used (in this image, 10 mL of contrast-containing solution), the injectate spreads extensively within the anterior and posterior epidural space and has a characteristic double line or railroad track appearance. (Adapted from Rathmell JP, Torian D, Song T. Lumbar epidurography. *Reg Anesth Pain Med* 2000;25:542, with permission.)

conditions, there is little space around the spinal nerve to accommodate the injected fluid, and paresthesia caused by the injected fluid causing some element of worsened nerve compression may occur. The spinal cord lies directly in front of the advancing needle during both transforaminal and interlaminar epidural injections carried out at the cervical level, and direct needle trauma to the cord can occur.[9] Patients with severe stenosis of the central spinal canal may be at particular risk for spinal cord injury, especially when using an interlaminar technique.[4]

Vascular Compromise

Evidence for vascular compromise has arisen in two areas: paraplegia following neurolytic celiac plexus block[15,16] and catastrophic neural injuries associated with injection of particulate steroid, particularly during cervical transforaminal injection.[17] Paraplegia following neurolytic celiac plexus block has been discussed in detail in Chapter 23. Briefly, celiac plexus block is commonly carried out at the T12/L1 vertebral level, and the injectate is placed over the anterolateral aspect of the vertebral bodies or around the anterolateral aspect of the aorta. The artery of Adamkiewicz, the largest spinal segmental artery, arises from the posterolateral aspect of the aorta, most often on the left between the T10 and L2 vertebral levels, in the precise vicinity where the injectate is placed for celiac plexus block. This artery is critical to providing adequate blood supply to the anterolateral spinal cord at the low thoracic level, and compromise of this vessel

can lead to spinal cord ischemia and/or infarction similar to that seen in patients undergoing surgical repair of the thoracic spinal cord for aneurysm or dissection. The injection of neurolytic solution in this region has been hypothesized to lead to spasm of this critical reinforcing artery, and there is at least one case of transient paraplegia.[15] More often, the neurologic insult is permanent. While the mechanism may by arterial spasm and resultant ischemia, as our understanding of the spinal cord injury that ensues after intra-arterial injection of particulate steroid into the same vessel, it seems more plausible that the spinal cord injury is the direct result of intra-arterial injection of the neurolytic solution.

Catastrophic neural injury following intra-arterial injection of particulate steroid has been well described in association with transforaminal injections,[17] stellate ganglion block,[9] and cervical facet injections.[18] Several mechanisms of injury have been postulated to lead to injury during these injections, including arterial spasm or dissection, but no evidence to support these alternate mechanisms has emerged. The likely mechanism is direct intra-arterial injection of minute steroid particles in suspension that occlude the end-arteriolar circulation of the vessel injected, leading to ischemia and infarction. During transforaminal injection, injection into the spinal medullary arteries can lead to spinal cord infarction, and injection into the vertebral artery can lead to occlusion of the end arterioles in the posterior cerebral circulation, resulting in cortical blindness, cerebellar infarction, and death from the resultant intracranial hypertension. Direct injection in to the vertebral artery can also occur with stellate ganglion block or high-cervical facet injections. This mechanism of injury is strongly supported by studies in experimental animals[19,20] and in case reports detailing the resultant injuries.[18] In an elegant study using anesthetized swine, injection of particulate steroid into the vertebral artery resulted in massive posterior circulation stokes on MRI and persistent coma without any spontaneous respiratory effort in these animals[19]; in contrast, intra-arterial injection of the nonparticulate steroid dexamethasone causes no apparent injury to the brain. In a detailed case report of a man receiving a C1/C2 intra-articular facet injection with particulate steroid, intra-arterial injection into the adjacent vertebral artery resulted in a massive, fatal posterior circulation stroke[18] (Fig. 30-6).

These publications strongly support the mechanism of injury of particulate steroid causing end-arteriolar occlusion; the alternate hypotheses of arterial spasm or dissection have no evidence to support them to date.

▶ PREVENTION

Prevention of Direct Trauma to Neural Structures

Neural structures cannot be directly visualized using fluoroscopy; thus, their position must be inferred based on their

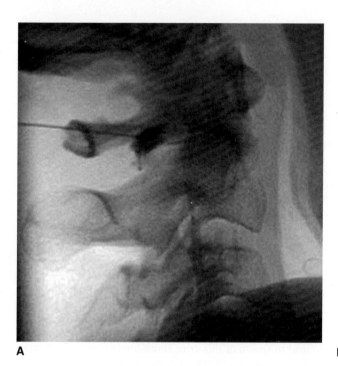

A

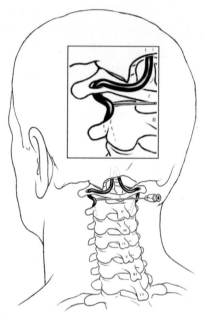

B

FIGURE 30-6. Massive posterior circulation stroke resulting from inadvertent injection of particulate steroid into the left vertebral artery during C1/2 intra-articular facet injection. This patient became comatose immediately after the intra-articular cervical facet steroid injection. **A:** Lateral x-ray shows needle posterior to the C1/2 joint, with radiographic contrast over the posterior portion of the joint. **B:** Schematic illustration, with inset highlighting the anatomic area of interest, demonstrates proximity of superior cervical portion of the vertebral artery to the injection site. **C:** Reformatted CT angiography of the left vertebral artery (posterior view), performed 5 hours after the cervical injection, does not reveal evidence of arterial dissection, vasospasm, or occlusion. *(Cont.)*

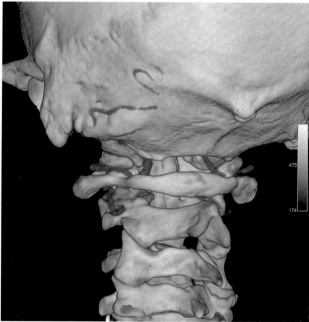

C

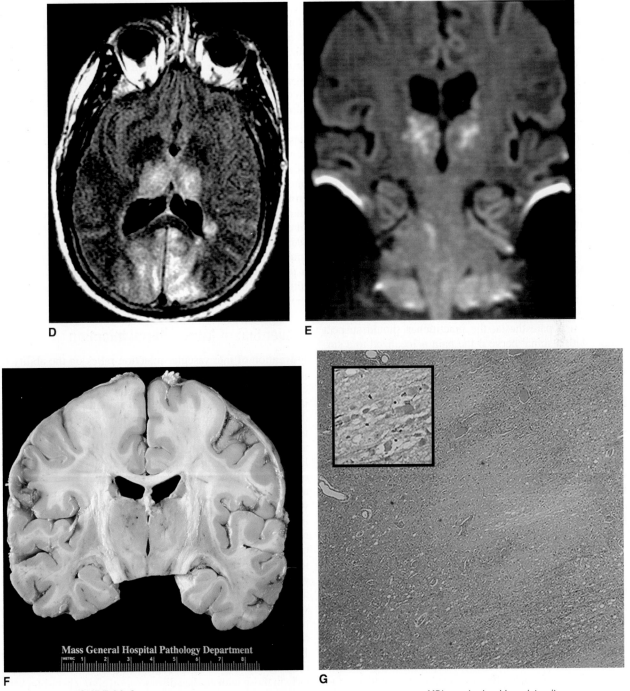

FIGURE 30-6. *(Continued)* **D:** Axial T2 fluid attenuated inversion recovery sequence MRI reveals signal hyperintensity within the posterior circulation territory. **E:** Coronal diffusion-weighted imaging sequence through the thalami demonstrates bithalamic diffusion restriction as well as right pontine. **F:** Fixed brain demonstrates gross evidence of bithalamic necrosis and microhemorrhages. **G:** Luxol fast blue with hematoxylin and eosin staining of thalamic section demonstrates small irregular discrete areas of acute infarction. **G, Inset:** Axonal spheroids are present in the surrounding thalamus adjacent to the lesions, consistent with ischemic injury. The combination of small, distinct regions of infarction with axonal spheroids confirms that the ischemic lesions occurred due to occlusion of distal vascular beds, consistent with the hypothesis of microembolization. (Adapted from Edlow BL, Wainger BJ, Frosch MP, et al. Posterior circulation stroke after C1-C2 intraarticular facet steroid injection: evidence for diffuse microvascular injury. *Anesthesiology* 2010;112:1532–1535, with permission.)

typical proximity to the bony structures that can be seen on fluoroscopy. Prevention of trauma begins with a review of any available diagnostic studies and careful planning of needle placement during the injection. Indeed, severe spinal stenosis caused by cervical spondyloarthropathy and or disc

herniation can lead to complete effacement of the epidural fat and spinal fluid surrounding the spinal cord. Needle entry into the spinal canal at such a severely stenotic level can result in direct trauma to the cord, even without trespass of the dura.[4] Interlaminar epidural injection at such severely stenotic levels should be avoided. In a similar fashion, severe spinal foraminal stenosis can lead to neural compression when even small volumes of any injectate are placed directly within the foramina. The only means to avoid neural injury is to carefully monitor any symptoms reported by the patient during injection and slow or halt the injection if radicular pain is reported.

The use of deep sedation of general anesthesia during the conduct of regional anesthesia and pain treatment techniques has been the subject of extensive debate.[21] Proponents state that sedation improves safety by assuring that the patient will remain relatively immobile when the needle is in close proximity to critical structures; opponents point out that deep sedation eliminates the ability of the patient to report contact with neural structures, eliminating any possibility of using the patient's early report of symptoms as an early warning sign, signaling potential neural injury. In the ASA Closed Claims study, the use of deep sedation or evidence that the patient was unresponsive at the time of injury was associated with a significant increase in the incidence of permanent spinal cord injury during the conduct of pain treatment at the cervical spinal level.[9] In the event that a patient does report a paresthesia, the practitioner should suspect contact with a spinal nerve if the pain is localized to a single extremity, and spinal cord contact or penetration should be suspected when the patient reports both upper and lower extremity pain during needle advancement. If this occurs, the needle should be withdrawn and redirected. The spinal cord can be entered without producing any neural injury; however, if the spinal cord is penetrated and *any* substance is injected, it is likely that severe neurologic injury will ensue. It appears to be the neuronal disruption caused by placing injectate into the substance of the cord that produces the most severe injury, rather than direct trauma caused by needle entry. Nonetheless, if an arterial structure within the cord is trespassed, bleeding into the cord can also produce significant injury.

Once the needle is in final position, it is critical to use images obtained in multiple planes to establish the final needle position. An AP image tells nothing about the needle depth, while a lateral image tells nothing about the medial-lateral placement of the needle. Combining the two images, an accurate measure of the needles position in three dimensions can be reconstructed (Figs. 30-3 and 30-4).

Use of ultrasound has gained widespread acceptance for performing peripheral nerve blocks to provide surgical anesthesia.[22] This is precisely because ultrasound can be used to directly visualize superficial neural structures, like the brachial plexus. Ultrasound has proven to increase the success rate of many peripheral nerve blocks. However, it is less clear if ultrasound will improve the safety of these techniques.[23] Indeed, direct intraneural injection and intravascular injection can still occur with the use of ultrasound guidance. In pain treatment, use of ultrasound has not advanced as quickly. There are likely two explanations for this slow penetration of ultrasound into the pain clinic setting: first, pain practitioners have been using fluoroscopy now for many years, and fluoroscopy allows direct and precise visualization of the bony elements of the neuraxis; second, use of ultrasound to image neuraxial structures is limited by the confines of the echogenic bony elements of the spine, which prevent direct visualization of many structures. Nonetheless,

the safety of several pain treatment techniques may well be improved by the use of ultrasound. Stellate ganglion block is foremost among these. The position of the great vessels of the neck, the thyroid gland, the esophagus, and the vertebral artery can only be inferred from the position of the bony elements of the spine when using fluoroscopy (Fig. 30-7A). In contrast, these structures can be directly visualized using ultrasound (Fig. 30-7B, C), and a number of techniques for using ultrasound to safely perform this block have been described. Indeed, the use of ultrasound is likely to quickly replace the use of fluoroscopy based on this superior visualization. Likewise, the position of the neurovascular bundle and the pleura during intercostal block can only be inferred from the position of the inferior margin of the rib during intercostal nerve block (Fig. 30-8A). In contrast, these structures can be seen directly using ultrasound (Fig. 30-8B, C), facilitating precise placement of the injectate adjacent to the intercostal nerve while avoiding penetration of the pleura. If a pneumothorax is suspected following injection, M-mode ultrasound provides a simple bedside means to detect even the smallest air collections (Fig. 30-8D).[24]

Prevention of Intra-arterial Injection

Prevention of intravascular injection relies on the ability to identify when the tip of a needle or catheter lies within a vascular structure *before* local anesthetic or particulate steroid is administered. The consequences of intravascular injection depend on the vascular structure into which the injectate is placed and the nature of the injectate. Local anesthetic and neurolytic solutions are often administered in relatively large doses for specific procedures—in pain treatment, doses of local anesthetic large enough to produce systemic toxicity are rarely employed, except during celiac plexus block or with intra-arterial injection. Conventional means for detecting intravascular injection rely on visual evidence of blood return when the needle or catheter is aspirated or the detection of signs and symptoms associated with intravascular injection. Local anesthetics can produce unique symptoms when injected into the blood stream: tinnitus, circumoral numbness, and metallic taste (see Chapter 7)—but these symptoms are not reliably produced, particularly with more potent agents like bupivacaine. The addition of epinephrine to the injectate in small concentrations, for example, 1:200,000, will lead to an increase in heart rate following intravascular injection, but again can be unreliable particularly in those with cardiac disease or receiving beta-blockers. Local anesthetic toxicity can occur after either intravenous or intra-arterial injection, and the recognition and treatment are discussed in detail in Chapter 7.

Intra-arterial injection of particulate steroid can lead to devastating neurologic injury. Radiographic guidance lends a unique and sensitive means to detect intravascular needle or catheter location, and this approach can be used to prevent inadvertent injection of local anesthetic or steroid into a vascular structure. It is critical to understand that injection of radiographic contrast into a vascular structure can only be detected reliably by using a live or real-time technique. If contrast is injected and then a single, static image is obtained at some point thereafter, any contrast that was injected intravascularly will likely have disappeared, as it will be diluted and carried away from the site of injection by

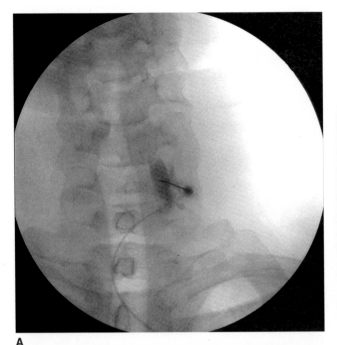

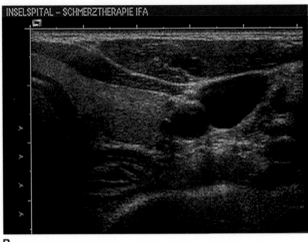

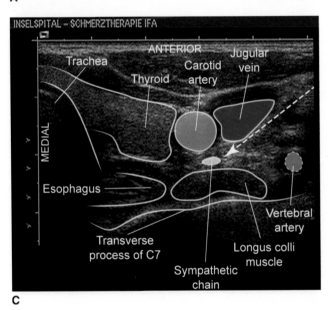

FIGURE 30-7 Stellate ganglion block. A: AP radiograph of the cervical spine during stellate ganglion block at C6. The needle is in position at the junction of the C6 transverse process and the vertebral body, just inferior to the uncinate process of C6. Radiographic contrast (1.5 mL of iohexol 180 mg per mL) has been injected and spreads along the anterolateral surface of C6 to reach the adjacent vertebra. Typically, 5 to 10 mL of volume is necessary to see spread to the level of the stellate ganglion at T1. **B:** Anatomy relevant to stellate ganglion block as seen on ultrasound. Transverse (short-axis) ultrasound view at the level of the transverse process of C7. **C:** Labeled image. Note that the vertebral artery can be seen anterior to the echogenic transverse process at the level of C7. The vertebral artery cannot be seen clearly at the C6 level on ultrasound, as it lies posterior to the echogenic transverse process within the foramen transversarium. At the level of C7, the superior margin of the thyroid is seen just lateral to the trachea. The *dashed arrow* indicates the optimal trajectory for placing a needle using an in-plane approach, for example, placing the needle in a lateral to medial direction with the shaft in the transverse plane of the ultrasound image. (Ultrasound image courtesy of Urs Eichenberger MD, PhD, University Department of Anesthesiology and Pain Therapy, University Hospital of Bern, Bern, Switzerland, 2011.)

the passing blood flow. Thus, the contrast must be injected under continuous x-ray exposure. The use of digital subtraction dramatically improves the visualization of vascular structures by subtracting the baseline image and leaving only those structures that are in motion as the image sequence is taken (Fig. 30-9). Using live fluoroscopy, with or without digital subtraction, markedly increases the sensitivity of detecting intravascular needle location. In one series, 20% of cervical transforaminal injections were seen with live fluoro,[10] while only 20% may have any evidence of blood return on aspiration.[11] The addition of digital subtraction appears to increase the sensitivity with which intravascular location can be seen.[13] Once intravascular needle position has been ruled out using contrast injection and a live x-ray technique, it is critical to assure that the needle position has not moved. Many practitioners recommend attaching a short, flexible extension tubing to the needle at the start of the pro-

cedure; this allows the practitioner performing the injection to attach and detach syringes to the catheter without touching the needle, thus reducing the chances of any change in needle position before the particulate steroid is administered. Indeed, using this combination of live x-ray and radiographic contrast, there have been no reported cases of neural injury attributed to particulate steroid. Nonetheless, it is important to remain vigilant, as patient movement and confusing patterns of contrast spread can easily be missed without close attention to the live x-ray sequence, and it is entirely feasible that intravascular needle position could be overlooked.

Prevention of Intrathecal Injection

Use of radiographic guidance and injection of small volumes of radiographic contrast can be used to identify when a needle has penetrated the dura. Injection of subarachnoid local

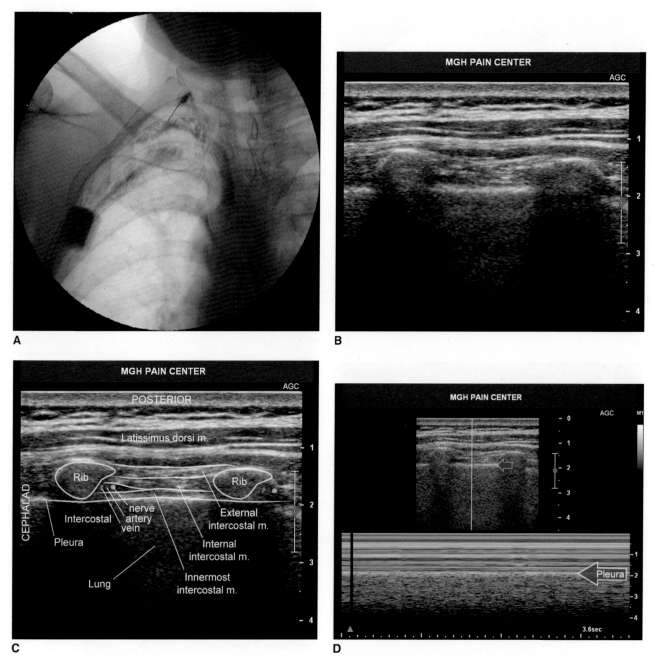

FIGURE 30-8. Intercostal nerve block. A: Anterior-posterior radiograph of the chest during intercostal nerve block. A needle is in position just inferior to the inferior margin of the second rib, approximately 5 cm from midline. Three milliliters of radiographic contrast containing phenol has been injected. The solution has spread along the course of the intercostal nerve, extending medially to the paravertebral space and several centimeters lateral from the point of injection. **B:** Ultrasound view in the sagittal plane near the mid-scapular line over the posterolateral chest wall at the level of eighth and ninth ribs. **C:** Labeled image. Note the clear delineation of adjacent muscular layers between adjacent ribs, the echogenic anterior surface of the two adjacent ribs, and the pleura. The neurovascular bundle lies just inferior to the inferior margin of each rib. **D:** M-mode (time-motion mode) ultrasound through the same region depicted in **(B, C)**. There is stark contrast in the ultrasound patterns seen using M-mode between the muscular layers and the pleura (*red arrow*). The appearance of the muscular layers on M-mode is a series of continuous parallel lines; in contrast, the lung has a speckled pattern owing to the constant movement of the alveoli during respiration. The pleural interface is easy to identify using M-mode and provides a simple tool for use in early detection of even the smallest pneumothoraces.

anesthetic can lead to a dense sensory and motor block when administered at the lumbar level and total spinal anesthesia with respiratory arrest when this occurs at the cervical level. While the topic remains the subject of significant debate, intrathecal injection of particulate steroid preparations may lead to neurotoxicity (see Chapter 27). Practitioners must learn to recognize the characteristic patterns of epidural (Fig. 30-10) and intrathecal (Fig. 30-11) contrast spread. It is also important to recognize unusual patterns of contrast spread like the loculated posterior contrast collections

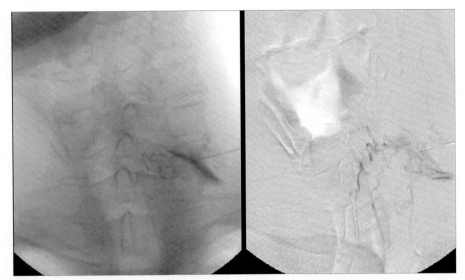

FIGURE 30-9. **Posterior-anterior view of the cervical spine during C7/T1 transforaminal injection, including a digital subtraction sequence after contrast injection.** An anteroposterior view of an angiogram obtained after injection of contrast medium, prior to planned transforaminal injection of corticosteroids. **A:** Image as seen on fluoroscopy. The needle lies in the left C7/T1 intervertebral foramen. Contrast medium outlines the spinal nerve. The radicular artery appears as a thin tortuous line of contrast passing medially from the site of injection. **B:** Digital subtraction angiogram reveals that the radicular artery extends to the midline to join the anterior spinal artery, and much of the contrast is located in the correct location surrounding the spinal nerve. (Reprinted from Rathmell JP, Aprill C, Bogduk N. Cervical transforaminal injection of steroids. *Anesthesiology* 2004;100:1597, with permission.)

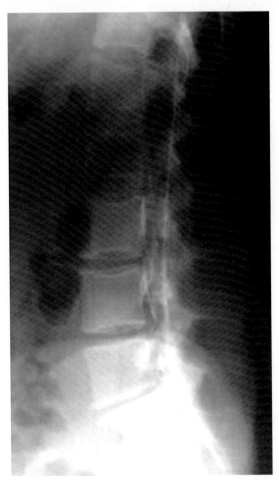

FIGURE 30-10. **Lateral radiograph of the lumbar spine after epidural placement of contrast media (epidurogram).** Contrast extends along both the anterior and posterior aspects of the epidural space on the lateral radiograph producing a "double line" or "railroad track" appearance characteristic of epidural localization of the contrast.

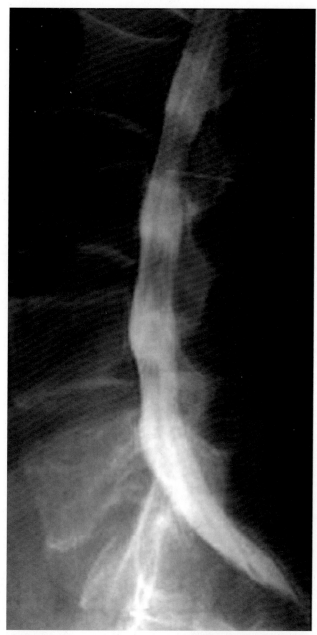

FIGURE 30-11. **Lateral radiograph of the lumbar spine after intrathecal placement of contrast media (myelogram).** The spinal needle enters via the L2/3 interspace. Contrast outlines the lumbar nerve roots within the thecal sac as they travel laterally toward the neural foramina.

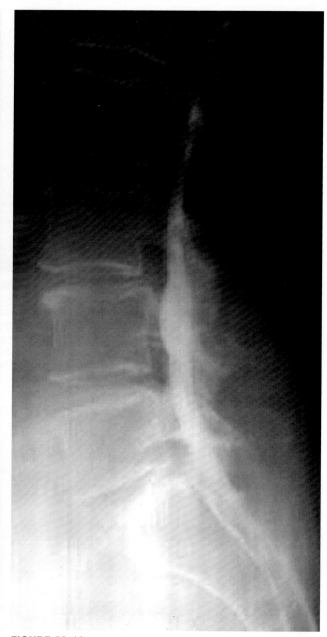

FIGURE 30-12. **Lateral radiograph of the lumbar spine with subdural contrast media.** The dense collection of contrast media is confined to the posterior aspect of the spinal canal. The posterior border of the fluid collection is linear (the dura mater) while the anterior border is somewhat more irregular (the arachnoid mater).

that signal subdural injection (Fig. 30-12). During epidural steroid injection, it is wise to abort the procedure before placing steroid when either subdural or intrathecal needle position is suspected.

▶ TREATMENT AND WHEN TO SEEK CONSULTATION

Prevention of injury is the only reliable means to assure the safety of image-guided interventions. Once neural injury has occurred, either via direct trauma to neural structures or following intra-arterial injection of particulate steroid,

there is no effective means to improve the subsequent outcome. Immediate, supportive care should be given, including airway management, resuscitation, and treatment of seizures. Diagnostic imaging should be obtained without delay to establish the nature and magnitude of the injury. Thereafter, transfer to the care of a neurologist or neurosurgeon for supportive care is likely the best avenue. In the case of spinal cord injury, there is some evidence that use of high-dose intravenous steroids following traumatic spinal cord transection can improve neurologic outcome,[25,26] and on this basis some advocate treatment of needle trauma and ischemic spinal cord injury in the same fashion. Permanent, disabling spinal cord injury is more the rule than the exception.[9] After acute stabilization, most patients will need significant rehabilitation aimed at regaining functional capacity.

► SUMMARY

The use of image guidance has rapidly developed into routine use in providing many pain treatment techniques, and there is insufficient scientific evidence to judge if this increased use has improved safety. Nonetheless, the logical appeal is overwhelming, so overwhelming that it is now unlikely that scientific comparisons of most techniques with and without radiographic guidance will ever be conducted. This chapter is meant to be a pragmatic discussion of what we do know about imaging and pain treatment with respect to improvement in safety. This same analysis can serve to guide future investigators who set out to better understand how to apply new imaging techniques and in the process how to evaluate rigorously their benefits.

References

1. Chou R, Atlas SJ, Stanos SP, et al. Nonsurgical interventional therapies for low back pain: a review of the evidence for an American Pain Society clinical practice guideline. *Spine (Phila Pa 1976)* 2009;34:1078–1093.
2. Sethee J, Rathmell JP. Epidural steroid injections are useful for the treatment of low back pain and radicular symptoms: pro. *Curr Pain Headache Rep* 2009;13:31–34.
3. Armon C, Argoff CE, Samuels J, et al.; Therapeutics and Technology Assessment Subcommittee of the American Academy of Neurology. Assessment: use of epidural steroid injections to treat radicular lumbosacral pain: report of the Therapeutics and Technology Assessment Subcommittee of the American Academy of Neurology. *Neurology* 2007;68:723–729.
4. Field J, Rathmell JP, Stephenson JH, et al. Neuropathic pain following cervical epidural steroid injection. *Anesthesiology* 2000;93:885–888.
5. White AH, Derby R, Wynne G. Epidural injections for the diagnosis and treatment of low back pain. *Spine* 1980;5:78–86.
6. Renfrew DL, Moore TE, Kathol MH, et al. Correct placement of epidural steroid injections: fluoroscopic guidance and contrast administration. *AJNR Am J Neuroradiol* 1991;12:1003–1007.
7. El-Khoury G, Ehara S, Weinstein JN, et al. Epidural steroid injection: a procedure ideally performed with fluoroscopic control. *Radiology* 1988;168:554–557.
8. Stevens DS, Balatbat GR, Lee FM. Coaxial imaging technique for superior hypogastric plexus block. *Reg Anesth Pain Med* 2000;25(6):643–647.
9. Rathmell JP, Michna E, Fitzgibbon DR, et al. Injury and liability associated with cervical procedures for chronic pain. *Anesthesiology* 2011;114:918–926.
10. Nahm FS, Lee CJ, Lee SH, et al. Risk of intravascular injection in transforaminal epidural injections. *Anaesthesia* 2010;65:917–921.
11. Kim do W, Han KR, Kim C, et al. Intravascular flow patterns in transforaminal epidural injections: a comparative study of the cervical and lumbar vertebral segments. *Anesth Analg* 2009;109: 233–239.
12. Rathmell JP. Toward improving the safety of transforaminal injection. *Anesth Analg* 2009;109:8–10.
13. McLean JP, Sigler JD, Plastaras CT, et al. The rate of detection of intravascular injection in cervical transforaminal epidural steroid injections with and without digital subtraction angiography. *PM R* 2009;1:636–642.
14. Manchikanti L, Pampati V, Boswell MV, et al. Analysis of the growth of epidural injections and costs in the Medicare population: a comparative evaluation of 1997, 2002, and 2006 data. *Pain Physician* 2010;13:199–212.
15. Wong GY, Brown DL. Transient paraplegia following alcohol celiac plexus block. *Reg Anesth* 1995;20:352–355.
16. Abdalla EK, Schell SR. Paraplegia following intraoperative celiac plexus injection. *J Gastrointest Surg* 1999;3:668–671.
17. Rathmell JP, Aprill C, Bogduk N. Cervical transforaminal injection of steroids. *Anesthesiology* 2004;100:1595–1600.
18. Edlow BL, Wainger BJ, Frosch MP, et al. Posterior circulation stroke after C1-C2 intraarticular facet steroid injection: evidence for diffuse microvascular injury. *Anesthesiology* 2010;112:1532–1535.
19. Okubadejo GO, Talcott MR, Schmidt RE, et al. Perils of intravascular methylprednisolone injection into the vertebral artery. An animal study. *J Bone Joint Surg Am* 2008;90:1932–1938.
20. Dawley JD, Moeller-Bertram T, Wallace MS, et al. Intra-arterial injection in the rat brain: evaluation of steroids used for transforaminal epidurals. *Spine (Phila Pa 1976)* 2009;34:1638–1643.
21. Bernards CM, Hadzic A, Suresh S, et al. Regional anesthesia in anesthetized or heavily sedated patients. *Reg Anesth Pain Med* 2008;33:449–460.
22. Sites BD, Chan VW, Neal JM, et al. The American Society of Regional Anesthesia and Pain Medicine and the European Society of Regional Anaesthesia and Pain Therapy joint committee recommendations for education and training in ultrasound-guided regional anesthesia. *Reg Anesth Pain Med* 2010;35(2 Suppl):S74–S80.
23. Neal JM. Ultrasound-guided regional anesthesia and patient safety: an evidence-based analysis. *Reg Anesth Pain Med* 2010;35 (2 Suppl):S59–S67.
24. Ueda K, Ahmed W, Ross AF. Intraoperative pneumothorax identified with transthoracic ultrasound. *Anesthesiology* 2011;115:653–655.
25. Delamarter RB, Coyle J. Acute management of spinal cord injury. *J Am Acad Orthop Surg* 1999;7:166–175.
26. Kwon BK, Tetzlaff W, Grauer JN, et al. Pathophysiology and pharmacologic treatment of acute spinal cord injury. *Spine J* 2004;4:451–464.

31

Complications Associated with Neurolytic Blocks

Honorio T. Benzon and Farooq Khan

▶ DEFINITION

Neurolytic blocks involve the destruction of a nerve and are commonly performed in patients with severe pain secondary to advanced cancer or occlusive vascular disease, while their use in chronic nonmalignant pain (e.g., chronic relapsing pancreatitis) is more limited. Raj recommended the following five criteria for neurolysis[1]: (i) the presence of severe pain, (ii) the failure of less invasive techniques to relieve the pain, (iii) the presence of well localized pain, (iv) the relief of pain with diagnostic local anesthetic blocks, and

(v) the absence of undesirable effects after diagnostic blocks (Box 31-1).

Neurolytic blockade carries significant risk of potentially devastating side effects and life-altering but predictable consequences that must be carefully weighed against the expected benefits of pain reduction. For this reason, neurolytic blocks are best suited to patients with a short life expectancy who experience severe pain despite aggressive conservative attempts to control the pain. For instance, neuraxial neurolysis can provide profound pain relief for patients with pain related to invasive tumors involving the pelvis, but

BOX 31-1 Criteria for Use of Neurolytic Blockade

- Pain is severe
- Pain persists after use of less invasive treatment
- Pain is well localized
- Pain is relieved with diagnostic blocks using local anesthetic
- No undesirable effects appear during local anesthetic blocks

Adapted from Raj PP. Peripheral neurolysis in the management of pain. In: Waldman SD, Winnie AP, eds. *Interventional Pain Management.* Philadelphia, PA: WB Saunders, 1996:392–400.

this approach often also leads to loss of bowel and/or bladder function and may well also produce weakness in the lower extremities. It should also be emphasized that relief from neurolytic blocks is usually not complete, since most patients with cancer pain have multiple sources of their pain.

Neurolytic blocks can be peripheral, neuraxial, or visceral. Of the three, visceral blocks are most commonly performed, while neuraxial and peripheral neurolytic blocks are performed less frequently for several reasons. In the case of peripheral neurolytic nerve blocks, blocking mixed motor and sensory nerves can cause motor deficit leading to loss of functionality for the patient. In addition, peripheral neuritis and deafferentation pain are potential painful consequences, while the block itself is not predictably permanent.[1] Finally, the patient may also be dissatisfied with the subsequent numbness of the area (Box 31-2).

Neuraxial neurolytic blocks, including both subarachnoid and epidural alcohol or phenol neurolytic blocks, are rarely used today because neuraxial opioids can effectively and safely be used in the treatment of cancer pain. Where an intrathecal drug delivery system can provide widespread pain relief that can be adjusted to accommodate many scenarios, a successful neurolytic block may have to be repeated with changes in pain pathology, such as the presence of new metastatic lesions. In such cases, it is impractical to perform subsequent subarachnoid neurolytic injections due to their attendant risks, while an indwelling intrathecal drug delivery

BOX 31-2 Limitations of Peripheral Neurolytic Blocks

- Motor deficits are likely when mixed sensory-motor nerves are blocked.
- Neuritis/deafferentation pain may occur and can be more severe than preexisting pain.
- Neurolytic blocks are not predictably long lasting or permanent.
- Sensory loss following peripheral neurolysis is often bothersome to the patient.

Adapted from Raj PP. Peripheral neurolysis in the management of pain. In: Waldman SD, Winnie AP, eds. *Interventional Pain Management.* Philadelphia, PA: WB Saunders, 1996:392–400.

system will cover new areas of pain and continue to be useful. Visceral neurolytic blocks are among the most useful neurolytic blocks and are still in common use today. The viscera are usually supplied by a plexus of sympathetic nerves (e.g., celiac plexus) that are amenable to neurolysis. Properly done, visceral neurolytic blocks have no attendant motor weakness and the effects are predictable and gratifying. This chapter reviews complications from neurolytic blocks related to the technical aspects of needle placement and those that may result from the actions of the neurolytic agent.

▶ COMPLICATIONS FROM NEUROLYTIC AGENTS: PHARMACOLOGY AND PATHOPHYSIOLOGY

The neurolytic agents commonly employed include ethyl alcohol, phenol, and, less commonly, glycerol. Ethyl alcohol causes neurolysis by extracting cholesterol, phospholipids, and cerebrosides from the nervous tissue and precipitating lipoproteins and mucoproteins.[2] Its injection into a peripheral nerve results in wallerian degeneration wherein the axon and the Schwann cell are damaged.[3] In wallerian degeneration, the axon breaks down and the myelin sheath retracts, forming ellipsoids of myelin.[4] The axoplasm gets enclosed within the ellipsoids of myelin, followed by hydrolysis within the ellipsoids by lysosomal enzymes. Regeneration occurs during the 1st week of injury when Schwann cells start to multiply and macrophages ingest debris.[4] By the end of the 1st week, Schwann cells may develop a chain within the endoneurium. Macrophages disappear after 2 weeks, whereas endoneurial tubes are filled with Schwann cells. When neurolytic agents are injected into the subarachnoid space, the changes occur in the dorsal roots, posterior portion of the spinal cord, and the Lissauer's tract.[5]

Alcohol is commercially available as a 95% concentration, which is more than adequate for neurolytic blocks since studies have shown that a concentration of 33% or greater is necessary to affect neurolysis.[6] Ethyl alcohol is used in a variety of neurolytic blocks, such as visceral sympathetic blocks (celiac plexus, superior hypogastric plexus), lumbar paravertebral sympathetic blocks, and injections into the subarachnoid space and the trigeminal ganglia. Some authors recommend injecting a local anesthetic before the alcohol injection, because it is an irritant and causes burning pain upon injection. Alcohol is injected undiluted when used for peripheral injections. In celiac plexus blocks, the alcohol is usually diluted with a local anesthetic to a concentration of 50% to diminish the pain upon injection. Alcohol is hypobaric with respect to the cerebrospinal fluid, and the patient has to be positioned with the painful side up when intrathecal injection is performed. Denervation and relief of pain usually occurs over a few days after injection and is complete after 1 week.[1] Intravascular injection of 30 mL of 100% ethanol will result in a blood ethanol level well above the legal limit for intoxication, but below the danger of severe alcohol toxicity. Intravenous injection may cause thrombosis of the vessel.[7] Complications of using ethanol for neurolytic blocks range from transient paraplegia to irreversible spinal cord damage.[8,9] Of note, ethanol has been increasingly used in the rehabilitation setting to treat spasticity in post stroke patients.[10,11]

Phenol, also known as carbolic acid, causes neurolysis by coagulating proteins within nerve tissue. There is minimal discomfort on injection since it acts as a local anesthetic at lower concentrations. It has a strong affinity for vascular tissue, and injury to the blood vessels at or near nervous tissues may contribute to its neurotoxicity.[12] For this reason, some clinicians prefer alcohol in celiac plexus blocks because the injection of phenol puts the nearby major blood vessels at risk. Five percent phenol is equivalent to 40% alcohol in neurolytic potency.[13] The intrathecal injection of phenol causes changes similar to that of alcohol, and there is degeneration of fibers in the posterior columns and posterior nerve roots. The degree of damage after peripheral injection is concentration-dependent, and the changes range from segmental demyelination to wallerian degeneration.[14]

The concentrations of phenol used for neurolysis range from 3% to 15%. The authors use a 6% aqueous solution. At lower concentrations, it acts as a local anesthetic, and as a result, there is minimal discomfort upon injection of the drug. Phenol is relatively insoluble in water and at concentrations above 6% has to be prepared with the addition of glycerin. At these concentrations, it is fairly viscous. Phenol has a clinical biphasic action, and the initial relief is secondary to its local anesthetic effect. This relief fades within the first 24 hours, and lasting analgesia occurs 3 to 7 days after the injection secondary to the neurolytic action of the drug. Phenol is hyperbaric with respect to cerebrospinal fluid, and the patient has to be positioned with the painful side down when subarachnoid injection is performed. The intravascular injection of phenol results in convulsions secondary to an increase in the excitatory transmitter acetylcholine in the central nervous system.[15] Large systemic doses of phenol (>8.5 g) cause effects similar to those seen with local anesthetic overdose: generalized seizures and cardiovascular collapse. Acute renal and pulmonary collapse requiring hemodialysis and ventilatory support has been reported with large systemic doses of phenol as well.[16] Clinical doses up to 1,000 mg are unlikely to cause serious toxicity. Like ethanol, it should be noted that phenol is not only used for the management of pain but in the treatment of spasticity.[17]

▶ COMPLICATIONS FROM SPECIFIC NEUROLYTIC BLOCKS

Neurolytic agents can be injected into peripheral nerves, along the neuraxis within the intrathecal or epidural spaces or adjacent to visceral sympathetic nerves. Each of these sites of injection is associated with specific complications. Peripheral neurolysis includes injection into the trigeminal ganglion, truncal, upper and lower extremities, trigger points, and neurolysis for spasticity.[1]

Neurolytic Blocks of the Head and Neck

Gasserian Ganglion Neurolysis

Blockade of nerves in the head and neck is performed for variety of reasons (Table 31-1). These include blockade of the trigeminal ganglion for trigeminal neuralgia that is not responsive to medical management and for relief of cancer pain secondary to invasive tumors of the orbit, maxillary sinus, and mandible; neurolysis of the pituitary for

TABLE 31-1 Indications and Complications from Neurolysis in the Head		
SITE OF NEUROLYSIS	**INDICATIONS**	**COMPLICATIONS**
Trigeminal ganglion	Trigeminal neuralgia	Hemorrhage into temporal fossa Mastication problems Corneal anesthesia/ulceration Nasal ulceration Permanent anesthesia of cheek and nose Abducens palsy Trophic disturbances Anesthesia dolorosa
Pituitary (chemical hypophysectomy)	Metastatic cancer	Endocrine complications (see text) CSF rhinorrhea Air embolism Visual field defects Ocular nerve palsy Meningitis

metastatic cancer (specifically breast and prostate cancer); and blockade of individual peripheral nerves in the head.

The gasserian ganglion is formed from two trigeminal roots that exit the ventral surface of the brain stem at the midpontine level.[18] The roots pass forward and in a lateral direction, in the posterior fossa of the cranium, across the border of the petrous temporal bone. It then enters the Meckel's cave in the middle cranial fossa. The gasserian ganglion contains the ophthalmic, maxillary, and mandibular divisions. A smaller motor root joins the mandibular division as it exits the foramen ovale. It should be noted that a dural pouch, the trigeminal cistern, lies behind the trigeminal ganglion. In gasserian ganglion block, the needle is inserted approximately 2.5 cm lateral to the side of the mouth and advanced, perpendicular to the middle of the eye (with the eye in the midposition), in a cephalad direction toward the auditory meatus.[19] When contact is made with the base of the skull, the needle is withdrawn and "walked" posteriorly toward the foramen ovale. A free flow of CSF is usually noted, and fluoroscopy is then used to confirm correct needle placement. Very small amounts (i.e., 0.1 mL increments) of local anesthetic or neurolytic agent are injected to a total of 0.4 to 0.5 mL. Either absolute alcohol or 6.5% phenol in glycerin is employed as the neurolytic agent. Due to their different baricities, the patient remains supine if alcohol is used but placed in a sitting position with the chin on the chest prior to the injection of phenol. This maneuver localizes the phenol around the maxillary and mandibular divisions of the trigeminal nerve, avoiding the ophthalmic division and the risk of keratitis from loss of the conjunctival reflex.

The pterygopalatine space is highly vascular, and significant hematoma of the face and subscleral hematoma of the eye can occur. Veins in the subtemporal region can be punctured, causing hemorrhage in the temporal fossa. Local anesthetic injection can lead to spinal anesthesia because the ganglion lies within the cerebrospinal fluid. Blockade of the motor fibers of the trigeminal nerve can interfere with mastication.[20] Oculomotor palsy, which results in diplopia and strabismus, is usually temporary. Abducens palsy is also temporary, although cases of permanent lateral rectus palsy have been reported.[7] Spread of the neurolytic agent into the facial nerve results in paralysis of the facial muscles and inability of the eyelid to close, resulting in keratitis or corneal ulceration. Blockade of the greater superficial petrosal nerve may result in lack of tear formation and conjunctivitis. Blockade of the acoustic nerve may result in deafness or dizziness. The delayed effects of gasserian ganglion neurolytic block include trophic problems such as keratitis, ulcerations in the nose, and erosions in the mouth. These disturbances usually occur after trauma to the area. Another delayed complication is anesthesia dolorosa. Since the neurolytic block of the gasserian ganglion is associated with myriad devastating complications, many neurosurgeons and pain medicine practitioners choose to perform radiofrequency rhizotomy of the ganglion instead.[7] The same approach is employed when radiofrequency needles are advanced to the ganglion. With stimulation, the nerve fibers coming from the region of the lancinating pain are localized and selectively destroyed with the radiofrequency current. Since no chemical neurolytic is used, spread of the neurolytic agent into the CSF and surrounding structures is not a consideration with radiofrequency rhizotomy. The complications of thermal radiofrequency rhizotomy of the trigeminal ganglion are related either to the placement of the needle or to thermal lesion to the surrounding tissue. Some common complications and their incidences include masseter weakness (18%), paresthesia/dysesthesia (20%), diplopia (1.5%), and keratitis (3%).[21] Other complications include inadvertent injury to the surrounding tissue (puncture of cavernous sinus, carotid artery, jugular foramen, or foramen magnum) or oculomotor, trochlear, and abducens nerve injury.[22] The incidences of the different complications with chemical neurolysis and radiofrequency rhizotomy of the gasserian ganglion are listed in Table 31-2. The technical difficulty and complications associated with gasserian ganglion block led some investigators to perform peripheral branch (supraorbital, infraorbital, and mandibular nerves) injections with 10% phenol to relieve the pain of tic douloureux.[23]

Pituitary Ablation

Chemical ablation of the pituitary with alcohol was widely used in the late 1970s and early 1980s, where it was recommended for the treatment of metastatic cancer pain, especially breast and prostate cancer.[24,25] Among this patient population, the results seemed to be better in patients with hormone-dependent tumor. Since that time, modifications of the original technique have been proposed to simplify the approach and to decrease the incidence and severity of cerebrospinal fluid leak.[24,26] The patient must be intubated and sedated for the procedure. A spinal needle is advanced, under biplanar fluoroscopic guidance, through the nose until the tip rests against the anterior wall of the sella turcica. Phenol or alcohol, in aliquots of 0.2 mL, is injected to a total of 4 to 6 mL. The pupils are monitored during the injection.

Papillary dilatation indicates spillage of the drug outside the sella and blockade of the oculomotor nerve. The injection is stopped if this occurs, and the needle is reinserted to a more anterior position. Cyanomethacrylate resin 0.5 mL is injected before the needle is withdrawn to prevent CSF leak. Cryoneurolysis and radiofrequency lesions have also been described.[27]

Most of the complications are related to the destruction of the pituitary gland, including diabetes insipidus, adrenal insufficiency, hypothyroidism, hypothermia, and lowering of libido.[24,25,28] Other complications include CSF rhinorrhea, impairment of consciousness, visual field defects, ocular nerve palsy, air embolism, and meningitis (Table 31-1). The incidences of these complications have been described by Swerdlow and Waldman[29] (Tables 31-2 and 31-3). Whereas Waldman found an incidence of 1% for CSF rhinorrhea, Swerdlow[7] noted a range of 1% to 20% in published reports. Swerdlow also noted an incidence of 1% to 10% for visual field defects, 1% to 32% for ocular nerve palsy, and 1% to 2% for meningitis. The endocrine complications cannot be prevented but are treated with replacement therapy. Fluoroscopic guidance and meticulous technique will help prevent some of the complications, and perioperative administration of antibiotics and sterile technique prevents the infectious complications.

Other Neurolytic Blocks of the Head and Neck

Neurolytic blocks of individual cranial nerves and their branches have also been performed, and complications are related to nerve location and the tissues innervated. Neurolytic block of the maxillary nerve at the foramen rotundum or of the infraorbital nerve may cause ulceration and sloughing of the ala of the nose and the cheek, ischemic necrosis of the palate, or sloughing of the posterior portion of the superior ridge of the maxilla.[7] Blockade of the mandibular nerve at the foramen ovale may result in weakness of the muscles of mastication in the blocked side, whereas blockade of the facial nerve causes weakness or paralysis of the facial muscles. Blockade of the glossopharyngeal nerve is rarely performed because of proximity of the nerve to the vagus, spinal accessory, and hypoglossal nerves. The close location of the other nerves led investigators to recommend blockade of the glossopharyngeal nerve under fluoroscopic control[30] or to use radiofrequency rhizotomy.[31] The sensory area of innervation of the glossopharyngeal nerve includes the nasopharynx, eustachian tube, uvula, tonsil, soft palate, base of the tongue, and part of the external auditory canal.[1] Paralysis of the pharyngeal muscles is a consequence of blockade of the glossopharyngeal nerve.

Stellate Ganglion Neurolysis

The cervical sympathetic trunk contains the superior, middle, and inferior cervical ganglia. In 80% of the population, the lowest cervical ganglion is fused with the first thoracic ganglion, forming the cervicothoracic (stellate) ganglion. The cervical sympathetic chain lies anterior to the prevertebral fascia, which encloses the prevertebral muscle. The sympathetic chain is enclosed within the alar fascia, a thin fascia that separates the cervical sympathetic chain from the retropharyngeal space. The carotid sheath is connected to the alar fascia by a mesothelium-like fascia. The fascial plane that encloses the sympathetic chain may be in direct

TABLE 31-2 Complications from Trigeminal Ganglion Neurolysis

COMPLICATION	ALCOHOL BLOCK (SWERDLOW)	RADIOFREQUENCY RHIZOTOMY COMPLICATION (LOESER)
Rhizotomy (Loeser)		
Abducens palsy (temporary)	2%	
Glossopharyngeal palsy (temporary)	1%	
Oculomotor palsy (temporary)	4%–6%	
Blindness	1%	
Corneal anesthesia	20%–69%	
Corneal ulceration	2%	
Nasal ulceration	2%–12%	
Anesthesia of cheek and nose	66%	
Trigeminal motor weakness	1%	
Paresthesias		12%–20%
Masseter weakness		5%–24%
Diplopia		0%–2%
Keratitis		1.6%–4%

The nerve palsies were temporary.

Adapted from (a) Swerdlow M. Complications of neurolytic neural blockade. In: Cousins MJ, Bridenbaugh PO, eds. *Neural Blockade in Clinical Anesthesia and Management of Pain.* 2nd ed. Philadelphia, PA: JB Lippincott, 1988:719–735. (b) Loeser JD, Sweet WH, Tew JM, et al. Neurosurgical operations involving peripheral nerves. In: Bonica JJ, ed. *The Management of Pain.* 2nd ed. Philadelphia, PA: Lea & Febiger, 1990:2044–2066.

TABLE 31-3 Incidence of Complications of Neuroadenolysis of the Pituitary

COMPLICATION	INCIDENCE (%)
Transient bilateral frontal headache	100
Diabetes insipidus	40
Hyperthermia	35
Increased pulmonary secretions	20
Transient visual disturbances	10
Permanent visual disturbances	5
Cerebrospinal fluid leakage	1
Pituitary hemorrhage	1
Infection	0.5

From Waldman SD. Neuroadenolysis of the pituitary: indications and technique. In: Waldman SD, Winnie AP, eds. *Interventional Pain Management.* Philadelphia, PA: WB Saunders, 1996:519–525 with permission.

communication with several spaces and structures, including the brachial plexus, vertebral artery, endothoracic fascia, and the thoracic wall muscle at T1-T2. At the C6 level, the cervical sympathetic trunk is located posterolaterally to the prevertebral fascia on the surface of the longus colli muscle.[32] The carotid vessels are anterior, whereas the nerve roots that contribute to the inferior portion of the brachial plexus are lateral to the ganglion. The vertebral artery passes over the ganglion and enters the vertebral foramen posterior to the anterior tubercle of C6. The communications of the fascia covering the stellate ganglion with several structures, as noted previously, and the proximity of the stellate ganglion to the vertebral and carotid vessels, phrenic nerve, and the recurrent laryngeal nerve explain some of the potential complications of the stellate ganglion block.[33]

Several techniques of stellate ganglion block have been described. These include insertion of the needle at the level of C6, placement of the needle at C7, and the posterior thoracic approach.[33] With C6 placement, the needle is in contact with either the C6 tubercle or the junction between the C6 vertebral body and the tubercle (Fig. 31-1). The needle is withdrawn 2 mm, an initial test dose of 0.5 to 1 mL is injected, and volumes of 5 to 10 mL have been injected. The injectate travels caudad and reaches the stellate ganglion and the upper thoracic sympathetic ganglia.[34] A smaller volume of drug is adequate when the needle is placed at the level of C7. However, there is increased incidence of vertebral artery injection with this approach because the artery lies anterior to the C7 transverse process. There is also an increased risk of pneumothorax because the dome of the lung is close to the injection site. The posterior thoracic approach requires fluoroscopic guidance to identify the lamina of T1 or T2, and dye injection is recommended to document the spread of the drug. In this approach, the needle contacts the lamina of T1 or T2, is moved laterally off the lamina, and is advanced to pass the costotransverse ligament at a depth of 2 cm beyond the lamina. Either loss of resistance is used or dye is injected to confirm proper needle placement.

A technique involving the use of ultrasound was described by Kapral.[35] Since the initial technique was developed, there have been many modifications made with the aim of increasing the safety, efficacy, and speed of the block.[32,36] The patient is positioned supine with the neck slightly hyperextended, and an ultrasound probe is placed at the level of C6, providing a cross section of the anatomy at this level.

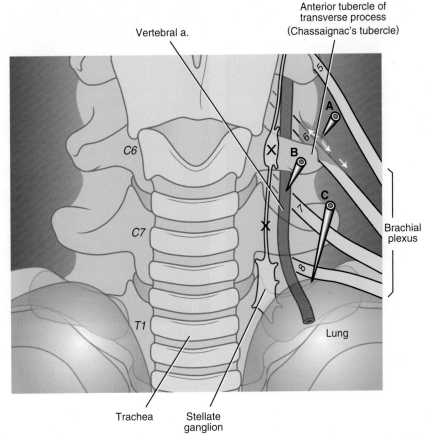

FIGURE 31-1. **Complications of stellate ganglion neurolysis.** The stellate ganglion conveys sympathetic fibers to and from the upper extremities and the head and neck. The ganglion is composed of the fused superior thoracic ganglion and the inferior cervical ganglion and is named for its fusiform shape (in many individuals, the two ganglia remain separate). The stellate ganglia lie over the head of the first rib at the junction of the transverse process and uncinate process of T1. The ganglion is just posteromedial to the cupola of the lung and medial to the vertebral artery, and these are the two structures most vulnerable. Stellate ganglion block is typically carried out at the C6 or C7 level to avoid pneumothorax, and a volume of solution that will spread along the prevertebral fascia inferiorly to the stellate ganglion is employed (usually 10 mL). When radiographic guidance is not used, the operator palpates the anterior tubercle of the transverse process of C6 (Chassaignac's tubercle), and a needle is seated in the location. With radiographic guidance, it is simpler and safer to place a needle over the vertebral body just inferior the uncinate process of C6 or C7 (locations of proper needle placement are marked X). Incorrect needle placement can lead to pneumothorax, damage to the vertebral artery or intra-arterial injection, or spread of the injectate adjacent to the exiting spinal nerves where they join to form the brachial plexus. Contrast can also course proximally along the spinal nerves to the epidural space. (Modified from Rathmell JP. Atlas of image-guided intervention in regional anesthesia and pain medicine. 2nd ed. Philadelphia, PA: Lippincott Williams & Wilkins, 2012, with permission.)

Visible are the trachea, esophagus, thyroid gland, carotid artery, jugular vein, longus colli muscle, and transverse process of C7 (Figure 31-2). A 25-gauge, 1½-inch needle can be advanced in plane with the ultrasound probe paratracheally toward the longus colli muscle, while avoiding the other structures, and stopping once the tip reaches the prevertebral fascia. At this point, 5 to 10 mL of local anesthetic is deposited under direct visualization and can be seen spreading along the prevertebral fascia.[37]

The complications of an intravascular injection of local anesthetic are well known. These include loss of consciousness, apnea, hypotension, and seizures. Local anesthetic blocks of the stellate ganglion have been performed for complex regional pain syndrome, vascular insufficiency of the upper extremities, and hyperhidrosis of the face and upper extremities. Neurolytic blockade of the stellate ganglion has been performed for complex regional pain syndrome when

there is consistent relief after diagnostic block with local anesthetic and without prolongation of the duration of pain relief. The overall incidence of complications is 0.17%.[38] The exact incidence of pneumothorax is not known. Aside from Horner's syndrome, hoarseness, blockade of the brachial plexus, subarachnoid and epidural spread, and cord infarction have been reported.[39] Brachial plexus block is secondary to the needle being inserted too posteriorly or from the spread of the drug along the prevertebral fascia. Ptosis can be corrected by suspension operation of the upper eyelid. Additionally, retropharyngeal hematomas have been reported ranging from minimal patient discomfort to complete loss of airway.[40,41] An unusual reported complication is transient locked-in syndrome, in which the patient is paralyzed and cannot breathe or speak, but can only move their eyes due to accidental intravascular anesthetic injection.[42] These complications led other investigators to use

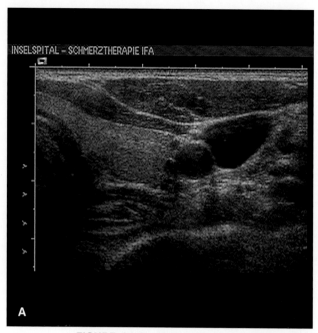

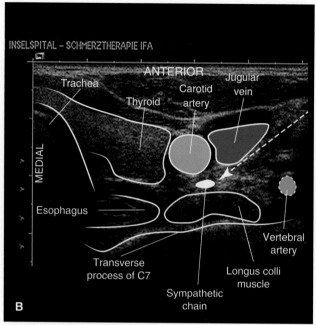

FIGURE 31-2. Anatomy relevant to stellate ganglion block as seen on ultrasound. A: Transverse (short-axis) ultrasound view at the level of the transverse process of C7. **B:** Labeled image. Note that the vertebral artery can be seen anterior to the echogenic transverse process at the level of C7. The vertebral artery cannot be seen clearly at the C6 level on ultrasound, as it lies posterior to the echogenic transverse process within the foramen transversarium. At the level of C7, the superior margin of the thyroid is seen just lateral to the trachea. The dashed arrow indicates the optimal trajectory for placing a needle using an in-plane approach, for example, placing the needle in a lateral to medial direction with the shaft in the transverse plane of the ultrasound image. (Ultrasound image courtesy of Urs Eichenberger MD, PhD, University Department of Anesthesiology and Pain Therapy, University Hospital of Bern, Bern, Switzerland, 2011. Reproduced from Rathmell JP. Atlas of image-guided intervention in regional anesthesia and pain medicine. 2nd ed. Philadelphia, PA: Lippincott Williams & Wilkins, 2012, with permission.)

alternative techniques to cervicothoracic sympathectomy, including radiofrequency rhizotomy and thoracoscopic sympathectomy.

For relief of craniocervical pain secondary to cancer, intraspinal opioid therapy through an implanted cervical epidural catheter has been recommended, especially in cases where neurolytic blockade of the nerve(s) is not feasible or is associated with serious side effects.

Neurolytic Blocks of the Trunk and Extremities

Intercostal and Thoracic Paravertebral Neurolysis

Intercostal blocks are used in the treatment of thoracic or abdominal wall pain and as adjunct in surgery.[43,44] Complications include pneumothorax, intravascular injection, intrapulmonary injection with consequent bronchospasm, and neuraxial spread (Figure 31-3 and Table 31-4). The incidence of pneumothorax detected by radiograph is 0.082% to 2%.[45] Clinically significant pneumothorax occurs at a low rate and chest tube insertion is rarely required. Another reported complication is total spinal anesthesia after intraoperative intrathoracic injection.[46] The intrathoracic injection at a medial location resulted in the injection of the local anesthetic into a dural cuff or into the nerve itself, with proximal spread of the drug. Bronchospasm from intrapulmonary injection of phenol has been reported.[47] Persistent paraplegia from intercostal block with 7.5% phenol has additionally been reported, with the authors suspecting

the damage occurred via absorption of phenol through the intervertebral foramen and subsequent destruction of motor and sensory nerve roots.[48] Similar to the advantages of its use in other peripheral nerve blocks, ultrasound has made intercostal nerve block a safer technique in that the pleura is visualized preventing its puncture and avoiding pneumothorax.[49]

Paravertebral somatic block is an alternative to intercostal or epidural blockade. Although most of the studies looked at the utility of paravertebral block for surgery, it is also a useful tool as a diagnostic and prognostic block in the pain clinic.[50,51] The authors employ it in patients with chest pain secondary to cancer and in patients with chronic chest pain. One advantage of paravertebral blockade over intercostal nerve block is the smaller number of injections, in that a single injection blocks several segments. The complications include pneumothorax, vascular injection, hypotension, and urinary retention (Table 31-4). The use of fluoroscopy is recommended when the procedure is performed in the pain clinic because the occurrence of pneumothorax is a big setback in this group of patients. The use of ultrasound has made the technique safer via real-time visualization of the paravertebral space, adjoining structures, and the needle.[52]

Ilioinguinal and Iliohypogastric Neurolysis

Ilioinguinal and iliohypogastric nerve blocks are used in the perioperative management of pain after inguinal

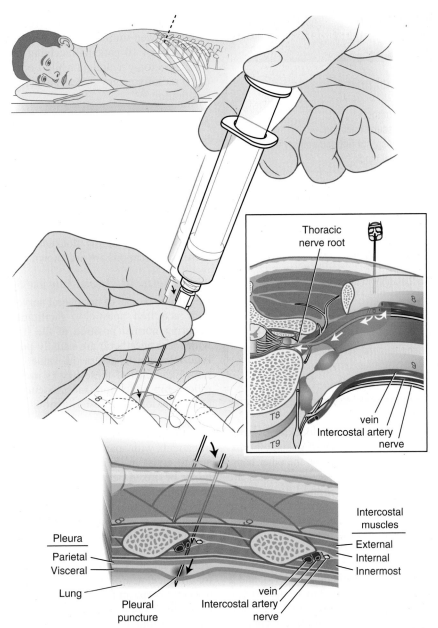

FIGURE 31-3. Complications of intercostal neurolysis. The thoracic nerve roots exit the spinal canal through the intervertebral foramina and divide into anterior and posterior primary rami. The anterior rami course laterally to enter a groove beneath the inferior margin of each rib, where they traverse laterally inferior to the intercostal vein and artery. Intercostal nerve block is carried out by inserting a needle just inferior to the rib margin. When the needle tip is directly adjacent to the intercostal nerve, the intercostal vessels lie in close proximity, and thus intravascular injection often occurs. Advancing the needle deep beyond the rib margin may result in pneumothorax. Proximal spread of injectate along the course of the intercostal nerve can result in epidural spread.

herniorrhaphy. Preoperative wound infiltration can decrease pain scores and analgesic requirements after inguinal herniorrhaphy. The preemptive analgesic effect of preincisional infiltration of local anesthetic before herniorrhaphy has not been firmly established. One study showed a beneficial effect,[53] whereas another study did not.[54] Bilateral ilioinguinal nerve blocks have also been shown to decrease pain after cesarean section.[55] In the pain clinic, ilioinguinal and iliohypogastric nerve blocks are performed in the diagnosis and treatment of inguinal and suprapubic pain after lower abdominal surgery or inguinal hernia repair. Complications of the block include unintentional blocks of the lateral

femoral cutaneous and femoral nerves. The incidences of these complications are not known. Neurolytic blocks of these nerves are presently being supplanted by pulsed radiofrequency rhizotomy.[56] Diagnostic blocks are obviously recommended before neurolytic injection or pulsed radiofrequency rhizotomy is performed.

Paravertebral Sympathetic Neurolysis

Paravertebral sympathetic blocks are performed for the treatment of complex regional pain syndromes, vascular insufficiencies of the lower extremities, phantom limb pain, and other conditions such as hyperhidrosis and trench

TABLE 31-4 Complications after Truncal Blocks

BLOCK	COMPLICATIONS
Intercostal	Pneumothorax Intravascular injection Bronchospasm (intrapulmonary injection) Neuraxial block
Thoracic	Pneumothorax
Paravertebral	Intravascular injection
Somatic	Hypotension Urinary retention
Lumbar	Subarachnoid injection
Paravertebral	Ureteral injury
Sympathetic	Nerve root block Genitofemoral nerve block Postsympathectomy dysesthesia Backache

foot. Thoracic paravertebral sympathetic blocks are rarely performed because of the high incidence of pneumothorax. Lumbar paravertebral sympathetic blocks, on the other hand, are frequently utilized. In this technique, the needles are placed in the anterolateral surface of L2 and L3.[57] Fluoroscopy is used to confirm vertebral level of placement, correct position of the needle tip, and adequate spread of the dye. Although a single needle technique has been proposed,[58] two needles (one at L2 and the other at L3) are recommended for chemical neurolysis so that a smaller volume can be injected per needle. One to 2 mL of local anesthetic is injected, and if it is followed by a temperature increase, 3 to 4 mL of 6% to 10% phenol is injected per needle. The reported complications of the block include subarachnoid injection secondary to injection near the dural cuff at the intervertebral foramen, sensory and motor block due to nerve root injury, paresthesias, and backache[7] (Fig. 31-4 and Table 31-4). The ureter can be injured from the needle or from phenol-induced thrombosis of the branch of the ovarian artery supplying the ureter. Genitofemoral neuralgia occurs in 7% to 20% of patients and may last 4 to 5 weeks.[59]

Postsympathectomy dysesthesia results in numbness and pain in the thigh and may last several months. The use of fluoroscopy is mandatory when neurolytic block of the sympathetic chain is performed. Radiofrequency rhizotomy of the lumbar sympathetic nerves has been employed to avoid the complications from spillage of the neurolytic agent.[60] Despite evidence of early sympathetic blockade, the use of radiofrequency rhizotomy did not result in long-term relief. Compared with phenol neurolysis, incomplete neurolysis appears to be more common with radiofrequency rhizotomy.[61] However, the incidence of postsympathectomy neuralgia is higher in the phenol group (33% vs. 11%). A randomized controlled double-blinded study on 20 patients evaluated phenol versus radiofrequency rhizotomy. The results showed similar improvement in pain scores and noted that 1 out of 10 patients receiving phenol developed postsympathectomy neuralgia while 1 out of 10 phenol and 2 out of 10 radiofrequency patients experienced pain with needle positioning.[62,63]

Neurolysis of Other Peripheral Nerves

Neurolysis of the nerves in the extremities is very rarely performed because of the attendant paralysis of the extremity. Mullin reported neurolytic blockade of the brachial plexus with 10 mL 10% phenol in a patient with a painful arm secondary to Pancoast tumor.[64] The patient had short-term pain relief with minimal motor blockade. The complications from neurolysis of peripheral nerves include painful dysesthesias and sensory and motor blockade. The exact incidences of these complications are not known.

Neurolysis for Myofascial Pain and Spasticity

Neurolytic blocks of peripheral nerves are useful in patients with acquired spasticity, facilitating rehabilitation and restoring normal position of the limb. Diagnostic blocks with local anesthetic are usually performed before neurolytic injection to assess the value of the neurolytic injection. Examples of these blocks include obturator block to relieve hip adduction, musculocutaneous nerve block for elbow flexion, and posterior tibial nerve block for plantar flexion.[65]

Peripheral nerve blocks with phenol have been performed in patients with spasticity to improve their gait and balance and to assist in their rehabilitation. In this technique, the motor or mixed nerves are targeted preferentially. A nerve stimulator is recommended for precise needle localization. Injections of small volumes of 3% to 5% phenol are effective in relieving motor points in affected muscles. Relaxation of the muscle usually lasts 2 months, and functional training of the limb is performed during this time. In a randomized controlled trial of 20 patients evaluating phenol versus alcohol for chemical neurolysis of the tibial motor branches for gastrocnemius spasm after stroke, alcohol maintained its effect for 6 months in nine patients, while phenol lasted the same amount of time in six patients.[66] The reported complications include focal motor weakness in 15% of patients and dysesthesias in 10% of patients. The motor weakness usually lasts 1 week, whereas the dysesthesias last several days to weeks. A rare complication after phenol block of the brachioradialis and musculocutaneous nerves is arterial occlusion of the patient's upper limb.[67]

Neurolytic injections have been reported to be useful in patients with palpable painful neuromas (0.2–0.5 mL of 5% phenol),[68] in patients with poststernotomy pain secondary to scar neuroma (2–3 mL of 6% phenol),[69] and patients with painful surgical scars (1 mL of absolute alcohol).[70] Neuritis has not been reported after these trigger-point injections.

Visceral Sympathetic Neurolysis

Neurolytic Celiac Plexus Block

Celiac plexus blocks are very effective in relieving pain from intra-abdominal cancer because the celiac plexus innervates the abdominal viscera except for the left side of the colon and

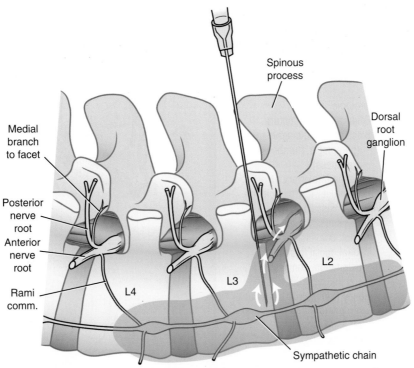

FIGURE 31-4. Complications of lumbar sympathetic neurolysis. During lumbar sympathetic block, injectate can spread from the correct location over the anterolateral surface of the lumbar vertebral bodies posteriorly to bathe the exiting spinal nerves and along the nerve roots to enter the epidural space. Neurolytic lumbar sympathetic block is typically carried out using multiple needles placed at L2, L3, and L4 to allow effective neurolysis using a small volume of injectate through each needle, thereby minimizing the risk of spread of the neurolytic solution. (Modified from Rathmell JP. Atlas of image-guided intervention in regional anesthesia and pain medicine. 2nd ed. Philadelphia, PA: Lippincott Williams & Wilkins, 2012, with permission.)

the pelvic viscera. The efficacy of neurolytic celiac plexus block (NCPB) has recently been shown in a randomized placebo-controlled study.[71] In this randomized controlled trial of 100 patients with unresectable pancreatic cancer, NCPB was compared with systemic analgesics. The patients who had analgesics had a sham injection, under fluoroscopy, with subcutaneous bupivacaine in the sites where the celiac plexus block needles are usually inserted. The patients were followed weekly for 1 year or until their death. The pain intensity and quality of life scores were improved 1 week after treatment in both groups, with a larger decrease in pain scores in the celiac plexus group. Pain was also lower over time in the NCPB group. However, opioid consumption, quality of life, and survival were not significantly different between the two groups.

Neurolysis of the celiac plexus can be performed through several approaches. These include the transaortic approach, transcrural approach, anterior approach, and via bilateral splanchnicectomy.[72] The three percutaneous NCPB techniques (the transcrural approach, transaortic approach, and the bilateral splanchnicectomy) were noted to be equally effective.[72] No statistical difference was noted in terms of the degree of pain relief, whether immediate or until the patient's death. Complications were minimal with all techniques, although the incidence of hypotension was less in the transaortic approach. Ultrasound-guided celiac plexus block has been described but there are no controlled studies on it.[73] Endoscopic ultrasound-guided celiac plexus block is performed by gastroenterologists but only a few well-controlled studies evaluated its efficacy.[74]

The complications of NCPB can be divided into neurologic, vascular, and visceral injuries; pneumothorax and pleural effusion; and metabolic complications[75] (Table 31-5). Neurologic complications include epidural and dural puncture, blockade of the somatic nerve roots (resulting in unilateral weakness or paraplegia or numbness of the thigh), and injection into the artery of Adamkiewicz, resulting in paraplegia.[76] Exposure to phenol or alcohol results in vasospasm of the segmental lumbar arteries in dogs,[77] and alcohol has been shown to have contractile effects in human aortic muscle cells by increasing the intracellular concentration of ionized calcium.[78] Vascular injury is quite common in this technique because the plexus is close to several blood vessels. It should be noted that one of the techniques of celiac plexus block is the transaortic approach. Intravascular injection of phenol results in convulsions,[15] whereas intravascular injection of alcohol usually does not result in intoxication because the resulting blood levels are low.[79] High levels of acetaldehyde may occur in Asians, who lack the enzyme aldehyde dehydrogenase, resulting in facial flushing, palpitations, and hypotension.[80]

Visceral injury usually involves the kidney, resulting in hematuria or even infarction when the neurolytic agent is injected into the renal parenchyma. Injury to the kidney occurs when the needle is inserted more than 7.5 cm from the midline, a higher vertebral body (T11) is targeted, and

TABLE 31-5	Complications of Visceral Sympathetic Blocks
BLOCK	**COMPLICATIONS**

Celiac plexus	Neurologic
	    Epidural/dural puncture
	    Block of somatic nerve roots
	        (paraplegia, numbness,
	        weakness)
	    Injection into artery of
	        Adamkiewicz (paraplegia)
	Vascular: vascular injury
	    Intravascular injection
	    Phenol: convulsions
	    Alcohol: facial flushing,
	        palpitation, convulsion
	Visceral injury
	    Kidney (hematuria, infarction)
	    Lung: pneumothorax, pleural
	        effusion
	Chylothorax
	Ejaculatory failure

Superior hypogastric plexus	Retroperitoneal hematoma Ischemia of foot

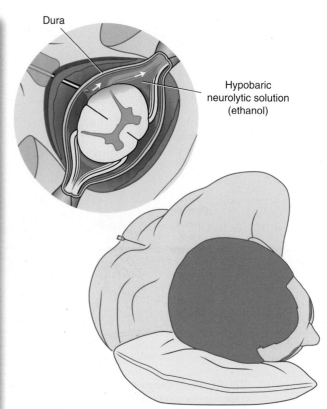

FIGURE 31-5. Complications of intrathecal neurolysis. Intrathecal neurolysis is performed infrequently for those who have intractable pain of the trunk or lower extremities associated with locally invasive cancer. When the block is performed using alcohol, a hypobaric solution, the patient is placed in the lateral position with the painful region upward or nondependent and the torso rotated 45 degrees anteriorly to bring the dorsal roots to the highest point within the CSF. The alcohol solution is then administered in small increments, and the hypobaric solution rises to bathe the dorsal roots. The neurolytic solution is placed directly adjacent to the spinal cord, and damage to the cord is a distinct possibility during intrathecal neurolysis.

when the needle tip rests excessively lateral to the vertebral body. Injury to the pancreas rarely occurs as shown by minimal, if any, changes in the amylase levels after celiac plexus block. Pneumothorax and pleural effusion have been reported after celiac plexus block. The mechanism of pleural effusion appears to be diaphragmatic irritation from overflow of the alcohol into the subdiaphragmatic space.[81] Acute pancreatitis and hemorrhage have also been proposed as possible mechanisms.[75] Other reported complications of NCPB include chylothorax[82] and ejaculatory failure.[83] In a study on 104 celiac plexus blocks, the reported complications and their incidences are weakness or numbness in the T10-L2 distribution (8%), lower chest pain (3%), postural hypotension (2%), failure of ejaculation (2%), urinary difficulty (1%), and warmth and fullness of the leg (1%).[83] Most of the complications of celiac plexus block can be avoided by the use of fluoroscopy or computed tomography and by meticulous technique. See Chapter 23 for a detailed discussion of the complications associated with celiac plexus block.

Neurolytic Superior Hypogastric Plexus and Ganglion Impar Block

Superior hypogastric plexus blocks are utilized in the management of pelvic pain secondary to cancer.[84–86] The superior hypogastric plexus lies in the retroperitoneum bilaterally, extending from the lower third of the fifth lumbar vertebra to the upper third of the first sacral vertebra. Complications include retroperitoneal hematoma and acute ischemia of the foot secondary to dislodgement of atherosclerotic plaques from the iliac vessels. No neurologic complications have been noted after 200 cases with this block.[86] Plancarte

performed 227 of these blocks on patients with a wide variety of abdominal complaints over a 3 year period, where he utilized a bilateral approach and injected phenol for neurolysis. He reported 159 (79%) positive responses with a 43% reduction in opioid use in 115 (72%) patients and no reported complications.[87]

Ganglion impar block lies at the sacrococcygeal junction and relieves perineal pain.[88] No complications have been reported with this technique, but the published experience with this block is minimal. See Chapter 24 for a detailed discussion of the complications associated with superior hypogastric and ganglion impar blocks.

Neuraxial Neurolysis

Subarachnoid neurolytic (Figures 31-5 and 31-6) blocks are utilized in patients with short-life expectancy, whose pain is somatic in origin and limited to two or three dermatomes, not completely relieved by analgesic and adjunctive medications, and completely relieved by prognostic local anesthetic blocks.[89] The recommended dose of subarachnoid alcohol and phenol is very small (0.1-mL increments are injected up to a total of 0.8 mL). The patient is to remain in position for at least 30 minutes after the injection, and air is injected

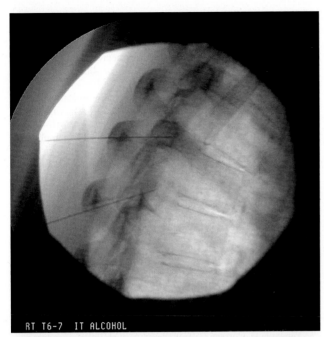

FIGURE 31-6. Intrathecal alcohol injection: Lateral view showing two needles in final position in the right posterolateral spinal canal within the subarachnoid space. The patient had severe postherpetic neuralgia and was previously unresponsive to medications and intrathecal methylprednisolone. She had excellent relief after an intrathecal alcohol injection.

TABLE 31-6	Complications of Subarachnoid Neurolytic Blocks
• Dural puncture headache
• Bowel paralysis
• Bladder paralysis
• Numbness
• Muscle weakness
• Dysesthesia

to clear the needle before it is withdrawn. Complications include meningeal puncture headache, aseptic meningitis, bowel and bladder dysfunction, numbness, muscle weakness, and dysesthesia[89] (Table 31-6). The incidences of these complications ranged from 1% to 26% for rectal and urinary dysfunction, 1% to 14% for lower extremity paresis, 1% to 21% for sensory loss, and 0.3% to 4% for paresthesia/neuritis.[90] The nature of the complication depends on the site of injection. Motor weakness is noted when the injection is at the lumbar or cervical area, whereas bladder complications usually occur when the level of injection is below the thoracic nerve roots. Because of the severity of the complications, it is important that patients be properly selected and informed of the complications. Patients should also be properly positioned and the needle inserted at the proper interspace.

The epidural approach to chemical neurolysis has been advocated for improved efficacy at the thoracic and cervicothoracic junction, increased safety, ease of repeated injections, and relief of bilateral pain.[91,92] The placement of a thoracic epidural catheter is less demanding than positioning of multiple needles just barely into the subarachnoid space but not within the spinal cord.[93] As stated previously, subarachnoid alcohol is injected with the painful side up, whereas phenol is injected with the painful side down. Positioning with respect to the baricity of the alcohol or phenol is not a consideration in epidural neurolysis. The epidural catheter is inserted at the vertebral level corresponding to the painful area. Confirmation of catheter placement with injection of a radiopaque dye is recommended to confirm the spread of the injectate. Three to 4 mL of local anesthetic is injected, and the patient's response is followed. The same volume (2–5 mL) of 5.5% phenol in saline, or ethyl alcohol

is injected over 20 to 30 minutes in 0.2-mL increments. The injections are given daily for up to 3 days,[91] or until the patient has significant pain relief.[92] Analgesia lasts 1 to 3 months. It should be noted that there has been no study that compared the efficacy of subarachnoid and epidural neurolysis. Although no serious complications were noted in previous publications, the safety of epidural neurolysis has been questioned. In primates, lower extremity weakness has been noted clinically, and posterior nerve root damage was demonstrated histologically.[94] Autopsy studies in a patient showed destruction at the outer third of the dura, with no abnormality of the spinal cord or the nerve roots.[95]

Subarachnoid neurolytic block for cancer pain is rarely used now because intrathecal opioid pumps have supplanted it. Intrathecal morphine pumps have the advantage of managing pain from progression of the disease or future sites of painful metastases, which are common occurrences in a patient with malignancy.

A case report of transforaminal 5% phenol injection has been published. Per the report, the patient had leiomyosarcoma that was metastatic to the epidural space, could not take narcotics due to constipation, and had severe unremitting flank and low back pain. Transforaminal approach to the epidural space was chosen due to the epidural tumor burden, and three levels (L3-4, L1-2, T12-L1) were performed in two stages. The patient reported complete pain relief, and no side effects were noted until the patient passed away 11 days later.[96]

▶ CRYONEUROLYSIS AND ITS COMPLICATIONS

Cryoanalgesia is a technique wherein peripheral nerves are destroyed by extreme cold to achieve pain relief.[97] After cryolesion, there is wallerian degeneration with axonal disintegration and breakup of the myelin sheaths, with minimal disruption of the endoneurium and other connective tissue elements. Recovery occurs after several weeks, and relief lasts 2 weeks to 5 months.[97] It has been used in the treatment of pain after surgery, including thoracotomy and inguinal herniorrhaphy.[98,99] For chronic pain management, cryoanalgesia has been employed in intercostal neuralgia, painful neuromas, and back pain secondary to facet syndrome. It has also been used for head and neck pain.[100] Virtually every peripheral somatic nerve can be lesioned. Complications are minimal and are largely related to the procedure itself, especially the location of the nerve to be blocked. A possible complication is the development of full thickness destruction of the skin secondary to freezing along the needle. The use of cryoanalgesia has declined over the last few years, partly because of the temporary nature of its effect. Thermal radiofrequency rhizotomy has gained widespread use in the management of facet syndrome,[101] whereas pulsed radiofrequency is gaining popularity in the rhizotomy of peripheral nerves.[102] See Chapter 32 for detailed discussion of radiofrequency treatment and its complications.

References

1. Raj PP. Peripheral neurolysis in the management of pain. In: Waldman SD, Winnie AP, eds. *Interventional Pain Management*. Philadelphia, PA: WB Saunders, 1996:392–400.
2. Rumsby MG, Finean JB. The action of organic solvents on the myelin sheath of peripheral nerve tissue-II (short chain and aliphatic alcohols). *J Neurochem* 1966;13:1509–1511.
3. Myers RR, Katz J. Neurolytic agents. In: Raj PP, ed. *Practical Management of Pain*. 2nd ed. St. Louis, MO: Mosby Year Book, 1992:701–712.
4. Jain S, Gupta R. Neurolytic agents in clinical practice. In: Waldman SD, Winnie AP, eds. *Interventional Pain Management*. Philadelphia, PA: WB Saunders, 1996:167–171.
5. Gallagher HS, Yonezawa T, Hoy RC, et al. Subarachnoid alcohol block. II: histological changes in the central nervous system. *Am J Pathol* 1961;35:679.
6. Labat G. The action of alcohol on the living nerve: experimental and clinical considerations. *Anesth Analg Curr Res* 1933;12:190–196.
7. Swerdlow M. Complications of neurolytic neural blockade. In: Cousins MJ, Bridenbaugh PO, eds. *Neural Blockade in Clinical Anesthesia and Management of Pain*. 2nd ed. Philadelphia, PA: JB Lippincott, 1988:719–735.
8. Wong GY, Brown DL. Transient paraplegia following alcohol celiac plexus block. *Reg Anesth* 1995 20:352–355.
9. McGarvey ML, Ferrante FM, Patel RS, et al. Irreversible spinal cord injury as a complication of subarachnoid ethanol neurolysis. *Neurology* 2000;54:1522–1524.
10. Kong KH, Chua KS. Intramuscular neurolysis with alcohol to treat post-stroke finger flexor spasticity. *Clin Rehabil* 2002;16:378–381.
11. Jang SH, Ahn SH, Park SM, et al. Alcohol neurolysis of tibial nerve motor branches to the gastrocnemius muscle to treat ankle spasticity in patients with hemiplegic stroke. *Arch Phys Med Rehabil* 2004;85:506–508.
12. Wood KM. The use of phenol as a neurolytic agent. *Pain* 1978;5:205–229.
13. Moller JE, Helweg-Larson J, Jacobson E. Histopathological lesions in the sciatic nerve of the rat following perineural application of phenol and alcohol solutions. *Dan Med Bull* 1969;16:116–119.
14. Schaumburg HH, Byck R, Weller RO. The effect of phenol in peripheral nerve: a histological and physiologic study. *J Neuropathol Exp Neurol* 1970;29:615–630.
15. Benzon HT. Convulsions secondary to intravascular phenol: a hazard of celiac plexus block. *Anesth Analg* 1979;58:150–151.
16. Gupta S, Ashrith G, Chandra D, et al. Acute phenol poisoning: a life-threatening hazard of chronic pain relief. *Clin Toxicol (Phila)* 2008;46:250–253.
17. Khalili AA, Betts HB. Peripheral nerve block with phenol in the management of spasticity: indications and complications. *JAMA* 1967;200:1155–1157.
18. Waldman SD. Blockade of the Gasserian ganglion and the distal trigeminal nerve. In: Waldman SD, Winnie AP, eds. *Interventional Pain Management*. Philadelphia, PA: WB Saunders, 1996:230–241.
19. Brown DL. Trigeminal (gasserian) ganglion block. In: Brown DL, ed. *Atlas of Regional Anesthesia*. Philadelphia, PA: WB Saunders, 1992:140.
20. Crimeni R. Clinical experience with mepivacaine and alcohol in neuralgia of the trigeminal nerve. *Acta Anaesthesiol Scand* 1966;10:173.
21. Loeser JD, Sweet WH, Tew JM, et al. Neurosurgical operations involving peripheral nerves. In: Bonica JJ, ed. *The Management of Pain*. 2nd ed. Philadelphia, PA: Lea & Febiger, 1990:2044–2066.
22. Ugur HC, Savas A, Elhan A, et al. Unanticipated complication of percutaneous radiofrequency trigeminal rhizotomy: rhinorrhea: report of three cases and a cadaver study. *Neurosurgery* 2004;54:1522–1524.
23. Wilkinson HA. Trigeminal nerve peripheral branch phenol/glycerol injections for tic douloureux. *J Neurosurg* 1999;90:828–832.
24. Katz J, Levin AB. Treatment of diffuse metastatic cancer pain by instillation of alcohol into the sella turcica. *Anesthesiology* 1977;46:115–121.
25. Corssen G, Holcomb MC, Moustapha I, et al. Alcohol induced adenolysis of the pituitary gland: a new approach to control of intractable cancer pain. *Anesth Analg* 1977;56:414–421.
26. Waldman SD, Feldstein GS. Neuroadenolysis of the pituitary: description of a modified technique. *J Pain Symptom Manage* 1987;2:45–49.
27. Yanagida H, Corssen G, Trouwborst A, et al. Relief of cancer pain in man: alcohol-induced neuroadenolysis vs. electrical stimulation of the pituitary gland. *Pain* 1984;19:133–141.
28. Katz J, Levin AB. Long-term follow-up study of chemical hypophysectomy and additional cases. *Anesthesiology* 1979;51:167–169.
29. Waldman SD. Neuroadenolysis of the pituitary: indications and technique. In: Waldman SD, Winnie AP, eds. *Interventional Pain Management*. Philadelphia, PA: WB Saunders, 1996:519–525.
30. Montgomery W, Cousins MJ. Aspects of the management of chronic pain illustrated by ninth cranial nerve block. *Br J Anaesth* 1972;44:383–385.
31. Pagura JR, Shnapp, M, Passarelli P. Percutaneous radiofrequency glossopharyngeal rhizotomy for cancer pain. *Appl Neurophysiol* 1983;46:154.
32. Gofeld M, Bhatia A, Abbas S, et al. Development and validation of a new technique for ultrasound-guided stellate ganglion block. *Reg Anesth Pain Med* 2009;34:475–479.
33. Nader A, Benzon HT. Peripheral sympathetic blocks. In: Benzon HT, Raja SN, Molloy RE, et al.,eds. *Essentials of Pain Medicine and Regional Anesthesia*. 2nd ed. Philadelphia, PA: Elsevier, 2005:689–693.
34. Christie JM, Martinez CR. Computerized axial tomography to define the distribution of solution after stellate ganglion nerve block. *J Clin Anesth* 1995;7:306–311.
35. Kapral S, Krafft P, Gosch M, et al. Ultrasound imaging for stellate ganglion block: direct visualization of puncture site and local anesthetic spread. A pilot study. *Reg Anesth* 1995;20:323–328.
36. Narouze S, Vydyanathan A, Patel N. Ultrasound-guided stellate ganglion block successfully prevented esophageal puncture. *Pain Physician* 2007;10:747–752.
37. Shibata Y, Fujiwara Y, Komatsu T. A new approach of ultrasound-guided stellate ganglion block. *Anesth Analg* 2007;105:550–551.
38. Marples IL, Atkin RE. Stellate ganglion block. *Pain Rev* 2001;8:3–11.
39. Keim HA. Cord paralysis following injection into traumatic cervical meningocele: complication of stellate ganglion block. *NY State J Med* 1970;70:2115–2116.
40. Higa K, Hirata K, Hirota K, et al. Retropharyngeal hematoma after stellate ganglion block: analysis of 27 patients reported in the literature. *Anesthesiology* 2006;105:1238–1245.
41. Takanami I, Abiko T, Koizumi S. Life-threatening airway obstruction due to retropharyngeal and cervicomediastinal hematomas following stellate ganglion block. *Thorac Cardiovasc Surg* 2009;57:311–312.

42. Dukes RR, Alexander LA. Transient locked-in syndrome after vascular injection during stellate ganglion block. *Reg Anesth* 1993;18:378–380.

43. Moore DC, Bridenbaugh LD. Intercostal nerve block in 4,333 patients: indications, techniques, and complications. *Anesth Analg* 1962;41:1–11.

44. Molloy RE. Truncal blocks: intercostal, paravertebral, interpleural, suprascapular, ilioinguinal, and iliohypogastric nerve blocks. In: Benzon HT, Raja S, Molloy RE, et al., eds. *Essentials of Pain Medicine and Regional Anesthesia.* 2nd ed. New York, NY: Elsevier/Churchill Livingstone, 2005:636–644.

45. Moore DC, Bridenbaugh LD. Pneumothorax: its incidence following intercostal nerve block. *JAMA* 1960;174:842.

46. Benumof JF, Semenza J. Total spinal anesthesia following intrathoracic intercostal nerve blocks. *Anesthesiology* 1975;43:124–125.

47. Atkinson GL, Shupack RC. Acute bronchospasm complicating intercostal nerve block with phenol. *Anesth Analg* 1989;68:400.

48. Kowalewski R, Schurch B, Hodler J, et al. Persistent paraplegia after an aqueous 7.5% phenol solution to the anterior motor root for intercostal neurolysis: a case report. *Arch Phys Med Rehabil* 2002;83:283–285.

49. Byas-Smith MG, Gulati A. Ultrasound-guided intercostal nerve cryoablation. *Anesth Analg* 2006;103:1033–1035.

50. Purcell-Jones G, Pither CE, Justins DM. Paravertebral somatic nerve block: a clinical radiographic, and computed tomographic study in chronic pain patients. *Anesth Analg* 1989;68:32–39.

51. Perttunen K, Nilsson E, Heinonen J, et al. Extradural, paravertebral and intercostal nerve blocks for post-thoracotomy pain. *Br J Anaesth* 1995;75:541–547.

52. Cowie B, McGlade D, Ivanusic J, et al. Ultrasound-guided thoracic paravertebral blockade: a cadaveric study. *Anesth Analg* 2010;110:1735–1739.

53. Ejlersen E, Andersen HB, Elaisen K, et al. A comparison between preincisional and postincisional lidocaine infiltration and postoperative pain. *Anesth Analg* 1992;74:495–498.

54. Dierking GW, Dahl JB, Kanstrup J, et al. Effect of pre-vs. postoperative inguinal inguinal field block on postoperative pain after herniorrhaphy. *Br J Anaesth* 1992;68:344–348.

55. Bunting P, McConachie I. Ilioinguinal nerve blockade for analgesia after cesarean section. *Br J Anaesth* 1988;61:773–775.

56. Cohen SP, Foster A. Pulsed radiofrequency as a treatment for groin pain and orchialgia. *Urology* 2003;61:645–647.

57. Umeda S, Arai T, Hatano Y, et al. Cadaver anatomic analysis of the best site for chemical lumbar sympathectomy. *Anesth Analg* 1987;66:643–646.

58. Hatangdi VS, Boas RA. Lumbar sympathectomy: a single-needle technique. *Br J Anaesth* 1985;57:285.

59. Cherry DA. Chemical lumbar sympathectomy. *Curr Concepts Pain* 1984;2:12–15.

60. Rocco AG. Radiofrequency lumbar sympatholysis: the evolution of a technique for managing sympathetically maintained pain. *Reg Anesth* 1995;20:3–12.

61. Haynsworth RF, Noe CE. Percutaneous lumbar sympathectomy: a comparison of radiofrequency denervation versus phenol neurolysis. *Anesthesiology* 1991;74:459–463.

62. Straube S, Derry S, Moore RA, et al. Cervico-thoracic or lumbar sympathectomy for neuropathic pain and complex regional pain syndrome. *Cochrane Database Syst Rev* 2010;(7):CD002918.

63. Manjunath PS, Jayalakshmi TS, Dureja GP, et al. Management of lower limb complex regional pain syndrome type 1: an evaluation of percutaneous radiofrequency thermal lumbar sympathectomy versus phenol lumbar sympathetic neurolysis—a pilot study. *Anesth Analg* 2008;106:647–649.

64. Mullin V. Brachial plexus block with phenol for painful arm associated with Pancoast syndrome. *Anesthesiology* 1980;53:341–342.

65. Garland DE, Lucie RS, Waters RL. Current uses of open phenol nerve block for adult acquired spasticity. *Clin Orthop Rel Res* 1982;165:217–222.

66. Kocabas H, Salli A, Demir AH, et al. Comparison of phenol and alcohol neurolysis of tibial nerve motor branches to the gastrocnemius muscle for treatment of spastic foot after stroke: a randomized controlled pilot study. *Eur J Phys Rehabil Med* 2010;46:5–10.

67. Gibson JM. Phenol block in the treatment of spasticity. *Gerontology* 1987;33:327.

68. Ramamurthy S, Walsh NE, Schenfeld LS, et al. Evaluation of neurolytic blocks using phenol and cryogenic block in the management of chronic pain. *J Pain Symptom Manage* 1989;4:72.

69. Todd DP. Poststernotomy neuralgia: a new pain syndrome. *Anesth Analg* 1989;69:691.

70. Defalque RJ. Painful trigger points in surgical scars. *Anesth Analg* 1982;61:518–520.

71. Wong GY, Schroeder DR, Carns PE, et al. Effect of neurolytic celiac plexus block on pain relief, quality of life, and survival in patients with unresectable pancreatic cancer: a randomized controlled trial. *JAMA* 2004;291:1092–1099.

72. Ischia S, Ischia A, Polati E, et al. Three posterior percutaneous celiac plexus block techniques. *Anesthesiology* 1992;76:534–540.

73. Bhatnagar S, Gupta D, Mishra S, et al. Bedside ultrasound-guided celiac plexus neurolysis with bilateral paramedian needle entry technique can be an effective pain control technique in advanced upper abdominal cancer pain. *J Palliat Med* 2008;11:1195–1199.

74. Kaufman M, Singh G, Das S, et al. Efficacy of endoscopic ultrasound-guided celiac plexus block neurolysis for managing abdominal pain associated with chronic pancreatitis and pancreatic cancer. *J Clin Gastroenterol* 2010;44:127–134.

75. Waldman SD, Patt RB. Celiac plexus block and splanchnic nerve block. In: Waldman SD, Winnie AP, eds. *Interventional Pain Management.* Philadelphia, PA: WB Saunders, 1996:360–373.

76. Galizia EJ, Lahiri SK. Paraplegia following coeliac plexus block with phenol. *Br J Anaesth* 1974;46:539–540.

77. Brown DL, Rorie DK. Altered reactivity of isolated segmental lumbar arteries of dogs following exposure to ethanol and phenol. *Pain* 1994;56:139.

78. Johnson ME, Sill JC, Brown DL, et al. The effect of neurolytic agent ethanol on cytoplasmic calcium in arterial smooth muscle and endothelium. *Reg Anesth* 1996;21:6–13.

79. Jain S, Hirsch R, Shah N, et al. Blood ethanol levels following celiac plexus block with 50% ethanol. *Anesth Analg* 1989;68:S135.

80. Noda J, Umeda S, Mori K, et al. Acetaldehyde syndrome after celiac plexus block. *Anesth Analg* 65:1300–1302.

81. Fujita Y, Takori M. Pleural effusion after CT-guided alcohol celiac plexus block. *Anesth Analg* 1987;66:911–912.

82. Fine PG, Bubela C. Chylothorax following celiac plexus block. *Anesthesiology* 1985;63:454–456.

83. Black A, Dwyer B. Coeliac plexus block. *Anaesth Intensive Care* 1973;1:315.

84. Plancarte R, Amezcua C, Patt RB, et al. Superior hypogastric plexus block for cancer pain. *Anesthesiology* 1990;73:236–239.

85. de Leon-Casasola OA, Kent E, Lema MJ. Neurolytic superior hypogastric plexus block for chronic pelvic pain associated with cancer. *Pain* 1993;54:145–151.

86. Rosenberg SK, Tewari R, Boswell MV, et al. Superior hypogastric plexus block successfully treats penile pain after transurethral resection of the prostate. *Reg Anesth Pain Med* 1998;23:618–620.

87. Plancarte R, de Leon-Casasola OA, El-Helaly M, et al. Neurolytic superior hypogastric plexus block for chronic pelvic pain associated with cancer. *Reg Anesth* 1997;22:562–568.

88. Wemm K, Saberski L. Modified approach to block the ganglion impar (ganglion of Walther). *Reg Anesth* 1995;20:544.

89. Winnie AP. Subarachnoid neurolytic blocks. In: Waldman SD, Winnie AP, eds. *Interventional Pain Management.* Philadelphia, PA: WB Saunders, 1996;401–405.

90. Cousins MJ. Chronic pain and neurolytic neural blockade. In: Cousins MJ, Bridenbaugh PO, eds. *Neural Blockade in Clinical Anesthesia and Management of Pain.* 2nd ed. Philadelphia, PA: JB Lippincott, 1988:1053–1084.

91. Korevaar WC. Transcatheter thoracic epidural neurolysis using ethyl alcohol. *Anesthesiology* 1988;69:989–993.

92. Racz GB, Sabongy M, Gintautas J, et al. Intractable pain therapy using a new epidural catheter. *JAMA* 1982;248:579–581.

93. Molloy RE. Intrathecal and epidural neurolysis. In: Benzon HT, Raja S, Molloy RE, et al.,eds. *Essentials of Pain Medicine and Regional Anesthesia*. 2nd ed. New York, NY: Elsevier/Churchill Livingstone, 2005:550–557.

94. Katz JA, Selhorst S, Blisard KS. Histopathological changes in primate spinal cord after single and repeated epidural phenol administration. *Reg Anesth* 1995;20:283–290.

95. Hayashi I, Odashiro M, Sasaki Y. Two cases of epidural neurolysis using ethyl alcohol and histopathologic changes in the spinal cord. *Masui* 2000;49:877–880.

96. Candido KD, Philip CN, Ghaly RF, et al. Transforaminal 5% phenol neurolysis for the treatment of intractable cancer pain. *Anesth Analg* 2010;110:216–219.

97. Lloyd JW, Barnard JDW, Glynn CJ. Cryoanalgesia: a new approach to pain relief. *Lancet* 1976;2:932–934.

98. Gough JD, Williams AB, Vaughan RS. The control of post-thoracotomy pain: a comparative evaluation of thoracic epidural fentanyl infusion and cryo-analgesia. *Anaesthesia* 1988;43:780–783.

99. Wood G, Lloyd J, Bullingham R, et al. Postoperative analgesia for day case herniorrhaphy patients: a comparison of cryoanalgesia, paravertebral blockade, and oral analgesia. *Anaesthesia* 1981;36:603–610.

100. Barnard D, Lloyd J, Evans J. Cryoanalgesia in the management of chronic facial pain. *J Maxillofacial Surg* 1981;9:101–102.

101. Rallo-Clemans R, Benzon HT. Facet joint pain: facet joint injections and facet rhizotomy. In: Benzon HT, Raja S, Molloy RE, et al.,eds. *Essentials of Pain Medicine and Regional Anesthesia*. 2nd ed. New York, NY: Elsevier/Churchill Livingstone, 2005:348–355.

102. Shah RV, Racz GB. Pulsed mode radiofrequency lesioning of the suprascapular nerve for the treatment of chronic shoulder pain. *Pain Physician* 2003;6:503–506.

32

Complications Associated with Radiofrequency Treatment for Chronic Pain

James P. Rathmell and Adam J. Carinci

Experimental attempts to use electricity to produce discrete tissue lesions were reported as early as the 1870s in animals and introduced into clinical practice in the 1930s.[1] Sweet and Mark[2] attempted to use direct current but found that this led to unpredictable and irregular lesions that varied in size by a factor of 4. Sweet and subsequent investigators suggested that use of a high-frequency current might produce more predictable lesions. From their experimental work on hemostasis, Aranow[3] adapted a radiofrequency (RF) technique for producing neural lesions in the 1950s. RF generators utilize high-frequency waves in the range of 300 to 500 kHz to produce tissue lesions via ionic means. Because high frequencies in this range were also used in radiotransmitters, the current was named RF current. Conventional RF treatment uses a constant output of high-frequency electric current, produces controllable tissue destruction surrounding the tip of the treatment cannula (Fig. 32-1), and, when placed at precise anatomic locations, has demonstrated success in reducing a number of different chronic pain states, including chronic neck pain after whiplash injury[4] and trigeminal neuralgia.[5]

Pulsed RF uses brief "pulses" of high-voltage RF-range (~300 kHz) electrical current that produce the same voltage fluctuations in the region of treatment that occur during conventional RF treatment but without heating to a temperature at which tissue coagulates (Box 32-1). The conceptual appeal of a minimally invasive nondestructive technique that is useful in treating chronic pain of any sort is compelling. In clinical practice, there has been a mass migration to the use of pulsed RF despite little data to support efficacy of this new technique. The modality has great appeal, specifically because it is not neurodestructive. With conventional RF, the thermal lesion occasionally leads to worsening pain and even new onset of neuropathic pain.[6] A small retrospective case series[7] and extensive clinical experience among practitioners suggest that pulsed RF results in neither increased pain nor any risk of neuropathic pain and that

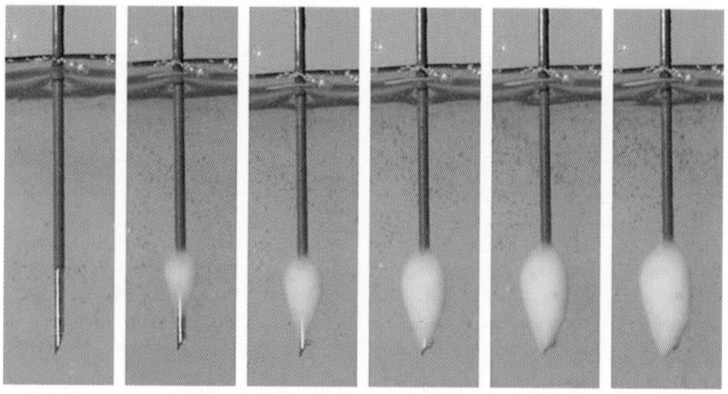

FIGURE 32-1. Conventional RF lesion. A 10-cm RF cannula with a 5-mm active tip is immersed in egg white and a lesion is carried out at 80°C for 90 seconds. The size of the lesion is maximal near the mid-portion of the active tip, with little coagulation at the tip of the needle. Thus, for optimal application of conventional RF treatment the shaft of the needle's active tip must be placed adjacent to the target. The size of the lesion is near maximal by 60 seconds of treatment, changing little in size thereafter. (Reproduced with permission from Rathmell JP. *Atlas of Image-guided Intervention in Regional Anesthesia and Pain Medicine.* 2nd ed. Philadelphia, PA: Lippincott Williams & Wilkins, 2012.)

it is very well tolerated by patients from treatment through recovery. This technique is in need of further study to validate its usefulness.

▶ DEFINITION

Conventional wisdom holds that the usefulness of RF stems from the ability to produce a small lesion of precise dimensions in a specific anatomic location.[10] Pulsed RF produces the same voltage fluctuations in the region of treatment as conventional RF but without tissue coagulation. Complications associated with RF treatment fall into two broad categories: those that arise during placement of the RF cannula and those that result from neural destruction during conventional RF neurotomy. As may occur with any technique that requires

needle placement, direct injury to neural or vascular structures in the vicinity of treatment can occur. Both conventional and pulsed RF treatment are associated with similar risk of injury during needle placement. Conventional RF neurotomy using a heat lesion that produces neural destruction is also associated with the sequelae of neural injury that follow placement of lesions. Even with proper technique, conventional RF lesions are associated with sensory loss and onset of neuropathic pain in a subset of patients. The frequency and severity of these neural changes vary with the specific site of treatment and are most common after intracranial RF lesioning of the trigeminal ganglion. Injury to adjacent nerves can also occur, and the frequency of these complications is minimized by the proper use of sensory and motor stimulation before lesioning.

▶ RADIOFREQUENCY TREATMENT FOR TRIGEMINAL NEURALGIA

Scope

Trigeminal neuralgia (tic douloureux) is a common idiopathic form of neuropathic pain that presents with paroxysms of pain involving one or more division of the trigeminal nerve (cranial nerve V). The disorder typically strikes those in the sixth decade of life, is of sudden onset without a precipitating event, and has a 2:1 predominance in females (Table 32-1).[11] Patients report episodic and severe pain involving one or more branches of the trigeminal nerve. The most commonly affected branches are the second and third divisions together, followed closely by involvement of either the second or third division alone. Those affected often describe a small area that "triggers" paroxysms of pain. Perhaps, pressure on an incisor or slight touch to the margins of the lip precipitates lancinating pains along the entire course of the involved division of the trigeminal nerve. The pain typically occurs in brief paroxysms lasting just seconds at a time, but may escalate to a frequency of many episodes daily.[12] The underlying etiology remains unknown, but experts have hypothesized that

---

BOX 32-1 How Is "Radiofrequency" Energy Used to Treat Pain?

RF generators produce high-frequency voltage fluctuations in the range of 300 to 500 kHz, the medium frequency range of the electromagnetic spectrum used in amplitude modulated broadcasting.

Conventional (*thermal*) RF *treatment* utilizes a continuous output of RF voltage fluctuations that produces movement of ions within the tissue adjacent to the uninsulated tip of the needle or "cannula." Movement of ions leads to heating within the tissue. The temperature at the tip of the cannula is measured continuously during treatment using a small wire probe inserted in the cannula, the thermocouple. The power output of the generator is adjusted to maintain a constant temperature at the tip of the cannula, typically 80°C. The size of the uninsulated or "active" tip of the cannula (typically ranging from 2 to 10 mm) and the temperature maintained during treatment determine the size of the lesion that results. Tissue coagulation begins above about 45°C; thus,

conventional RF treatment has also been termed "neurolysis," "neurotomy," or "ablation."

Pulsed RF treatment uses brief "pulses" of the same range (~300 kHz) of RF voltage fluctuations, using cannula and thermocouple identical to those used during conventional RF treatment. The energy is applied intermittently, typically in pulses of energy lasting 20 to 30 milliseconds and repeated twice each second (2 Hz). The power output and the duration of the pulses are varied automatically by the RF generator to assure that the tip temperature does not rise above a set temperature point, most often 42°C, to assure that no tissue coagulation occurs. It has been demonstrated that applying such pulses of energy adjacent to specific neural structures can produce changes in gene expression within neurons in the dorsal horn of the spinal cord.[8] However, how or if these changes in gene expression relate to reduction in pain and the clinical utility of pulsed RF treatment awaits further validation.[9]

TABLE 32-1 Characteristics of 154 Consecutive Patients with Trigeminal Neuralgia Treated with RF Rhizotomy

CHARACTERISTIC	15-YEAR FOLLOW-UP (100 PATIENTS)	<15-YEAR FOLLOW-UP (54 PATIENTS)
Age (y)	63 (range 35–82)	62 (range 44–4)
Sex		
Male	35 (35%)	19 (35%)
Female	65 (65%)	35 (65%)
Mean pain	6.4 y (range 3 mo–21 y)	7 y (range 6 mo–16 y)
Side of pain		
Right	35 (35%)	15 (28%)
Left	65 (65%)	39 (72%)
Pain distribution		
CN V1	2 (2%)	1 (2%)
CN V2	15 (15%)	10 (19%)
CN V3	17 (17%)	13 (24%)
CNs V1, V2	20 (20%)	9 (17%)
CNs V2, V3	42 (42%)	20 (37%)
CNs V1, V2, V3	4 (4%)	1 (2%)

CN, cranial nerve.
Adapted from Taha JM, Tew JM Jr, Buncher CR. A prospective 15-year follow up of 154 consecutive patients with trigeminal neuralgia treated by percutaneous stereotactic radiofrequency thermal rhizotomy. *J Neurosurg* 1995;83:989–993.

second-order neurons within the trigeminal ganglion become sensitized, and following sensory input from the trigger area seizure-like hyperactivity is triggered in adjacent sensory neurons and is manifested as pain. Recurrent trauma due to pulsatile compression of the ganglion caused by the small branch vessels from the adjacent carotid siphon has been postulated as the underlying cause of neural injury that leads to trigeminal neuralgia,[13,14] and from this hypothesis treatment via posterior craniotomy and microvascular decompression has evolved as a successful treatment.[15]

Upon initial presentation, patients should undergo a thorough neurologic examination to exclude other causes that might precipitate similar symptoms, such as an intracranial tumor or demyelinating disease. In the majority of cases, no underlying etiology can be clearly identified, and treatment begins with antiepileptic drugs. Carbamazepine has long been the drug of first choice and is successful in controlling the pain in the majority of patients.[16] Indeed, early practitioners often regarded response to carbamazepine as diagnostic for this disorder. At the current time, owing to the appearance of blood dyscrasias and hepatotoxicity in a minority of those receiving carbamazepine, newer antiepileptic drugs (including lamotrigine, oxcarbazepine, gabapentin, pregabalin, and duloxetine) are often used prior to treatment with carbamazepine.

Invariably, a proportion of patients will continue to experience debilitating pain despite drug treatment or their pain will recur and become refractory to pharmacologic management, and this group will seek further treatment. A wide range of neuroablative techniques have been developed, all aimed at destroying a small number of cells within the affected area of the trigeminal ganglion and thereby eliminating the neuronal excitability.[17] Available techniques range from chemical destruction with glycerol to focused external-beam radiotherapy (radiosurgery), and among these neuroablative techniques the most widely used has been percutaneous RF ablation of the trigeminal ganglion (Table 32-2).[17] The use of high-resolution magnetic resonance imaging (MRI) and radiosurgery has rapidly evolved in recent years, and many experts place this treatment modality foremost among available treatment options.[18] Choosing among the available treatment techniques can be difficult, but most experts currently recommend microvascular decompression via a posterior fossa approach for those patients without coexisting medical illness that would make the risk of this major surgery unacceptable.[17] All of the available neuroablative techniques will produce some degree of sensory and/or motor loss. Microvascular decompression is the only treatment approach associated with a high success rate without creating neurologic deficits and without the need for ongoing pharmacologic therapy. However, because this is a major intracranial surgery, there is a small but significant risk of major neurologic injury and death.

RF ablation of the trigeminal ganglion has been in use for decades, and there are large retrospective series conducted in a similar fashion to guide our understanding of the usefulness and complications associated with this approach. In current times, the use has declined and is now limited·to those patients who have failed pharmacologic therapy and are not deemed medically fit or decline to undergo microvascular decompression.[17] The initial success rates for all surgical interventions range from 92% to 98% (Table 32-2). The rate of pain recurrence among percutaneous techniques is lowest with RF rhizotomy (20% in 9 years) when compared with glycerol rhizotomy (54% in 4 years) and balloon compression (21% in 2 years).[17] The most common complications and adverse effects (some of which are an expected part of the treatment) include facial numbness (98%), dysesthesia (24%), anesthesia dolorosa (1.5%), corneal anesthesia (7%), keratitis (1%), and trigeminal motor dysfunction (24%) (Table 32-2). A recent review details the range of incidence of complications from the published literature (Table 32-3).[19]

Mechanism of Injury

The mechanism of injury during RF rhizotomy for trigeminal neuralgia may be related to injury caused during placement

TABLE 32-2 Results of Percutaneous Techniques and Posterior Fossa Exploration for Patients Treated for Trigeminal Neuralgia

	PATIENTS (%)				
	PERCUTANEOUS TECHNIQUES			POSTERIOR FOSSA EXPLORATION	
	RF RHIZOTOMY ($n = 6{,}205$)	GLYCEROL RHIZOTOMY ($n = 1{,}217$)	BALLOON COMPRESSION ($n = 759$)	MICROVASCULAR DECOMPRESSION ($n = 1{,}417$)	PARTIAL TRIGEMINAL RHIZOTOMY ($n = 250$)
Procedure completed	100	94	99	85	100
Initial pain relief	98	91	93	98	92
Success of procedure	98	85	92	83	92
Pain recurrence	23	54	21	15	18
Facial numbness	98	60	72	2	100
Minor dysesthesia	14	11	14	0.2	5
Major dysesthesia	10	5	5	0.3	5
Anesthesia dolorosa	1.5	1.8	0.1	0	1
Corneal anesthesia	7	3.7	1.5	0.05	3
Keratitis	1	1.8	0	0	0
Trigeminal motor dysfunction	24	1.7	66	0	0
Permanent cranial nerve deficit	0	0	0	3[a]	
Perioperative morbidity	1.2	1	1.7	10[a]	
Intracranial hemorrhage or infarction	0	0	0	1[a]	
Perioperative mortality	0	0	0	0.6[a]	

[a]Combined values for microvascular decompression and partial trigeminal rhizotomy.
Adapted from Taha JM, TewJM. Comparison of surgical treatments for trigeminal neuralgia reevaluation of radiofrequency rhizotomy. *Neurosurgery* 1996;38:865–871.

of the cannula or injury that results from the thermal destruction during RF treatment. The RF cannula is inserted through the skin just adjacent to the lateral margin of the mouth and cephalad via the foramen ovale in the base of the skull until the active tip lies adjacent to or within the trigeminal ganglion. Placement of the cannula generally requires brief intervals of deep sedation. En route to the trigeminal ganglion, the cannula courses medial to the body of the mandible just beneath the oral mucosa, and there is significant risk of piercing the oral mucosa and dragging bacteria into the cranium. Meningitis is a rare complication, and the exact portal of bacterial entry is usually uncertain.[20,21] Within the skull, the trigeminal ganglion lies lateral to the posterior clinoid process of the sella turcica, just lateral to the internal carotid artery, anterior to the pons, and medial to the inferomedial aspect of the temporal lobe of the brain (Fig. 32-2). Excessive advancement of the needle risks injury to these structures. Indeed, case reports of brain stem injury have appeared.[22] Excessive anterior angulation of the advancing cannula can lead it through the pterygopalatine fossa up through the inferior orbital fissure and into the optic canal, where optic nerve injury and monocular blindness have occurred.[23] In addition, toward its posterior aspect, the trigeminal ganglion is enveloped closely within dural reflections, and even proper placement of the cannula often results in the appearance of cerebrospinal fluid (CSF) flowing freely from the cannula. This rarely creates any long-term sequelae, but may lead to reports of CSF rhinorrhea,[24] believed to be retrograde flow of CSF through the foramen ovale and into the auditory (Eustachian) tube through an opening in the canal created during needle placement.

Neural injury during RF ablation of the trigeminal ganglion is universal and is indeed the goal of this treatment modality. Direct destruction of a small area of neurons within the distal portion of the ganglion or the nerve rootlets is believed to be the mechanism that interrupts the episodic pain. To target the RF treatment area, the cannula is advanced until a low-voltage high-frequency current produces a paresthesia within the area where the patient typically experiences pain. Thereafter, heat lesioning is begun for 60-second intervals at 60°C under brief periods of general anesthesia. Between treatments, the patient is allowed to recover enough to allow sensory testing within the cutaneous distribution where the pain is localized. Repeated lesions are created at gradually increasing temperatures (typically 2°C increments) to increase the degree of neural destruction until the patient reports the appearance of slight hypesthesia in the affected region. The most common adverse effects of this approach are related to the size and location of the thermal lesion (Tables 32-2 and 32-3). Judging the extent of the sensory change following each lesion can be quite difficult and is often clouded by effects of the anesthetic. If the extent of the lesion is excessive, the area of sensory loss can extend to the ophthalmic division of the trigeminal nerve (V1) and can result in loss of the corneal reflex and corneal anesthesia, and keratitis may ensue. The majority of patients (98%)[17] will report some detectable degree of sensory loss within the region treated, and this loss of sensation can be bothersome to some. Others have reported dense sensory anesthesia and ongoing neuropathic pain in the region of treatment (anesthesia dolorosa). Treatment of the mandibular division of the trigeminal nerve (V3) involves motor fibers to the masseter muscle and weakness during mastication is common. Finally, direct heating of the trigeminal rootlets can lead to dramatic rises in blood pressure and intracranial bleeding.[25] In a recent large review examining 6,205 patients treated with RF rhizotomy for trigeminal neuralgia, this complication has not been reported.[17] Perhaps due to the advent of more rapidly acting sedative hypnotics and meticulous intraoperative monitoring, such dangerous swings in blood pressure have become less common.

Diagnosis

Diagnosis of adverse effects and complications associated with RF treatment for trigeminal neuralgia is usually self-evident. Masticatory weakness, variable degrees of hypesthesia, and anesthesia dolorosa occur with sufficient frequency that they should be expected and patients should be counseled regarding each as a part of the informed consent process prior to treatment. CSF rhinorrhea is typically painless and self-limited. New onset of a focal neurologic deficit or headache after treatment warrants immediate

TABLE 32-3 Complications of RF Rhizotomy for Trigeminal Neuralgia	
COMPLICATION	**ESTIMATED INCIDENCE (%)**
Attributable to lesions of the trigeminal nerve	
Numbness	71–98
Dysesthesia	11–27
Anesthesia dolorosa	0.2–7.9
Corneal anesthesia	1–21
Keratitis	0.2–20
Masseter weakness (motor root)	1–25
Due to inclusion/injury of adjacent nerves	
Optic nerve lesion	0.001
Diplopia (CN III, IV, or VI)	0.5–2
Hearing problems	0.01–2
Due to injury of other adjacent structures	
Carotid-cavernous fistula	0.1
Subdural, infratemporal hemorrhage	0.0002
Intracerebral hemorrhage (needle puncture)	0.0006
Other	
Intracerebral hemorrhage (not due to needle)	0.002
Subdural hemorrhage	0.0007
Seizure	0.0002
Hemiparesis	0.0003
Perioperative mortality (all causes)	0.0006–0.0026

Adapted from Lord SM, Bogduk N. Radiofrequency procedures in chronic pain. *Best Pract Res Clin Anesthesiol* 2002;16:597–617.

imaging of the brain using MRI to rule out hematoma formation with reversible compression of neural elements. Although direct neural injury is by far the more common cause leading to new focal deficits, a reversible cause should be ruled out. Indeed, this technique has been largely performed by neurosurgeons. Ongoing and close collaboration with a neurosurgeon is warranted for anesthesiologists

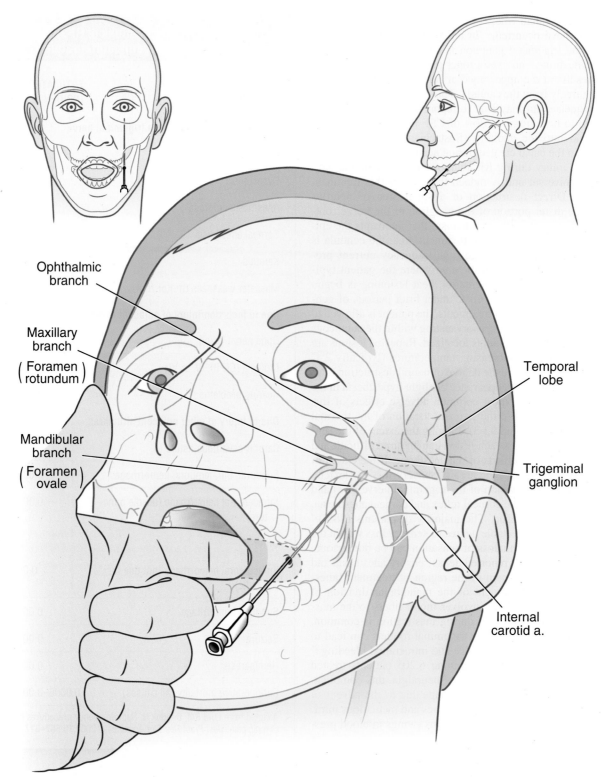

FIGURE 32-2. **Mechanism of complications that arise during RF treatment for trigeminal neuralgia.** The RF cannula is inserted just lateral to the lateral margin of the lips and advanced medial to the mandible and lateral to the oral mucosa. The index finger of the operator is placed in the patient's mouth to ensure that the tip of the cannula does not penetrate the oral mucosa en route to the foramen ovale. Note the close proximity of the carotid artery, the temporal lobe, and the brain stem to the final position of the cannula (**insets**). The proper trajectory of the needle and final needle position are shown in the frontal and axial planes.

and others who perform the technique independently, and immediate neurosurgical consultation should be readily available whenever the technique is used. For those patients who develop corneal anesthesia following the procedure, consultation with an ophthalmologist should be arranged to guide treatment aimed at preventing keratitis.

Treatment

Treatment of the most common adverse effects associated with RF treatment for trigeminal neuralgia is symptomatic. Most problems are self-limited. Like other forms of neuropathic pain stemming from neural injury, anesthesia dolorosa is difficult to treat. The use of antiepileptic and antidepressant drugs is the cornerstone of management for this problem. In the immediate time interval following RF treatment, the pain can be extreme, and use of opioid analgesics (often in high doses) is the only available means of temporizing. Onset of a new focal neurologic deficit may herald significant direct neural trauma. Therapy is guided by diagnostic imaging. In the event that significant intracranial bleeding occurs, immediate surgical decompression may be warranted.

Prevention

Central to successful application of RF treatment for trigeminal neuralgia is the use of meticulous image-guided placement of the RF cannula and creation of the smallest anatomically correct lesion that will produce mild hypesthesia in the region affected. Correct needle placement begins with advancing the needle over the medial aspect of the mandible beneath the oral mucosa. Penetration of the oral mucosa and further advancing the needle risks seeding the intracranial vault with oral bacteria. This can be avoided by placing a gloved hand in the patient's mouth and palpating the needle beneath the oral mucosa as it is advanced. Once the needle has been advanced beyond the posterior extent of the mandible toward the base of the skull, there is no further risk of penetrating the oral mucosa. Trauma to extracranial vascular structures near the skull base, including the carotid artery as it enters the carotid canal, is minimized by use of fluoroscopic guidance. The foramen ovale should be identified near the base of the lateral pterygoid plate, and excessive deviation from this location should be avoided. Once the needle has entered the foramen ovale, fluoroscopic images in the AP and lateral planes should be used to avoid excessive cranial advancement. The needle tip should not be inserted beyond a line drawn between the superior aspects of the anterior and posterior clinoid processes in a lateral radiograph to avoid direct trauma to the temporal lobe and brain stem (Fig. 32-2). Sensory stimulation should then be carried out just after traversing the foramen. Repeated sensory stimulation after each small (2- to 3-mm) advance of the needle will ensure that the needle reaches the proper position without excessive advancement within the cranium.

For those patients with involvement of the ophthalmic division of the trigeminal nerve (V1), many experts question the usefulness of RF treatment.[17] Because thermal injury to the ganglion to the point of sensory loss is required for successful treatment, some degree of corneal anesthesia is to be expected if the lesion is targeted to this region of the ganglion. Nonetheless, when other treatment options are not available even those with involvement of V1 have been successfully treated, albeit at a heightened risk of corneal anesthesia and subsequent keratitis.

▶ RADIOFREQUENCY TREATMENT FOR FACET-RELATED PAIN

Scope

Neck and low back pain are ubiquitous and have many causes. Each element of the spine can give rise to distinct pain syndromes. Facet-related pain has been recognized as a common cause of axial neck and low back pain (i.e., pain that is primarily along the spinal axis as opposed to radicular pain that extends into the extremities and suggests neural compression).[26] The diagnosis of facet-related pain is made on the basis of symptoms. There are no definitive diagnostic studies, and, thus, the diagnosis is imprecise at best. Patients with facet-related pain typically report deep aching pain that predominantly overlies the spinal axis. The pain may be unilateral or bilateral. The most common causes of facet-related pain appear to be degenerative changes within the facet joints, most often osteoarthritis ("spondylosis"). There may be some history of trauma, particularly in facet-related neck pain. The most common injuries are sudden twisting or flexion-extension injuries (e.g., whiplash). Symptoms are usually exacerbated by extension. There are well-documented patterns of referred pain arising from various facet joints that help with deciding where treatment should be focused.[27–29] Imaging studies (CT, MRI) may be completely normal, even though facet arthropathy of varying degrees is quite common. Most clinicians rely on diagnostic injections to guide patient selection for RF facet denervation. Intra-articular facet injections or blocks of the medial branch nerves to the facet using local anesthetic should produce transient relief of the symptoms before proceeding with RF treatment.

Despite widespread use of RF thermoablation for facet-related pain, there is limited data regarding the safety of this technique and its associated complications. No formal safety assessment has been performed.[30] In the absence of such formal assessment, knowledge must be gleaned from review of published studies. Attempts to evaluate incidence and severity of complications are frustrated by variability in the published literature. Authors have differed widely regarding the detail with which complications have been reported, and some authors have neither reported complications nor remarked on their absence. Nonetheless, numerous reports have confirmed the safety of RF facet denervation. Several large series of patients treated with lumbar RF denervation have been reported without major complications.[31] Notably, there have been few reports of major neurologic injury resulting from this technique, and it is rare to see anything more than transient exacerbation of symptoms following RF facet denervation. The primary limitations of this technique are the rate of failure and return of pain after treatment.

It is clear that less than half of reported patients that undergo diagnostic blocks proceed to neurolysis. Of those undergoing lumbar facet denervation, about half of patients obtain good to excellent pain relief. In a summary report of numerous uncontrolled studies, the proportion of patients achieving >50% pain relief varied from 17% to 82%, with a mean success rate of 48%. However, the proportion of patients obtaining complete relief was unstated, and the duration of follow-up was often less than a year.[32] In contrast, more recent studies have incorporated rigorous patient selection criteria and sham controls. Among the best designed and conducted of trials was a recent prospective, randomized, placebo- (sham) controlled study of patients with cervical pain (whiplash) that demonstrated 50% pain reduction for a median of 9 months after facet denervation versus 8 days in the sham-treated group.[33] A recent systematic review concluded that percutaneous RF neurolysis of the sensory nerves to the facet joints is a safe and modestly effective treatment for facet-related pain.[34] While dozens of observational or retrospective studies have reported varying clinical results with the use of pulsed RF treatment, only one, small well-controlled randomized trial has appeared in recent years. Van Zundert et al.[35] and his colleagues randomized 23 patients with chronic cervical radicular pain to receive either pulsed RF treatment for the dorsal root ganglion (DRG) at the painful level or sham treatment and showed superior pain reduction lasting to 6-month follow-up in those receiving active treatment.[35] This technique is in need of further study to validate its usefulness.

A recent review details the adverse effects and complications associated with cervical RF neurotomy (Table 32-4).[17] In a series of 28 patients who received cervical RF treatment, McDonald et al.[36] reported no complications. In a comment on this article, Burchiel[37] asserted the importance of warning patients about the possibility of both cutaneous dysesthesia and postoperative pain and numbness that could last between 2 and 34 months,[37] both of which are common sequelae of cervical RF neurotomy that are often considered expected outcomes rather than complications. The most common complications associated with cervical medial branch neurotomy include postoperative pain (97%); ataxia, unsteadiness, and spatial disorientation (23%); and vasovagal syncope (2%) (Table 32-4). Lord et al.[38] found that brief postoperative pain was the only side effect of lower cervical procedures, but ataxia occurred when the third occipital nerve was treated. Because the third occipital nerve carries a large proportion of fibers involved in cutaneous innervation, numbness routinely accompanies lesioning of this nerve. In patients whose treatment was successful, this numb patch regressed over 1 to 3 weeks and was replaced by dysesthesia and pruritis, followed by the return of normal cutaneous sensation and pain. Unsuccessful treatment was characterized by the loss of numbness and return of pain within 1 week.

The incidence of expected treatment-related adverse effects and complications associated with lumbar RF medial branch neurotomy is markedly lower than that observed following treatment at cervical levels. Postoperative pain has emerged as the most prevalent complication of RF medial branch neurotomy. This pain is usually transient, although neuritic pain may occasionally last for months to years. Information related to RF complications was contained mainly in anecdotal reports (Box 32-2), with most large series reporting no complications.[31,39–41] In a contemporary retrospective study designed to assess that frequency of complications, Kornick et al.[42] found that 92 patients who received 616 lumbar RF lesions in 116 procedures performed over a 5-year period had a 1% incidence of postoperative pain. Only one-half of those affected experienced pain for >2 weeks. There were no major complications such as infection or new

neurologic deficit. In 122 patients who received lumbar, cervical, or thoracic RF treatment with a minimum follow-up of 1 year, 22% reported transient discomfort and burning pain. Universally, resolution occurred within 1 month.[43]

Major complications have been acknowledged mainly in the form of case reports. Serious complications appear to be rare, and the available data prevent meaningful systematic analysis. Kornick et al.[30] noted minor burns due to insulation breaks in electrodes, improper function of grounding pads, or unexplained reasons. There is no evidence of any significant risk of infection or hemorrhage. RF ablation is also used as a minimally invasive means for local treatment of several types of solid malignancies.[48] Three cases of lumbosacral radiculopathy were reported following RF ablation of intra-abdominal metastases, suggesting that when RF thermocoagulation is applied directly to a lumbosacral nerve root thermal injury is likely.[49]

Separate consideration should be given to the emerging use of pulsed RF techniques that do not cause neurodestruction. Mungliani[50] noted that this technique produces no clinical evidence of neural damage and minimal postoperative soreness. Manchikanti[51] asserted that this technique "may be used in neuropathic pain without adverse sequelae and safely

TABLE 32-4 Observed Complications of Cervical Medial Branch Neurotomy

COMPLICATION	OBSERVED FREQUENCY (%)	95% CI (%)
Vasovagal syncope	2	0–6
Postoperative pain	97	94–100
Ataxia, unsteadiness, spatial disorientation	23	14–32
Cutaneous numbness		
TON procedures	88	75–100
C3/4 procedures	80	55–100
Lower levels	19	8–30
Dysesthesias		
TON procedures	56	37–75
C3/4 procedures	30	2–58
Lower levels	17	6–27
Dermoid cyst	1	0–4
Transient neuritis	2	0–6

CI, confidence interval; TON, third occipital nerve.
Modified from Lord SM, Bogduk N. Radiofrequency procedures in chronic pain. *Best Pract Res Clin Anesthesiol* 2002;16:597–617.

BOX 32-2 Anecdotal Reports of Complications Following Lumbar RF Medial Branch Neurotomy

Complications that have not been reported

- Allergic reaction to local anesthetic
- Hematoma
- Infection

Complications appearing in unpublished medicolegal proceedings:

- One patient with coagulation of the lumbar ventral ramus when the procedure was carried out under general anesthesia. General anesthesia rendered the patient unable to report pain in the lower extremity when the lesion was being produced.
- One patient with full-thickness burns through skin and muscle when an uninsulated spinal needle was used in place of the dispersive ground pad. The burns occurred directly around the entire course of the uninsulated spinal needle.

Complications appearing in published case reports:

- Four cases of small superficial burns due to breaks in the insulation along the cannula.[44]
- Two cases of burns at the dispersive ground pas adhesion site due to malfunction of the RF generator.[45]
- One unexplained burn.[46]

Adapted from Standards Committee of the International Spine Intervention Society. Percutaneous lumbar radiofrequency medial branch neurotomy. In: Bogduk N, ed. Practice Guidelines: *Spinal Diagnostic and Treatment Procedures*. San Francisco, CA: International Spine Intervention Society, 2004:195–196. (Ref. 47.)

in CRPS." Despite the enthusiasm for pulsed RF, precisely because it does not appear to be neurodestructive, the nature and extent of lesions made by these methods have not been described, and little evidence has been published to demonstrate efficacy.[19]

Mechanism of Injury

Similar to RF treatment of trigeminal neuralgia, complications during RF ablation of the medial branch nerves may be related to injury caused during placement of the cannula and injury that results from the thermal destruction during RF treatment. The anatomic configuration of the sensory nerves to the facet joints allows safe destruction without damage to the sensory and motor nerves to the extremities. The spinal nerve roots exit the spinal canal via the intervertebral foramina and divide into anterior and posterior primary rami (Fig. 32-3). The anterior ramus supplies sensory and motor innervation to the trunk and extremities according to the spinal level of the nerve root. The posterior primary ramus divides again into medial and lateral branches. The lateral branch of the posterior primary ramus provides motor innervation to the spinal erector muscles and a small variable area of cutaneous sensory innervation to the area directly overlying the spinous processes. The medial branch

of the posterior primary ramus supplies sensory innervation to the facet joints. The medial branch, or nerve to the facet, travels along the base of the superior articular process of the facet joint of each vertebra, where it joins with the medial-most portion of the transverse process. In this location, radiographic guidance allows precise placement of the RF cannula, and lesions can be produced without affecting the anterior primary ramus (i.e., without risk of unwanted damage to the sensory or motor nerves to the trunk and extremities).

Direct injury to soft tissues and periosteum during traumatic needle placement can lead to transient local pain for several days following treatment. The needle can also be advanced anteriorly and cause direct injury to the exiting spinal nerve. More likely is that the patient will report a transient paresthesia extending to the peripheral distribution of the nerve contacted as the needle contacts the spinal nerve. Paresthesia is not uncommon and typically resolves immediately with needle repositioning. However, persistent paresthesia may occur.

Thermal injury caused by incorrect position of the RF cannula has also been reported.[49] The precise anatomic location of the bifurcation of the posterior primary ramus of the spinal nerve into medial and lateral branches is variable, and often the cannula cannot be positioned at a point that allows close enough proximity to the medial branch without the lesion also engulfing the lateral branch (Figs. 32-3 and 32-4). The lateral branch supplies some motor innervation to the lumbar paraspinous musculature. Electromyography studies of these muscle groups following RF medial branch neurotomy at a single level have indicated denervation potentials (positive sharp waves and fibrillation potentials), and adjacent muscle segments have demonstrated polysegmental innervation from each spinal level.[52] This polysegmental innervation likely accounts for the lack of significant clinically detectable weakness following RF medial branch neurotomy. Indeed, many practitioners view motor stimulation in the paraspinous muscle groups without motor stimulation in the lower extremities as a reliable sign of good position of the cannula. The lateral branch also carries a small and variable number of sensory fibers that supply sensation to a small area overlying the spinous processes. Transient hyperesthesia manifested as a sunburn-like sensation has been reported after lumbar RF treatment and more commonly after cervical RF treatment.[19] The large sensory distribution of the cervical medial branch nerves is responsible for the high incidence of cutaneous sensory loss and dysesthesias, particularly with treatment of the third occipital nerve and the medial branch nerves at C3 and C4.

More concerning is a cannula position that is so far anterior to the transverse process that the active tip lies in contact with the spinal nerve (Figs. 32-3 and 32-4). This position should be easily detected during sensory and motor stimulation prior to lesion creation (see further discussion following under Prevention). However, once local anesthetic has been placed through the cannula prior to lesion creation if the cannula is moved anteriorly spinal nerve injury can occur. Despite this theoretic concern, not even a single case report of new onset radicular pain following RF treatment has appeared.

Diagnosis

Reports of new onset radicular pain following RF medial branch neurotomy are typically self-limited. Physical

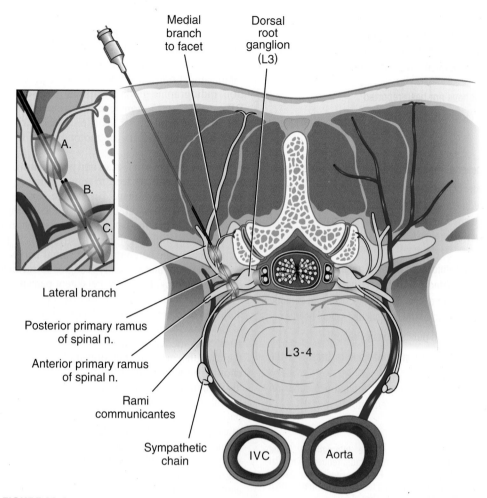

FIGURE 32-3. **Mechanism of complications that arise during lumbar RF medial branch neurotomy.** Axial diagram of lumbar RF medial branch neurotomy. A 22-gauge 10-cm RF cannula with a 5-mm active tip is advanced just anterior to the base of the transverse process where it joins with the superior articular process. **A:** An RF cannula in correct position for lumbar RF medial branch neurotomy. The point of bifurcation of the posterior primary ramus of the spinal nerve into medial and lateral branches is variable and conventional RF treatment commonly destroys both nerves. The medial branch supplies sensation to the facet joint and the lateral branch provides motor innervation to the paraspinous musculature and a small and variable patch of sensory innervation to the skin overlying the spinous processes. **B:** Neurolysis of the lateral branch does not have any demonstrable effect on strength of the paraspinous muscles. However, cutaneous hyperesthesia and/or hypoesthesia do occur infrequently. **C:** Placement of the RF lesion directly on the anterior primary ramus of the spinal nerve can cause severe and persistent radicular pain.

examination is likely to reveal a limited area of sensory loss or allodynia without any motor deficit. Large fibers within the spinal nerve are resistant to destruction during RF treatment. Thus, diagnosis relies on familiarity with the technical aspects of cannula placement during a particular treatment and physical examination alone. If a large sensory deficit is present or discernable focal weakness is apparent, neurologic consultation and consideration of diagnostic imaging to rule out other causes of nerve compression (e.g., herniated nucleus pulposus or localized hematoma) are warranted.

Treatment

Most sequelae following RF medial branch neurotomy are self-limited and require nothing more than reassurance and time to resolve. Patients should be warned to expect a transient increase in pain for several days to weeks following treatment. Providing a brief course of oral analgesics can

obviate unnecessary return visits. If new onset radicular pain with or without allodynia appears, spinal nerve injury should be suspected, and oral neuropathic pain treatment with a tricyclic antidepressant or anticonvulsant should be started. Localized allodynia described as a "sunburn" sensation is common, particularly following RF treatment of the high cervical medial branch nerves (TON, C3, and C4). Topical 5% lidocaine patch (Lidoderm, Endo Pharmaceuticals, Chadds Ford, PA) can prove invaluable for symptomatic management in these cases, which also tend to resolve within days to weeks of treatment. Persistent numbness is also common and rarely requires specific treatment.

Prevention

Injury to the spinal nerves during lumbar RF medial branch neurotomy is best avoided by precise anatomic placement of the RF cannula using fluoroscopic guidance. The cannula

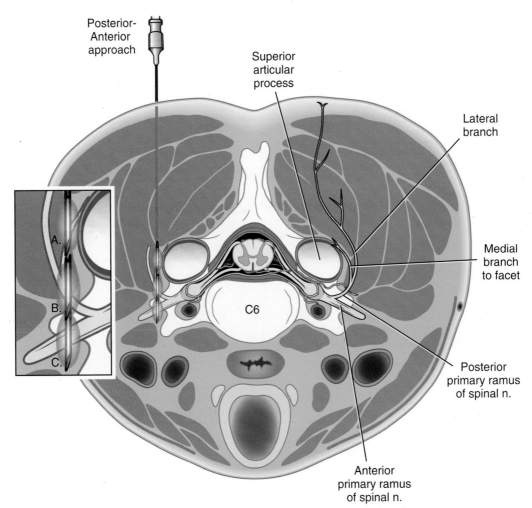

FIGURE 32-4. **Mechanism of complications that arise during cervical RF medial branch neurotomy.** Axial diagram of cervical RF medial branch neurotomy. When a posterior approach is used, the needle is first seated on the lateral margin of the facet column and then walked off the lateral margin of the facet column and advanced 2 to 3 mm to place the active tip along the course of the medial branch nerve. **A:** An RF cannula in correct position for cervical RF medial branch neurotomy. The point of bifurcation of the posterior primary ramus of the spinal nerve into medial and lateral branches is variable and conventional RF treatment commonly destroys both nerves. The medial branch supplies sensation to the facet joint and the lateral branch provides motor innervation to the paraspinous musculature and a small and variable patch of sensory innervation to the skin overlying the spinous processes. **B:** Neurolysis of the lateral branch does not have any demonstrable effect on strength of the paraspinous muscles. However, cutaneous hyperesthesia and/or hypoesthesia do occur infrequently. This is particularly frequent following conventional RF treatment of the third occipital nerve and the C3 and C4 medial branch nerves owing to their large cutaneous sensory components. **C:** Placement of the RF lesion directly on the anterior primary ramus of the spinal nerve can cause severe and persistent radicular pain.

should be gently advanced to contact the superior margin of the transverse process precisely where it joins the superior articular process of the facet and then advanced no more than 2 to 3 mm further over the superior margin of the transverse process to lie along the course of the medial branch nerve (Fig. 32-3). By contacting the transverse process, the depth of the advancing cannula is assured before it approaches the more anterior spinal nerve within the intervertebral foramen.

Similarly, the spinal cord and great vessels of the neck can be avoided during cervical RF medial branch neurotomy by careful patient positioning and use of radiographic guidance. The medial branch nerves to the facets course across the articular pillar, midway between the superior and inferior articular processes. The nerves can be anesthetized

by placing a needle from a posterior approach (Fig. 32-4) or a lateral approach (Fig. 32-5). The lateral approach is more comfortable for the patient, as they can lie on one side rather than face down, and the needle must traverse less tissue en route to the target. However, when the needles are inserted from a lateral approach, they are directed toward the spinal cord. Even slight rotation of the neck can lead to confusing the left and right articular pillars and lead to cannula entry into the spinal canal or anteriorly toward the vertebral artery within the foramen transversarium (Fig. 32-5).

The physiologic testing conducted after placement of RF cannula and prior to lesion generation is likely the factor that makes complications so uncommon and has assured clinicians that this neuroablative technique is so safe. Once the

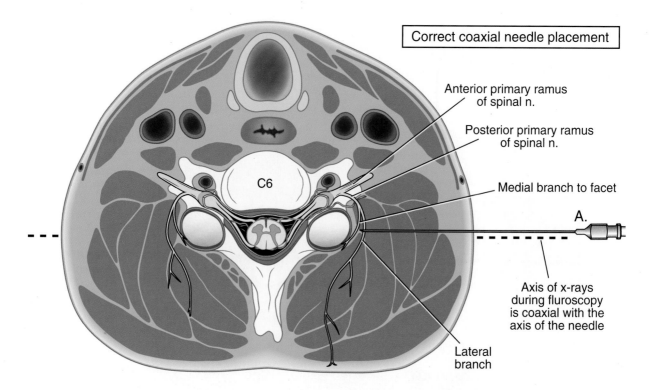

Correct coaxial needle placement

Anterior primary ramus of spinal n.

Posterior primary ramus of spinal n.

Medial branch to facet

C6

A.

Axis of x-rays during fluroscopy is coaxial with the axis of the needle

Lateral branch

Incorrect needle placement resulting from failure to align the left and right articular pillars during fluroscopy

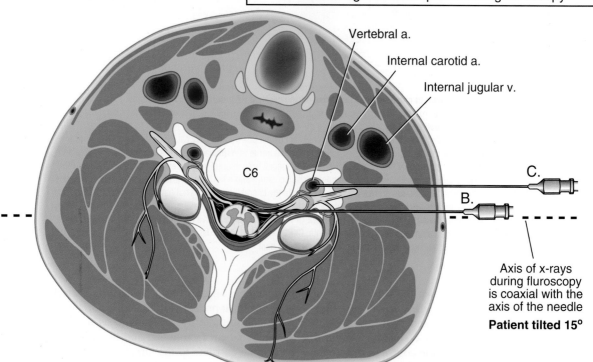

Vertebral a.

Internal carotid a.

Internal jugular v.

C6

C.

B.

Axis of x-rays during fluroscopy is coaxial with the axis of the needle

Patient tilted 15°

FIGURE 32-5. **Mechanism of complications that arise during cervical pulsed RF medial branch treatment using a lateral approach.** Axial diagram of cervical RF medial branch treatment using a lateral approach. Many practitioners carry out pulsed RF treatment using a lateral approach for needle placement. When needles are placed from a lateral approach, they are directed toward the spinal canal, and care must be taken to keep the needle tip over the bony facet target at all times as the needle is advanced. The top panel shows proper positioning of the RF cannula from a lateral approach **(A)** using a coaxial technique with good alignment of the left and right articular pillars during fluoroscopy. Poor alignment on radiography can easily lead the practitioner to confuse the left and right articular pillars. The bottom panel shows a patient positioned 15 degrees off axis, with the left and right articular pillars not aligned. This can easily occur with seemingly small rotations of the cervical spine that occur when the patient turns the head to one side. With such poor alignment, the path of the needle can **(B)** traverse the neural foramen and enter the substance of the spinal cord or **(C)** stray anterior to the foramen and penetrate the vertebral artery.

cannulae have been positioned using radiographic guidance, their proper position is confirmed using electrical stimulation similar to that used for nerve localization using a nerve stimulator to conduct peripheral nerve blocks. Proper testing for sensory-motor dissociation is conducted (the patient should report pain or tingling during stimulation at 50 Hz at <0.5 V and have no motor stimulation to the affected myotome at 2 Hz at no less than three times the sensory threshold or 3 V). Thereafter, great care must be taken to prevent any movement of the cannulae. Each level is anesthetized with 0.5 mL of 2% lidocaine, and lesions are created at 80°C for 60 to 90 seconds.

▶ WHEN TO SEEK CONSULTATION

RF medial branch neurotomy is safe and modestly effective for treatment of facet-related pain. The most common adverse effect is a transient increase in pain following treatment. Consultation should be sought whenever unexpected sequelae ensue. The most common would be the appearance of a previously undetected focal neurologic deficit following RF treatment. Although most will be in the form of a transient radicular pain or area of cutaneous hyperesthesia, the appearance of a previously undetected motor deficit or a progressive deficit warrants immediate neurologic consultation. Direct injury to the spinal cord or vertebral artery may prove catastrophic, indicating immediate neurosurgical consultation with diagnostic evaluation guided by the presenting signs and symptoms and the suspected injury.

▶ OTHER RADIOFREQUENCY PROCEDURES IN CHRONIC PAIN

A number of other procedures for RF treatment for pain have been described, including lesions of the dorsal root entry zone (DREZ), dorsal rhizotomy and DRG procedures, thoracic medial branch nerves, splanchnic nerves, and sacroiliac (SI) joints. DREZ lesions have been used to treat patients with intractable deafferentation pain.[10] The procedure involves general anesthesia and surgical exposure via laminectomy. The involved spinal segments are located using electrophysiologic testing, and an RF lesion is placed within the DREZ to interrupt cells within the substantia gelatinosa as well as nociceptive fibers traveling to adjacent segments within Lissauer's tract. The indications for this procedure remain unclear, and claims of efficacy are based on small uncontrolled case series. A recent review reported the total complication rates following DREZ lesioning from 0% to 60%, with a mean of 38%.[53] The proximity of the lateral corticospinal tract and dorsal columns to the site of the DREZ lesion is an inherent problem with the procedure, and unwanted neurologic deficits occur in 12% to 40% of cases.[54,55] The potential for incurring neurologic deficits is high, yet DREZ lesions may have a role—particularly for the treatment of intractable deafferentation pain in those with previous neurologic deficits (e.g., brachial plexus avulsion or spinal cord transection).[10]

Despite extensive application of dorsal rhizotomy and DRG procedures, evidence supporting the safety and clinical utility of this approach remains scant.[19] Thermal[55] and pulsed[35] RF treatment of the DRG for treatment of cervicobrachial pain has been examined in randomized controlled trials, revealing modest success rates. Patients treated with thermal RF lesions adjacent to the cervical DRG experienced rates as high as 10% troublesome burning pain, 50% vague burning sensation, and 35% hyposensibility in the treated dermatome,[56,57] while those treated with pulsed RF had no sequelae.[35]

RF treatment has been adapted for the treatment of pain related to SI dysfunction, and several new devices have appeared in recent years. SI joint syndrome is described as mechanical pain generated at the SI joint with or without appreciable lesions on imaging.[58] SI joint pain represents one of the more common causes of axial low back pain, comprising between 15% and 25% of cases.[59,60] SI joint syndrome is often considered a difficult clinical entity to accurately diagnose by physical exam, and some studies have suggested that a diagnostic injection of local anesthetic in to the joint may be the only way to diagnose the condition.[61] The pain generated from the SI joint can be the result of sprain injury, fracture, diastasis, pyogenic or crystal arthropathy, and spondyloarthropathy.[62]

Periarticular and intra-articular corticosteroid injections in patients suspected of having SI joint pain are widely used; however, the results are divided as to whether or not they afford any long-term benefit.[63] In recent years, RF denervation has emerged as a potential alternative to steroid injections for severe or refractory cases of SI joint pain.

Denervation of the posterior portion of the joint can be affected by producing a strip-like lesion along the posterior aspect of the joint, from the posterior-inferior portion of the joint cephalad to the posterior-superior iliac spine, the point above which access to the joint is obstructed by the overlying iliac crest. Using the bipolar lesion technique, denervation is accomplished by creating a strip lesion along the posterior aspect of the joint capsule. This is done by using two RF cannulae positioned parallel to one another, no more than 5 to 6 mm apart along the posterior aspect of the joint. One of the two cannulae is attached to the electrode port of the RF generator, and the other cannula is attached to the ground (reference) port. The resulting lesion extends between the two cannulae (Fig. 32-6). By placing the cannulae sequentially

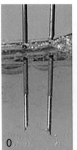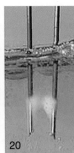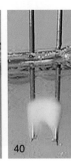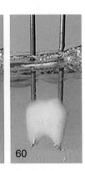

FIGURE 32-6. Bipolar RF lesion. Two 10-cm SMK RF cannulae with 5-mm active tips are immersed in egg white, and a lesion is carried out at 90°C for 90 seconds. The lesion is maximal in size by 90 seconds of treatment and bridges between the two cannulae only if they remain <6 mm apart. If the cannulae are spaced more than 6 mm apart, two discrete unipolar lesions are created. (Full data appear in Pino C, Hoeft M, Hofsess C, et al. Morphologic analysis of bipolar radiofrequency lesions: implications for denervation of the sacroiliac joint. *Reg Anesth Pain Med* 2005;30:335–338.)

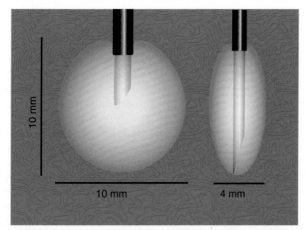

FIGURE 32-7. Diagram demonstrating the difference in lesion size and shape between cooled (*left*) and conventional RF probes (*right*).

one above the other along the posterior portion of the SI joint, a strip lesion is created. Denervation of the posterior portion of the joint can also be affected by placing specific lesions to directly treat the medial branch nerves at the L4 and L5 levels as well as the lateral branch nerves at the S1, S2, and S3 levels using a new water-cooled RF device that produces larger lesions of significantly different geometry than conventional lesions (Fig. 32-7). In small case series and one controlled trial, this treatment has shown significant efficacy (about one-third of patients will receive 50% or greater pain reduction lasting an average of 12 months).[64]

Numerous uncontrolled and controlled studies have been published on the efficacy of the procedure, and a recent meta-analysis[65] synthesizes this body of work to date. Ultimately, meta-analysis is limited by the available literature, and strength of that literature incorporated into the study. Therefore, the small number of trials included (10 total) and lack of randomized controlled trials present (only a single study) limit the strength of the pooled analysis. Nonetheless, the meta-analysis indicates that RF is an effective treatment for SI joint pain as 60.1% of the patients had improvement of pain of more than 50% at 3 months and 49.9% showed more than 50% pain reduction at 6 months. Future, randomized-controlled studies will provide further insight into the efficacy of this treatment.

Complications specific to SI joint RF treatment have not been fully described in the literature. As with any RF procedure, there is always the possibility of postprocedure exacerbation of pain. Since up to 10 separate denervation sites are required for SI joint RF and the lesions encompass a significantly larger volume of tissue than other RF techniques, postprocedure pain flares may be more likely than with RF treatment in other regions. There are anecdotal reports of abscess formation in the presacral soft tissues following RF treatment of the SI joint (Fig. 32-8). Additionally, inadvertent advancement of the RF canula through the sacral foramen could potentially lead to neuritis, vascular puncture, or injury to lower abdominal/pelvic viscera. Radiographic guidance, in both the AP and lateral projections, assists the guidance of proper RF cannula placement. As the technique gains popularity, more potential unforeseen complications may arise in clinical practice and, subsequently, in the literature.

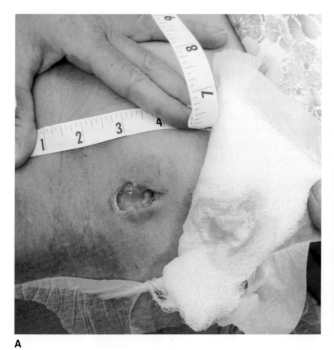

A

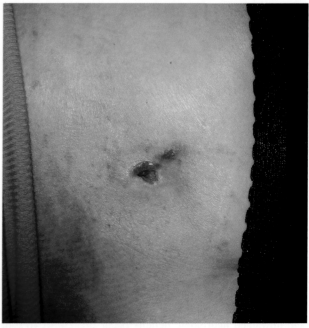

B

FIGURE 32-8. Presacral soft tissue abscess and skin breakdown following thermal RF treatment of the sacroiliac joint. A middle-aged woman underwent thermal RF treatment to the right sacroiliac joint for treatment of chronic right lumbosacral pain. Five separate lesions were placed using 22-gague, 100 cm RF cannulae with 10 mm active tips placed perpendicular to the posterior plane of the sacrum (L5, S1, S2, S3, and S4 levels). The patient presented 1 week later with obvious skin burns at each of the treated levels without fluctuance or discharge and was managed expectantly. **A:** Six weeks following treatment, despite ongoing wound care by a burn specialist, she presented with breakdown of the skin overlying the area of treatment and purulent discharge requiring surgical debridement. **B:** Over the following 6 months, the wound slowly closed by secondary intention with ongoing wound care using a vacuum wound dressing. (Images provided by author.)

► SUMMARY

In the 1960s, White and Sweet[66] first used electrical stimulation for guidance of needle placement followed by the use of RF energy to produce a thermal destructive neural lesion controlled by temperature monitoring. Since then, a range of RF procedures has been introduced for treatment of chronic pain. Among the most common are RF rhizotomy for trigeminal neuralgia and RF medial branch neurotomy for facet-related pain. Although they are by definition destructive to neural tissue, these procedures have proven to be safe and effective across a wide variety of treatment settings. No systematic evaluation of safety has been performed, and there is marked variability in the thoroughness and detail with which complications have been reported. Nonetheless, complications are possible, but remain distinctly uncommon and are generally self-limiting. It is also apparent that different procedures are associated with different sets of complications. By far the most frequently encountered complication is transient postprocedure pain. More serious complications do occur, but are uncommon.

Improved knowledge regarding the effectiveness of RF treatment for specific conditions and the associated expected adverse events and complications would be facilitated by standardization of reporting regarding procedures and outcomes. Particular attention should be paid to exact report of the lesion type, location, and number with a careful description of technique, and meticulous detailing of outcome measures beyond pain reduction (e.g., improvement in function, return to work, and so on). Before meaningful and systematic evaluation of complications can begin, there must be consensus regarding their definition, evaluation, and reporting in future clinical studies.

References

1. Kirschner M. Zur elektrochirurgie. *Arch Klin Chir* 1931;161: 761–766.
2. Sweet WH, Mark VH. Unipolar anodal electrolyte lesions in the brain of man and rat: report of five human cases with electrically produced bulbar or mesencephalic tractotomies. *AMA Arch Neurol Psychiatry* 1953;70:224–234.
3. Aranow S. The use of radiofrequency power in making lesions in the brain. *J Neurosurg* 1960;17:431–438.
4. Lord SM, Barnsley L, Wallis BJ, et al. Percutaneous radiofrequency neurotomy for chronic cervical zygapophyseal-joint pain. *N Engl J Med* 1996;335:1721–1726.
5. Kanpolat Y, Savas A, Bekar A, et al. Percutaneous controlled radiofrequency trigeminal rhizotomy for the treatment of idiopathic trigeminal neuralgia: 25-year experience with 1,600 patients. *Neurosurgery* 2001;48:524–532.
6. Kornick C, Kramarich SS, Lamer TJ, et al. Complications of lumbar facet radiofrequency denervation. *Spine* 2004;29:1352–1354.
7. Mikeladze G, Espinal R, Finnegan R, et al. Pulsed radiofrequency application in treatment of chronic zygapophyseal joint pain. *Spine J* 2003;3:360–362.
8. Van Zundert J, de Louw AJ, Joosten EA, et al. Pulsed and continuous radiofrequency current adjacent to the cervical dorsal root ganglion of the rat induces late cellular activity in the dorsal horn. *Anesthesiology* 2005;102:125–131.
9. Richebe P, Rathmell JP, Brennan TJ. Immediate early genes after pulsed radiofrequency treatment: neurobiology in need of clinical trials. *Anesthesiology* 2005;102:1–3.
10. Lord SM, Bogduk N. Radiofrequency procedures in chronic pain. *Best Pract Res Clin Anesthesiol* 2002;16:597–617.
11. Taha JM, Tew JM Jr, Buncher CR. A prospective 15-year follow up of 154 consecutive patients with trigeminal neuralgia treated by percutaneous stereotactic radiofrequency thermal rhizotomy. *J Neurosurg* 1995;83:989–993.
12. Eller JL, Raslan AM, Burchiel KJ. Trigeminal neuralgia: definition and classification. *Neurosurg Focus* 2005;18:E3.
13. Dandy WE. Concerning the cause of trigeminal neuralgia. *Am J Surg* 1934;24:447–455.
14. Gardner WJ, Sava GA. Hemifacial spasm: reversible pathophysiologic state. *J Neurosurg* 1962;21:240–247.
15. Janetta P. Treatment of trigeminal neuralgia by micro-operative decompression. In: Youmans J, ed. *Neurological Surgery*. Philadelphia, PA: WB Saunders, 1990:3928–3942.
16. Canavero S, Bonicalzi V. Drug therapy of trigeminal neuralgia. *Expert Rev Neurother* 2006;6:429–440.
17. Taha JM, Tew JM. Comparison of surgical treatments for trigeminal neuralgia reevaluation of radiofrequency rhizotomy. *Neursurgery* 1996;38:865–871.
18. Aryan HE, Nakaji P, Lu DC, et al. Multimodality treatment of trigeminal neuralgia: impact of radiosurgery and high resolution magnetic resonance imaging. *J Clin Neurosci* 2006;13: 239–244.
19. Lord SM, Bogduk N. Radiofrequency procedures in chronic pain. *Best Pract Res Clin Anesthesiol* 2002;16:597–617.
20. Mitchell RG, Teddy PJ. Meningitis due to Gemella haemolysans after radiofrequency trigeminal rhizotomy. *J Clin Pathol* 1985;38:558–560.
21. Göçer AI, Çetinalp E, Tuna M, et al. Fatal complication of the radiofrequency trigeminal rhizotomy. *Acta Neurochir (Wien)* 1997;139:373–374.
22. Berk C, Honey CR. Brain stem injury after radiofrequency trigeminal rhizotomy. *Acta Neurochir (Wien)* 2004;146:635–636.
23. Egan RA, Pless M, Shults WT. Monocular blindness as a complication of trigeminal radiofrequency rhizotomy. *Am J Ophthalmol* 2001;131:237–240.
24. Ugur HC, Savas A, Elhan A, et al. Unanticipated complication of percutaneous radiofrequency trigeminal rhizotomy rhinorrhea report of three cases and a cadaver study. *Neurosurgery* 2004;54:1522–1526.
25. Sweet WH, Poletti CE, Roberts JT. Dangerous rises in blood pressure upon heating of the trigeminal rootlets: increased bleeding times in patients with trigeminal neuralgia. *Neurosurgery* 1985;17:843–844.
26. Cavanaugh JM, Lu Y, Chen C, et al. Pain generation in lumbar and cervical facet joints. *J Bone Joint Surg Am* 2006;88(suppl 2): 63–67.
27. Bogduk N, Marsland A. The cervical zygapophyseal joints as a source of neck pain. *Spine* 1988;13:610–617.
28. Boas RA. Facet joint injections. In: Stanton-Hicks MA, Boas RA, eds. *Chronic Low Back Pain*. New York, NY: Raven Press, 1982:199–211.
29. Dreyfuss P, Tibiletti C, Dreyer SJ. Thoracic zygapophyseal joint pain patterns. *Spine* 1994;19:807–811.
30. Kornick C, Kramarich SS, Lamer TJ, et al. Complications of lumbar facet radiofrequency denervation. *Spine* 2004;29:1352–1354.
31. North RB, Han M, Zahurak M, et al. Radiofrequency lumbar facet denervation: analysis of prognostic factors. *Pain* 1994;57: 77–83.
32. North RB, Misop H, Zahurak M, et al. Radiofrequency lumbar facet denervation: analysis of prognostic factors. *Pain* 1994;57:77–83.
33. Lord SM, Barnsley L, Wallis BJ, et al. Percutaneous radiofrequency neurotomy in the treatment of cervical zygapophyseal joint pain. *N Engl J Med* 1996;335:1721–1726.
34. Guerts JW, van Wijk RM, Stolker RJ, et al. Efficacy of radiofrequency procedures for the treatment of spinal pain: a systematic review of randomized clinical trials. *Reg Anesth Pain Med* 2001;26:394–400.

35. Van Zundert J, Patijn J, Kessels A, et al. Pulsed radiofrequency adjacent to the cervical dorsal root ganglion in chronic cervical radicular pain: a double blind sham controlled randomized clinical trial. *Pain* 2007;127:173–182.

36. McDonald GJ, Lord SM, Bogduk N. Long-term follow-up of patients treated with cervical radiofrequency neurotomy for chronic neck pain. *Neurosurgery* 1999;45:61–67.

37. Burchiel KJ. Comments. *Neurosurgery* 1999;45:67–68.

38. Lord SM, Barnsley L, Bogduk N. Percutaneous radiofrequency neurotomy in the treatment of cervical zygapophysial joint pain: a caution. *Neurosurgery* 1995;36:732–739.

39. Dreyfuss P, Halbrook B, Pauza K, et al. Efficacy and validity of radiofrequency neurotomy for chronic lumbar zygapophysial joint pain. *Spine* 2000;25:1270–1277.

40. van Kleef M, Barendse GA, Kessels A, et al. Randomized trial of radiofrequency lumbar facet denervation for chronic low back pain. *Spine* 1999;24:1937–1942.

41. Leclaire R, Fortin L, Lambert R, et al. Radiofrequency facet joint denervation in the treatment of low back pain: a placebo-controlled clinical trial to assess efficacy. *Spine* 2001;26:1411–1416.

42. Kornick C, Kramarich SS, Lamer TJ, et al. Complications of lumbar facet radiofrequency denervation. *Spine* 2004;29: 1352–1354.

43. Pevsner Y, Shabat S, Catz A, et al. The role of radiofrequency in the treatment of mechanical pain of spinal origin. *Eur Spine J* 2003;12:602–605.

44. Shealy CN. Percutaneous radiofrequency denervation of spinal facets. Treatment for chronic back pain and sciatica. *J Neurosurg* 1975;43:448–451.

45. Ogsbury JS III, Simon RH, Lehman RA. Facet "denervation" in the treatment of low back syndrome. *Pain* 1977;3:257–263.

46. Katz SS, Savitz MH. Percutaneous radiofrequency rhizotomy of the lumbar facets. *Mt Sinai J Med* 1986;53:523–525.

47. Standards Committee of the International Spine Intervention Society. Percutaneous lumbar radiofrequency medial branch neurotomy. In: Bogduk N, ed. *Practice Guidelines: Spinal Diagnostic and Treatment Procedures*. San Francisco, CA: International Spine Intervention Society, 2004:195–196.

48. Dupuy DA, Goldberg SN. Image-guided radiofrequency tumor ablation challenges and opportunities. *J Vasc Interv Radiol* 2001;12:1135–1148.

49. Coskun DM, Gilchrist J, Dupuy D. Lumbosacral radiculopathy following radiofrequency ablation therapy. *Muscle Nerve* 2003;28:754–756.

50. Mungliani R. The longer term effect of pulsed radiofrequency for neuropathic pain. *Pain* 1990;80:437–439.

51. Manchikanti L. The role of radiofrequency in the management of complex regional pain syndrome. *Curr Rev Pain* 2000;4:437–444.

52. Wu PB, Date ES, Kingery WS. The lumbar multifidus muscle in polysegmentally innervated. *Electromyogr Clin Neurophysiol* 2000;40:483–485.

53. Fazl M, Houlden DA. Dorsal root entry zone localization using direct spinal cord stimulation: an experimental study. *J Neurosurg* 1995;82:592–594.

54. Nashold BS Jr, Ostdahl RH. Dorsal root entry zone lesions for pain relief. *J Neurosurg* 1979;51:59–69.

55. Thomas DG, Jones SJ. Dorsal root entry zone lesions (Nashold's procedure) in brachial plexus avulsion. *Neurosurgery* 1984;15: 966–968.

56. van Kleef M, Liem L, Lousberg R, et al. Radiofrequency lesion adjacent to the dorsal root ganglion for cervicobrachial pain: a prospective double blind randomized study. *Neurosurgery* 1996;38:1127–1131.

57. van Kleef M, Spaans F, Dingemans W, et al. Effects and side effects of a percutaneous thermal lesion of the dorsal root ganglion in patients with cervical pain syndrome. *Pain* 1993;52:49–53.

58. McKenzie-Brown AM, Shah RV, Seghal N, et al. A systematic review of sacroiliac joint interventions. *Pain Phys* 2005;8:115–125.

59. Cohen SP. Sacroiliac joint pain: a comprehensive review of anatomy, diagnosis, and treatment. *Anesth Analg* 2005;101:1440–1453.

60. Dreyfuss P, Dreyer SJ, Cole A, et al. Sacroiliac joint pain. *J Am Acad Orthop Surg* 2004;12:255–265.

61. Dreyfuss P, Michaelsen M, Pauza K, et al. The value of medical history and physical examination in the diagnosis of sacroiliac joint pain. *Spine* 1996;21:2594–2602.

62. Ferrante FM, King LF, Roche EA, et al. Radiofrequency sacroiliac joint denervation for sacroiliac syndrome. *Reg Anesth Pain Med* 2001;26:137–142.

63. Cohen SP, Hurly RW, Buckenmaier CC, et al. Randomized placebo-controlled study evaluating lateral branch radiofrequency denervation for sacroiliac joint pain. *Anesthesiology* 2008;109:279–288.

64. Dreyfuss P, Henning T, Malladi N, et al. The ability of multi-site, multi-depth sacral lateral branch blocks to anesthetize the sacroiliac joint complex. *Pain Med* 2009;10:679–688.

65. Aydin SM, Gharibo CG, Mehnert M, et al. The role of radiofrequency ablation for sacroiliac joint pain: a meta-analysis. *PM R* 2010;9:842–851.

66. White JC, Sweet WH. *Pain and the Neurosurgeon*. Springfield, MA: Charles C. Thomas, 1969.

33

Complications Associated with Lysis of Epidural Adhesions and Epiduroscopy

Gabor B. Racz and James E. Heavner

Lysis of epidural adhesions is an interventional pain management technique that has evolved over time.[1] The goal of lysis of epidural adhesions is to break down barriers in the epidural space that are thought to contribute to painful processes and prevent delivery of pain relieving drugs to target sites. The technique that was first described and is still most commonly used relies on introduction of a navigable catheter into the epidural space. More recently, epiduroscopy was introduced as an alternative or complementary approach to the catheter technique. The lysis procedure is conducted throughout the spinal axis but epiduroscopy assisted lysis is generally limited to the lumbar and sacral regions. This chapter focuses on complications associated with lysis to treat upper cervical and low back pain, lower extremity radiculopathy, and spinal stenosis.

The goal during lysis of epidural adhesions is to reduce mechanical barriers preventing medications from reaching the dorsal root ganglion. The technique emerged from observations during image-guided injection. It was obvious that in some patients scar tissue formation prevented fluid injection or catheter placement adjacent to the spinal nerves. The sensory block that develops when epidural local anesthetic is administered to produce surgical anesthesia or analgesia or anesthesia for childbirth is typically symmetric, suggesting that the spread of local anesthetic in this population is relatively uniform. However, in those with chronic back pain, the spread of contrast was irregular, with large filling defects seen in many patients. Fluid placed in the epidural space will follow the path of least resistance and will not spread to locations where there is obstruction caused by scar tissue. If a catheter was placed in the vicinity of the observed scar tissue and a local anesthetic, radio-opaque contrast, and other fluids injected, pain relief often followed, and the duration of the pain relief was far beyond the duration of the local anesthetic effect. Placement of large-volume injections into the epidural space often resulted in prolonged pain relief and more uniform spread of contrast throughout the epidural space. This suggested that placement of fluid within the epidural space could lead to reduction in or elimination of mechanical barriers caused by scarring.

In 1991, Kuslich et al.[2] delineated the pain-sensitive structures in the spinal canal while doing surgical laminectomies under local anesthesia.[2] Using mechanical as well as electrical stimulation, they found that pain-sensitive structures included the annulus, nerve roots, facet joints, posterior longitudinal ligament, tendinous insertion of muscles (but not the muscles themselves), ligaments, and fascia. They also found that nerve roots are painful if they are compressed, swollen, inflamed, or restricted by scar tissue. Nerves are 3.2 times more likely to produce radicular pain if they are surrounded by scar tissue.[3] The lateral recess area is where nerve roots exit the vertebral canal. These roots are subjected to trauma from scar formation, hypertrophic facet joints, bulging discs, and numerous surgical- and injection-technique-related complications.[1] Beginning with the observations made by Kuslich et al., the ventrolateral epidural space has gradually come to be recognized as the target site for treatment during lysis of epidural adhesions. The development of a navigable radio-opaque kink-resistant soft-tipped catheter has allowed placement at or near this target site in most patients. However, there have been a number of complications associated with lysis of epidural adhesions. In some cases, the use of large volumes within the epidural space has produced barotrauma to the spinal canal contents, including the spinal cord, nerve roots, and blood supply to the cord. Here we review the complications that have been reported during lysis of epidural adhesions, discuss possible mechanisms for each complication, and suggest means of preventing these complications.

▶ THE TECHNIQUE OF EPIDURAL LYSIS OF ADHESIONS

Our discussion is limited mostly to the procedure that involves accessing the epidural space via the sacral hiatus. This is similar to the approach used for caudal epidural anesthesia. Radiography is used to guide needle and catheter placement and to perform epidurograms. When epiduroscopy is performed, radiography is also used to guide movement of the epiduroscope. For the catheter technique, the sacral hiatus is approached with a 15- to 16-gauge epidural needle with a curved tip (RX-Coude needle, Epimed International, Johnstown, NY; Fig. 33-1) about 2 to 3 cm off midline and 4 to 5 cm inferior to the sacral hiatus. To avoid penetration of the dural sac, the needle tip is advanced no further than to the S3 neural foramen. Epidurography is performed using 10 mL

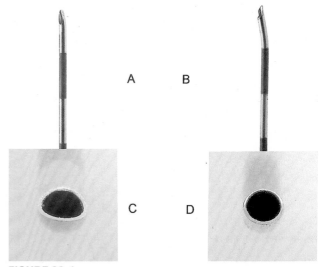

FIGURE 33-1. A: Tuohy needle tip. Note curved sharp tip. B: RX Coude needle tip. Note open tip-curve moved more proximally. **C:** Tuohy needle tip, end-on view. Note oval-shaped opening. **D:** RX Coude needle tip end-on view. Note round-shaped opening.

of nonionic radiographic contrast material to detect the presence of any filling voids (Fig. 33-2). Next, a steerable catheter is advanced into the void and 2 to 5 mL of contrast is injected as a marker, followed by 10 mL of 0.9% saline and hyaluronidase injection to remove the defect. Contrast is injected again to confirm filling of the void. Then, corticosteroid and local anesthetic are injected in small aliquots to a total volume of 10 mL. Thirty minutes later, 10% (hypertonic) saline is infused through the catheter and may be repeated two more times at 12- to 24-hour intervals. Then the catheter is removed. Precautions to prevent infection include aseptic technique, sterile dressing of the catheter entry site, and systemic antibiotics. A bacterial filter is attached to catheters after steroid injection as long as the catheter is in place. All fluids except steroid are injected through the filter.

Skill in threading the catheter to the target site improves with learning and experience. It is helpful for steering to make a 15-degree bend in the catheter about 1 inch from the tip. Thread the catheter near the midline to just above S3. Then rotate the tip so it dives to the ventrolateral target near the involved nerve root. Steer with both the needle and catheter

When epiduroscopy is performed, the same approach used for the catheter technique is employed with two notable modifications: (i) the method used to access the epidural space and (ii) the use of 0.9% saline to open the epidural space to aid visualization and to wash away material that limits visualization. Access to the space is attained using the Seldinger technique. First, an epidural needle is placed on midline, a guidewire inserted, and a stab wound made with a scalpel blade. A 10-F dilator and sheath are then inserted. The guidewire and dilator are removed, and the epiduroscope is inserted through the sheath. We use a 20-mL syringe to manually inject 0.9% saline as needed to aid visualization.

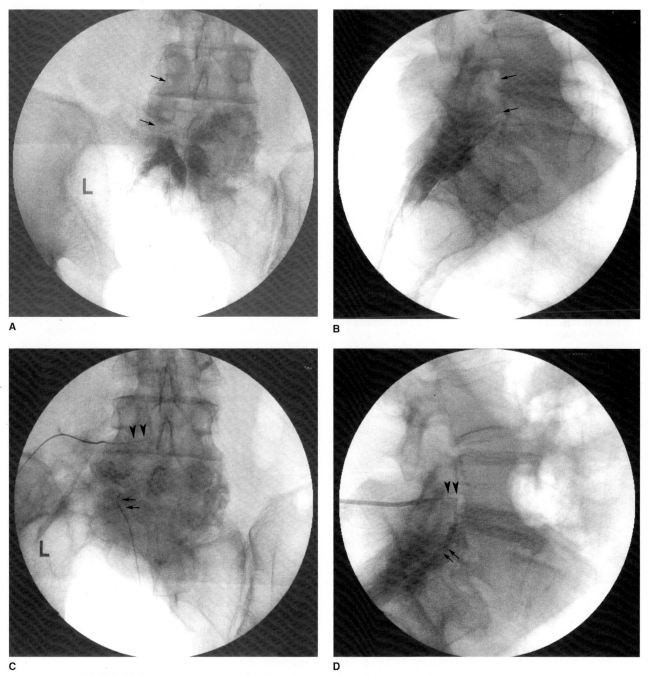

FIGURE 33-2. A patient with chronic back pain and radiculopathy. AP **(A)** and lateral **(B)** radiographs after contrast injection. Marked scarring is evidenced by lack of anterior spread (*L*, left; *arrows* indicate filling defects caused by scarring). AP **(C)** and lateral **(D)** radiographs after epidural lysis of adhesions demonstrating contrast spread to the anterior epidural space. Two catheters have been advanced to the left lateral epidural space at the L5/S1 level (*L*, Left; *arrowheads* indicate the transforaminal catheter; *arrows* indicate the tip of the caudal catheter).

▶ DEFINITION AND SCOPE

As experience with the lysis procedure increased and the technique was refined, complications were recognized. The likelihood of complications was found to be greater if pathologic processes are present, particularly arachnoiditis and extensive epidural scarring (as often found in patients with chronic pain following prior spine surgery; i.e., failed back surgery syndrome). Types of complications related to lysis of epidural adhesions are listed in Table 33-1, and the causes of complications are listed in Table 33-2. As is the case with many technically demanding techniques, the incidence of problems declines with increased operator experience. In our training program, fellows must be supervised closely for about 5 to 7 months.

TABLE 33-1 Complications Related to Lysis of Epidural Adhesions
• Allergic reactions
• Headache
• Iatrogenic-Cushingoid syndrome
• Macular hemorrhage[a]
• Somatosensory and somatomotor dysfunction
• Bowel, bladder, sexual dysfunction
• Infection
• Pain at epidural entry site
• Local anesthetic toxicity: CNS, cardiovascular

[a]Has been reported after an epiduroscope is used but not following use of a steerable catheter.

COMPLICATIONS INDUCED BY MEDICATIONS

Allergic Reactions

Classes of diagnostic and therapeutic agents used during epidural lysis that have allergenic potential include iodine-containing radiographic contrast agents, surgical disinfectants, antibiotics, local anesthetics, and hyaluronidase. It is important to obtain an accurate history to identify patients predisposed to allergic reactions. In certain cases, prophylactic use of corticosteroid and antihistamine may allow the use of allergens in susceptible patients. Documented anaphylactic reactions to local anesthetics and hyaluronidase are rare.[4]

Hyaluronidase has been documented to be effective in reducing failure from the lysis procedure from 18% to 6%.[5] Use of hyaluronidase appears to facilitate the spread of injected solutions and opening of the lateral recesses. This helps to prevent loculation of the injectate and compression of nerves, spinal canal structures, and the blood supply to the spinal cord. Based on outcomes of a large number of epidural hyaluronidase injections, Moore[4] suggested that the incidence of anaphylactic or sensitivity reactions may be 3%. Hyaluronidase is a proteinaceous substance, and, therefore, repeat administration could theoretically lead to sensitization. However, we have not seen a single serious sensitivity reaction following administration. Hyaluronidase is commonly injected with local anesthetic to produce retrobulbar nerve block, and allergic reactions in this setting are also rare. Nevertheless, caution must be advised because of the potential for an anaphylactic reaction. Appropriate treatment, including injectable epinephrine, must be readily available. A purified form of hyaluronidase, rHuPH20, synthesized in vitro, was introduced in 2005. The purified form does not contain extraneous allergenic material as do animal-derived crude extracts.[6]

TABLE 33-2 Causes of Complications Related to Lysis of Epidural Adhesions	
REACTION TO DRUGS (ETC.)	PROCEDURE RELATED
• Allergic	• Procedure pain at epidural access site
• Antibiotic	• Due to aggravation of inflammation
• Iodine-containing substances	• Due to hypertonic saline
• Radio-opaque contrast	• Excess fluid volume reinjected (relative, absolute)
• Disinfectants	• Barotrauma
• Local anesthetics	• Ischemia of nerves or cord
• Hyaluronidase	• Retinal hemorrhage
• Toxicity due to absolute or relative overdose	• Nonsterile technique
• Local anesthetics	• Epidural hematoma
• Corticosteroids	• Catheter shearing
	• Misplaced catheters or needles
	• Wrong tissue planes, structures

Hypertonic Sodium Chloride

Hypertonic saline was originally injected intrathecally into patients under general anesthesia in efforts to treat pain associated with cancer.[7] However, evidence from laboratory studies indicated that epidural administration might be safer and more effective. Thus, we began to use epidural hypertonic saline in our practice.[8]

Hypertonic sodium chloride injection is usually safe if at least 20 to 30 minutes have lapsed between local anesthetic and steroid injection and the subsequent injection of the hypertonic solution. In patients suffering from a demyelinating disease such as multiple sclerosis, we do not use hypertonic saline. We fear that the demyelination found in those with multiple sclerosis could well result in exaggerated effects, perhaps leading to direct neuronal injury. Indeed, King et al.[9] demonstrated that hypertonic saline produces persistent block of unmyelinated nerves (C-fibers) in dorsal rootlets of cats in vitro.

During epidural lysis, intrathecal injection can occur if the needle or catheter unknowingly traverses the dura. Undesirable effects observed following intrathecal injection of hypertonic saline include severe pain and muscle cramps in affected segments, hypertension, cardiac arrhythmias, pulmonary edema, and cerebral infarction. Localized paresis lasting many hours, paresthesias sometimes persisting for weeks, transient hemiplegia, and permanent loss of sphincter control with sacral anesthesia have been reported as complications following intrathecal injection of hypertonic saline.[10] Depending on the injection volume, these neurologic sequelae are often temporary and may be treated symptomatically. Subarachnoid injection is avoided only by strict adherence to technique. Injection of hypertonic saline through sharp needles where the needle tip may migrate through tissue planes should be avoided. The use of a spring-tip catheter reduces intrathecal migration and makes exact catheter localization with site-specific injection possible. Waiting 20 to 30 minutes after injecting local anesthetic (0.2% ropivacaine or 0.25% bupivacaine) to be sure motor block due to subdural spread does not develop also promotes site specific injection.

Steroids

Epidural steroid injection has been used to treat radiculopathy since the 1950s.[11] The issues are how much and which type of steroid one should use and whether the preservative may be cytotoxic and produce adhesive arachnoiditis. The fact that steroids will precipitate and form a sludge-like material is also a concern (see Chapter 27 for a discussion of epidural steroid injection). There is growing concern that intra-arterial injection of particulate steroid may produce vascular occlusion with subsequent devastating neurologic damage (see Chapter 26 for a discussion of transforaminal injection of steroids). In our current practice, we typically use 4 mg of dexamethasone because it is not particulate and 10 mL of 0.2% ropivacaine or 0.25% bupivacaine administered in 2- to 3-mL increments. During prior years, we have used triamcinolone acetate as well as methylprednisolone acetate. Betamethasone is preferred by some clinicians based on the belief that its aqueous vehicle is safer than the organic vehicle and other additives to formulations of triamcinolone and methylprednisolone. Steroid-related adverse effects are rare in the setting of epidural lysis of adhesions. Adverse effects of longer-term use of corticosteroids are discussed in Chapter 32. In a review of complications associated with epidural steroid injections, Abram and O'Connor[12] concluded that all reports of neurologic sequelae following neuraxial steroid injections involved subarachnoid injections or attempted epidural injections in which subarachnoid placement could not be ruled out. These complications included arachnoiditis and aseptic meningitis. Increased susceptibility to epidural infection (epidural abscess) has also been associated with epidural steroid injection especially if chronic distal site infection is not recognized.

Radiographic Contrast

Before the advent of water-soluble agents, oil-based agents were used and produced numerous cases of arachnoiditis when administered intrathecally. Thereafter, ionic agents became widely used, but generalized seizures and a number of fatal outcomes were reported after injection of ionic contrast media with inadvertent spread from the epidural space to the subarachnoid space.[13] These observations have led to the near-universal use of nonionic contrast agents for spinal injections of all types, the most common agent being iohexol. Common ionic agents that should be avoided in the epidural space are meglumine diatrizoate and sodium diatrizoate. Other frequently used ionic agents are diatrizoate, iothalamate, and metrizoate. Nonionic agents, such as iohexol, are the agents of choice for diagnostic myelography and are safe and effective for both epidural and intrathecal use. The most common nonionic agents in clinical use include iohexol, iopamidol, and ioversol. The most common reactions to these are anaphylactoid, and there are some high-risk groups that should be recognized (e.g., those with previous contrast reactions). Less common are osmotically-mediated toxic reactions, including acute renal failure, and rare are reactions such as arachnoiditis. If the wrong contrast is injected, for example, an ionic contrast agent like diatrizoate, after 20 to 30 minutes, blood pressure, and heart rate increase and the patient may report a sensation of heat associated with tonic-clonic, seizure-like twitching down the torso, and extremities. Upon verification that wrong agent was injected, aspiration of cerebrospinal fluid (CSF) from the subarachnoid space and irrigation and barbotage with copious preservative-free saline has been recommended by some experts. Administration of systemic steroids and treatment of seizures as needed with anticonvulsant medication is warranted.

Local Anesthetics

We typically inject 10 mL of 0.25% bupivacaine or 0.2% ropivacaine during the procedure for lysis of epidural adhesions. Before doing so, fluoroscopic imaging with contrast injection is done to confirm epidural location of the catheter (not intravascular, subdural, substance, or subarachnoid). If a vein is entered, the catheter is moved to a different site. Intravenous injection of bupivacaine can lead to cardiac toxicity, but the use of contrast should detect intravascular injection before local anesthetic is administered. The small dose of local anesthetic used during this procedure is unlikely to produce cardiac toxicity even in the event it is all given intravascularly. A detailed description of the presentation of local anesthetic-related complications appears in Chapter 7.

▶ COMPLICATIONS INDUCED BY FLUID INJECTION AND NEEDLE AND CATHETER PLACEMENT

Fluid Injection into a Confined Space: Barotrauma and Ischemia

Epidural scarring can lead to confined compartments within the epidural space. Injection of fluid into one of these compartments or into the subdural space can have the net effect of creating a space-occupying lesion that causes direct barotrauma to underlying tissue and/or blocks blood flow to the spinal cord or cauda equina—producing ischemic injury. The term loculation is used for this phenomenon. In 1997, Rocco et al.[14] elucidated the concept of compartmental filling in the diseased epidural space. They described the presence of epidural compartments that are sequentially filled during fluid injection. The fluid first fills one compartment and depending on the pattern and degree of epidural scarring fluid then overflows into adjacent compartments.

Injection of hypertonic saline solution into a closed loculated compartment within the epidural space can produce direct trauma by pressing on adjacent neural structures. Hypertonic saline is hyperosmolar and will also cause fluid shifts that will further increase the volume and pressure within loculated compartments as osmosis draws fluid into the space. To reach equilibrium, the 10% sodium chloride must reach 0.9% sodium chloride, and in the process the volume expands 11 times over the injected volume. Normally, fluid placed within the lateral recesses of the epidural space flows freely through the neuroforamen to the paraspinous region outside the spinal canal. To avoid barotrauma, it is important to document free flow of contrast from the epidural space to prevent excess pressure buildup that may compress the nerves, the spinal cord, or the nerve roots through which blood supply is carried to the spinal cord. Severe neurologic sequelae ranging from temporary sensory or motor deficits to complete paraplegia can follow barotrauma. The manifestations are variable and are dependent on the exact structure or structures compromised. The only means of preventing such injury is by ensuring that any visible areas of loculation are opened during the lysis procedure in order to establish drainage during the lysis procedure, before hypertonic saline is administered.

Figure 33-3 illustrates the appearance of loculation in the cervical area of a patient and subsequent relief by additional fluid injection and flexion-rotation or chin to shoulder movement of the patient's head. The patient had a prior C5-6, C6-7 cervical fusion for chronic neck pain following a whiplash-type injury. Subsequent to fusion, the patient was involved in another motor vehicle accident that caused hyperextension of the neck and developed left-sided severe facial pain. The patient had severe allodynia in the temporal area, the ear, and just in front of the ear spreading down toward the ramus of the mandible. The differential diagnosis was atypical facial pain versus C3 radiculopathy, and the patient was scheduled for cervical epidural neurolysis. Contrast was injected and a Racz Stim Cath (Epimed International, Johnstown, NY) was threaded through the left

side of the C4 area laterally. Considerable difficulty was encountered in advancing the catheter. Following multiple attempts, there was a clear pop, and the catheter could then be threaded cephalad to the C3 nerve root. Injected contrast remained primarily on the left side and tracked across to the right side at the C2-3 area (Figs 33-3A, B). This tracking has been recognized recently as perivenous counter spread (PVCS), that is, spread of contrast within the epidural space preferentially along the course adjacent to venous structures suggesting extensive scarring and restriction of contrast spread. PVCS is a danger sign indicating pressure build up.[15] To open a runoff pathway, flex the neck, which enlarges the neural foramen. Rotation of the head further facilitates the sliding of the inferior articulating process over the superior articulating process making the neural foramen larger.[16] The patient immediately reported bilateral arm and neck pain with the injection of only 2 mL of iohexol (240 mg/mL). The absence of lateral spread was recognized, and hyaluronidase (1,500 U in 10 mL) was slowly injected through the catheter. The patient was asked to rotate the head left to right. During the slow injection, the contrast was suddenly seen to be displaced through the neuroforamina to the outside of the spinal canal, releasing pressure on the spinal cord (Fig. 33-3C, D). The patient's pain rapidly subsided. Direct stimulation of the C3 nerve root reproduced the patient's pain, suggesting the diagnosis of posttraumatic C3 neuropathic pain. Toward the conclusion of the lysis procedure, the C2 through C4 area had clear runoff on fluoroscopy (Fig. 33-3E). At this point, local anesthetic and steroids (0.2% ropivacaine-containing 4 mg dexamethasone diluted in a total volume of 6 mL was injected in 1-mL increments to a total of 4 mL). The facial pain stopped and the catheter was fixed in place and connected to a bacterial filter. Thirty minutes later, 3 mL of 10% sodium chloride was infused with the patient in the left lateral dependent position. On the 2nd day, the catheter was injected with 5 mL of 0.2% ropivacaine through the bacterial filter, followed by 4 mL of 10% sodium chloride. This was repeated the same day a second time, and the catheter was removed. At the time of discharge, the facial pain was not

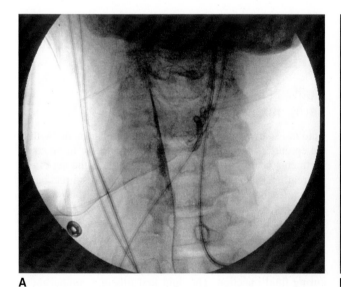

A

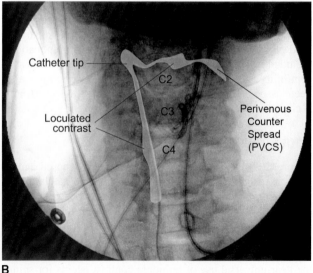

B

FIGURE 33-3. A: Cervical AP radiograph of patient following contrast injection demonstrates restricted spread (loculation); B: Labeled image. (*Cont.*)

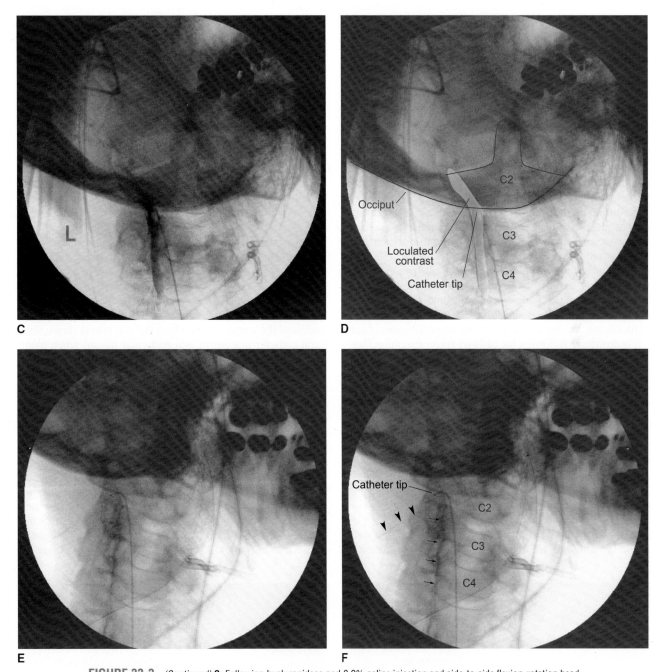

FIGURE 33-3. *(Continued)* **C:** Following hyaluronidase and 0.9% saline injection and side-to-side flexion-rotation head movement contrast can be seen entering the neural foramen; **D:** Labeled image. **E:** Contrast runoff in the C2, 3, 4 area; **F:** Labeled image.

present. The patient remains pain free 6½ years later without additional interventions.

We have reviewed several cases of cord injury where the cervical injection (usually single shot) was followed by onset of pain, numbness, and motor block involving the ipsilateral lower extremity or both lower extremities with or without bladder dysfunction. It is our belief that movement of the head from side to side during the procedure causes the fluid, which is under pressure within an area of loculation, to open a path for lateral runoff. This leads to reduction of the pressure on the spinal cord, the nerve roots, and their blood supply. We have developed this method over the past 20 years, and it is used when loculation and pain are noted particularly during

cervical lysis of adhesions. A small amount of contrast is used as a marker to be displaced by the lower-viscosity hyaluronidase solution. The pain reported by the patient is most likely related to ischemia caused by the pressure from the initial injection. When loculation is suspected, time should not be wasted on magnetic resonance imaging (MRI) and surgical consultation. Immediate action as described above is required to prevent serious morbidity or death. Important to note that signs and symptoms of loculation disappear after successful treatment in the same order that they appear, that is, pain is the first symptom to appear and the first to disappear.

Suspected loculation of non–contrast-containing fluids may be confirmed by injecting water-soluble contrast into the suspected site. The injection expectedly will aggravate symptoms, but will allow documentation and drainage of the loculation.

Large-volume Epidural Injections

Uncontrolled injections of relatively large volumes of fluid into the epidural space can lead to retinal hemorrhage. There is no exact volume known to produce retinal hemorrhage, but volumes <65 mL are thought to be safe.[17] Our experience is that larger volumes (up to 100 mL) can be used safely if the injection rate is not rapid, and flow from the epidural space (absence of loculation) is documented. The volumes used during the lysis procedure done with a catheter usually do not reach 65 mL. Lateral catheter placement where the fluid escapes from the spinal canal through the intervertebral foramen reduces the likelihood of a pressure increase and consequently minimizes the risk of retinal hemorrhage. If the catheter is in the midline or if it is within the subdural or subarachnoid space, injection of even modest volumes can result in a significant rise in CSF pressure and lead to retinal hemorrhage. We are not aware of any recorded cases of retinal hemorrhage following the catheter lysis procedure. However, 12 cases of visual impairment following epiduroscopy or epidural fluid injection have been reported.[18] The impairment was due to retinal hemorrhage characteristic of venous origin. Complete recovery of vision typically occurred over a period of days to months. There is no specific treatment for retinal hemorrhage unless there is extension of blood into the vitreous humor. In such cases, vitrectomy may help to restore vision.

Misplaced Catheters and Needles: Subdural, Intrathecal, and Intraneural Injection

The most common problem with the lysis procedure is unfamiliarity with the technique. Inexperienced practitioners often place the catheter in the midline for lysis of adhesions. In a prospective randomized study, Manchikanti et al.[19] showed that non–site-specific catheter placement is completely ineffective, as is single caudal epidural injection. In addition, the midline catheter is more likely to enter the subdural space (Fig. 33-4). If the patient suffers from coexisting arachnoiditis, bowel and/or bladder dysfunction may result. Subdural contrast spread must be recognized before subsequent injection. Subdural injection of local anesthetic and steroid will result in motor block. Subdural injection of hypertonic saline can give rise to loss of bowel and bladder function.[1] The only means of preventing these devastating complications is through strict attention to detail: the catheter must be in the ventrolateral epidural space and should never be in the midline.

Subdural injections are usually recognized during the injection of radiographic contrast. Contrast spread in the subdural space produces a railroad-track–like pencil outline of the dura in anterior-posterior (AP) and lateral x-ray views. The contrast spread is extensive. If the cause is subdural catheter placement, the catheter most likely will be in the middle of the spinal canal on both AP and lateral views. Subdural catheter placement is a particular hazard when using cutting needles such as the Husted, Tuohy, and R-K needles. The tip of the needle, although in the epidural space, can cut through the dura—producing a flap-like hole. When the catheter is inserted, it enters the subdural space through this opening. Threading of the catheter is remarkably easy, but it can be recognized to be subdural because the catheter cannot be directed to the target area, which is the lateral epidural space. On the lateral view, the catheter will be in the mid spinal canal, rather than either in a dorsal or ventral location typical of an epidural catheter position. Subdural catheter and scope placement in the midline can lead to increased pressure interrupting blood supply to the spinal cord. Sedation is a serious issue. One needs to be able to communicate with the patient. An example of the importance of

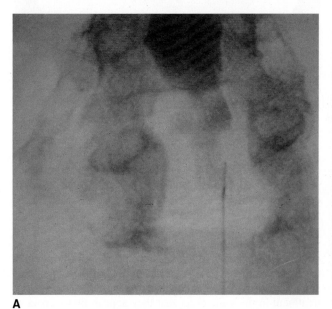

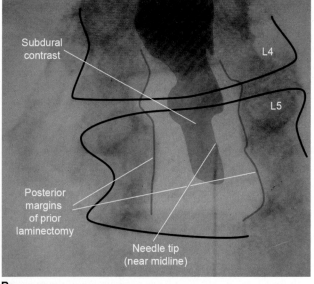

A
B

FIGURE 33-4. **A: Anteroposterior radiograph of the lumbar spine during epidural lysis of adhesions.** This patient had previous laminectomy. The catheter is located in the midline, where penetration of the dura mater is more likely. Contrast is seen extending into the subdural compartment. **B:** Labeled image.

communication is a patient who complained of bilateral leg pain upon injection of radiopaque contrast followed by hyaluronidase, total volume 20 mL. A 22-gauge spinal needle was inserted via the interlaminar approach, and 13 mL of contrast containing fluid was aspirated from the subdural space. The patient immediately reported relief of pain. This technique has been used by others also who recognize the importance of lateral as well as AP views to diagnose the cause of pain in these cases. In another case, subdural placement during epiduroscopy was not recognized in a sedated patient. The patient developed bowel, bladder, and sexual dysfunction and pursued litigation.

Subdural injection is not generally a problem if there is no resistance to dye spread within the subdural space. Restricted spread of fluid produces pressure that compresses blood supply traversing the subdural space toward the spinal cord. As a result, the cord becomes ischemic. Measures of preventing subdural injections include recognition of the characteristic contrast spread and use of small volumes of local anesthetic. Subarachnoid injections should be recognized, particularly if one always aspirates between injection and uses test doses of local anesthetics. Bupivacaine 0.25% or ropivacaine 0.2% will give a significant sensory and motor block within 15 to 20 minutes following injection when sudden respiratory motor block and arrest occur. Therefore, postinjection monitoring in a safe setting is essential.

Sheared Catheters

Avoidance of shearing catheters requires skill and the use of appropriate equipment, especially the appropriate epidural needle and catheter. In our training program with five pain fellows, we find that if fellows shear catheters, they usually do so during the first 4 months of training. Usually the shearing is a consequence of using Husted, Touhy, or R-K needles. All are needles with a cutting edge (Fig. 33-1), as are the needles supplied with spinal cord stimulator implant kits. Using a needle that is too small also increases the risk of shearing.

Prevention of catheter shearing requires attention to the direction of the catheter and the direction of the needle tip. The direction of the catheter and the direction on the tip of the needle must be similar. If the direction of the catheter is different from the opening of the needle, the sharp edge of the needle will cut into the outer plastic coating of the spring wire or the plastic catheter if the catheter is withdrawn through the needle. The cut creates a fishhook-like defect in the catheter coating. As soon as one recognizes that the catheter is caught on the needle tip, the needle and catheter should be removed simultaneously. If difficulty in withdrawing a catheter is noted after the needle has been removed, a method proven successful for us is to wait a few minutes and then disengage the fishhook-like effect by pushing and twisting the catheter prior to pulling. The hole created by the needle is bigger than the catheter, and thus this push-and-twist motion often allows for easy removal of the catheter. If there is a hang-up, one should not forcibly pull the catheter, as this will cause separation of the catheter at the cut. There are reports of placing an R-K needle over the catheter through the original puncture site and successfully removing the partially cut catheter.

As a part of the informed consent, we include a discussion that catheter shearing is a possibility, and in the event that we shear a catheter it will be surgically removed. The available literature focuses primarily on the fate of catheters sheared in the course of acute pain management (surgical, labor, and delivery) rather than chronic pain management. In the setting of acute pain treatment, most authors recommend[20] that sheared catheters be left in place, unless the catheter's location is causing pain or radiculopathy. However, in our experience, patients with chronic pain where a catheter is sheared often believe that the retained catheter piece is contributing to their ongoing pain. We are aware of several medico-legal filings arising when sheared catheters were left behind. Therefore, we arrange for surgical consultation and removal of sheared catheters. Individual practitioners need to make decisions about removal of sheared catheters on a case-by-case basis.

Both the Husted and Touhy needles have an oval-shaped opening (Fig. 33-1). The tips of these needles are sharp, predisposing to cutting into the outer plastic wall of catheters. The RX-Coude needle (Epimed International, Johnstown, NY) has a wider tip, is not as sharp, and has the curvature further back on the shaft of the needle than the Husted and Touhy needles. This design allows directional assistance in guiding the catheter to the appropriate site. It is our opinion that the RX-Coude needle is far superior for directing the catheter and reducing shearing. However, movement of the needle may cut the dura once the tip enters the epidural space. A recent development is the use of a RX-Coude needle with an interlocking blunt stylet that protrudes 1 mm beyond the needle tip. This pushes the dura away and allows rotation of the needle so a catheter can be directed to the desired location. Similarly, a 14 gauge needle and blunt stylet can be used to place spinal cord stimulation leads.

Other

Perineal numbness is probably one of the most common symptoms following the epidural lysis procedure performed via a caudal approach though the sacral hiatus. It is usually self-limited and is likely the consequence of neuropraxia produced by pressure from the needle and the catheter on the S5 nerve roots as they exit near the sacral hiatus. In rare instances, the sacral hiatus area may remain painful after the procedure. This may be due to neuroma formation and usually responds to injection of local anesthetics into the painful neuroma site. In rare instances, one of the S5 nerves may be cut by the needle tip, and prolonged or permanent perineal numbness can occur. We have observed no hematomas and no loculation in the sacral canal. Fluid nearly always escapes through the S3 foramen and usually by other routes into the pelvis.

Patients with syrinx within the spinal cord appear to be at risk for injury caused by increases in pressure within the epidural space. For example, we are aware of a case of paralysis that developed following nothing more than the loss of resistance induced pressure change used for spinal cord stimulator electrode placement (personal communication). We are not aware of any pressure induced complications during epidural lysis of adehesions or epiduroscopy in patients with spinal cord syrinx. However, caution should be exercised when performing these procedures on any patient with a known syrinx or any other intrinsic abnormality of the spinal cord.

► INFECTION, HEMATOMA, AND OTHER COMPLICATIONS

Infection

The possibility of infection must be kept in mind anytime the epidural space is entered. Careful history must be taken to rule out purulent sinusitis, bladder infection, pneumonia, or periodontal infection. Any evidence of preexisting chronic infection puts the patient at risk, particularly if steroids are administered into the epidural space. Delayed overwhelming infection (sepsis) has been seen after epidural injection in patients with preexisting chronic infection. This usually occurs on the 12th to 13th day and patients present with surprisingly few symptoms. Rarely, these patients may die from the multisystem complications that ensue. Epidural infection more typically presents with symptoms including increased pain, neck pain, headache, photophobia, numbness, or weakness. The signs are elevated temperature, meningismus, and some neural deficits. Abnormalities in the laboratory findings include elevated white blood counts, elevated erythrocyte sedimentation rate, and spinal fluid abnormalities. Epidural infections usually respond to antibiotic treatment administered for 5 to 10 days (see Chapter 5 for a detailed discussion of epidural abscess.)

Our approach for preventing infection includes a systematic approach to placing the catheter. The patient is given intravenous prophylactic antibiotic before the procedure is begun. We insert the needle 2 inches distal to the sacral hiatus, 1 inch off midline so that a length of the catheter is tunneled through tissue. Prior to placement, the catheter is soaked in saline with 50 U/mL of bacitracin (50,000 U diluted in 1 L), and when steroid is administered through the catheter, it is done in the operating room using full sterile precautions. Upon completion of the steroid injection, a bacterial filter is placed on the catheter. The bacterial filter is not removed during the remainder of the treatment, and no further steroids are administered. In the event the bacterial filter or the connector becomes disconnected, the catheter is removed. We apply antibiotic ointment at the puncture site. The site is covered by two split venous dressing gauze sponges surrounded by adhesive and covered by a transparent occlusive dressing. A pressure dressing is applied over the occlusive dressing and fixed with adhesive tape. Oral antibiotics are given for 5 days. With this approach, we have not seen a single infection necessitating surgical drainage.

Hematoma

The incidence of hematoma formation in the vertebral canal produced by the lysis procedure is rare. This may well be because high-pressure veins are converted to low-pressure veins by the lysis procedure, a concept discussed further in material following. Most of the bleeding is venous bleeding following placement of the catheter or needle. Preoperative assessment of the patient must include a careful drug history and evaluation of platelet function, as patients may take one or more of the numerous drugs that inhibit platelet function and interfere with normal coagulation. Prevention and management of epidural hematoma are discussed in detail in Chapter 4.

During upper thoracic needle placement for cervical lysis catheter placement there have been epidural hematomas related to needle placement where complete recovery ensued following MRI diagnosis and surgical evacuation. Patients reported back pain, bladder problems and lower extremity weakness. There have also been several cases where, instead of evacuation, observation was chosen and resulted in permanent cord injury. In addition, we are aware of a single case where thoracic injection induced loculation and subdural spread of contrast, saline and steroid mixture (total volume 5 mL) causing thoracic pain, lower extremity paresthesia and weakness that was reversed by repetitive flexion rotation of the thoraco-lumbar torso. Follow up MRI was negative for hematoma as an explanation (personal communications).

Harry Crock, world-renowned spine surgeon, documented that there are high-pressure veins in failed back surgery patients (personal communication). He suggested that these high-pressure veins are the consequence of occluded venous runoff through the neural foramina. He documented that by doing a single surgical foraminotomy he was able to convert the high-pressure veins to low-pressure veins and thus reduce the likelihood of high-pressure venous bleeding. The phenomenon is analogous to deflating a tourniquet on an arm. Our experience is that the lysis procedure as we perform it is equivalent to a fluid foraminotomy. Evidence for this is secondary. We have done over 8,000 lysis procedures in over 20+ years, yet not a single epidural hematoma occurred where surgical intervention was necessary to drain the hematoma. Hematomas, we are aware of, are usually caused by single-needle epidural steroid injection via interlaminar epidural approaches, usually in failed back surgery patients.

Identifying High-risk Patients

Myelopathy may be produced by midline needle injection or midline or near-midline catheter placement and small-volume injections. The injected volume is insufficient to reach the lateral epidural space and open a neuroforamen. As a result, there is loculation with sustained pressure on the spinal cord.

Clinical examples of loculation come from personal experience, either in the clinical setting or in the medical-legal arena. The combined hazard of unrecognized or preexisting arachnoiditis in the presence of extensive epidural scarring in failed back patients with radiculopathy was reported in our first publication on epidural adhesiolysis. Because of extensive hardware, a preprocedure MRI or CT scan was not done. The patient had severe pain and radiculopathy together with foot drop. The lysis of adhesions procedure was recommended. Contrast, local anesthetic (10 mL of 0.25% bupivacaine) and steroid were injected. Postprocedure motor block was noted in the recovery room. At this point, the procedure was abandoned and the motor block proceeded to recover. However, there was a permanent loss of bowel and bladder function. Unfortunately, the pain continued. A myelogram revealed severe arachnoiditis, likely a result of the previous multiple surgeries and diagnostic studies. Spinal opioid infusion was started and provided long-standing pain relief. This was reported to highlight to the risk associated with doing epidural adhesiolysis in patients with arachnoiditis and epidural scarring. Unfortunately, this story has reoccurred a

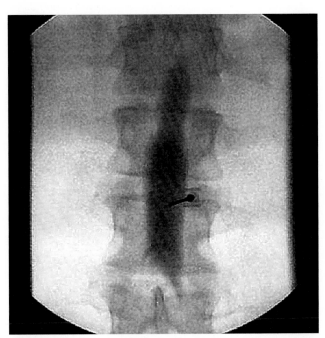

FIGURE 33-5. AP radiograph of the lumbosacral spine near the lumbosacral junction showing loculation and subdural spread of contrast. Extensive subdural spread of the radiographic contrast can be seen extending over more than two vertebral levels. This pattern can be distinguished from intrathecal injection, as the spread of intrathecal contrast would not be limited superiorly or inferiorly and would also spread laterally to fill the dural cuffs.

attention must be paid to the history and the examination of the patient. Practitioners must recognize the patient who has preexisting arachnoiditis and epidural scarring as at high risk for subdural spread that can lead to loculation and secondary ischemia of the cauda equina and the spinal cord. Loculation and the described concepts of fluid spread within the epidural space must be kept in mind at all times. The technique is effective, not only in the lumbar and sacral areas but in the thoracic and the cervical areas. The target site has to be site specific to the ventrolateral epidural space to have maximum efficacy. It is effective with radiculopathy and with some of the back pain syndromes where the sinuvertebral system is involved. It also is more effective in the treatment of spinal stenosis than are single-shot epidural steroid injections.[8]

As a conservative estimate, the technique has been done in numerous centers worldwide over 1.7 million times since the initial technique was reported. The incidence of complications is low. Infection and bleeding should be extremely rare. Shearing of catheters is uncommon among experienced practitioners and with improved needle and equipment design.

number of times in other physician practices with results of not only bowel and bladder function loss but also resulting in paraplegia. The best way to deal with this problem is to be highly aware of the danger of subdural spread in the presence of arachnoiditis. Both epidural scarring and arachnoiditis are particularly common in the patient who has one or more prior spinal surgeries. In such patients, even a single needle injection can produce permanent paralysis as the fluid dissects through a surgical scar into the subdural space and cuts off crucial circulation to the spinal cord.

Prolonged ischemia can be prevented by detecting loculation and moving volume away from the subdural space to the epidural space (Fig. 33-5). The problem is rare and motor block typically resolves without intervention. The question remains: at what point in time should the practitioner who recognizes that loculation of fluid within the subdural space has occurred either place multiple needle sticks to drain the loculated fluid or consider surgical intervention for decompression?

▶ SUMMARY

Lysis of epidural adhesions for treating chronic low back pain and radiculopathy is markedly effective on short-term follow-up and moderately effective on long-term (i.e., 12 months follow-up), as demonstrated by prospective randomized studies.[21,22] There are numerous retrospective studies and clinical reports that demonstrate similar results. Prospective randomized studies showed that catheter placement, if it is not site specific, to be ineffective. The technique is technically challenging and requires a significant learning period. Careful

References

1. Racz GB, Holubec JT. Lysis of adhesions in the epidural space. In: Racz GB, ed. *Techniques of Neurolysis*. Boston, MA: Kluwer, 1989:57–72.
2. Kuslich SD, Ulstrom CL, Michael CJ. The tissue origin of low back pain and sciatica. *Orthop Clin North Am* 1991;22:181–187.
3. Ross JS, Robertson JT, Frederickson RC, et al. Association between peridural scar and recurrent radicular pain after lumbar discectomy: magnetic resonance evaluation. *Neurosurgery* 1996;38:855–861.
4. Moore DC. The use of hyaluronidase in local and nerve block analgesia other than spinal block: 1520 cases. *Anesthesiology* 1951;12:611–626.
5. Heavner JE, Racz GB, Raj PP. Percutaneous epidural neuroplasty: prospective evaluation of 0.9% NaCl vs. 10% NaCl with or without hyaluronidase. *Reg Anesth Pain Med* 1999;24:202–207.
6. Dunn A, Heavner JE, Racz GB, et al. Hyaluronidase: a review of approved formulations, indications and off label use in chronic pain management. *Expert Opin Biol Ther* 2010;10:127–131.
7. Hitchcock ER. Hypothermic-saline subarachnoid injection. *Lancet* 1970;1:843.
8. Racz GB, Heavner JE, Singleton W, et al. Hypertonic saline and corticosteroid injected epidurally for pain control. In: Racz GB, ed. *Techniques for Neurolysis*. Boston, MA: Kluwer Academic Publisher, 1989:73–86.
9. King JC, Jewett DL, Sundberg HR. Differential blockade of cat dorsal root c-fibers by various chloride solutions. *J Neurosurg* 1972;36:569–583.
10. Swerdlow M. Complications of neurolytic neural blockade. In: Cousins MJ, Bridenbaugh PO, eds. *Neural Blockade*. Philadelphia, PA: Lippincott, 1980:543–553.
11. Larkin TM, Carragee E, Cohen S. A novel technique for delivery of epidural steroids and diagnosing the level of nerve root pathology. *J Spinal Disord Tech* 2003;16:186–192.
12. Abram SE, O'Connor TC. Complications associated with epidural steroid injection. *Reg Anesth* 1996;21:149–162.
13. Junck L, Marshall WH. Neurotoxicity of radiological contrast agents. *Ann Neurol* 1983;13:469–484.
14. Rocco AG, Philip JH, Boas RA, et al. Epidural space as a starling resistor and elevation of inflow resistance in a diseased epidural space. *Reg Anesth* 1997;22:167–177.
15. Racz GB, Heavner JE. Cervical spinal canal loculation and secondary ischemic cord injury—PVCS—perivenous counter spread—danger sign! *Pain Pract* 2008;8:399–403.

16. Kitogawa T, Fujiwara A, Kobayashi N, et al. Morphologic changes in the cervical neural foramen due to flexion and extension (*in vitro* imaging study). *Spine* 2004;29:2821–2825.

17. Saberski LR, Brull SJ. Epidural endoscopy-aided drug delivery: a case report. *Yale J Biol Med* 1995;68:7–15.

18. Gill JBV, Heavner JE. Visual impairment following epidural fluid injections and epiduroscopy: a review. *Pain Med* 2005;6:367–374.

19. Manchikanti L, Rivera JJ, Pampati V, et al. One-day lumbar epidural adhesiolysis and hypertonic saline neurolysis in treatment of chronic low back pain: a randomized, double-blind trial. *Pain Physician* 2004;7(2):177–186.

20. Bromage PR. *Epidural Analgesia*. Philadelphia, PA: WB Saunders, 1978:664–665.

21. Boswell MV, Shah RV, Everett CR, et al. Interventional techniques in the management of chronic spinal pain: evidence-based practice guidelines. *Pain Physician* 2005;8:1–47.

22. Hayek SM, Helm S, Benjamin RM, et al. Effectiveness of spinal endoscopic adhesiolysis in post lumbar surgery syndrome. *Pain Physician* 2009;12:419–435.

34

Complications Associated with Chronic Opioid Therapy

Richard Rosenquist

The search for a rapid and reliable means of providing pain control has vexed humanity for all of recorded history. Opium's analgesic and mind-altering properties have been known for centuries. In 1805, the German pharmacist Friedrich W. Serturner isolated and described the principal alkaloid and powerful active ingredient in opium, which he named "morphium" after Morpheus, the Greek god of dreams. We know it today as morphine. This was soon followed by the discovery of other alkaloids of opium: codeine in 1832 and papaverine in 1848. By the 1850s, these pure alkaloids (rather than the earlier crude opium preparations) were being commonly prescribed for the relief of pain, cough, and diarrhea. Subsequent research into this class of compounds has produced numerous opioid analgesic compounds and delivery systems. In recent decades, numerous organizations have promoted the importance of effective pain treatment, ongoing research has provided greater insight into the types and causes of pain, and demand for pain treatment has grown. In the absence of well-designed and well-validated treatments for the wide variety of chronic pain conditions, attention turned toward opioid analgesics as the obvious choice for treating all chronic pain complaints. The use of opioids for treatment of chronic noncancer pain has experienced a meteoric rise, and many patients have had great relief of pain and improvement in function.

However, increased use has been accompanied by a marked increase in the number of patients experiencing both anticipated and unanticipated complications. In many cases, patients were informed only of the common side effects of therapy and otherwise led to believe that there was little long-term consequence to the use of this class of medications. In addition, there has been a dramatic increase in the number of fatalities related to the use of prescription opioids leading to the development of a variety of new abuse-resistant drug formulations and legislative remedies applied to the problem. This chapter seeks to dispel some myths and address complications related to chronic opioid therapy.

► COMMON OPIOID-RELATED ADVERSE EFFECTS

Common opioid-related adverse effects include constipation, urinary retention, sedation, delirium, dry mouth, respiratory depression, hyperhidrosis, pruritus, muscular spasm, tremor, nausea, and vomiting. The use of opioid analgesics is associated with these side effects, which are so common they are considered an expected part of therapy. In some cases, tolerance develops and side effects diminish. In others, side effects persist for the duration of therapy. Some or all of these side effects are present in almost all patients receiving chronic opioid therapy. The exact group of side effects and their relative severity is highly variable, individual, and drug and dose dependent.

In a systematic review of 34 randomized trials, Moore and McQuay[1] examined the prevalence of adverse events related to oral opioid administration. The trials were of relatively short duration, with only two trials longer than 4 weeks and only one as long as 8 weeks. Although the trials are of relatively short duration, they are characteristic of the vast majority of literature used to support the use of opioids in treating chronic pain. The authors found that 51% of all patients taking oral opioids experienced at least one adverse event and that 22% of patients discontinued therapy due to adverse events, including dry mouth, nausea, constipation, dizziness, drowsiness or somnolence, pruritus, or vomiting (Box 34-1). The pathophysiology of these side effects is related to direct effects on opioid receptors in the brain, spinal cord, peripheral nervous system, and gut.

Constipation

Scope

Constipation related to the use of opioid analgesics is the most common adverse effect of chronic opioid therapy and usually requires some form of treatment, either dietary or

---

BOX 34-1 Common Opioid-related Adverse Effects and Their Estimated Incidence During Oral Administration

- 22% of patients discontinued therapy due to adverse events
- 25% dry mouth
- 21% nausea
- 15% constipation
- 14% dizziness
- 14% drowsiness or somnolence
- 13% pruritus
- 10% vomiting

From Moore RA, McQuay HJ. Prevalence of opioid adverse events in chronic non-malignant pain: systematic review of randomized trials of oral opioids. *Arthritis Res Ther* 2005;7:R1046–R1051.

medical.[2] In the rare circumstance in which chronic diarrhea is present, reduction in bowel motility may be a welcome relief. However, in most cases, this is an undesirable side effect that should be anticipated and requires active treatment.

Pathophysiology

Opioids impair normal bowel function by binding to intestinal μ-opioid receptors and interrupting the normal coordinated rhythmic contractions required for intestinal motility. Opioids can also alter intestinal fluid secretion by a direct effect on the enteric nervous system. These actions are often accompanied by decreased gastric emptying, abdominal cramping, spasm, and bloating, and usually result in decreased frequency of bowel movements, formation of hard, dry stools, painful defecation, and incomplete bowel evacuation. In addition, peripheral actions of opioids on the gut may contribute to nausea and vomiting.

Diagnosis

Constipation is typically diagnosed on the basis of history alone. In some cases, constipation may be severe and evidence gathered through the use of abdominal x-ray, but this is the exception rather than the rule. Finally, the use of the hydrogen breath test to assess gastrointestinal transit time has been used in the research setting and in advanced gastrointestinal evaluations, but does not have wide use as a means of diagnosing constipation in the clinical setting.[3]

Prevention/Treatment

In the case of opioid-induced constipation, prevention and treatment are almost simultaneous. When chronic opioid therapy is initiated, it should be assumed that constipation is likely to occur and treatment should be initiated. Initial treatment may be limited to dietary changes such as increased liquid, dietary fiber, and fruit intake. If dietary changes are insufficient, use of a stool softener such as docusate sodium, promotility compounds such as senna, osmotic agents such as polyethylene glycol, and bulk agents such as methylcellulose may be used alone or in combination to reduce constipation.[2,4,5]

Future treatments using opioid antagonists such as alvimopan and methylnaltrexone that act to block opioid receptors in the gut without affecting opioid analgesia may offer improved treatment of this side effect. In a study by Paulson et al.[6] examining the use of alvimopan in a 21-day trial of treatment for opioid-induced bowel dysfunction, the authors demonstrated significant efficacy in the management of opioid-induced bowel dysfunction. Over the 21-day treatment period, 54%, 43%, and 29% had a bowel movement within 8 hours of administration of 1.0 or 0.5 mg of alvimopan versus placebo. A more recent study by Jansen et al. examined the use of alvimopan in a randomized, placebo-controlled trial for opioid-induced bowel dysfunction in patients with noncancer pain. The primary efficacy endpoint was the proportion of patients experiencing at least three spontaneous bowel movements (SBMs; bowel movements with no laxative use in the previous 24 hours) per week over the treatment period and an average increase from baseline of at least one SBM per week. A significantly greater proportion of patients in the alvimopan 0.5 mg twice-daily group met the primary endpoint compared with placebo (72% vs. 48%, $p < 0.001$). Treatment with alvimopan twice daily also improved other symptoms such as stool consistency, straining, incomplete evacuation, abdominal bloating, abdominal pain, and decreased appetite compared with placebo. The opioid-induced bowel dysfunction Symptoms Improvement Scale (SIS) responder rate was 40.4% in the alvimopan 0.5 mg twice daily group, versus 18.6% with placebo ($p < 0.001$). Active treatment with alvimopan did not increase the requirement for opioid medication or increase average pain intensity scores.[7]

Sedation/Delirium

Scope

Sedation is commonly observed during initiation of opioid therapy or when significant dose increases are made.[8] It is often associated with transient drowsiness or cognitive impairment. These symptoms usually resolve after a few days, and reassurance and recommendation to avoid alcohol or driving at the initiation of therapy are sufficient. In most cases, patients receiving stable doses of medication do not have significant impairment in cognitive or driving ability compared to patients not taking opioids.[9,10] However, in some cases, symptoms persist and may be related to other comorbidities or the concomitant use of other sedating medications. Delirium is an acute confusional state that leads to a disturbance of consciousness and comprehension. Although sedation, mild cognitive impairment (or even hallucinations) frequently occur when opioids are started or when significant dose increases are implemented, the differential diagnosis of opioid-induced delirium is often complicated.

Pathophysiology

The pathophysiology of sedation or delirium occurring with opioid administration is related to the effects of opioids and their metabolites on receptors in the brain and spinal cord. Factors such as renal dysfunction, hepatic dysfunction, chronic high-dose opioids, preexisting cognitive impairment, dehydration, concurrent administration of other psychoactive drugs, smoking cessation, or terminal illness may all contribute to the development of delirium.

Risk Factors

Risk factors for sedation associated with the use of opioid analgesics include opioid naiveté, rapid dose increases, renal insufficiency, hepatic insufficiency, administration with other sedative medications, and concurrent metabolic disorders (Box 34-2). The relative risk of one opioid producing delirium over another is not well documented, although

---

BOX 34-2 Risk Factors for Sedation in Association with the Use of Opioid Analgesics

- Opioid naiveté
- Rapid dose escalation
- Renal insufficiency
- Hepatic insufficiency
- Administration with other sedative medications
- Concurrent metabolic disorders

meperidine (with its toxic metabolite normeperidine) has been singled out as a particularly dangerous compound. The route of administration and the lipophilicity of the opioid have been suggested as potential risk factors.

Diagnosis

Diagnosis of the causes of sedation, cognitive dysfunction, or delirium should include a careful history to elicit the temporal relationship between opioid administration and altered mental function. In addition, assessment should include evaluation of potential coexisting conditions such as dementia, renal insufficiency, metabolic encephalopathies, brain metastases, and concurrent administration of other pharmacologic agents with central nervous system activity. For instance, undesirable effects following acute overdose, after a significant dose increase and after changing to a new drug, may be related to the drug itself. In contrast, gradual onset of sedation or delirium in the setting of worsening renal insufficiency may be the result of toxic metabolite accumulation.

Prevention

Prevention of sedation/delirium may be accomplished by limiting the initial dose and rate of dose escalation and avoiding administration of these compounds to patients with limited ability to metabolize them or excrete the metabolites. In addition, choosing agents with less risk of toxic metabolite accumulation may be beneficial. Opioids may be excreted in the parent form by the kidneys. However, those that are not readily eliminated in this fashion are metabolized to form more water-soluble metabolites. Those patients with impaired renal function, including most elderly individuals and those receiving high-dose or long-term opioid therapy, are at particular risk. Normeperidine, a metabolite of meperidine, causes neurotoxicity—especially in elderly patients and those with poor renal function. Its use for acute pain should be limited to 1 to 2 days, and it should be avoided in the management of chronic pain.

Morphine-3-glucuronide and morphine-6-glucuronide are the two major water-soluble morphine metabolites dependent on renal elimination.[11] Morphine-3-glucuronide has antinociceptive properties and has been associated with hyperalgesia and myoclonus.[12,13] Morphine-6-glucuronide is a potent analgesic and may be more potent than morphine.[14] Normorphine is another metabolite produced and may contribute to analgesic and toxic effects. The major hydromorphone metabolite is hydromorphone-3-glucuronide. This compound does not have analgesic properties, but is a more potent neuroexcitant than morphine-3-glucuronide.[15] Oxycodone is metabolized to hydromorphone and has been suggested as a potentially safer alternative in some elderly or renally impaired patients, although there is no solid data to support this assertion.

Treatment

Treatment should proceed from conservative measures such as opioid reduction or rotation and reducing or discontinuing other sedative medications to addition of a psychostimulant if necessary. As with other opioid-induced side effects, dose reduction, drug rotation, evaluation for active metabolite retention, and reduction or elimination of other psychoactive substances have been suggested as initial treatment steps.

Dry Mouth

Scope

Dry mouth is an extremely common complication of chronic opioid administration and has been associated with severe dental problems. In one study, 84% of patients experienced this symptom either temporarily or throughout the entire study period, and reports of dry mouth were present in 65% of the assessments.[16]

Pathophysiology

This side effect appears to be the result of a direct action of opioids and their metabolites.[16] The exact mechanism has not been described, but it is thought that this may be related to interference with nerve-mediated mechanisms and parasympathetic impulses activating glandular muscarinic or adrenergic receptors.[17]

Risk Factors

The risk of this side effect appears to be directly related to dose and in the case of morphine directly related to the amount of morphine-6-glucuronide.[16] This symptom can be exacerbated by other compounds with anticholinergic effects.

Diagnosis

There are no specific diagnostic studies recommended for this side effect.

Prevention

There are no specific preventive measures for this side effect.

Treatment

Treatment can consist of opioid reduction or rotation, elimination of anticholinergic or anticonvulsant compounds with xerostomic effects, or symptomatic treatment by encouraging liquid intake. Symptomatic treatment such as fluid intake, artificial saliva, or encouraging the patient to use chewing gum or hard candy to promote saliva release may be helpful. In addition, agents that promote salivary excretion such as pilocarpine and bethanechol chloride have been advocated.[17]

Respiratory Depression

Scope

Respiratory depression is a very real concern to all physicians prescribing opioid analgesics and is potentially the most dangerous side effect. This side effect, like many others related to the administration of opioid analgesics, is of most concern during initiation of therapy, with significant dose increases, or when the potential for active metabolite accumulation is present. Tolerance to the respiratory depressant effects of opioids usually develops over the course of days to weeks. True respiratory depression is rare in patients who have been receiving opioids chronically.[18] When it does occur, it is often related to a recent dose increase or conversion from one opioid to another. If the dose of opioid has been stable, an alternative explanation such as pneumonia, pulmonary embolism, cardiomyopathy, or recent coadministration of another sedating medication should be considered.[19,20]

The use of opioids in the treatment of those with severe pain near the end of life is often considered controversial due to the very real potential for a "double effect." The moral doctrine of double effect is roughly defined as follows: Double effect provides that it can be morally good to shorten a patient's life as a foreseen and accepted but unintended side effect of an action undertaken for a good reason, even if it is agreed that intentionally killing the patient or shortening the patient's life is wrong. The use of sedation in the terminal setting to control the sometimes intense pain of dying patients may have the effect of shortening the patient's life. This creates concern that the provision of appropriate palliative care mandates actions that may be indistinguishable from euthanasia, which is illegal in most places and morally objectionable to many. Invoking double effect addresses these worries: the intent of the physician is to control the suffering, not to shorten life. Evidence of physician intent should be found in notations on the patient's chart and in the recorded dosages and titration of the opioid analgesics. Consequently, the action is not euthanasia but appropriate palliative care.[21]

Pathophysiology

High concentrations of opioid receptors are present in many supraspinal brain respiratory centers, including the nucleus solitarius, the nucleus retroambigualis, and the nucleus ambiguous.[22] In addition, there are specific chemosensitive brain areas that mediate opioid-induced respiratory effects. Opioids interfere with pontine and medullary respiratory centers that regulate respiratory rhythmicity (Fig. 34-1). The μ-receptor action of opioids on respiratory centers in the brain stem produces dose-dependent depression by direct action on brain stem respiratory centers to the point of apnea with sufficient doses.

There is also controversy regarding the role of different subclasses of μ-opioid receptors in producing these effects. The exact mechanism by which the various respiratory centers involved in ventilatory drive, respiratory rhythm generation, chemoreception, and neural integration remains unclear. The net result is that the stimulatory effect of CO_2 in ventilation is significantly reduced. This decreases the slopes of the ventilatory and occlusion pressure response to CO_2 and minute ventilatory responses to increases of $PaCO_2$ are shifted to the right (Fig. 34-1, inset). In addition, the resting end-tidal PCO_2 and apneic thresholds are increased. Opioids also decrease hypoxic ventilatory drive.[23,24] Carotid body chemoreception and hypoxic drive are blunted or eliminated by low doses of opioid analgesics. Opioids reduce the increase in respiratory drive normally associated with increased loads such as increased airway resistance.[23] Opioids exert effects on control of respiratory rhythm and pattern and produce increased respiratory pauses, delays in expiration, irregular and/or periodic breathing, and decreased, normal, or increased tidal volume.[25–27] The prolongation of expiratory time usually produces a greater effect on respiratory rate than on tidal volume. In most cases, although therapeutic doses may reduce respiratory rate, the resultant increase in CO_2 stimulates central chemoreceptors and produces a compensatory increase in respiratory rate.

Risk Factors

Respiratory depression is a relatively rare complication in patients receiving long-term opioids. Although the role of opioids cannot be excluded in patients receiving long-term

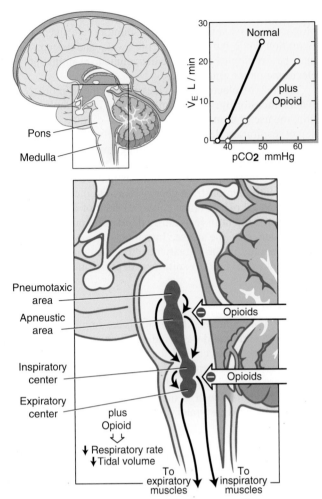

FIGURE 34-1. The pathophysiology of opioid-induced respiratory depression. Opioids bind to and inhibit respiratory centers within the medulla and pons responsible for the rate of respiration (pneumotaxic and apneustic centers) as well as the control of the muscles of inspiration and expiration that govern tidal volume. The inset is a graphic representation of the ventilatory response to progressive hypercapnia. The slope of the ventilatory response is reduced in the presence of opioids. The apneic threshold (the intercept on the x axis or the pCO2 value where apnea ensues) is shifted to the right. (**Inset** adapted from Bailey PL, Egan TD, Stanley TH. Intravenous opioid anesthetics. In: Miller RD, ed. *Anesthesia.* 5th ed. Philadelphia, PA: Churchill Livingstone, 2000:294, with permission.)

opioid therapy, alternate causes such as pneumonia, pulmonary embolism, cardiac dysfunction, or the coadministration of another sedating medication should be considered. In addition, patients with sleep apnea are at higher risk for developing altered respiratory patterns or complications related to the use of opioids.[28]

Diagnosis

Diagnosis of respiratory depression may be made when acquiring vital signs. However, respiratory rate is not always a reliable index of the magnitude of opioid-induced respiratory depression. High doses of opioids often eliminate spontaneous respirations, but do not necessarily produce unconsciousness. In this setting, patients may still be responsive to verbal commands and may breathe when directed to do so. Another clinical sign of opioid effect that may be observed is the presence of pupillary constriction. In the clinical setting, the most common method of evaluating respiratory depression is measuring respiratory rate and oxygen saturation while the patient is both awake and asleep. This may be accomplished with either clinical examination or electronic monitoring devices.

The use of electronic devices may provide more consistent monitoring, but alarms may be ignored. In addition, the use of monitoring such as pulse oximetry may not detect respiratory depression immediately because oxygen saturation may fall long after the beginning of respiratory depression and decreased respiratory rate. In the acute overdose situation, blood gas analysis may be required and subsequently demonstrate decreased PaO_2, increased CO_2, and decreased pH. In some cases, reversal of opioid effect with improvement in respiratory depression provides indirect evidence of the cause. In patients receiving chronic opioid therapy in the outpatient setting, monitoring is not employed, and mild respiratory depression may occur undetected.

Prevention

Prevention of respiratory depression is accomplished by limiting initial and total dose, avoiding situations in which significant metabolite accumulation may occur, reducing doses in patients with concurrent medications that may exacerbate respiratory depression, and adjusting doses for patients with medical conditions such as sleep apnea that increase the risk of opioid-induced respiratory depression.

Treatment

Treatment consists of opioid dose reduction, elimination or reduction of other medications with respiratory depressant or sedative effects, and in rare cases the administration of opioid antagonists. The administration of opioid antagonists should be reserved for severe respiratory depression because acute withdrawal or untoward physiologic responses to naloxone administration can occur. These include the development of increased pain, nausea, vomiting, shivering, metabolic stress, hypertension, tachycardia, pulmonary edema, cerebrovascular accident, cardiac arrhythmia, cardiac arrest, and death. In addition, due to its short half-life, if naloxone is not continued respiratory depression may recur.[29-35]

Hyperhidrosis

Hyperhidrosis (excessive sweating) is an adverse effect commonly reported by patients receiving oral opioids, but has received little attention in the medical literature. In one study of patients receiving methadone, the incidence of excessive sweating was 45%.[36] This is thought to be related to mast cell degranulation and has been successfully controlled with antihistamines. In most cases, this is not excessively troubling to the patient and rarely requires treatment.[37,38]

Myoclonus

Scope

Muscular spasm (myoclonus) and tremor can occur with opioid administration. Myoclonus is often mild and self-limited, but in some cases can persist and become severe, producing distresses for both the patient and the family. Symptoms range from mild twitching to generalized spasms

and can exacerbate pain due to involuntary movement. This symptom tends to occur more frequently with high doses of opioids and when patients are drowsy or entering light sleep.

Pathophysiology

The pathophysiology of myoclonus is not well characterized, but may be related to accumulation of metabolites. Following administration, opioids such as morphine and hydromorphone are metabolized primarily to morphine-3-glucuronide or hydromorphone-3-glucuronide. The 3-glucuronide metabolites are devoid of analgesic activity and have been theorized to play a role in antagonizing the antinociceptive effects of the parent compound and the active 6-glucuronide metabolite.[39] It has also been implicated in potentially playing a role in the development of tolerance.

Several rodent studies have demonstrated that morphine-3-glucuronide and high-dose morphine administered by the intracerebroventricular and intrathecal routes produce symptoms of altered pain behavior such as hyperalgesia, allodynia, motor excitation, seizures, and even death.[39-46] The mechanisms of these neurotoxic phenomena are not fully elucidated. There have been conflicting results in animal studies regarding the reversibility of opioid-induced neuroexcitation by naloxone, and a nonopioid receptor mechanism has been theorized.[42-46] The behavioral excitation of high-dose morphine and morphine-3-glucuronide can be mimicked by the glycine antagonist strychnine.[44] However, an *in vitro* study was unable to demonstrate inhibition of H-strychnine binding by morphine or morphine-3-glucuronide.[47] Administration of *N*-methyl-D-aspartate (NMDA) antagonists causes a reduction of behavior excitation produced by high-dose morphine and morphine-3-glucuronide.[41,48]

Risk Factors

The risk of myoclonus is increased by the use of large doses of opioid analgesics and/or the accumulation of toxic metabolites and has been reported with multiple delivery routes including oral, subcutaneous, intravenous, epidural, and intrathecal. There does not seem to be a specific route of administration that is more likely to produce this side effect. The use of large doses and the accumulation of metabolites appear to play the largest role. The most common metabolites associated with this side effect are the 3-glucuronides. In addition, metabolites such as normeperidine and normorphine have been implicated.

Diagnosis

There are no specific diagnostic tests available. Although drug and metabolite levels may be obtained, levels associated with the development of symptoms in humans have not been well described. As a result, diagnosis is primarily made on the basis of history and physical examination alone.

Prevention

There are no specific preventive measures. Choosing the most appropriate compound to avoid toxic metabolite accumulation may be helpful in some cases. In other cases, switching to another opioid analgesic, opioid rotation, maximizing nonopioid analgesics, or using other interventional pain-relieving techniques may reduce the frequency and severity of symptoms.

Treatment

There are no prospective randomized trials that detail effective treatment for myoclonus. Empiric treatment usually consists of opioid dose reduction, rotation to a different opioid, or use of adjuvant analgesics. If myoclonus is persistent and other causes have been eliminated, treatment with benzodiazepines, skeletal-muscle relaxants, clonidine, acetylcholinesterase inhibitors, valproic acid, baclofen, or dantrolene has been recommended.[49–60]

Nausea and Vomiting

Scope

The presence of nausea and vomiting in association with opioid administration is common. Reports of the incidence of nausea in association with opioid administration range from 9% to 98%.[1,18,61] Vomiting is less common and has been reported from 0% to 39%.[1,18,61]

Pathophysiology

Nausea and vomiting are produced by the direct effects of opioids on the chemoreceptor trigger zone in the area postrema of the medulla, possibly through the activation of δ-receptors.[62] This effect, in combination with opioid-induced alterations in gastrointestinal motility, contributes to symptoms of nausea and vomiting.

Risk Factors

There are no specific risk factors for nausea and vomiting, and no specific opioid has been identified as being more emetogenic than another. These side effects, as with many others, are more common when the drug is initiated than after tolerance to the medication has developed.

Diagnosis

This diagnosis is made on the basis of history or direct observation. There are no laboratory tests to make the diagnosis of nausea.

Prevention

There is little that can be done to prevent nausea and vomiting. In some cases, one opioid may cause more nausea and vomiting for a given patient than another, and this drug should be avoided. As is commonly recommended in the treatment of chronic pain, the use of nonopioid analgesic adjuvants should be encouraged in general and as a potential means of decreasing this undesirable side effect. Avoiding opioid ingestion on an empty stomach may reduce these symptoms in some patients. There is no evidence from prospective trials to recommend the prophylactic use of antiemetics in the treatment of opioid-induced nausea and vomiting.

Treatment

Treatment of nausea may incorporate the use of a variety of compounds. However, it should be noted that recommendations for the use of these agents in the setting of chronic opioid therapy is unsupported by prospective study or systematic evaluation of retrospective data. Agents such as ondansetron, granisetron, metoclopramide, phenergan, prochlorperazine, dimenhydrate, phenothiazine, transdermal scopolamine, cisapride, and dexamethasone have all been suggested. In several case reports, the prevalence and severity of nausea and vomiting were reduced by rotation to another opioid.[63–65] There are two small studies demonstrating a reduction in nausea and vomiting by converting from oral to subcutaneous administration.[66,67] Data regarding the use of rectal administration is conflicting.[68,69] In rare cases, the use of an opioid antagonist or discontinuation of the opioid altogether may be required to eliminate nausea and vomiting.

► ENDOCRINE EFFECTS OF CHRONIC OPIOID THERAPY

Scope

Adverse effects of opioids on the endocrine system have been observed for almost a century, but are often not presented during medical education or in discussions with patients regarding the risk of using opioid analgesics. These complications include central hypogonadism, adrenocortical deficiency, and growth hormone deficiency (Box 34-3). Symptoms of hypogonadism include loss of libido, impotence, infertility (males and females), depression, anxiety, fatigue, loss of muscle mass and strength, amenorrhea, irregular menses, galactorrhea, osteoporosis, and fractures.[70–80] Symptoms of adrenocortical deficiency include insidious onset of slowly progressive fatigability, weakness, anorexia, nausea and vomiting, weight loss, cutaneous and mucosal pigmentation, hypotension, and occasional hypoglycemia.[81–83] The spectrum may vary depending on the duration and degree of adrenal hypofunction and may range from mild chronic

---

BOX 34-3 Endocrine Effects of Chronic Opioid Therapy

- Central hypogonadism
- Loss of libido
- Impotence
- Infertility (males and females)
- Depression
- Anxiety
- Fatigue
- Loss of muscle mass and strength
- Amenorrhea, irregular menses
- Galactorrhea
- Osteoporosis and fractures
- Adrenocortical deficiency
- Insidious onset of slowly progressive fatigability
- Weakness
- Anorexia
- Nausea and vomiting
- Weight loss
- Cutaneous and mucosal pigmentation
- Hypotension
- Occasional hypoglycemia
- Growth hormone deficiency
- Growth hormone deficiency in adults is of uncertain consequence

fatigue to fulminating shock. Symptoms of growth hormone deficiency in adults are uncertain.[83]

Pathophysiology

The pathophysiology of these complications is related to effects of opioids on the hypothalamic-pituitary-gonadal process of controlling secretion of gonadal hormones (Fig. 34-2). The normal process begins with secretion of gonadotropin-releasing hormone (GNRH). This hormone causes the pituitary gland to secrete luteinizing hormone (LH) and follicle stimulating hormone (FSH). These hormones are released into the circulation and cause the testes and ovaries to secrete testosterone or estrogen, respectively. These hormones in turn affect the hypothalamus and pituitary, forming a complex feedback loop.

Opioids (endogenous and exogenous) bind to receptors in the hypothalamus, pituitary, and testes to modulate gonadal function.[72,84–87] Decreased or altered release of GNRH at the hypothalamus with resultant alterations in LH and FSH release from the pituitary has been documented.[84,85,87] Opioids also have a direct effect on the testes and produce decreased secretion of testosterone and testicular interstitial fluid.[70] The clinical effects of these interactions have been demonstrated in opioid addicts, methadone maintenance patients, and those receiving oral, transdermal, and intrathecal opioids for noncancer pain. In studies examining narcotic-induced hypogonadism during heroin use and addiction treatment with methadone, significant reductions in total testosterone levels have been demonstrated to occur as soon as 4 hours after ingestion.[88,89] In addition, there appears to be a close dose relationship in which increasing doses of opioids are associated with greater reductions in total testosterone.

In patients receiving intrathecal opioids for chronic noncancer pain, studies have documented hypogonadism associated with low LH values and normal or low FSH levels in both males and females.[73–75,83,90,91] These hormonal abnormalities are accompanied by decreased libido or impotence in males and irregular or absent menses in females.[92] Several studies have been published on the long-term effects of oral opioid therapy in males. In a study by Daniell,[93] endocrine function was measured in 54 patients on sustained-release opioids and compared to 27 healthy controls. Total testosterone levels were reduced below normal in 74% of the opioid group. Severe erectile dysfunction or diminished libido was present in 87% of opioid-ingesting men who had normal erectile function prior to opioid use.

Rajagopal et al.[79] reported a case series of cancer survivors taking opioids (morphine equivalent daily dose of 200 mg for at least 1 year) for chronic pain and compared them to matched controls not using opioids. In the opioid group, 90% exhibited hypogonadism. Sexual desire, anxiety and depression, and overall quality of life were significantly lower in the opioid group than in the controls. In addition to diminished sexual function, hypogonadism in males is associated with the development of significant reductions in bone density.[76,77,80] This can occur in males without other risk factors for reduced bone density. The relationship between chronic opioid administration and adrenocortical deficiency is not as clear, but direct opioid inhibition of hormone release at the level of the hypothalamus, the pituitary, and the adrenal cortex occurs (Fig. 34-3).

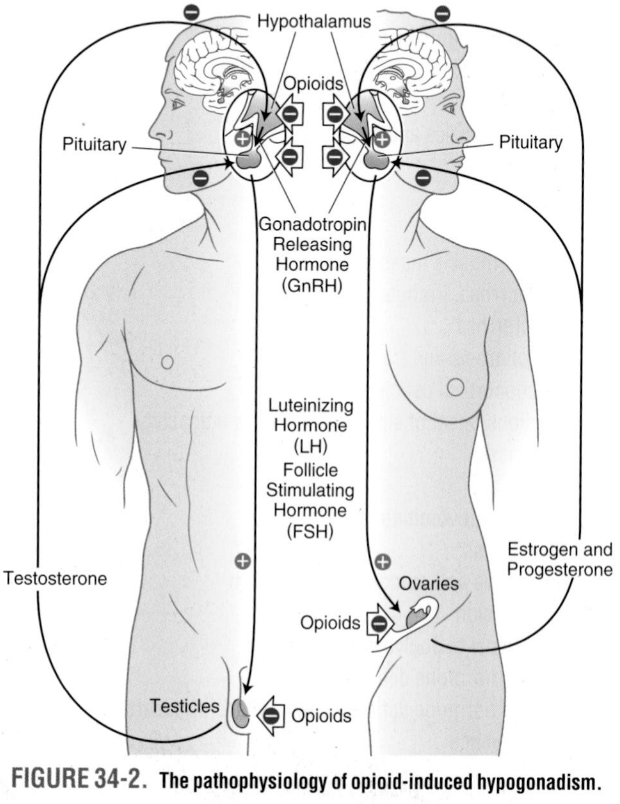

FIGURE 34-2. The pathophysiology of opioid-induced hypogonadism.

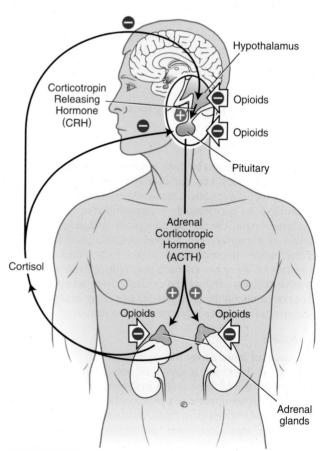

FIGURE 34-3. The pathophysiology of opioid-induced adrenal cortical insufficiency.

In one study evaluating long-term consequences of intrathecal opioid administration, 15% of patients developed hypocorticism.[83] Several other studies have demonstrated the ability of opioids to decrease cortisol levels as well as cortisol responses to adrenocorticotropin challenges.[94,95] The long-term clinical significance of these findings is unclear, but at least one case report of clinically significant adrenocortical insufficiency attributed to opiate-induced suppression of the hypothalamic-pituitary-adrenal axis has been reported. Growth hormone deficiency in association with chronic opioid administration has been reported, although the clinical significance remains unclear.[83] It does not appear that opioids have any significant effect on thyroid function.[96,97] The signs and symptoms of hypogonadism are well known. However, many of these symptoms are also common in patients with chronic pain conditions.

Risk Factors

All patients taking chronic opioid therapy are at risk of this side effect. The relative risk of one opioid versus another in the development of this complication has not been described. There appears to be a relationship of this complication to dose, and therefore those taking higher doses of opioids are at increased risk of developing endocrine complications.

Diagnosis

All patients receiving opioid therapy for chronic pain should be assessed prospectively for symptoms of hypogonadism. At present, there are no published standards for laboratory monitoring of patients receiving opioids for chronic pain. However, the extremely high incidence of hypogonadism associated with chronic opioid administration suggests that endocrine monitoring should be routine, especially for those receiving higher doses of opioids (Box 34-4).

Laboratory studies should include total testosterone, free testosterone, estradiol, LH, and FSH. In addition, monitoring of bone density should be considered in patients receiving chronic opioid therapy. This is especially important in at-risk patients because patients with fractures due to hypogonadism may have no other symptoms of hypogonadism.[80] The evidence to support routine monitoring of adrenocortical function is absent at present. This testing should only be performed in patients with symptoms of adrenal suppression. In those cases where this is questioned, a dexamethasone suppression test may be appropriate.

Prevention

There are no specific prevention strategies for opioid-induced hypogonadism, adrenal insufficiency, or growth hormone deficiency aside from avoiding opioid use altogether. There appears to be a dose-related relationship, with higher doses being associated with a greater prevalence and degree of hormonal suppression. As such, it is important to use the lowest effective dose in order to minimize adverse effects.

Treatment

Treatment of opioid-induced hypogonadism is in its nascency. There are no published standards, and clinical judgment must be relied onto balance choices among opioid dose reduction, opioid rotation, or elimination as a means of treatment versus hormone replacement. If patients have clinically relevant effects relating to sexual function or mood, or other symptoms and/or laboratory testing reveal hypogonadism, treatment should be considered. This may consist of a trial of opioid rotation, increased emphasis on nonopioid analgesics, or techniques that may allow dose reduction or eliminating the use of opioids altogether. If opioid rotation, dose reduction, or opioid elimination do not rectify the problem, testosterone supplementation is appropriate.

The goal of therapy should be to increase total serum testosterone concentrations to within the normal physiologic range of 300 to 1,200 ng/dL.[98–100] This can be accomplished with a variety of formulations, including intramuscular injections, transdermal patches, and transdermal gel. The transdermal preparations are a reasonable means of beginning, with intramuscular injections reserved for those who fail to respond to more conservative therapies. A study by Aloisi et al. examining hormone replacement therapy in morphine-induced hypogonadism in male chronic pain patients demonstrated significant improvements across a range of measurements over a 1-year observation period. These included total and free testosterone and dihydrotestosterone, pain-rating indices, SF-36, and sexual dimension of the Aging Males Symptom Scale.[101] Testosterone supplementation is not free of adverse effects. Common adverse effects associated with this therapy include local site reactions, sleep apnea, and hematologic abnormalities (particularly polycythemia). Menstrual irregularities and virilization may occur in women, whereas oligospermia, priapism, baldness, and gynecomastia may occur in men. A more severe risk in men is the potential for growth (benign or malignant) of the prostate gland. Although a clear link between exogenous testosterone and prostate cancer has not been established, patients receiving supplemental testosterone must be monitored with rectal examinations and prostate-specific antigen.

BOX 34-4 Endocrine Monitoring in Patients Receiving Chronic Opioids

There are no published standards for laboratory monitoring of patients receiving opioids for chronic pain. However, the extremely high incidence of hypogonadism associated with chronic opioid administration suggests that endocrine monitoring should be routine, especially for those receiving higher doses of opioids. Laboratory studies should include total testosterone, free testosterone, estradiol, LH, and FSH. Monitoring of bone density should be considered in patients receiving chronic opioid therapy. This is especially important in at-risk patients because patients with fractures due to hypogonadism may have no other symptoms of hypogonadism. The evidence to support routine monitoring of adrenocortical function is absent at present. This testing should only be performed in patients with symptoms of adrenal suppression. In those cases where this is questioned, a dexamethasone suppression test may be appropriate.

▶ IMMUNOSUPPRESSION

Scope

Opioids can produce immunosuppression through neuroendocrine effects or via a direct effect on the immune system. There is an abundance of evidence in the laboratory setting of this phenomenon on the basis of animal studies, but its importance as an adverse effect of opioid therapy is not fully understood.[102–106] In the clinical setting, there is both increased prevalence and severity of bacterial and viral infections in intravenous drug users with increased morbidity and mortality.[107–110]

The exact role of opioid-induced immunosuppression in this population is difficult to determine because this high-risk population often has other confounding variables such as hepatitis, human immunodeficiency virus (HIV), and malnutrition that produce immunomodulatory effects of their own. There have been no prospective or retrospective reviews of patients receiving chronic opioid therapy to examine whether or not they have an increased incidence of infectious disorders. There is no definitive information available to determine if one opioid has greater immunosuppressive effects than another.

Pathophysiology

The effects of opioids on immunomodulatory function have been described in a number of human volunteer studies.[111,112] Individuals chronically exposed to opioids demonstrate a series of changes in their ability to respond to immunological challenges. These include decreased natural killer cell cytolytic activity, blood lymphocyte proliferation responses to mitogen, and alterations in complex immune responses, including antibody-dependent cell-mediated cytotoxicity and antibody production.[103,107–109,113,114] Opioids also suppress hematopoietic cell development, producing atrophy of the thymus and spleen and reduced number of macrophages and B cells in the murine spleen.[104–106,115] In patients with HIV infection, there is a significant correlation between drug abuse and HIV infection.[110,116] In human peripheral blood mononuclear cell cultures, morphine promotes HIV-1 growth.[117,118]

Opioids have also been demonstrated to have a direct effect on CCR5 turnover, and methadone in clinically relevant doses significantly enhances HIV infection of macrophages with the upregulation of expression of CCR5, a primary co-receptor for macrophage-tropic HIV entry into macrophages.[119] Animal studies have also clearly demonstrated that opioids alter development, differentiation, and function of immune cells. Hamra and Yaksh[120] demonstrated that morphine inhibits lymphocyte proliferation, decreased splenic lymphocyte number, and altered phenotypic expression of cell surface markers.

Risk Factors

Long-term exposure to opioids appears more likely to suppress immune function than short-term exposure, and withdrawal may also induce immunosuppression in animal studies. Evidence for immunosuppression in humans is limited, although opioids have been shown to increase immunosuppression in patients infected with HIV and may increase the viral load.[116–119] Clear evidence from human studies in patients taking long-term opioids is lacking, and some opioids may be less immunosuppressive than others. This concern is compounded by the fact that pain itself can impair immune function. Therefore, patients receiving high-dose opioids with poor pain control may be at the greatest risk of this complication.

Diagnosis

Although opioid-induced immunosuppression has been demonstrated in a research setting, there are no currently accepted or recommended clinical laboratory testing methods for evaluation of opioid-induced immunosuppression.

Prevention

There are no known means of preventing the development of opioid-induced immunosuppression.

Treatment

At present, the only currently available therapy is to rotate opioids, reduce total dose, or eliminate the use of opioid analgesics altogether.

▶ HYPERALGESIC EFFECTS OF CHRONIC OPIOID THERAPY

Although chronic opioids are prescribed for the treatment of pain, there is a growing body of evidence that their use may be associated with the development of abnormal sensitivity to pain.[121] This may explain situations in which failure to relieve pain occurs in some patients despite increases in the opioid dose. The incidence of this adverse response to opioid analgesics is not well described, but should be considered whenever increased pain is present with opioid administration and dose escalation is not associated with improved pain control.

Opioid-induced alterations in pain sensitivity have been observed in patients treated for pain as well as those with opioid addiction.[122–125] Preclinical and clinical studies suggest that opioid-induced abnormal pain sensitivity shares common characteristics with the cellular mechanisms of neuropathic pain.[126,127] Mao et al.[128] have demonstrated that repeated exposure to opioids can produce NMDA receptor-mediated changes in the spinal cord dorsal-horn cells that cause abnormal pain sensitivity.[128] They have also demonstrated neuronal apoptosis associated with morphine tolerance with evidence for an opioid-induced neurotoxic mechanism. Consistent use of opioids may result not only in the development of tolerance, but may produce a pronociceptive state. Although it is relatively weak, there is both animal and human evidence that reducing testosterone levels may contribute to increased pain sensitivity.

The contribution of each of these processes to the clinical picture of pharmacologic tolerance has not been clarified by animal or human studies. As a result, both desensitization and sensitization occurring during prolonged opioid therapy may contribute to apparent decreases in analgesic efficacy and create a confusing clinical picture. There are no well-described diagnostic tests to determine if increased pain sensitivity in patients receiving treatment with opioid analgesics represents disease progression, tolerance, or opioid-induced abnormal sensitivity. Evaluation may require opioid reduction, rotation, or elimination. There are no well-defined methods of preventing opioid-induced hyperalgesia. There may be a role for NMDA antagonists in the prevention of opioid tolerance and opioid-induced hypersensitivity, but this remains to be clarified. As with other opioid-induced adverse effects, dose limitation may be helpful in maintaining efficacy and limiting hyperalgesia.

▶ ACUTE PAIN MANAGEMENT IN THE OPIOID-TOLERANT PATIENT

Treatment of acute pain in the opioid-tolerant patient can be extremely challenging and can be a problem in any patient taking chronic opioids prior to an acutely painful event such as surgery or a motor vehicle accident (Box 34-5). This problem occurs whether the opioid was being taken for legitimate or illegitimate purpose prior to the acute event. Opioid tolerance is a pharmacologic phenomenon related to the consistent use of opioids and is associated with the need to increase the dose to maintain equipotent analgesic effects.

Tolerance can be a learned phenomenon associated with environmental clues and psychological factors. It can also be an adaptive process involving downregulation, desensitization of opioid receptors, or increased pain sensitivity. Regardless of the exact pathophysiology, the net result is that these patients can be extremely challenging to treat for acute pain conditions. There is little in the way of diagnostic evaluation or prevention that can be accomplished in the acute pain setting. It is vital to determine how much opioid was being consumed prior to the acute painful event and ensure that the patient's baseline is maintained to prevent withdrawal. It is important to determine if alternate nonopioid analgesic techniques may be used to produce analgesia. This circumvents the problems of opioid tolerance and frequently allows the delivery of excellent analgesia. Regional analgesia using local anesthetics in the epidural space or along peripheral nerves is one means of producing analgesia in the opioid-tolerant patient.

Other nonopioid analgesics such as nonsteroidal anti-inflammatory drugs (NSAIDs), ketamine, and anticonvulsants should be considered as well. If opioid analgesics are the only alternative, the selection of an opioid analgesic other than is the one that is taken on a daily basis may offer some benefit. The potential requirement of a markedly increased dose of opioid analgesic to achieve adequate analgesia in the opioid-tolerant patient should be anticipated and prescriptions written to accommodate these requirements. These dose requirements may approach 300% to 350% of the preoperative chronic opioid dose.[129–131] As a result, patients with preexisting tolerance are often undermedicated and never receive adequate analgesia. The potential to produce hyperalgesia should always be considered as well.

BOX 34-5 Acute Pain Management in the Patient with Opioid Tolerance or a History of Opioid Addiction

Two groups of patients present particular challenges to the clinician in the perioperative period: those who have been taking large doses of opioids for chronic pain and those with current or previous addiction. Simple rules of thumb for managing the opioid-tolerant patient or those with a history of addiction include the following.

- Consider regional analgesic techniques (spinal opioids, epidural infusions) to improve analgesia and minimize systemic opioid effects. Keep in mind that higher-than-usual doses of neuraxial opioid may be required in those with significant tolerance.
- Use adjunctive analgesics (e.g., NSAIDs) whenever possible to reduce total opioid requirements.
- Administer opioid analgesics liberally to control pain in the immediate postoperative period. Do not attempt to limit the opioid dose or wean opioid analgesics in the immediate postoperative period. Those with significant tolerance will invariably require higher-than-average doses to control acute pain.
- Use the preoperative opioid doses as a baseline requirement and administer additional doses beyond this to control acute pain. This baseline requirement can be administered as a continuous intravenous infusion as part of patient-controlled analgesia (PCA) or by continuing the preoperative long-acting opioid in addition to use of PCA.
- Consider consultation with a substance-abuse specialist during hospitalization for those with ongoing opioid abuse or a history of addiction.
- Closely coordinate (communicate) the plan for pain management with the patient's primary care provider before hospital discharge. Although acute escalation in the opioid requirement is often necessary in the perioperative period, a plan for weaning the opioids to their previous levels should be established before the patient is discharged from the hospital.

▶ ADDICTION, PHYSICAL DEPENDENCE, TOLERANCE, ABUSE, DIVERSION, AND WITHDRAWAL

Scope

Opioid analgesics are commonly prescribed to reduce pain. When used appropriately, they provide significant relief of pain and improvement in function in some patients. However, despite their potential for good, there is a dark side to opioid analgesics. The dark side consists of addiction, physical dependence, tolerance, abuse, diversion, withdrawal, and, in some cases, death. Addiction is designated as a process whereby a behavior that can function both to produce pleasure and to provide escape from internal discomfort is employed in a pattern characterized by (i) recurrent failure

---

BOX 34-6 Defining Opioid Addiction,
Dependence, and Tolerance

- Opioid addiction: This formal definition is similar to the popular conception of addiction as a compulsion or overpowering drive to obtain a drug in order to experience its psychological effects. Addiction is not synonymous with physical dependence. Although all individuals who are taking opioids for an extended period of time will exhibit withdrawal symptoms if the drug is abruptly discontinued, few will exhibit the compulsive behavior and psychological dependence characteristic of addiction. Opioid addiction rarely occurs iatrogenically.
- Physical dependence: This has been defined as a state of adaptation that is manifested by a drug-class-specific withdrawal syndrome that can be produced by abrupt cessation, rapid dose reduction, decreasing blood level of the drug, and/or administration of an antagonist.
- Tolerance: This has been defined as a state of adaptation in which exposure to a drug induces changes that result in a diminution of one or more of the drug's effects over time.

From American Psychiatric Association. *DSM IV.* 4th ed. Arlington, VA: American Psychiatric Publishing, 2000:182–183.

---

to control the behavior (powerlessness) and (ii) continuation of a behavior despite significant negative consequences (unmanageability; Box 34-6). The exact incidence of this disorder in association with the use of prescription opioids is not known, but the nonmedical use or abuse of prescription drugs has been labeled as a serious and growing public health problem.[132,133]

A report by the National Institute on Drug Abuse (NIDA) estimates that 48 million people age 12 and older have used prescription drugs for nonmedical reasons in their lifetimes.[134] This represents approximately 20% of the U.S. population. Even more alarming is the fact that the 2004 NIDA's monitoring the future survey of eighth-, tenth-, and twelfth-graders found that 9.3% of twelfth-graders reported having used Vicodin (hydrocodone bitartrate and acetaminophen tablets, USP; Abbott Laboratories, North Chicago, IL) without a prescription in the past year and 5% reported having used OxyContin (controlled release oxycodone hydrochloride; Purdue Pharma, L.P., Stamford, CT) without a prescription, making these medications among the most commonly abused prescription drugs by adolescents.[134]

Gilson et al.[135] published a reassessment of trends in the medical use and abuse of opioid analgesics and implications for diversion control looking at the years 1997 to 2002 as a follow-up to a previous article published by Joranson et al.[136] 4 years earlier. They evaluated trends in the medical use and abuse of fentanyl, hydromorphone, meperidine, morphine, and oxycodone and the abuse trend for opioid analgesics as a class compared to trends in the abuse of other drug classes. Results of their study demonstrated a marked increase in medical use and abuse of four of the five studied opioid analgesics. In 2002, opioid analgesics accounted for 9.85% of all drug abuse, up from 5.75% in 1997. In the United States in 2007, unintentional poisonings were the second leading cause of injury death with approximately 93% of all unintentional poisoning deaths caused by drug poisoning. This unfortunate circumstance has been particularly notable in several states, with Florida representing the most dramatic. The Centers for Disease Control and Prevention (CDC) Morbidity and Mortality Weekly Report of July 8, 2011 summarizes the results of a CDC analysis of the Florida Medical Examiners Commission. This analysis found that from 2003 to 2009, the number of annual deaths in which medical examiner testing showed lethal concentrations of one or more drugs increased 61.0%, from 1,804 to 2,905, and the death rate increased 47.5%, from 10.6 to 15.7 per 100,000 population. During 2003 to 2009, death rates increased for all substances except cocaine and heroin. The death rate for prescription drugs increased 84.2%, from 7.3 to 13.4 per 100,000 population. The greatest increase was observed in the death rate from oxycodone (264.6%), followed by alprazolam (233.8%) and methadone (79.2%). By 2009, the number of deaths in Florida involving prescription drugs was four times the number involving illicit drugs.[137]

Although the exact reasons for growing abuse of prescription drugs is unclear, accessibility is likely a contributing factor. Drug diversion can be best defined as the diversion of licit drugs for illicit purposes.[138]

Pathophysiology

The pathophysiology of opioid addiction appears to be neurophysiologic reinforcement (reward). At least one mesolimbic "reward pathway" has been identified, and others may exist. This pathway involves dopaminergic neurons originating in the ventral tegmental area (VTA) and projecting into the forebrain, particularly the nucleus accumbens. The dopaminergic neurons are probably continuously inhibited in the VTA, perhaps by gamma-aminobutyric acid (GABA). Release of dopamine from these neurons onto dopamine receptors in the nucleus accumbens produces positive reinforcement.[139]

Physical dependence has been defined as a state of adaptation that is manifested by a drug-class-specific withdrawal syndrome that can be produced by abrupt cessation, rapid dose reduction, decreasing blood level of the drug, and/or administration of an antagonist. Withdrawal is defined as a clinical syndrome produced by withdrawal of an opioid drug from an opioid-dependent individual by (i) the cessation or abrupt reduction in dosage of an opioid or (ii) the administration of an opioid antagonist. This clinical syndrome will occur in all patients taking significant doses of opioid analgesics for an extended period upon acute withdrawal.

The duration and degree of withdrawal will be dependent both on the amount of drug being taken and the reason for acute withdrawal. Symptoms may occur immediately after administration of an opioid antagonist or up to 48 hours after cessation or reduction of opioid dose. Initial symptoms include restlessness, mydriasis, lacrimation, rhinorrhea, sneezing, piloerection, yawning, perspiration, restless sleep, and aggressive behavior. Severe symptoms include muscle spasms, back aches, abdominal cramping, hot and cold flashes, insomnia, nausea, vomiting, diarrhea, tachypnea, hypertension, hypotension, tachycardia, bradycardia, and cardiac dysrhythmias.

Although there is no specific test for opioid withdrawal, administration of an opioid antagonist or agonist/antagonist preceding the onset of symptoms should be taken as presumptive evidence. If the symptoms come on gradually, history of opioid use or the presence of a positive urine drug screen may be helpful. In addition, withdrawal from other substances such as alcohol or benzodiazepines as well as psychiatric disease or other toxic states should be considered. Laboratory testing of electrolytes, blood glucose, hemoglobin and hematocrit, renal function, arterial blood gas, and electrocardiogram may all be appropriate. Following a full evaluation, treatment of withdrawal may include restoration of the opioid dose or substitution with an alternate opioid, after which gradual dose reduction may be implemented if desired. Tolerance has been defined as a state of adaptation in which exposure to a drug induces changes that result in a diminution of one or more of the drug's effects over time.

Risk Factors

Unlike many of the side effects observed with opioids, addiction is not a predictable drug effect but rather represents an idiosyncratic adverse reaction in biologically or psychosocially vulnerable individuals. The presence of a history of early substance abuse, a family or personal history of substance abuse, or the presence of comorbid psychiatric disorders are good predictors of potentially problematic prescription opioid use.[140]

Diagnosis

Diagnosis of drug abuse and diversion can be made by a variety of methods. There are many common characteristics or behaviors observed in patients with drug abuse disorders (Box 34-7).

Prevention

Prevention of drug abuse and addiction is an ongoing process that must be employed in all patients receiving opioid analgesics. Primary prevention involves helping at-risk individuals from developing addictive behaviors. Secondary prevention requires uncovering potentially harmful substance abuse prior to the onset of overt symptoms or problems. Tertiary prevention involves treating the medical consequences of drug abuse and facilitating entry into formalized treatment so that disability is minimized followed by ongoing maintenance of remission achieved by formal treatment.

In addition, the use of a formal consent for opioid management helps to outline expectations regarding refills, taking drugs as prescribed, urine drug screening, and consequences for violation of the agreement.[142,143] Urine drug screens prior to initiating opioid therapy may reveal the use of other prescription or nonprescription drugs. In addition, random urine drug screening during therapy may reveal the presence of nonprescribed drugs, illegal drugs, or complete absence of the prescribed opioid in some cases of drug diversion.[144]

BOX 34-7 Characteristics and Behaviors Associated with Drug Abuse and Diversion

- Use of prescription opioids in unapproved or inappropriate fashion
- Obtaining opioids outside of medical settings
- Repeated requests for dose increases or early refills despite adequate analgesia
- Multiple episodes of prescription "loss" or special trips
- Repeated episodes of seeking or obtaining prescriptions from other clinicians or emergency departments without informing primary prescriber or after warnings to desist
- Evidence of deterioration in function at work, at home, or socially that appears related to drug use
- Repeated resistance to changes in therapy despite clear evidence of adverse physical or psychological effects of the drug
- Positive urine drug screen for other substances of abuse such as cocaine, marijuana, amphetamines, or alcohol
- Meets Diagnostic and Statistical Manual (DSM) IV criteria for substance abuse[141]
- A maladaptive pattern of substance use leading to clinically significant impairment or distress, as manifested by one (or more) of the following, occurring within a 12-month period:
  1. Recurrent substance use resulting in a failure to fulfill major role obligations at work, school, or home (e.g., repeated absences or poor work performance related to substance use; substance-related absences, suspensions, or expulsions from school; neglect of children or household)
  2. Recurrent substance use in situations in which it is physically hazardous (e.g., driving an automobile or operating a machine when impaired by substance use)
  3. Recurrent substance-related legal problems (e.g., arrests for substance-related disorderly conduct)
  4. Continued substance use despite having persistent or recurrent social or interpersonal problems caused or exacerbated by the effects of the substance (e.g., arguments with spouse about consequences of intoxication, physical fights)
- The symptoms have never met the criteria for substance dependence for this class of substance.

Treatment and Rehabilitation

Once a diagnosis of drug abuse or addiction is made, some form of treatment or counseling should be initiated as soon as possible. Decisions regarding how aggressively to respond will be determined on an individual basis. In some cases, counseling may be employed as an initial approach. The importance of taking the medication as prescribed and a reiteration of the rules regarding prescription refills may be sufficient. Other cases may require cessation of drug therapy or referral to a substance abuse program. If a decision is made to withdraw the patient from chronic opioid therapy, this may be accomplished in several ways.

A slow and gradual reduction can be performed to minimize symptoms of withdrawal. Symptoms of withdrawal typically have their onset approximately 12 hours after the last dose of morphine. Symptoms of withdrawal will peak within 48 to 72 hours and resolve over a period of days. Shorter-acting opioids will have a more rapid onset and more intense clinical syndrome, and long-acting opioids will have a delayed onset, milder symptoms, and more prolonged duration of symptoms. If an aggressive approach to withdrawal is taken, symptoms may be controlled to some degree by the use of clonidine and/or benzodiazepines. In some cases, the use of anticholinergic compounds such as propantheline to reduce stomach cramps or atropine to control diarrhea may be necessary. In many cases, hospital admission for acute withdrawal is appropriate. Symptoms related to opioid withdrawal should usually abate within 1 to 2 weeks, and the adjuvant medications should be gradually reduced over that period.

► SUMMARY

The use of opioid analgesics is associated with significant complications ranging from constipation, sedation, and myoclonus to hypogonadism, immunosuppression, addiction, and death. In most cases, conservative measures such as opioid dose reduction, opioid rotation, minimizing concurrent drug administration, or using adjuvant analgesics are sufficient to decrease the severity of the complications. However, in some cases, hormone replacement, opioid discontinuation, or addiction treatment is necessary. It is important that these complications be considered prior to prescribing opioid analgesics and that there remain a high index of suspicion for their development throughout the time of their use.

References

1. Moore RA, McQuay HJ. Prevalence of opioid adverse events in chronic non-malignant pain: systematic review of randomized trials of oral opioids. *Arthritis Res Ther* 2005;7:R1046–R1051.
2. Fallon M, O'Neill B. ABC of palliative care: constipation and diarrhoea. *BMJ* 1997;315:1293–1296.
3. Yuan CS, Foss JF, Osinski J, et al. The safety and efficacy of oral methylnaltrexone in preventing morphine-induced delay in oral-cecal transit time. *J Clin Pharmacol* 1997;137:25–30.
4. Agra Y, Sacristan A, Ganzalez M, et al. Efficacy of senna versus laculose in terminal cancer patients treated with opioids. *J Pain Symptom Man* 1998;15:1–7.
5. Freedman MD, Schwartz HJ, Roby R, et al. Tolerance and efficacy of polyethylene glycol 3350/electrolyte solution versus lactulose in relieving opiate induced constipation: a double-blinded placebo-controlled trial. *J Clin Pharmacol* 1997;37:904–907.
6. Paulson DM, Kennedy DT, Donovick RA, et al. Alvimopan: an oral, peripherally acting, μ-opioid receptor antagonist for the treatment of opioid-induced bowel dysfunction, a 21-day treatment-randomized clinical trial. *J Pain* 2005;6:184–192.
7. Jansen JP, Lorch D, Langan J, et al. A randomized, placebo-controlled phase 3 trial (study SB-767905/012) of alvimopan for opioid-induced bowel dysfunction in patients with non-cancer pain.*J Pain* 2011;12:185–193.

8. Bruera E, Macmillan K, Hanson J, et al. The cognitive effects of the administration of narcotic analgesics in patients with cancer pain. *Pain* 1989;39:13–16.
9. Vainio A, Ollila J, Matikainen E, et al. Driving ability in cancer patients receiving long-term morphine analgesia. *Lancet* 1995;346:667–670.
10. Tassain V, Attal N, Fletcher D, et al. Long term effects of oral sustained release morphine on neuropsychological performance in patients with chronic non-cancer pain. *Pain* 2003;104:389–400.
11. Anderson G, Christrup L, Sjøgren P. Relationships among morphine metabolism, pain and side effects during long-term treatment: an update. *J Pain Symptom Manage* 2003;25:74–90.
12. Christrup L. Morphine metabolites. *Acta Anaesthesiol Scand* 1997;41:116–122.
13. Sjøgren P, Jensen N, Jensen T. Disappearance of morphine-induced hyperalgesia after discontinuing or substituting other opioid agonists. *Pain* 1994;59:313–316.
14. Hanna MH, Elliott KM, Fung M. Randomized, double-blind study of the analgesic efficacy of morphine-6-glucuronide versus morphine sulfate for postoperative pain in major surgery. *Anesthesiology* 2005;102:815–821.
15. Murray A, Hagen NA. Hydromorphone. *J Pain Symptom Manage* 2005;5:57–66.
16. Andersen G, Sjøgren P, Hansen SH. Pharmacological consequences of long-term morphine treatment in patients with cancer and chronic non-malignant pain. *Eur J Pain* 2004;8:263–271.
17. Götrick B, Åkerman S, Ericson D, et al. Oral pilocarpine for treatment of opioid-induced oral dryness in healthy adults. *J Dent Res* 2004;83:393–397.
18. McNicol E, Horowicz-Mehler N, Fisk RA, et al. Management of opioid side effects in cancer-related and chronic noncancer pain: a systematic review. *J Pain* 2003;4:231–256.
19. Lyss AP, Portenoy RK. Strategies for limiting side effects of cancer pain therapy. *Semin Oncol* 1997;24:516–534.
20. O'Mahony S, Coyle N, Payne R. Current management of opioid-related side effects. *Oncology* 2000;15:61–77.
21. Boyle J. Medical ethics and double effect: the case of terminal sedation. *Theor Med Bioeth* 2004;25:51–60.
22. Wamsley JK. Opioid receptors: autoradiography. *Pharmacol Rev* 1983;35:69–83.
23. Weil JV, McCullough RE, Kline JS, et al. Diminished ventilatory response to hypoxia and hypercapnia after morphine in normal man. *N Engl J Med* 1975;292:1103–1106.
24. Kryger MH, Yacoub O, Dosman J, et al. Effect of meperidine on occlusion pressure responses to hypercapnia and hypoxia with and without external respiratory resistance. *Am Rev Respir Dis* 1976;114:333–340.
25. Forrest WH, Bellville JW. The effect of sleep plus morphine on the respiratory response to carbon dioxide. *Anesthesiology* 1964;25:137–141.
26. Rigg JRA, Rondi P. Changes in rib cage and diaphragm contribution to ventilation after morphine. *Anesthesiology* 1981;55:507–514.
27. Arunasalam K, Davenport HT, Painter S, et al. Ventilatory response to morphine in young and old subjects. *Anaesthesia* 1983;38:529–533.
28. Farney RJ, Walker JM, Cloward TV, et al. Sleep-disordered breathing associated with long-term opioid therapy. *Chest* 2003;123:632–639.
29. Estilo AE, Cottrell JE. Naloxone, hypertension and ruptured cerebral aneurysm. *Anesthesiology* 1981;54:352.
30. Flacke JW, Flacke WE, Williams GD. Acute pulmonary edema following naloxone reversal of high-dose morphine anesthesia. *Anesthesiology* 1977;47:376–378.
31. Prough DS, Roy R, Bumgarner J, et al. Acute pulmonary edema in healthy teenagers following conservative doses of intravenous naloxone. *Anesthesiology* 1984;60:485–486.

32. Michaelis LL, Hickey PR, Clark TA, et al. Ventricular irritability associated with the use of naloxone hydrochloride. *Ann Thorac Surg* 1974;18:608–614.

33. Partridge BL, Ward CF, Lienhart A. Pulmonary edema following low-dose naloxone administration. *Anesthesiology* 1986;65:709–710.

34. Just B, Delva E, Camus Y, et al. Oxygen uptake during recovery following naloxone. *Anesthesiology* 1992;76:60–64.

35. Estilo AE, Cottrell JE. Hemodynamic and catecholamine changes after administration of naloxone. *Anesth Analg* 1982;61:349–353.

36. Yaffe GJ, Strelinger RW, Parwatikar S. Physical symptom complaints of patients on methadone maintenance. *Proc Natl Conf Methadone Treat* 1973;1:507–514.

37. Gutstein HB, Akil H. Opioid analgesics. In: Hardman JG, Limbird LE, eds. *Goodman and Gilman's the Pharmacological Basis of Therapeutics*. Ohio: McGraw-Hill International, 2001:586.

38. Quigley CS, Baines M. Descriptive epidemiology of sweating in a hospice population. *J Palliat Care* 1997;13:22–26.

39. Smith MT, Watt JA, Cramond T. Morphine-3-glucuronide: a potent antagonist of morphine analgesia. *Life Sci* 1990;47:579–585.

40. Labella FS, Pinsky C, Havlicek V. Morphine derivatives with diminished opiate receptor potency show enhanced central excitatory activity. *Brain Res* 1979;174:263–271.

41. Barlett SE, Cramond T, Smith MT. The excitatory effects of morphine-3-glucuronide are attenuated by LY274614, a competitive NMDA receptor antagonist, and by midazolam, an agonist at the benzodiazepine site on the GABA$_A$ receptor complex. *Life Sci* 1994;54:687–694.

42. Snead OC. Opiate-induced seizures: a study of μ and δ specific mechanisms. *Exp Neurol* 1986;93:348–358.

43. Woolf CJ. Intrathecal high dose morphine produces hyperalgesia in the rat. *Brain Res* 1981;209:491–495.

44. Yaksh TL, Harty GJ, Onofrio BM. High doses of spinal morphine produce a nonopiate receptor-mediated hyperesthesia: clinical and theoretic implications. *Anesthesiology* 1986;64:590–597.

45. Yaksh TL, Harty GJ. Pharmacology of the allodynia in rats evoked by high dose intrathecal morphine. *J Pharmacol Exp Ther* 1988;244:501–507.

46. Shohami E, Evron S, Weinstock M, et al. A new animal model for action myoclonus. *Adv Neurol* 1986;43:545–552.

47. Barlett SE, Dodd PR, Smith MT. Pharmacology of morphine and morphine-3-glucuronide at opioid, excitatory amino acid, GABA and glycine binding sites. *Pharmacol Toxicol* 1994;75:73–81.

48. Lufty K, Woodward RM, Keana JFW, et al. Inhibition of clonic seizure-like excitatory effects induced by intrathecal morphine using two NMDA receptor antagonists: MK-801 and ACEA-1011. *Eur J Pharmacol* 1994;252:261–266.

49. McClain BC, Probst LA, Pinter E, et al. Intravenous clonidine use in a neonate experiencing opioid-induced myoclonus. *Anesthesiology* 2001;95:549–550.

50. Slatkin N, Rhiner M. Treatment of opioid-induced delirium with acetylcholinesterase inhibitors: a case report. *J Pain Symptom Manage* 2004;27:268–273.

51. Krames ES, Gershow J, Glassberg A, et al. Continuous infusion of spinally administered narcotics for the relief of pain due to malignant disorders. *Cancer* 1985;56:696–702.

52. Parkinson SK, Bailey SL, Little WL, et al. Myoclonic seizure activity with chronic high-dose spinal opioid administration. *Anesthesiology* 1990;72:743–745.

53. Glavina MJ, Robertshaw R. Myoclonic spasms following intrathecal morphine. *Anaesthesia* 1998;43:389–390.

54. De Conno F, Caraceni A, Martini C, et al. Hyperalgesia and myoclonus with intrathecal infusion of high-dose morphine. *Pain* 1991;47:337–339.

55. Eisele JH Jr, Grigsby EJ, Dea G. Clonazepam treatment of myoclonic contractions associated with high-dose opioids: case report. *Pain* 1992;49:231–232.

56. Obeso JA. Therapy of myoclonus. *Clin Neurosci* 1995;3:253–257.

57. Caviness JN. Myoclonus. *Mayo Clin Proc* 1996;71:679–688.

58. Holdsworth MT, Adams VR, Chavez CM, et al. Continuous midazolam infusion for the management of morphine-induced myoclonus. *Ann Pharmacother* 1995;29:25–29.

59. Hagen N, Swanson R. Strychnine-like multifocal myoclonus and seizures in extremely high-dose opioid administration: treatment strategies. *J Pain Symptom Manage* 1997;14:51–58.

60. Mercadante S. Dantrolene treatment of opioid-induced myoclonus. *Anesth Analg* 1995;81:1307–1308.

61. Cherny N, Ripamonti C, Pereira J, et al. Strategies to manage the adverse effects of oral morphine: an evidence-based report. *J Clin Oncol* 2001;19:2542–2554.

62. Wang SC, Glaviano VV. Locus of emetic action of morphine and hydergine in dogs. *J Pharmacol Exp Ther* 1954;111:329.

63. de Stoutz ND, Bruera E, Suarez-Almazor M. Opioid rotation for toxicity reduction in terminal cancer patients. *J Pain Symptom Manage* 1995;10:378–384.

64. Maddocks I, Somogyi A, Abbott F, et al. Attenuation of morphine-induced delirium in palliative care by substitution with infusion of oxycodone. *J Pain Symptom Manage* 1996;12:182–189.

65. Ashby MA, Martin P, Jackson KA. Opioid substitution to reduce adverse effects in cancer pain management. *Med J Aust* 1999;170:68–71.

66. McDonald P, Graham P, Clayton M, et al. Regular subcutaneous bolus morphine via an indwelling cannula for pain from advanced cancer pain. *Palliat Med* 1991;5:323–329.

67. Drexel H, Dzien A, Spiegel RW, et al. Treatment of severe cancer pain by low-dose continuous subcutaneous morphine. *Pain* 1989;36:169–176.

68. De Conno F, Ripamonti C, Saita L, et al. Role of rectal route in treating cancer pain: a randomized crossover clinical trial of oral versus rectal morphine administration in opioid-naïve cancer patients with pain. *J Clin Oncol* 1995;13:1004–1008.

69. Babul N, Provencher L, Laberge F, et al. Comparative efficacy and safety of controlled-release morphine suppositories and tablets in cancer pain. *J Clin Pharmacol* 1998;38:74–81.

70. Cicero TJ, Bell RD, West WG, et al. Function of the male sex organs in heroin and methadone users. *N Engl J Med* 1975;292:882–887.

71. Yen SSC, Quigley ME, Reid RL, et al. Neuroendocrinology of opioid peptides and their role in the control of gonadotropin and prolactin secretion. *Am J Obstet Gynecol* 1985;152:485–493.

72. Cicero T. Effects of exogenous and endogenous opiates on the hypothalamic-pituitary-gonadal axis in the male. *Fed Proc* 1980;39:2551–2554.

73. Paice JA, Penn RD, Ryan WG, et al. Altered sexual function and decreased testosterone in patients receiving intraspinal opioids. *J Pain Symptom Manage* 1994;9:126–131.

74. Paice JA, Penn RD. Amenorrhea associated with intraspinal morphine. *J Pain Symptom Manage* 1995;10:582–583.

75. Doleys DM, Dinoff BL, Page L, et al. Sexual dysfunction and other side effects of intraspinal opiate use in the management of chronic non-cancer pain. *AJPM* 1998;8:5–11.

76. Ebeling PR. Osteoporosis in men: new insights into aetiology, pathogenesis, prevention and management. *Drugs Aging* 1998;13:421–434.

77. Jackson JA, Riggs MW, Spiekerman AM. Testosterone deficiency as a risk factor for hip fractures in men: a case-control study. *Am J Med Sci* 1992;304:4–8.

78. Rajagopal A, Vassilopoulou-Sellin R, Palmer JL, et al. Hypogonadism and sexual dysfunction in male cancer survivors receiving chronic opioid therapy. *J Pain Symptom Manage* 2003;26:1055–1061.

79. Rajagopal A, Vassilopoulou-Sellin R, Palmer JL, et al. Symptomatic hypogonadism in male survivors of cancer with chronic exposure to opioids. *Cancer* 2004;100:851–858.

80. Anderson FH, Francis RM, Selby PL, et al. Sex hormones and osteoporosis in men. *Calcif Tissue Int* 1998;62:185–188.

81. Allolio B, Deuss U, Kaulen D, et al. FK33-824, a met-enkephalin analog, blocks corticotropin-releasing hormone-induced adrenocorticotropin secretion in normal subjects, but not in patients with cushing's disease. *J Clin Endocrinol Metab* 1986;63: 1427–1431.

82. Taylor T, Dluhy RG, Williams GH. Beta-endorphin suppresses adrenocorticotropin and cortisol levels in normal human subjects. *J Clin Endocrinol Metab* 1983;57:592–596.

83. Abs R, Verhelst J, Maeyaert J, et al. Endocrine consequences of long-term intrathecal administration of opioids. *J Clin Endocrinol Metab* 2000;85:2215–2222.

84. Genazzani AR, Genazzani AD, Volpogni C, et al. Opioid control of gonadotrophin secretion in humans. *Hum Reprod* 1993;8 (suppl 2):151–153.

85. Grossman A, Moult PJ, Gaillard RC, et al. The opioid control of LH and FSH release: effects of a met-enkephalin analogue and naloxone. *Clin Endocrinol (Oxf)* 1981;14:41–47.

86. Jordan D, Tafani JAM, Ries C, et al. Evidence for multiple opioid receptors in the human posterior pituitary. *J Neuroendocrinol* 1996;8:883–887.

87. Veldhuis JD, Rogol AD, Samojlik E, et al. Role of endogenous opiates in the expression of negative feedback actions of androgen and estrogen on pulsatile properties of luteinizing hormone secretion in man. *J Clin Invest* 1984;74:47–55.

88. Woody G, McLellan T, O'Brien C, et al. Hormone secretion in methadone-dependent and abstinent patients. *NIDA Res Monogr* 1988;81:216–223.

89. Mendelson JH, Inturrisi CE, Renault P, et al. Effects of acetylmethadol on plasma testosterone. *Clin Pharmacol Ther* 1976;19: 371–374.

90. Finch PM, Roberts LJ, Price L, et al. Hypogonadism in patients treated with intrathecal morphine. *Clin J Pain* 2000;16:251–254.

91. Winkelmuller M, Winkelmuller W. Long-term effects of continuous intrathecal opioid treatment in chronic pain of nonmalignant etiology. *J Neurosurg* 1996;85:458–467.

92. Pelosi MA, Sama JC, Caterini H, et al. Galactorrhea-amenorrhea syndrome associated with heroin addiction. *Am J Obstet Gynecol* 1974;118:966–970.

93. Daniell HW. Hypogonadism in men consuming sustained-action oral opioids. *J Pain* 2002;3:377–384.

94. Oltmanns KM, Fehm HL, Peters A. Chronic fentanyl application induces adrenocortical insufficiency. *J Intern Med* 2005;257: 478–480.

95. Facchinetti F, Volpe A, Farci G, et al. Hypothalamus-pituitary-adrenal axis of heroin addicts. *Drug Alcohol Depend* 1985;15: 361–366.

96. Chan V, Wang C, Yeung RT. Effects of heroin addiction on thyrotrophin, thyroid hormones and prolactin secretion in men. *Clin Endocrinol (Oxf)* 1979;10:557–565.

97. Rasheed A, Tareen IA. Effects of heroin on thyroid function, cortisol and testosterone level in addicts. *Pol J Pharmacol* 1995; 47:441–444.

98. Gooren LJ, Bunck MC. Androgen replacement therapy: present and future. *Drugs* 2004;64:1861–1891.

99. Behre HM, Kliesch S, Leifke E, et al. Long-term effect of testosterone therapy on bone mineral density in hypogonadal men. *J Clin Endocrinol Metab* 1997;82:2386–2390.

100. BMcClure RD, Oses R, Ernest ML. Hypogonadal impotence treated by transdermal testosterone. *Urology* 1991;37:224–228.

101. Aloisi AM, Ceccarelli I, Carlucci M, et al. Hormone replacement therapy in morphine-induced hypogonadic male chronic pain patients. *Reprod Biol Endocrinol* 2011;9:26–35.

102. Eisenstein TK, Hillburger ME. Opioid modulation of immune responses: effects on phagocyte and lymphoid cell populations. *J Neuroimmunol* 1998;83:36–44.

103. Molitor TW, Morilla A, Risdahl JM. Chronic morphine administration impairs cell-mediated immune responses in swine. *J Pharmacol Exp Ther* 1991;260:581–586.

104. Bryant HU, Bernton EW, Holaday JW. Immunosuppressive effects of chronic morphine treatment in mice. *Life Sci* 1987;41: 1731–1738.

105. Freier DO, Fuchs BA. Morphine-induced alterations in thymocyte subpopulations of B6C3F1 mice. *J Pharmacol Exp Ther* 1993;265:81–88.

106. Singhal P, Sharma P, Kapasi A. Morphine enhances macrophage apoptosis. *J Immunol* 1998;60:1886–1893.

107. Layon J, Idris A, Warzynski M, et al. Altered T-lymphocytes subsets in hospitalized intravenous drug abusers. *Arch Intern Med* 1984;144:1376–1380.

108. Nair MPN, Laing TJ, Schwartz SA. Decreased natural and antibodydependent cellular cytotoxic activities in intravenous drug abusers. *Clin Immunol Immunopathol* 1986;38:68–78.

109. Brown SM, Stimmel B, Taub RN, et al. Immunological dysfunction in heroin addicts. *Arch Intern Med* 1974;134:1001–1006.

110. Donahoe RM, Falek A. Neuroimmunomodulation by opiates and other drugs of abuse: relationship to HIV infection and AIDS. *Adv Biochem Psychopharmacol* 1988;44:145–158.

111. Crone LL, Conly JM, Clark KM, et al. Recurrent herpes simplex virus labialis and the use of epidural morphine in obstetric patients. *Anesth Analg* 1988;67:318–323.

112. Biagini RE, Henningsen GM, Klincewicz SL. Immunological analysis of peripheral leukocytes from workers at an ethical narcotics manufacturing facility. *Arch Environ Health* 1995;50:7–12.

113. Morgan EL. Regulation of human B lymphocyte activation by opioid peptide hormones: inhibition of IgG production by opioid receptor class (m-, k-, and d-) selective agonists. *J Neuroimmunol* 1996;65:21–30.

114. Palm S, Lehzen S, Mignat C, et al. Does prolonged oral treatment with sustained-release morphine tablets influence immune function? *Anesth Analg* 1998;86:166–172.

115. Hilburger ME, AdlerMW, Rogers TJ, et al. Morphine alters macrophage and lymphocyte populations in the spleen and peritoneal cavity. *J Neuroimmunol* 1997;80:106–114.

116. Centers for Disease Control. *HIV/AIDS surveillance report, Vol. 7, No. 2.* Atlanta, GA: US Department of Health and Human Services, 1996.

117. Peterson PK, Sharp BM, Gekker G, et al. Morphine promotes the growth of HIV-1 in human peripheral blood mononuclear cell cocultures. *AIDS* 1990;4:869–873.

118. Chao CC, Gekker G, Hu S, et al. Upregulation of HIV-1 expression in cocultures of chronically infected promonocytes and human brain cells by dynorphin. *Biochem Pharmacol* 1995;50:715–722.

119. Li Y, Wang X, Tian S, et al. Methadone enhances human immunodeficiency virus infection of human immune cells. *J Infect Dis* 2002;185:118–122.

120. Hamra JG, Yaksh TL. Equianalgesic doses of subcutaneous but not intrathecal morphine alter phenotypic expression of cell surface markers and mitogen-induced proliferation in rat lymphocytes. *Anesthesiology* 1996;85:355–365.

121. Ballantyne JC, Mao J. Opioid therapy for chronic pain. *N Engl J Med* 2003;349:1943–1953.

122. Brodner RA, Taub A. Chronic pain exacerbated by long-term narcotic use in patients with non-malignant disease: clinical syndrome and treatment. *Mt Sinai J Med* 1978;45:233–237.

123. Taylor CB, Zlutnik SI, Corley MJ, et al. The effects of detoxification, relaxation and brief supportive therapy on chronic pain. *Pain* 1980;8:319–329.

124. Savage SR. Long-term opioid therapy: assessment of consequences and risks. *J Pain Symptom Manage* 1996;11:274–286.

125. Compton MA. Cold-pressor pain tolerance in opiate and cocaine abusers: correlates of drug type and use status. *J Pain Symptom Manage* 1994;9:462–473.

126. Mao J, Price DD, Mayer DJ. Thermal hyperalgesia in association with the development of morphine tolerance in rats: roles of excitatory amino acid receptors and protein kinase C. *J Neurosci* 1994;14:2301–2312.

127. Mao J, Price DD, Mayer DJ. Mechanisms of hyperalgesia and opiate tolerance: a current view of their possible interactions. *Pain* 1995;62:259–274.

128. Mao J, Price DD, Mayer DJ. Experimental mononeuropathy reduces the antinociceptive effects of morphine: implications for common intracellular mechanisms involved in morphine tolerance and neuropathic pain. *Pain* 1995;61:353–364.

129. Peacock JE, Wright BM, Withers MR, et al. Evaluation of a pilot regimen for postoperative pain control in patients receiving oral morphine pre-operatively. *Anaesthesia* 2000;55:1192–1212.

130. Carroll IR, Angst MS, Clark JD. Management of perioperative pain in patients chronically consuming opioids. *Reg Anesth Pain Med* 2004;29:576–591.

131. Mitra S, Sinatra RS. Perioperative management of acute pain in the opioid-dependent patient. *Anesthesiology* 2004;101:212–227.

132. Kouyanou K, Pither CE, Wessely S. Medication misuse, abuse and dependence in chronic pain patients. *J Psychosom Res* 1997;43:497–504.

133. Compton WM, Thomas YF, Conway KP, et al. Developments in the epidemiology of drug use and drug use disorders. *Am J Psychiatry* 2005;162:1494–1502.

134. NIDA Research Report. Prescription drugs: abuse and addiction. NIH Publication No. 01-4881, printed 2001, revised August, 2005.

135. Gilson AM, Ryan KM, Joranson DE, et al. A reassessment of trends in the medical use and abuse of opioid analgesics and implications for diversion control: 1997–2002. *J Pain Symptom Manage* 2004;28:176–188.

136. Joranson DE, Ryan KM, Gilson AM, et al. Trends in medical use and abuse of opioid analgesics. *JAMA* 2000;283:1710–1714.

137. Centers for Disease Control and Prevention (CDC). Drug overdose deaths–Florida, 2003–2009. *Morb Mortal Wkly Rep* 2011;60:869–872.

138. American Pain Society. Definitions related to the use of opioids for the treatment of pain. Consensus Document from the American Academy of Pain Medicine, American Pain Society and American Society of Addiction Medicine, 2001.

139. Koob GF. Neuroadaptive mechanisms of addiction: studies on the extended amygdala. *Eur Neuropsychopharmacol* 2003;13:442–452.

140. Nedeljkovic SS, Wasan A, Jamison RN. Assessment of efficacy of long-term opioid therapy in pain patients with substance abuse potential. *Clin J Pain* 2002;18(suppl):S39–S51.

141. American Psychiatric Association. *DSM IV*. 4th ed. Arlington, VA: American Psychiatric Publishing, 2000:182–183.

142. Jacobson PL, Mann JD. The valid informed consent-treatment contract in chronic non-cancer pain: its role in reducing barriers to effective pain management. *Compr Ther* 2004;30:101–104.

143. Fishman SM, Mahajan G, Jung SW, et al. The trilateral opioid contract: bridging the pain clinic and the primary care physician through the opioid contract. *J Pain Symptom Manage* 2002;24:335–344.

144. Katz NP, Sherburne S, Beach M, et al. Behavioral monitoring and urine toxicology testing in patients receiving long-term opioid therapy. *Anesth Analg* 2003;97:1097–1102.

35

Complications Associated with Chronic Steroid Use

All substances are poisons; there is none which is not a poison.
The right dose differentiates a poison and a remedy.
—*Paracelsus (1493–1541)*

Marc A. Huntoon and Halena M Gazelka

Endogenous steroids are involved in a large number of physiologic processes, including modulating immune function, behavior, cardiovascular function, growth, metabolism, and inflammatory responses.[1] In regional anesthesia and pain medicine, exogenous glucocorticosteroids (GCS) are some of the most common pharmacologic agents in clinical use. Building on the initial work of Hench et al.,[2] steroids were first injected into arthritic joints by Thorn (unpublished) and then by Hollander et al.[3] These potent intermediate to long-acting GCS are now used to promote predominantly anti-inflammatory effects on target tissues. Routes of administration include oral, injectable, and transdermal. Injections are by far the most commonly used approach in pain medicine. Specifically, intermediate to long-acting corticosteroids administered for spinal/epidural use, intra-articular joint injections, periarticular joint injections, tendon sheath or ligamentous injections, trigger-point injections, neuroma or scar injections, and muscle injections are some of many potential targets.[4–9]

In spite of many known targets and the frequent use of these GCS, there is little consensus on the dose, frequency of use, or methodology appropriate to monitor activity, management, or prevention of long-term toxicity. Many toxicities known to be related to GCS use are delayed (often by months or even years), and thus many practitioners are unaware of the potential for serious complications related to the steroids or prevalence of these complications.[10]

▶ OVERALL SCOPE

Exogenous administration of GCS leads to suppression of the hypothalamic-pituitary axis (decreased plasma cortisol, decreased plasma adrenocorticotropic hormone [ACTH], and adrenal atrophy), and a number of other potential toxic effects (Table 35-1). In addition, other side effects may be specific to the site of injection (e.g., spinal arachnoiditis after intrathecal injection[11] and tendon rupture after tendon sheath injection[12]).

This chapter focuses on complications related to chronic steroid use. Transient elevations of blood glucose and impaired immune function are known and expected. Many possible complications are of little clinical significance for the average patient. Those complications, which may have prolonged clinical consequences, include steroid-induced osteoporosis, myopathy, collagen atrophy, avascular osteonecrosis, and spinal arachnoiditis. Because up to 82% of patients treated with long-term glucocorticoids (GC) will report some adverse event, this topic is pertinent to providers involved in their care.[13]

▶ GLUCOCORTICOSTEROID PHYSIOLOGY

GCS exert their effects by binding to a cytoplasmic GC receptor within target cells (Fig. 35-1). The GC receptor is expressed by part of a gene family, which includes cytosolic receptors for other hormones such as progesterone, estrogen, thyroid hormone, retinoic acid, and vitamin D. GC receptors are expressed in almost every type of cell, although density varies.

TABLE 35-1 Potential Toxic Effects of Exogenous Corticosteroids
• Hyperglycemia
• Lipogenesis, increased circulating fatty acids
• Muscle catabolism, myopathy
• Skin atrophy
• Telangiectasia
• Steroid-induced osteoporosis
• Lymphoid tissue proliferation
• Growth retardation
• Peptic ulcer
• Infection susceptibility
• Electrolyte imbalance
• Psychosis, depression
• Aseptic osteonecrosis
• Cataract formation
• Lipomatosis
• Truncal obesity, fat redistribution
• Cushingoid features (edema, buffalo hump, moon-facies, stria)

The inactive GC receptor is bound to a large protein complex that includes two subunits of the heat shock protein HSP90. HSP90 may facilitate a receptor conformation optimal for binding. Once the GC binds to the GC receptor, HSP90 dissociates to allow nuclear entry and binding to DNA. Steroids produce their effect by activating GC receptors to regulate the transcription of certain target genes. GC receptors form a dimer that binds to DNA at sites called GREs in the target genes, either inducing or suppressing gene function.[13] Steroids inhibit transcription of several cytokines (e.g., IL-1, TNFα, and IL-6). Steroids are potent inhibitors of cytokine-mediated inflammation. Transcription factor activator protein (AP-1) binding, normally activated by cytokines such as TNFα, may be inhibited by steroids.[14]

Besides their effects on inflammatory mediators, steroids may provide analgesia through several other routes, including blockade of nociceptive C-fiber conduction, interacting with norepinephrine and 5-hydroxytryptamine (5-HT) neurons in the dorsal horn substantia gelatinosa, counteracting the substance P suppression of naturally produced steroids in the spinal cord, and promoting favorable functional alterations within the spinal cord.[15]

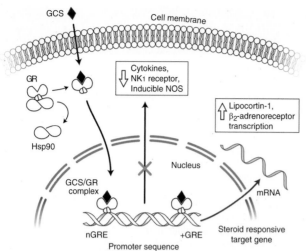

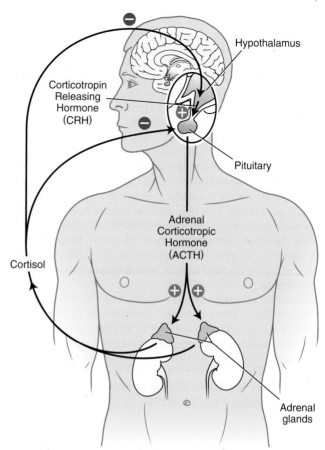

FIGURE 35-1. Glucocorticosteroids (GCS) pass through the cell membrane into the cytosol, where they interact with glucocorticoid receptors (GRs). A 90-kDa heat shock protein normally associated with the GR is split off, and the GCS/GR complex interacts with nuclear DNA glucocorticoid response elements (GRE and nGRE), which either promote or inhibit gene transcription. Cytokines: TNFa (tumor necrosis factor alpha), IL-1, IL-3, IL-4, IL-5, IL-6, and IL-8 (interleukins) transcription may be inhibited. Cytokine-induced NOS (nitric oxide synthase) is potently inhibited, as are effects on NK1 (neurokinin-1) transcription and other proinflammatory substances. Increased synthesis of lipocortin-1 may decrease lipid mediators of inflammation (leukotrienes, prostaglandins, and platelet-activating factor). Increased β2-adrenoceptor transcription may also occur.

FIGURE 35-2. The normal Hypothalamic-Pituitary-Adrenal (HPA) axis.

► HYPOTHALAMIC-PITUITARY-ADRENAL AXIS SUPRESSION

Scope

The propensity of exogenous corticosteroids to suppress the hypothalamic-pituitary-adrenal (HPA) axis has been recognized for decades.

Pathophysiology

Normally, secretion of cortisol by the adrenal glands exerts a negative feedback on the hypothalamus and pituitary gland. Rising cortisol levels in the plasma cause a decrease in the secretion of corticotropin releasing factor from the hypothalamus and a decrease in secretion of ACTH from the pituitary, resulting in a reduction in cortisol secretion by the adrenal glands. Exogenous steroids are capable of causing the same suppression (Fig. 35-2).

Risk Factors

There is little known regarding what quantity of steroids is "safe" (or even effective) to inject. Early studies of epidural or intrathecal corticosteroids used one to four doses of 80 mg methylprednisolone over the course of days to weeks until symptomatic improvement occurred.[4]

Many pain practitioners have patients in their practice who achieve time-limited relief of pain, but repeat doses are arbitrarily limited due to concerns of steroid complications. Recommendations still persist to give no more than three doses in 6 months.[16] Recommendations for a ceiling of 3 mg/kg methylprednisolone were based on a study of high-dose (280–600 mg) methylprednisolone used through an epidural catheter for 2 to 3 days.[17] An animal study revealed the effects of a single 2-mg/kg dose of triamcinolone on serum cortisol. Adrenal suppression was evident for up to 4 weeks.[18] In a large literature review of the safety of epidural steroids, Abrams and O'Connor[19] noted the safety of using smaller doses and the lack of major complications overall.

Urine GC screening tests have revealed measurable levels of triamcinolone up to 9 months after the patients last received injectable steroid, with HPA suppression evident for up to 5 months after injection.[20]

Diagnosis

Patients may present with the stigmata of Cushing's syndrome, including weight gain, fragile skin, easy bruising, lethargy, hirsutism, and skin striae. Cushing's syndrome represents the presence of excessive systemic GC. Although these patients resemble those with hypercortisolism, they will have suppression of the HPA axis on testing.

Low plasma cortisol, decreased urine cortisol excretion, low ACTH levels, and diminished response to cosyntropin stimulation are indicative of HPA suppression. Furthermore, exogenous corticosteroid levels can be measured in urine or serum.

More frequently, patients will have HPA suppression that is clinically detectable without evidence of Cushing's.[21]

Prevention

Currently, there is no consensus on the effective dose of steroids or the maximum cumulative allowable dose of steroids, although recommendation for doses not to exceed 3 mg/kg/y total has been published in the literature.[22] Even this does not guarantee safety. HPA axis suppression has been reported after a single epidural steroid injection.[23]

Treatment

Patients exhibiting evidence of hypercortisolism or of HPA suppression need to be closely monitored until normal physiologic activity has returned. They may not require GC supplementation, but this should be considered. Referral to an endocrinologist for appropriate diagnosis and management should be considered. Certainly, further administration of exogenous GC by injection should be limited.

Summary

In summary, HPA axis suppression is a relatively common complication of GC administration. There is no established guideline for the effective dose or the maximal cumulative dose of steroids that should be allowed. Further, the lack of information sharing amongst practitioners can lead to patients receiving excessive cumulative doses secondary to use of GC for multiple medical and pain conditions.

▶ GLUCOCORTICOSTEROID-INDUCED AVASCULAR NECROSIS

Scope

Avascular necrosis (AVN), also known as aseptic necrosis or osteonecrosis, is a condition in which the vascular supply to bone is compromised, leading to bone cell death. GC-induced AVN can occur at any bony location within the body. However, AVN of the hip produces particularly devastating functional consequences. GC-induced AVN can occur at any age and is often seen in individuals in their 30s and 40s. AVN typically occurs only after long-term GC administration, but may develop within as little as 2 to several weeks of initiating GC therapy.[24]

Pathophysiology

Hypotheses for the development of AVN include microvascular occlusion due to marrow lipid in the femoral head and resultant hypertension, fat emboli, and impaired repair of fatigue fractures. It is also thought that AVN may be caused by osteoblast or osteocyte apoptosis (programmed cell death).[25] Weinstein et al. demonstrated that subchondral fracture sites in GC-induced AVN patients were rich in apoptotic osteocyte lining cells. Conversely, femoral heads from AVN patients with alcoholism or sickle cell disease were devoid of this feature. Therefore, they proposed that AVN is not the appropriate term for this GC-induced condition, as the bone is not truly necrotic. Instead, bone microfractures are not repaired, because the osteocytes do not properly sense the need to do so.[25]

Risk Factors

In a review of the literature, Clinkscales and Cleary[26] found that for AVN the average cortisol equivalent doses were 17.5 g per patient, with an average time to symptom onset of 60 weeks. In one case, a 42-year-old patient received a total of 16 injections of either 40 mg of triamcinolone or 80 mg of methylprednisolone for treatment of hay fever. The patient subsequently developed AVN in both hips, which was related to his GC use.[24] Socie et al.[27] reviewed 4,388 patients treated with bone marrow transplant. Seventy-seven of these patients developed AVN, and only two did not receive GC therapy. Steroids were used to treat graft versus host disease (GvHD), and patients received them for a mean of 15 months. Older age increased the risk for AVN.[27] In a similar fashion, Marsh et al.[28] described a 21% incidence of AVN after doses of 5 mg/kg/d methylprednisolone to treat serum sickness over a 2- to 4-week period.

In contrast to chronic steroids, their utilization for acute injury has provided no conclusive evidence that short-term use (even in large doses) contributes to the development of AVN. In response to the National Acute Spinal Cord Injury Study-2 (NASCIS-2),[29] Wing et al.[30] studied 59 spinal cord injured patients who had received the high-dose spinal cord injury protocol dosing (methylprednisolone 30 mg/kg followed by 5.4 mg/kg/h for 23 hours) and compared them to 32 patients who had not received steroids. In spite of such large doses, there were no reported cases of AVN in these patients with a mean age of 32 years. Thus, it does not appear that short-term 23-hour very high-dose therapy has higher than a 5% risk of AVN.

Diagnosis

Diagnosis of AVN is made through the use of imaging studies. Magnetic resonance imaging (MRI) may show earlier changes than plain x-ray (Fig. 35-3). Large weight-bearing joints are the most likely to be involved. Clinical suspicion regarding the onset of new pain or functional aberration should

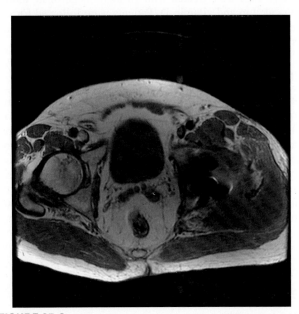

FIGURE 35-3. MRI illustrating avascular necrosis (AVN) in the left hip. Axial T1-weighted MRI demonstrating area of necrosis in the left femoral head.

be investigated as early as possible. Patients may present with an antalgic gait or frank limp, but may be asymptomatic early in the course of AVN. Diagnostically, it is known that up to two-thirds of patients can have bilateral involvement, and thus any asymmetry in exam should be noted. When the hip is involved, the patient may have significant pain if the examiner abducts and internally rotates the hip.

Prevention

Prevention of AVN is difficult due to the large variation in steroid doses that can lead to this complication and a lack of specific identifiable risk factors. However, available evidence suggests that the incidence of AVN increases with both the dose of GCS administered as well as the duration of exposure. Thus, using the smallest possible therapeutic GC dose for the shortest interval is likely to decrease the incidence of AVN.

Treatment and Rehabilitation

Patients should initially be managed with restriction or elimination of weight-bearing activities to avoid risk of pathologic fracture. Consultation with specialists in Orthopedics and Physical Medicine and Rehabilitation departments is necessary to implement proper therapy and prevent further damage. Treatment of AVN often requires joint replacement, and because of the relatively young age of some AVN patients, there may be a poorer long-term prognosis. Joint replacements have a finite life span, and thus younger patients may be advised to consider more conservative management initially. Other operative solutions, such as the use of vascularized fibular grafts, have been used but are not uniformly successful. If patients are not successfully treated by surgical means, they may develop chronic pain. Failed surgical patients may have substantial and ongoing ambulatory difficulties. Bisphosphonates can be considered. Agarwala et al.[31] studied the possible beneficial effect of bisphosphonate therapy in AVN patients. Sixty total patients with 100 affected hips were treated with 10 mg/d alendronate along with calcium and vitamin D. Patients were followed for an average of 37 months. Significant increases in functional status were seen. Surgery was avoided in all but six patients.

Summary

It appears that avascular osteonecrosis is a condition commonly seen with GC use, but although does seem to be variable, higher doses are more commonly associated. It may be that patients post–organ transplantation or with GvHD are more susceptible to the complication. A high clinical suspicion for AVN, particularly in younger patients with new functional limitations and pain, should be investigated early with imaging studies. Early consultation should be sought to initiate proper therapies.

▶ STEROID MYOPATHY

Definition

Chronic steroid myopathy is the most common form of drug-induced myopathy and is more prevalent with fluorinated compounds such as dexamethasone and triamcinolone.[32] Steroid myopathies take two major forms: (i) an acute corticosteroid myopathy (ACM), with rapid presentation of proximal and distal limb weakness, diaphragmatic weakness, and both type I and II muscle fiber necrosis, and (ii) chronic steroid myopathy with insidious onset and late findings of proximal limb muscle weakness and atrophy.[32,33]

Pathophysiology

The presumed pathophysiology of steroid myopathy is a direct toxic effect on sarcomeres that causes disruption, loss of myosin-thick filaments, and early cell death. It is thought that growth hormone (GH) or insulin-like growth factor-I (IGF-I) may have beneficial effects relative to the development of steroid myopathy.[34] Furthermore, glutamine synthetase is important in the development of myopathy secondary to steroids. GH and IGF-I decrease steroid-induced glutamine synthetase activity in skeletal muscle.[34,35] IGF-I is part of a family of anabolic hormones that affect muscle fibers capable of overcoming catabolic stressors, such as GCS. These anabolic effects of IGF-I are signaled via the enzymatic function of phosphatidyl inositol 3-kinase (PI3K). Under noncatabolic stress, PI3K activates a protein kinase reaction that increases muscle glucose uptake and protein synthesis and antagonizes protein catabolism.

PI3K is normally produced as a heterodimer on the insulin receptor substrate-1. GCS, such as dexamethasone, induce upregulation of a P85 alpha subunit. This P85 alpha monomer subunit then competes with the heterodimer for binding sites, leading to decreased PI3K activity. Apoptosis (programmed cell death) is likewise decreased after exposure to PI3K.[33]

At the mitochondrial level, it is known that GCS trigger changes in mitochondrial size (enlargement) and morphology. Mitochondrial damage may be related to reactive oxygen species (ROS). Mitochondrial dysfunction is selectively associated with damage caused by impaired oxidative capacity, rendered through overproduction of ROS. Dexamethasone increased mitochondrial membrane potentials, generation of ROS, and apoptosis. Treatment with superoxide dismutase muted these effects on ROS generation and apoptosis, but not the mitochondrial membrane potential, implying a major role for ROS generation in causing myopathy.[36]

Risk Factors

Patients on mechanical ventilation with critical illnesses such as sepsis, electrolyte imbalance, endocrine dysfunction, starvation, and hepatic and renal disorders have multiple catabolic stressors. These patients are more susceptible to ACM. An association with ACM and nondepolarizing neuromuscular blocking agents often presents as ventilatory weaning failure.[33]

Steroids are often used in cancer patients for the treatment of brain edema or cord compression, but also for cachexia, nausea, and bone pain. Batchelor[37] described the effects of GCS in adult cancer patients. In 15 patients, 9 (60%) were found to have muscle weakness in proximal limbs that interfered with normal daily activities. In eight of nine weak patients, the process manifested within 15 days of initiation of GCS treatment. Dyspnea was also present in these patients, indicating possible involvement of the respiratory muscles. These effects were seemingly correlated with cumulative steroid dose and were often reversible with drug cessation.

Diagnosis

Diagnosis of chronic steroid myopathy is dependent on its presentation and unfortunately may occur late in the treatment cycle. Laboratory findings are often only minimally abnormal or overlooked. Myotubular necrosis may demonstrate increases in serum creatine phosphokinase (CPK) as well as elevated urine creatine excretion. Electromyographic evidence of abnormal spontaneous discharges or small, short, motor-unit action potentials may also be found (which are commonly normal early). Muscle biopsy may reveal only nonspecific type II fiber atrophy.[32]

Prevention

Chronic use of corticosteroids may have deleterious effects on muscle and may be dose related. Exercise is not contraindicated and may be helpful. Braith et al.[38] studied a group of male heart transplant recipients that received GCS as part of their immune suppression protocol. Fourteen of these patients were randomly assigned to lumbar extension exercises 1 day per week plus Nautilus resistance exercises 2 days per week versus a control group without programmed exercise. After 6 months, fat-free mass had been restored to 3.9 ± 2.9% greater than before exercise therapy. The fat-free mass of the control group declined progressively over 6 months to 7 ± 4.4% lower than pre-exercise therapy. In another study, lung transplant patients received lumbar extensor muscle resistance training, which lessened their vertebral bone loss compared to nonexercising controls.[39] Similarly, Chromiak and Vandenburgh[40] demonstrated that *in vitro* skeletal muscle atrophy was attenuated with repetitive muscle stimulation. In this study, GCS induced rapid atrophy of fast-twitch skeletal muscle fibers. Repetitive 10% muscle stretch for 60 seconds every 5 minutes over 3 to 4 days decreased atrophy.[40]

Treatment

Treatment of steroid-induced myopathy involves decreasing drug dosage or discontinuation. There is evidence of benefit of resistance exercises such as weight lifting. Indeed, many pain management programs use injections to relieve pain, closely followed by therapeutic exercise or physical therapy.

Summary

In summary, it appears that GCS induce changes in mitochondrial ROS production, increase myoblast apoptosis, and decrease anabolic effects of gene transcription of protein kinases involved in IGF-1–mediated protein synthesis. The doses that cause these effects appear variable, and exercise may have beneficial effects. Adverse effects may be minimized by screening patients for subtle muscle weakness at regular intervals during GCS treatment. Drug cessation or reduction in dosage may improve the resultant myopathy.

▶ GLUCOCORTICOID-INDUCED OSTEOPOROSIS

Definition of the Complication

Glucocorticoid-induced osteoporosis (GIOP) is the most common drug-induced cause of osteoporosis and can be a significant cause of fractures in at-risk groups.

Scope

GIOP may occur in over 50% of long-term GCS users.[41] Fracture risk commences early (first 12 months) in the course of GCS dosing and may stabilize over time. Serious fractures may include vertebral body, trochanteric, or sacral/pelvic insufficiency fractures (Fig. 35-4). Fracture prevention is the most important factor in any therapeutic strategy for GIOP.

Pathophysiology

Two major pathways by which GCS lead to abnormalities in bone metabolism are (i) reduction in bone formation and (ii) increase in bone resorption. A direct inhibition of osteoblastic activity by GCS is the most agreed-upon mechanism. This is reported in the literature as reduced trabecular wall thickness because of a decrease in absolute number of osteoblasts and their premature death by apoptosis. Osteoblast dysfunction results in incomplete repair of the bone remodeling lacunae.[42]

Bone resorption caused by GCS appears to be related to the balance between osteoprotegerin (OPG) and OPG ligand (OPG-L). OPG, a TNFα-like cytokine receptor, promotes increased bone mass (osteopetrosis) in transgenic mice. Genetic knockout mice without the OPG gene have severe osteoporosis. In contrast, OPG-L stimulates osteoclastogenesis and therefore increased osteoclast resorptive activity. GCS appear to strongly influence this critical OPG/OPG-L balance. By affecting OPG and OPG-L m-RNA production, the OPG-L/OPG ratio is increased by GCS 20- to 40-fold.[42] GCS also appear to prevent osteoclast apoptosis. This indicates that early bone loss of GC-treated patients may be

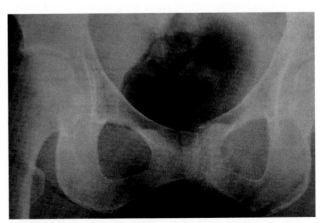

FIGURE 35-4. A pelvic fracture is noted (*arrow*) in a postmenopausal female after 3 weeks of high-dose corticosteroid therapy for newly diagnosed collagen-vascular disease. The fracture was quite painful and occurred without incident trauma.

due to extension of life span of preexisting osteoclasts (not prevented by bisphosphonates). Long-term beneficial bisphosphonate effects are thus likely due to prolonged life span of osteoblasts.[43]

Dovio et al.[44] studied 13 young multiple sclerosis patients receiving high-dose short-term GCS therapy and found an immediate and persistent decrease in bone formation and rapid and transient increase in bone resorption. Discontinuation was followed by a high bone turnover phase. They also noted that osteocalcin and procollagen a-1 gene expression was downregulated by GCS as evidenced by decreased levels of serum osteocalcin.

Risk Factors

Population groups at risk for GIOP would certainly include postmenopausal osteoporosis patients, but virtually any patient can be at risk. Patients at increased risk other than postmenopausal women include those with family history, men over age 50, those with prolonged immobilization, low weight, previous or suspected current vertebral fractures, smokers, and concomitant rheumatic illness.[45] Risk stratification to determine which patients are at risk, how to monitor at-risk patients, and when to institute appropriate treatment strategies have not been performed for any interventional pain injection series.

Given the fact that GCS are used by an estimated 1% to 3% of the population,[41] it is likely that the number of patients potentially at risk is huge. As the population of Americans over the age of 50 continues to increase, this number is quite likely to increase. Therapies for prevention of bone loss are already underutilized in our society.[46] Therefore, specific therapies for treatment of GIOP are needed.

Clues to the prevalence of steroid-induced side effects could be drawn from studies of inhaled steroids. A recent study reviewed 412 patients receiving 1.2 mg/d of inhaled triamcinolone for the treatment of chronic obstructive pulmonary disease.[47] Doses used were similar to that used in four to five epidural injections per year. Measures of bone mineral density (BMD) at the femoral neck and lumbar spine all declined in years 1 through 3, but not in the 1st year. Serum osteocalcin was not a useful marker in predicting those at risk for corticosteroid-induced osteoporosis. Age >56 and corticosteroid medication were associated with increased risk of bone loss, but sex, smoking history, exercise, or calcium and vitamin D intake were not.

Diagnostic Evaluation

Patients who are thought to be at risk (i.e., low weight, male over 50, previous fractures, and so on) should have BMD measured by an accepted technique such as dual energy x-ray absorptiometry scanning. It should be remembered that patients on GCS may fracture at relatively higher BMDs.

Prevention

Recommendations from the American College of Rheumatology Ad Hoc Committee on Corticosteroid-Induced Osteoporosis seem reasonable for those on chronic steroids[48] (Table 35-2). In general, patients receiving >5 mg/d prednisone equivalence, with plans to treat >3 months, should

---

TABLE 35-2 Recommendations for the Prevention and Treatment of Glucocorticoid-induced Osteoporosis

Patient beginning therapy with glucocorticoid (prednisone equivalent of ≥5 mg/d) with plans for treatment duration of ≥3 mo:

- Modify lifestyle risk factors for osteoporosis.
- Initiate smoking cessation or avoidance.
- Initiate reduction of alcohol consumption if excessive.
- Instruct in weight-bearing physical exercise.
- Initiate calcium supplementation.
- Initiate supplementation with vitamin D (plain or activated form).
- Prescribe bisphosphonate (use with caution in premenopausal women).

Patient receiving long-term glucocorticoid therapy (prednisone equivalent of ≥5 mg/d):

- Modify lifestyle risk factors for osteoporosis.
- Initiate smoking cessation or avoidance.
- Initiate reduction of alcohol consumption if excessive.
- Instruct in weight-bearing physical exercise.
- Initiate calcium supplementation.
- Initiate supplementation with vitamin D (plain or activated form).
- Prescribe treatment to replace gonadal sex hormones if deficient or otherwise clinically indicated.
- Measure BMD at lumbar spine and/or hip.

If BMD is not normal (i.e., T-score below −1):

- Prescribe bisphosphonate (use with caution in premenopausal women).
- Consider calcitonin as second-line agent if patient has contraindication to or does not tolerate bisphosphonate therapy.

If BMD is normal:

- Follow up and repeat BMD measurement either annually or biannually.

---

follow the panel recommendations. The earliest changes of corticosteroid-induced osteoporosis are commonly seen in trabecular bone such as the spine. Doses >10 mg/d may be associated with more significant bone loss. Bisphosphonates are the standard for initiation of preventive therapy, but PTH 1-34 (teriparatide) appears to be an emerging therapy. A study of 51 postmenopausal women on hormone replacement therapy (HRT) found significant increases in BMD at the lumbar spine when receiving teriparatide.[49] Teriparatide is an anabolic agent as opposed to the anticatabolic effects of the bisphosphonates. Van Staa et al.[50] pooled data from clinical trails of risedronate and placebo groups. The placebo patients' risk factors included their lumbar spine BMD values and the *daily dose* of corticosteroid as opposed to the cumulative dose. Nevertheless, patients on GCs had higher risk of fracture in spite of their younger age and higher bone density. This implies that the microarchitecture of the trabecular bone may be of significance in corticosteroid-induced osteoporosis.[50]

Treatment

Cessation of the GCS agent (or prophylactic treatment with bisphosphonates, calcium, and vitamin D supplementation) may be helpful. When administered over 1 or 2 years to patients on GCS for a variety of chronic disorders, etidronate, pamidronate, alendronate, and risedronate are efficacious in preventing or treating bone loss at spine and hip locations.[51–53] In a study by Adachi et al.[51] cyclical etidronate was instituted within 100 days of prednisone initiation in 141 men and women. The placebo group had decreased BMD measurements by 3.2%, and the treatment group showed an increase of BMD by 0.6% at 1 year.[51] A combined report of multicenter studies of 477 new and chronic GC users, including men and pre- and postmenopausal women, demonstrated significant improvement with alendronate.[52] While on 10 mg alendronate therapy, the BMD showed an increase by 2.9%, whereas the placebo group showed a 0.4% decrease in BMD of the spine. In another study, similar gains were seen at the trochanter as well as a small but significant improvement at the femoral neck. There was also a 90% reduction in the number of vertebral fractures observed. A 5-mg dose of alendronate was compared to 10 mg and found to be statistically equivalent except in postmenopausal women, in which the 10-mg dose resulted in significantly greater increases in lumbar spine BMD.[53]

▶ ARACHNOIDITIS

Definition

Arachnoiditis describes an inflammatory reaction of the arachnoid membrane that can occur as a result of invasion (surgery), neuraxial injections, certain myelograms, infections, blood, or other trauma.[54] It is thought that the injurious event (whether it be needle/surgical trauma, irritant substance, infectious, or other) induces a local inflammatory tissue reaction in the arachnoid or associated tissues. Many of these cases with subtle, often patchy, dysesthetic pain; poorly defined nondermatomal neurologic changes; and bowel/bladder functional changes are labeled chronic nerve irritation, "failed back surgery syndrome," cauda equina syndrome, and other nonspecific terms that lead to confusion about the true underlying cause. Unfortunately, although imaging can be helpful (see material following) physical examination likely does not differentiate what is causing the problem, and tissue biopsies are not feasible.[55]

Scope arachnoiditis has been reportedly present for over a century, coinciding with the introduction of cocaine intrathecal injections. Caution regarding the use of all intraspinal steroids has been advocated by Nelson et al.[11] and Nelson and Landau.[56] The incidence appears to be increasing, with an increase in spinal surgery frequency in the United States and the popularity of neural blockade.[55]

Pathophysiology

The arachnoid, pia, and adjacent neural structures may respond to injury or invasion by initiating an inflammatory response. This tissue reaction can then evolve, based on patient predisposition and immune factors, into a proliferative phase that leads to permanent adhesion, scarring, and fibroplastic reaction.[55]

Risk Factors

Cases of arachnoiditis have been reported after oil-based, myelogram injection, predominantly Pantopaque (iophendylate, Lafayette Pharmaceuticals, Lafayette, IN, introduced in 1944, but no longer manufactured). Unintentional injection of subarachnoid blood, chemical irritants, or toxins; abscesses or other infectious (tuberculosis) causes; neurolytics; surgical or needle neural trauma; intrathecal corticosteroids; and multiple other causes.[55] As pertaining to the cause of cases of arachnoiditis, there are no specific long-term data, and tracking is made difficult by the characterization of some cases of probable arachnoiditis under other neurologic condition headings. A large retrospective review of complications in Sweden over the last decade noted a total of 127 severe neurologic conditions after spinal and epidural blockade.[57] Interestingly, the incidence of subarachnoid needle complications was lower than the epidural rate, and obstetric cases were smaller compared to orthopedic cases. Osteoporosis was proposed as a previously unknown risk factor. In a large review of the literature by Abram and O'Connor,[19] they found a remarkable safety profile for epidural corticosteroid injections. Most of the cases with arachnoiditis involved multiple intrathecal injections, and others had disc disease or prior laminectomies. The authors found no cases attributable to epidural steroid injections alone. Latham et al.[58] found that intrathecal injections of betamethasone in sheep were safe in the equivalent concentrations used in humans, but larger doses could produce arachnoid changes. A recent large series of intrathecal methylprednisolone injections for the treatment of postherpetic neuralgia was surprisingly not associated with any reported arachnoiditis complications.[59]

Diagnostic Evaluation

Patients report a variety of symptoms that aid in the diagnosis of this condition. There may be any number of presentations (e.g., severe burning pain in the low back that persists at rest, neurologic deficits, perineal/saddle numbness, sympathetic or vascular changes, skin rashes, and itching[55,60]). MRI fast-spin axial T2 images may demonstrate characteristic empty sac with nerve root clumping (chain of pearls)[55] and adherence to the outer dural sac.[61] Myelogram may also demonstrate the presence or absence of pseudomeningocele, pachymeningitis, arachnoid ossification, syringomyelia, and other specific patterns. These imaging features allow more precise terminology and characterization of the true pathology instead of imprecise definitions such as "cauda equina syndrome."[55] Computer-assisted tomography with intravenous contrast dye may also be helpful in diagnosis, particularly if the patient is unable to tolerate MRI. Myelograms could potentially cause exacerbation of symptoms.

Prevention

Avoidance of intrathecal steroid injections, particularly in large doses, is most likely to reduce complications. Development of new neurologic changes should be promptly investigated. Consultation with neurology, neurosurgery, and diagnostic radiology colleagues is indicated.

Treatment

Treatment of arachnoiditis is difficult and limited and should focus on symptom management. Pain is treated with narcotic medications, oral steroids, or spinal cord stimulation. Surgical treatment is considered as a last resort and consists of scar tissue lysis, laminectomy, dural decompressive grafting, or posterolateral fusion with instrumentation.[60]

Summary

Epidural GCS injections have been implicated in the development of adhesive arachnoiditis, but it appears from reviewing the literature that intrathecal injections are most likely to be causative. MRI will help accurately diagnose the problem. Treatment is speculative and symptom oriented.

References

1. Chrousos GP. Adrenocorticosteroids and adrenocortical antagonists. In: Katzung BG, ed. *Basic and Clinical Pharmacology.* 9th ed. New York, NY: Lang Medical Books/McGraw-Hill, 2004: 641–660.
2. Hench PS, Kendall EC, Slocumb CH, et al. The effect of a hormone of the adrenal cortex (17-hydroxy-11-dehydrocorticosterone): compound E and of pituitary adrenocorticotropic hormone on rheumatoid arthritis. *Mayo Clin Proc* 1949;24:181–197.
3. Hollander JL, Brown EM, Jessar RA, et al. Hydrocortisone and cortisone injected into arthritic joints. *JAMA* 1951;147:1629–1635.
4. Winnie AP, Hartman JT, Meyers HL Jr, et al. Pain Clinic II: intradural and extradural corticosteroids for sciatica. *Anesth Analg* 1972;51:990–999.
5. Jacoby RK. The effect of hydrocortisone acetate on adult human articular cartilage. *J Rheumatol* 1976;3:384–389.
6. Friedman DM, Moore ME. The efficacy of intraarticular steroids in osteoarthritis: a double blind study. *J Rheumatol* 1980;7: 850–856.
7. Devor M, Govrin-Lippmann R, Raber P. Corticosteroids suppress ectopic neural discharge originating in experimental neuromas. *Pain* 1985;22:127–137.
8. Anderson B, Kaye S. Treatment of flexor tenosynovitis of the hand ("trigger finger") with corticosteroids: a prospective study of the response to local injection. *Arch Intern Med* 1991;151:153–156.
9. Williams JM, Brandt KD. Triamcinolone hexacetonide protects against fibrillation and osteophyte formation following chemically induced cartilage damage. *Arthritis Rheum* 1985;28:1267–1274.
10. Buckley LM, Marquez M, Hudson J, et al. Variations in physician's judgment about corticosteroid induced osteoporosis by physician specialty. *J Rheumatol* 1998;25:2195–2202.
11. Nelson DA, Vates TS, Thomas RB. Complications from intrathecal steroid therapy in patients with multiple sclerosis. *Acta Neurol Scand* 1973;49(2):176–188.
12. Bedi SS, Ellis W. Spontaneous rupture of the calcaneal tendon in rheumatoid arthritis after local steroid injection. *Ann Rheum Dis* 1970;29(5):494–495.
13. Curtis JR, Westfall J, Allison J, et al. Population based assessment of adverse events associated with long term glucocorticoid use. *Arthritis Rheum* 2006;55(3):420–426.
14. Barnes PJ, Adcock I. Anti-inflammatory actions of steroids: molecular mechanisms. *Trends Pharmacol Sci* 1993;14:436–441.
15. Baqui A, Bal R. The mechanism of action and side effects of epidural steroids. *Tech Reg Anesth Pain Manage* 2009;13: 205–211.
16. DeSio JM. Epidural steroid injections. In: Warfield CA, Bajwa ZH, eds. *Principles and Practice of Pain Medicine.* 2nd ed. New York, NY: McGraw-Hill, 2004:655–656.
17. Knight CL, Burnell JC. Systemic side effects of extradural steroids. *Anaesthesia* 1980;35:593–594.
18. Gorski DW, Rao TK, Glisson SN, et al. Epidural triamcinolone and adrenal response to stress. *Anesthesiology* 1981;55:A147.
19. Abrams SE, O'Connor TC. Complications associated with epidural steroid injections. *Reg Anesth* 1996;21:149–162.
20. Lansang MC, Farmer T, Kennedy L. Diagnosing the unrecognized systemic absorption of intra-articular and epidural steroid injections. *Endocr Pract* 2009;15(3):225–228.
21. Kay J, Findling J, Raff H. Epidural triamcinolone suppresses the pituitary-adrenal axis in human subjects. *Anesthesia Analg* 1994;79:501–505.
22. Deer T, Ranson M, Kapural L, et al. Guidelines for the proper use of epidural steroid injections for the chronic pain patient. *Tech Reg Anesth Pain Manage* 2009;13:288–295.
23. Horani MH, Siverberg AB. Secondary Cushing's syndrome after a single epidural injection of a corticosteroid. *Endocr Pract* 2005;11(6):408–410.
24. Nasser SMS, Ewan PW. Depot corticosteroid treatment for hay fever causing avascular necrosis of both hips. *BMJ* 2001;322: 1589–1591.
25. Weinstein RS, Nicholas RW, Manolagas SC. Apoptosis of osteocytes in glucocorticoid-induced osteonecrosis of the hip. *J Clin Endocrinol Metab* 2000;85:2907–2912.
26. Clinkscales A, Cleary JD. Steroid-induced avascular necrosis. *Ann Pharmacother* 2002;36:1105.
27. Socie G, Cahn JY, Carmelo J, et al. Avascular necrosis of bone after allogenic bone marrow transplantation: analysis of risk factors for 4388 patients by the Societe Francois de Griffe de Moelle. *Br J Haematol* 1997;97:865–870.
28. Marsh JCW, Zomas A, Hows JM, et al. Avascular necrosis after treatment of aplastic anemia with anti-lymphocyte globulin and high dose methylprednisolone. *Br J Haematol* 1993;84:731–735.
29. Bracken MB, Shepard MJ, Collins WF, et al. A randomized controlled trial of methylprednisolone or naloxone in the treatment of acute spinal cord injury: results of the Second National Acute Spinal Cord Injury Study. *N Engl J Med* 1990;322:1405–1411.
30. Wing PC, Nance P, Connell DG, et al. Risk of avascular necrosis following short term megadose methylprednisolone treatment. *Spinal Cord* 1998;36:633–636.
31. Agarwala S, Jain D, Joshi VR, et al. Efficacy of alendronate, a bisphosphonate, in the treatment of AVN of the hip: a prospective open-label study. *Rheumatology* 2005;44:352–359.
32. Wald JJ. The effects of toxins on muscle: clinical neurobehavioral Toxicology. *Neurol Clin* 2000;18(3):695–717.
33. Singleton JR, Baker BL, Thorburn A. Dexamethasone inhibits insulin-like growth factor signaling and potentiates myoblast apoptosis. *Endocrinology* 2000;141:2945–2950.
34. Kanda F, Takatani K, Okuda S, et al. Preventive effects of insulinlike growth factor-1 on steroid-induced muscle atrophy. *Muscle Nerve* 1999;22:213–217.

35. Kanda F, Okuda S, Matsushita T, et al. Steroid myopathy: pathogenesis and effects of growth hormone and insulin-like growth factor-1 administration. *Horm Res* 2001;56(Suppl 1):24–28.

36. Oshima Y, Kuroda Y, Kunishige M, et al. Oxidative stress associated mitochondrial dysfunction in corticosteroid-treated muscle cells. *Muscle Nerve* 2004;30:49–54.

37. Batchelor TT, Taylor LP, Thaler HT, et al. Steroid myopathy in cancer patients. *Neurology* 1997;48:1234–1238.

38. Braith RW, Welsch MA, Mills RM, et al. Resistance exercise prevents glucocorticoid-induced myopathy in heart transplant recipients. *Med Sci Sports Exerc* 1998;30:483–489.

39. Mitchell MJ, Baz MA, Fulton MN, et al. Resistance training prevents vertebral osteoporosis in lung transplant recipients. *Transplantation* 2003;76:557–562.

40. Chromiak JA, Vandenburgh HH. Glucocorticoid-induced skeletal muscle atrophy in vitro is attenuated by mechanical stimulation. *Am J Physiol* 1992;262:C1471–C1477.

41. Ettinger B, Pressman A, Shah HA. Who bears responsibility for glucocorticoid-exposed patients in a large health maintenance organization? *J Manag Care Pharm* 2001;7:228–232.

42. Hofbauer LC, Gori F, Riggs L. Stimulation of OPG ligand and inhibition of OPG production by glucocorticoids in human osteoblastic lineage cells: potential paracrine mechanisms of glucocorticoid-induced osteoporosis. *Endocrinology* 1999;140:4382–4389.

43. Weinstein RS, Chen JR, Powers CC, et al. Promotion of osteoclast survival and antagonism of bisphosphonate-induced osteoclast apoptosis by glucocorticoids. *J Clin Invest* 2002;109:1041–1048.

44. Dovio A, Perazzolo L, Giangiacomo O, et al. Immediate fall of bone formation and transient increase of bone resorption in the course of high-dose, short term glucocorticoid therapy in young patients with multiple sclerosis. *J Clin Endocrinol Metab* 2004;89:4923–4928.

45. Sambrook PN. How to prevent steroid induced osteoporosis. *Ann Rheum Dis* 2004;64:176–178.

46. Cohen D, Adachi JD. The treatment of glucocorticoid induced osteoporosis. *J Steroid Biochem Mol Biol* 2004;88:337–349.

47. Scanlon PD, Connett JE, Wise RA, et al. Loss of bone density with inhaled triamcinolone in lung health study II. *Am J Respir Crit Care Med* 2004;170:1302–1309.

48. American College of Rheumatology Ad Hoc Committee on Glucocorticoid-Induced Osteoporosis. Recommendations for the prevention and treatment of glucocorticoid-induced osteoporosis. *Arthritis Rheum* 2001;44:1496–1503.

49. Lane NE, Sanchez S, Modin GW, et al. Parathyroid hormone treatment can reverse corticosteroid-induced osteoporosis: results of a randomized controlled clinical trial. *J Clin Invest* 1998;102:1627–1633.

50. Van Staa TP, Laan RF, Barton IP, et al. Bone density threshold and other predictors of vertebral fracture in patients receiving oral glucocorticoid therapy. *Arthritis Rheum* 2003;48:3224–3229.

51. Adachi JD, Bensen WG, Brown J, et al. Intermittent etidronate therapy to prevent corticosteroid-induced osteoporosis. *N Engl J Med* 1997;337:382–387.

52. Saag KG, Emkey R, Schnitzer T, et al. Alendronate for the treatment and prevention of glucocorticoid-induced osteoporosis. *N Engl J Med* 1998;339:292–299.

53. Adachi R, Saag K, Delmas P, et al. Two-year effects of alendronate on bone mineral density and vertebral fractures in patients receiving glucocorticoids. *Arthritis Rheum* 2001;44:202–211.

54. Aldrete JA. Chronic adhesive arachnoiditis (Letter to the editor). *Br J Anaesth* 2004;93:301–303.

55. Aldrete JA. Neurological deficits and arachnoiditis following neuroaxial anesthesia. *Acta Anaesthesiol Scand* 2003;47:3–12.

56. Nelson DA, Landau WM. Intraspinal steroids: history, efficacy, accidentality, and controversy with review of United States Food and Drug Administration reports. *J Neurol Neurosurg Psychiatry* 2001;70:433–443.

57. Moen V, Dahlgren N, Irestedt L. Severe neurological complications after central neuraxial blockades in Sweden 1990–1999. *Anesthesiology* 2004;101:950–959.

58. Latham JM, Fraser RD, Moore RJ, et al. The pathologic effects of intrathecal betamethasone. *Spine* 1997;22:1558–1562.

59. Kotani N, Kushikata T, Hashimoto H, et al. Intrathecal methylprednisolone for intractable postherpetic neuralgia. *N Engl J Med* 2000;343:1514–1519.

60. Wright MH, Denney LC. A comprehensive review of spinal arachnoiditis. *Orthop Nurs* 2003;22(3):215–219.

61. Gundry CR, Fritts HM. Magnetic resonance imaging of the musculoskeletal system: the spine: part 8, section 3. *Clin Orthop Relat Res* 1998;346:262–278.

SECTION III

Medicolegal Perspective

Findings from the ASA Closed Claims Project

Lorri A. Lee, Dermot Fitzgibbon, Linda S. Stephens, and Karen B. Domino

Regional anesthesia and chronic pain management are frequently considered high risk in terms of liability. Despite numerous studies demonstrating the benefits of regional anesthesia,[1–3] many anesthesiologists view it as a less desirable alternative to general anesthesia because of the potential for direct injury to nerves caused by needle trauma. The use of ultrasound-guided anesthesia has been proposed as a potentially safer method of performing regional anesthesia, though class I evidence is not yet available.[4–6] Similarly, invasive pain management procedures utilize therapeutic and diagnostic techniques that are perceived by some practitioners to have a low benefit to risk ratio because of the potential for nerve injury and the refractory nature of chronic pain. Noninvasive pain management with opioids is also associated with significant risk as reports in the lay press and medical journals regarding deaths associated with prescription opioids have escalated over the last decade[7] (Chapters 34, 37). To assess the pattern of injuries and liability associated with regional anesthesia and chronic pain management, we used the American Society of Anesthesiologists (ASA) Closed Claims Database.

This database contains detailed information on adverse anesthetic outcomes obtained from the closed anesthesia malpractice insurance claim files of U.S. professional liability companies that cover approximately 60% of practicing anesthesiologists. The data collection process has been previously described in detail.[8,9] Anesthesiologist-reviewers visited insurance company sites and reviewed files from closed anesthesia claims. Injuries (complications) and mechanisms of injuries (damaging events) were assessed for each claim and information was entered on detailed data instrument collection forms. Injuries were designated with nerve damage if objective clinical, anatomic, or laboratory findings consistent with spinal cord or peripheral nerve damage were present.[10] Pain syndromes such as low back pain or muscle aches that could not be correlated with specific neuroanatomic lesions were designated as other complications, and not nerve damage. For purposes of this chapter, regional anesthesia data were obtained from a database of 6,894 claims, excluding obstetric and both acute and chronic pain management claims. Chronic pain management data were obtained from a subset of claims between 2005 and 2008 with detailed information on pain management from a database of 8,954 claims, previously described in detail elsewhere.[11,12]

Interpretation of data obtained from the ASA Closed Claims Database must be done with knowledge of its limitations.[9,13] Previous studies have shown that as few as 1 in 25 adverse events result in a malpractice claim being filed and that there is a tendency for higher severity injury claims to be filed compared to no or low severity injuries. Thus, incidence of complications cannot be determined because of a lack of a denominator for all adverse anesthetic outcomes in the United States and all anesthetics administered in the United States. Bias in description of events may be introduced by retrospective collection of data with partial reliance on direct participants. Finally, changes in practice patterns over time and knowledge of severity of outcome can lead to bias in determination of standard of care.[14] Despite these significant limitations, the ASA Closed Claims Database does provide useful information on rare adverse events that would be difficult to study prospectively, and it provides an overview of the medical liability for anesthesiologists.

▶ REGIONAL ANESTHESIA

Neuraxial Blocks for Regional Anesthesia Claims

A total of 443 claims associated with nonobstetric neuraxial (epidural/spinal blockade) anesthesia in the surgical setting were identified in the ASA Closed Claims Database from 1990 or later out of a total of 652 nonobstetric regional anesthesia claims (excluding acute and chronic pain claims). Mean age in the nonobstetric neuraxial anesthesia group was 57 years (range, 0.25–94), and approximately half (52%) of patients were ASA physical status 1 to 2 and half (48%) were ASA physical status 3 to 4. No patients with an ASA physical status 5 were present in this dataset. Neuraxial anesthetic claims were evenly split between male and female gender (51% vs. 49%) and one-third (31%) of patients were considered obese. The type of anesthetic technique with these claims included 45% subarachnoid blocks, 45% lumbar epidural blocks, 1% caudal epidural blocks, 5% thoracic epidural blocks, and 2% combined subarachnoid/epidural blocks. Although temporary injury accounted for the largest proportion of neuraxial anesthetic claims (45%), over

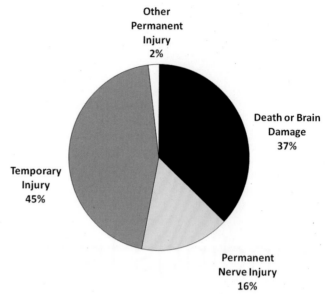

FIGURE 36-1. Outcomes in neuraxial regional anesthetics (*n* = 443). Neuraxial blocks for obstetrics and acute and chronic pain were excluded from this analysis.

one-third of claims were associated with high severity injuries (death or permanent brain damage, 37%) and 16% of claims with permanent nerve injury (Fig. 36-1).

Block-related mechanisms of injury were associated with 41% of all neuraxial anesthesia claims with the remaining 59% of claims including (in decreasing percentages of claims) no event (9%), other anesthetic events (6%), cardiovascular events (14%), respiratory events (9%), unknown events (4%), surgical events or patient condition (8%), medication problems (4%), and equipment problems (7%). Block technique (50%, *n* = 88), neuraxial cardiac arrest (21%, *n* = 37), dural puncture (9%, *n* = 17), and high spinal/epidural block (8%, *n* = 14) were the most common causes of block-related injury and accounted for 87% of claims in this category. Block technique referred to a complication thought to be caused by the technical performance of the block and most commonly was associated with needle or catheter damage to nerves or surrounding structures.

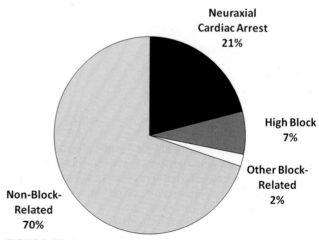

FIGURE 36-2. Mechanism of injury for neuraxial claims associated with death or brain damage (*n* = 163).

Block-related mechanisms of injury accounted for more than one quarter ($n = 48$, 29%) of the high severity claims associated with death or brain damage ($n = 163$). Neuraxial cardiac arrest ($n = 34$, 21%) and high spinal/epidural block ($n = 11$, 7%) were the most common block-related causes of death or brain damage (Fig. 36-2). Non–block-related mechanisms of injury for the high severity claims associated with death or brain damage were most commonly associated with cardiovascular events (e.g., air/fat pulmonary emboli, stroke, hypotension, and myocardial infarction, 33%) and respiratory events (e.g., inadequate ventilation, airway obstruction, bronchospasm, and aspiration, 20%). Other events including surgical events or patient condition, wrong drug or dose, unknown events, multiple events, and no event accounted for the remainder of non–block-related events.

Neuraxial Cardiac Arrest in Regional Anesthesia Claims

Neuraxial cardiac arrest (Box 36-1) accounted for 21% of all block-related causes of injury, and it was associated with the largest proportion of neuraxial anesthesia claims with death or brain damage ($n = 34$). Outcomes with neuraxial cardiac arrest in the ASA Closed Claims Database are predominately high severity with >90% resulting in death or brain damage. Mean age in these claims was 54 years, and 30% were ASA physical status 1 to 2, 54% were ASA physical status 3, and 8% were ASA physical status 4.

Neuraxial cardiac arrest claims were examined for associated factors as both capnography and pulse oximetry were widely available from 1990 onward (Table 36-1). Two-thirds occurred following subarachnoid block and 11% were after epidural anesthesia with accidental subarachnoid block (Table 36-1). Sedation was frequently utilized in these cases (76%) from the 1990s, and it has previously been implicated with neuraxial cardiac arrest with inadequate oxygenation and/or ventilation.[15] However, hypoxia and inadequate ventilation were not noted to precede these arrests as 81% of claims were associated with the use of pulse oximetry and 32% with capnography. Cardiac arrest was frequently identified by the presence of cyanosis, but there is little evidence to suggest that inadequate oxygenation and/or ventilation is a common event preceding neuraxial cardiac arrest.[16,17]

TABLE 36-1 Associated Factors for 1990s Neuraxial Cardiac Arrest Claims ($n = 37$) in Regional Anesthesia Claims	
	n (% OF 37 CLAIMS)
Subarachnoid block	24 (65)
Lumbar epidural block	13 (35)
Accidental subarachnoid block	4 (11)
Inadequate test dose	1 (3)
Pulse oximetry	30 (81)
Capnography	12 (32)
Sedation	28 (76)
Resuscitation delay	18 (49)
Cardiac arrest in prone position	6 (16)
Repositioning on table	7 (18)
Epinephrine not administered	2 (5)

BOX 36-1 Neuraxial Cardiac Arrest

1. Risk factors:
   - Mid- to upper thoracic block
   - Baseline bradycardia
   - Male gender
2. Occurs with spinal or epidural blockade at any time during the operation.
3. May be preceded by sudden bradycardia or may present as sudden asystole.
4. Neuraxial block patients must be monitored with EKG and pulse oximetry.
5. Vigilance should be heightened during the prone position or during positioning changes on the table.
6. Resuscitation drugs and airway equipment must be immediately available throughout case.

Monitoring with electrocardiogram and pulse oximetry is useful for providing immediate warning of bradycardia that may precede asystole in neuraxial cardiac arrest.

Unfortunately, half of these claims (49%) were associated with delays in resuscitation and were caused by delay in recognition of the event and/or delay in administration of appropriate resuscitation drugs. Six cases were in the prone position when cardiac arrest developed. Seven cases were in the midst of a position change on the OR table or moving between the OR table and the patient gurney when cardiac arrest developed. It is unclear if these position changes worsened a precarious physiologic state, or if they caused a delay in recognition of the cardiac arrest because of distraction or missing monitors, or delay in treatment for returning to the supine position. Anesthesiologists must be vigilant for this complication and promptly utilize resuscitative maneuvers if monitors are to be effective at prevention.

However, monitoring may not be as useful at preventing neuraxial cardiac arrest when there is a rapid and sudden onset of bradycardia/asystole that may not allow adequate time for treatment before cardiac arrest ensues.[16,17] Despite appropriate and timely resuscitative efforts, 17 of 19 claims resulted in death or brain damage. These poor outcomes may be explained by Rosenberg et al.[18] study that demonstrated that cardiac arrest in dogs during total spinal anesthesia is difficult to treat because of the presence of intense sympathetic blockade, which decreases circulating blood volume, reduces coronary perfusion pressure, and renders cardiopulmonary resuscitation (CPR) ineffective.[18] Additionally, other studies from this group in dogs have demonstrated that spinal anesthesia prevents a rise in epinephrine and norepinephrine catecholamine levels during cardiac arrest compared to controls without spinal anesthesia.[19] Therefore, both severe vasodilation and a defective neuroendocrine response to stress are thought to contribute to the poor outcome during neuraxial cardiac arrest. Cases of neuraxial cardiac arrest that promptly respond to therapy and result in no sequelae have been reported, but are unlikely to result in claims.[16,20] Consequently, the success and failure rates of prompt resuscitation, specific resuscitation drugs, and types of monitoring cannot be determined from this database.

The two most commonly proposed mechanisms to explain neuraxial cardiac arrest are (i) low-filling of the left ventricle causing a paradoxical bradycardic response via stretch/mechanoreceptors, commonly referred to as the Bezold-Jarisch reflex, and (ii) blockade of the cardiac accelerator fibers with sympathetic blockade >T4.[17] Patients with baseline bradycardia and male gender have been shown to have an increased occurrence of severe bradycardia (<40 beats per minute) under neuraxial blockade, and the bradycardic episodes are widely distributed throughout the time course of cases of variable duration.[17] Monitoring of electrocardiogram and pulse oximetry should be utilized for patients with neuraxial anesthetics for the entire duration of the case, and resuscitation drugs and equipment should be immediately available.

High Spinal/Epidural Block

High spinal/epidural blocks accounted for 2% (*n* = 14) of all nonobstetric neuraxial anesthesia claims in 1990 or later and 8% of the 180 neuraxial anesthesia claims associated with a block-related mechanism of injury. An outcome of death or brain damage was associated with 79% (*n* = 11) of these high block claims. Five of these 14 claims were associated with subarachnoid blockade, and 9 claims with epidural blockade (7 lumbar, 1 thoracic, and 1 caudal). An accidental subarachnoid block was thought to be associated with all of the epidural claims. There was no significant association with a specific local anesthetic. Mean age of patients was 52 years (range, 0.25–76 years), and no difference was observed with respect to gender (7 female: 7 male). The type of surgery associated with high spinal/epidural blocks included eight lower extremity procedures, two urologic procedures, two gynecologic procedures, and two abdominal operations. CPR was utilized in six claims.

Aspiration of the epidural catheter and use of a 3 mL test dose of local anesthetic with epinephrine should be utilized with epidural anesthetics to rule out both intravascular and intrathecal injections. Failure to wait the appropriate amount of time after the test dose may lead to a falsely negative result. Injection of a test dose of local anesthetic through the epidural needle prior to catheter placement is not adequate for testing the placement of the catheter. Increased vigilance for an accidental intrathecal injection during the entire course of an epidural anesthetic is essential for prompt diagnosis and resuscitation to avoid hypoxia and/or cardiovascular collapse.

Permanent Nerve/Spinal Cord Injuries in Neuraxial Regional Anesthesia Claims

Permanent nerve injuries were associated with 16% (*n* = 71) of the neuraxial anesthesia claims. Of these 71 permanent nerve injuries, 77% (*n* = 55) were judged as block-related mechanisms of injury, 8% (*n* = 6) related to surgical technique, 4% (*n* = 3) related to patient condition, and 10% (*n* = 7) related to other or unknown mechanisms (Fig. 36-3). Damage to the lumbosacral nerve roots and thoracolumbar spinal cord accounted for 93% of the permanent nerve injuries. The two most common causes of block-related permanent

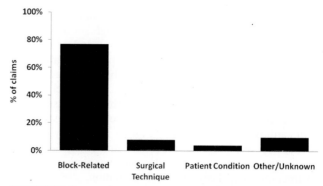

FIGURE 36-3. Permanent nerve damage in neuraxial anesthesia claims (*n* = 71).

nerve damage to the neuraxis (*n* = 55) were hematoma with or without block needle trauma (*n* = 27) and anterior spinal artery syndrome/infarct (*n* = 8). There were 15 neuraxial claims associated with cauda equina symptoms, of which 13 utilized lidocaine, 1 chloroprocaine, and 1 without injection of local anesthetic caused by block needle trauma. Blocks associated with permanent cauda equina injury were subarachnoid (*n* = 8), combined spinal-epidural (*n* = 2), unintentional intrathecal injection (*n* = 1), and lumbar epidural without evidence of intrathecal injection (*n* = 3).

Intrathecal lidocaine has been reported to cause either transient neurologic symptoms or persistent cauda equina symptoms since the early 1990s.[21,22] Lidocaine has also been shown to cause dose-related neurotoxicity when infused epidurally in a rat model in concentrations as low as 2%, though a strong clinical association has not been detected.[23] Recent experimental evidence indicates that low concentrations of lidocaine induce apoptosis, a form of programmed cell death in cell cultures, via the mitochondrial pathway.[24] At higher concentrations, toxicity is caused by cell necrosis in cell cultures.

Neuraxial Hematoma in Neuraxial Regional Anesthesia Claims

Surgical procedures for the 27 neuraxial hematoma claims were vascular (48%, *n* = 13), orthopedic (33%, *n* = 9), and abdominopelvic (19%, *n* = 5; Box 36-2). Not surprisingly, the most common associated factor for epidural/spinal hematoma was the presence of either preoperative (iatrogenic or intrinsic), intraoperative, or postoperative coagulopathy in 59% (*n* = 16) of these claims. Other associated factors included needle trauma to the spinal cord/conus medullaris (22%, *n* = 6) and catheter removal on anticoagulation (15%, *n* = 4). Of the cases with data available, symptom onset was postoperative day 0 in 33% (*n* = 9), postoperative day 1 in 19% (*n* = 5), and later than postoperative day 1 in 19% (*n* = 5) of patients (eight cases without symptom onset data). There was a delay of 1 or more days from symptom onset to diagnosis/treatment in at least 41% (*n* = 11) of cases. The most common symptom was failure of the block to resolve in the recovery room or ward after surgery (33%, *n* = 9) or increased motor block (22%, *n* = 6). Back pain was present in only 19% (*n* = 5) of claims.

Previous studies have shown that neuraxial anesthesia for vascular surgery has been associated with significant patient benefits including reduced graft thrombosis and improved graft blood flow.[25–27] However, a recent review in the Cochrane Database examining four randomized controlled trials of neuraxial anesthesia compared to general anesthesia for

BOX 36-2 Neuraxial Hematoma in Regional Anesthesia Claims

1. Risk factors:
   - Perioperative coagulopathy, usually iatrogenic
   - Vascular surgery
   - Needle trauma at or above the L1 level
2. Symptoms:
   - Failure of block to resolve or increased motor block out of proportion to local anesthetic (most common)
   - Increased sensory block
   - Back pain (least common)
3. Diagnosis:
   - MRI–T2 weighted image (most sensitive and specific)
   - CT Myelography[a]
4. Treatment:
   - Prompt surgical evacuation
   - Time interval from onset of symptoms to decompression and neurologic deficits prior to decompression predict neurologic recovery.

[a]CT of the spine without myelography is not recommended for detection of spinal epidural hematoma.

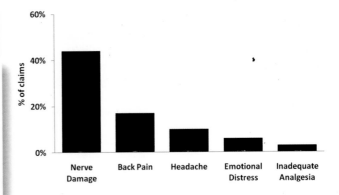

FIGURE 36-4. Temporary injuries associated with neuraxial anesthesia claims ($n = 198$).

was the most common cause of temporary injury (44%) followed by back pain (17%), headache (10%), emotional distress (6%), and inadequate analgesia (3%, Fig. 36-4).

Standard of care associated with nonobstetric neuraxial anesthetic claims was judged as less than appropriate in 45% of death or brain damage claims, 34% of permanent nerve injury claims, and only 18% of temporary injury claims. Payments also trended with severity of injury as death or brain damage claims had a median payment (in 2008) of $536,000 (range $3,350–$8,220,000); permanent nerve injury claims had a median payment of $457,000 ($7,000–$2,647,000); and temporary injury claims had a median payment of $63,700 (range $1,000–$1,876,000).

Peripheral Nerve Blocks in Regional Anesthesia Claims

Peripheral nerve blocks for surgical anesthesia were associated with 135 claims in 1990 or later excluding acute and chronic pain claims and accounted for 21% of all nonobstetric regional anesthesia claims ($n = 652$). Axillary blocks were the most common peripheral nerve block (36%) followed by interscalene blocks (30%), intravenous regional blocks (15%), ankle blocks (6%), supraclavicular blocks (4%), and miscellaneous blocks (10%). Outcome severity for peripheral nerve blocks was associated with death or brain damage in only 16% of claims, with permanent nerve damage in 13% of claims, and with temporary injury in 70% of claims.

The mechanism of injury for claims associated with death or brain damage ($n = 22$) was block-related in only five claims (23%), all related to intravascular injection/absorption. Non–block-related events included cardiovascular ($n = 10$, 45%), respiratory ($n = 3$, 9%), medication ($n = 2$, 9%), and other ($n = 2$, 9%). Regional techniques utilized in these claims were interscalene block ($n = 10$), axillary blocks ($n = 6$), ankle block ($n = 2$) intravenous regional blocks ($n = 1$), and miscellaneous blocks ($n = 3$).

Permanent nerve damage associated with peripheral nerve blocks occurred in 17 of 135 claims (13%, Table 36-2). Temporary injuries accounted for the majority of peripheral nerve block claims ($n = 95$) and included nerve damage ($n = 46$), pneumothorax ($n = 8$), emotional distress/fright ($n = 7$), and miscellaneous causes ($n = 34$). The mechanism of injury was designated as block-related in 44% of all peripheral nerve

lower limb revascularization found no significant differences between groups for mortality rate, myocardial infarction, or amputation.[28] In this review, patients in the neuraxial anesthesia group did have a significantly lower incidence of pneumonia compared to the general anesthesia group. Prospective studies of complications associated with neuraxial anesthetics and vascular surgery have demonstrated a very low incidence of epidural/spinal hematoma.[29–31] Consequently, regional anesthesia for vascular surgery will continue to be used, but anesthesiologists and other health care providers should have increased vigilance for neuraxial hematomas in these patients. Patients with neuraxial blocks out of proportion to the local anesthetic being utilized (especially increased motor block) should be evaluated immediately for the presence of a neuraxial hematoma. Magnetic resonance imaging (MRI) is the most useful radiologic study for detecting these lesions. Epidural hematomas may also be detected by CT myelography, but CT of the spine without myelography can easily miss a spinal epidural hematoma. Neurologic recovery from epidural/spinal hematomas is thought to be partially dependent on time to decompression so prompt diagnosis and treatment are essential to a good outcome. Injuries from neuraxial hematoma caused by the wrong level of needle insertion during subarachnoid block may partially be caused by the anatomic variability among patients in the end of the spinal cord and in the alignment of the iliac crests with lumbar interspaces.[32,33] Needle insertion at the most caudad suitable interspace may reduce these types of complications, particularly in obese patients where landmarks may be difficult to palpate.

Temporary Injuries in Neuraxial Regional Anesthesia Claims

Temporary injuries accounted for the largest proportion of neuraxial anesthesia claims (45%, $n = 198$). Nerve damage

TABLE 36-2 Permanent Nerve Injuries Associated with Peripheral Nerve Blocks for Surgical Anesthesia (n = 17)

	n (% OF 17 CLAIMS)
Brachial plexus	6 (35)
Median nerve	6 (35)
Ulnar nerve	3 (18)
Radial nerve	2 (12)
Spinal cord	3 (18)
Sciatic nerve	2 (12)

Total sums to >17 and >100% due to multiple nerve injuries in some claims.

brain damage group. Overall, permanent nerve injury claims had a 41% payment rate with only 12% judged to be less than appropriate care and a median payment of $290,000 (range $74,000–$990,000). Temporary injury claims had a 24% payment rate with only 14% of claims judged with less than appropriate care and a median payment of $31,000 ($600–$636,500).

Summary for Regional Anesthesia Claims

Over one-third of the neuraxial regional anesthesia claims in the nonobstetric surgical anesthesia were associated with death or brain damage, and 16% with permanent nerve damage. Block-related mechanisms of injury accounted for over one-quarter of death or brain damage claims, with neuraxial cardiac arrest and high block as the two most common causes. Outcome after neuraxial cardiac arrest in this database remains poor despite the use of pulse oximetry and capnography, although successful resuscitations would be less likely to result in claims. Occurrence of neuraxial cardiac arrest in the prone position or during position changes on the table was associated with one third of these claims. Accidental intrathecal blocks comprised over half of the high spinal/epidural block claims. Although neuraxial hematoma is rare based on large prospective studies, this complication continues to occur in association with either intrinsic or iatrogenic anticoagulation and usually results in permanent damage to the neuraxis. Outcome from these three complications may be improved with heightened vigilance and rapid diagnosis and treatment.

Claims associated with peripheral nerve blocks are predominately of temporary severity of injury. Permanent nerve injury occurred in only 13% of the peripheral nerve block claims, and <4% of claims associated with death or brain damage were associated with a block-related mechanism of injury. Large randomized trials will need to determine if the use of ultrasound for peripheral nerve blocks will decrease the number of permanent nerve injuries compared to conventional techniques.

block claims (27% block technique, 6% unintentional intravenous injection/absorption, 6% pneumothorax, 2% needle trauma to nerve, 1% high block from unintentional intrathecal injection, 1% inadequate analgesia, and 3% unexplained block-related).

These results are consistent with data from prospective studies that have demonstrated relatively few high severity injuries associated with peripheral nerve blocks.[34–36] The voluntary reporting system established by Auroy et al.[34] over a 10-month period in France found only 7 high severity injuries out of 23,784 upper extremity blocks, and no cases were associated with death.[34] Lower extremity blocks were associated with slightly more high severity injuries in this study with 15 complications out of 20,162 blocks. It is unclear why there are so few claims associated with lower extremity blocks compared to upper extremity blocks in the Closed Claims Database, but it may be attributable to different practice patterns between France and the United States (e.g., possibly more neuraxial anesthetics are used for lower extremity procedures in the United States).

As almost half of the peripheral nerve block claims were associated with block technique as the mechanism of injury, improved tools or techniques to more accurately locate nerves and avoid surrounding tissues are needed. Several small studies have demonstrated the benefits of ultrasound in performance of peripheral nerve blocks, including reduced onset time for block and improvement in quality and duration of block.[37,38] It remains unclear if ultrasound-guided regional anesthesia will reduce the incidence of significant block-related injuries as randomized controlled trials are lacking (Chapter 17).[6,39]

Liability associated with peripheral nerve blocks was similar to neuraxial anesthetics and was related to severity of injury. The highest percentage of less than appropriate care (41%), the highest percentage of claims with payment (86%), and the highest median payments ($543,750—range $18,000–$1,875,000) were associated with the death or

▶ CHRONIC PAIN MANAGEMENT

Cervical Interventional Procedures—Review of the Literature

The role of interventional procedures for chronic pain management is controversial and efficacy is not well defined.[40,41] There is no strong evidence to support the use of any type of injection therapy (epidural, facet joint, or local sites) for subacute or chronic low back pain in patients without radicular pain.[42] Most common among interventional therapeutic pain treatments are the use of epidural injection of steroids to treat acute radicular pain often associated with disk herniation or spinal stenosis and facet injections to treat chronic neck or low back pain usually associated with facet degeneration. Increased utilization of interventional therapies and surgeries has not been associated with improved health status among patients with low back pain.[43] Evidence from randomized, placebo-controlled trials showing benefits of most nonsurgical interventional therapies for back pain is limited.[44] Despite the lack of proven efficacy, Medicare data demonstrated that overall growth in interventional techniques from 1998 to 2005 was 179%.[45] Between 1994 and 2001, there was a 271% increase in lumbar epidural steroid injections and a 231% increase in facet injections in a Medicare population.[46]

Transforaminal epidural steroid injections or selective nerve root blocks are frequently used both in the treatment of cervical radiculopathy and for diagnostic purposes. With increased utilization of interventional pain treatments, unanticipated complications have been reported, particularly an increase in neurologic injuries, including spinal cord infarction and stroke, which have been associated with interventional pain treatment.[47–50] Serious reported complications include anterior spinal artery syndrome,[51,52] quadriplegia,[53] ischemic stroke,[54,55] and death.[56] Catastrophic neurologic complications may occur as a result of radicular arterial uptake of injectate, arterial perforation leading to dissection/thrombosis, and needle-induced vasospasm.[48] Nahm et al.[57] reported that the highest incidence of intravascular injection during transforaminal injections was at the cervical level. This may occur because of differences in the content of the vessels in the intervertebral foramina resulting from different types of arterial supply to the spinal cord at various spinal levels. In the thoracolumbar levels, spinal arterial branches arise from the aorta and iliac vessels while in the cervical spine, arterial branches to the cord arise from the vertebral, ascending cervical, superior intercostals, and deep cervical arteries (see Figure 12-2).

Anterior spinal artery syndrome and cerebellar ischemia are devastating complications of cervical transforaminal injections. Reports of anterior spinal artery syndrome or brain injury occurring during cervical transforaminal steroid injections raise safety concerns.[50,51,56,58–61] A potential hazard to the safe performance of cervical transforaminal injections would be the presence of a vessel that communicates with the anterior spinal artery in the posterior aspect of the foramen. Ascending and deep cervical arterial branches enter the external opening of the posterior intervertebral foramen near the classic target area for transforaminal epidural injections.[62] These branches occasionally supply anterior radicular and segmental medullary arteries to the spinal cord. Because these arteries are contributors to anterior spinal artery flow, injection into or injury to these vessels may explain the occurrence of ischemic neurologic events (Chapter 28).

Although interlaminar cervical injections are generally considered safer than transforaminal injections, serious complications can also occur with the interlaminar approach.[63] Cervical spine anatomy is not analogous to the lumbar spine, and the distance to the dura and the dimensions of the cervical epidural space varies.[64,65] Some authors recommend not injecting higher than C6-7 interspace as the epidural space is largest in this area[66] and, if a preprocedure MRI shows significant canal narrowing at the level of pathology, performing the injection below that level or avoiding the injection entirely.[53] Epidural procedures in the cervical region may be more prone to complications because of the narrow distance between the ligamentum flavum and the spinal cord.[63] Severe neurologic injuries have been reported after interlaminar injections, caused by needle trauma to the spinal cord or nerves.[67–71] Fluoroscopic guidance is widely used and advocated to obtain accurate needle positioning but cannot guarantee prevention of dural puncture or spinal cord penetration either by the interlaminar[72] or transforaminal approach.[73]

Cervical Interventional Procedures: ASA Closed Claims Analysis

Summary of Results

A second analysis of the 294 chronic pain malpractice claims collected between 2005 and 2008 by the ASA Closed Claims Project was published in *Anesthesiology* in 2011.[12] This work compared 64 claims for cervical procedures (22%) to all other chronic pain claims collected during this period. Most (83%) of the claims related to cervical procedures that occurred between 2000 and 2006.

The mechanism of injury in these claims and the use of sedation in spinal cord injury claims were of particular interest in this analysis. Neuraxial injury was defined by the anatomic location where the injury occurred (including epidural, intrathecal, or other areas) and by the mechanism of the injury. Injuries may result from compressive lesions, ischemia/infarction, direct trauma, or other mechanisms. Clinical manifestations of neuraxial injuries consisted of quadriplegia or quadriparesis, paraplegia or paraparesis, unilateral tract signs unilateral (including corticospinal tract as manifested by ipsilateral hemiparesis, spinothalamic tract manifested by contralateral pain or temperature loss, or dorsal column usually manifesting as ipsilateral proprioception), bilateral tract signs, reticulospinal, and gray matter injuries.

Of the 64 cervical procedures involved in these claims, almost all were blocks or injections (91%) with four claims (6%) for radiofrequency ablation. Forty-three of the 58 blocks (67%) were epidurals (of which 41 were steroid injections—12 transforaminal and 28 interlaminar), seven (11%) were stellate ganglion blocks, and six (9%) were trigger point injections. The indication for these procedures was cervical radicular pain in 50%, neck pain of musculoskeletal origin in 28%, complex regional pain syndrome in 11%, and spinal stenosis in 5%. Patients in malpractice claims who underwent a cervical procedure were more likely to be women (73%; $p < 0.011$) and healthier ($p < 0.001$) than other chronic pain patients.

Almost 60% of patients who had cervical procedures experienced spinal cord injuries compared to 11% of those receiving other chronic pain treatment ($p < 0.001$, Fig. 36-5) with the majority (91%) occurring during epidural procedures (20 of these were interlaminar injections and 10 were transforaminal injections). Of interest, other procedures such as trigger-point injections, stellate ganglion block, and facet injection were also associated with spinal cord injury. The majority of the 38 spinal cord injuries (87%) resulted in permanent

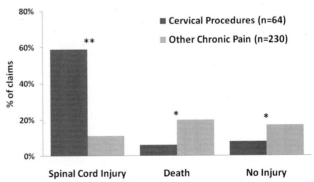

FIGURE 36-5. Cervical procedure outcomes compared to other chronic pain treatment. *$p < 0.01$; **$p < 0.001$.

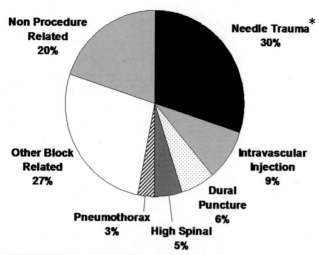

FIGURE 36-6. Mechanism of injury associated with cervical procedures (n = 64). Eighty percent of damaging events were procedure-related. *More likely to be associated with general anesthesia or sedation (p < 0.01).

disabling injuries and manifested as quadriplegia/quadriparesis (27%), paraplegia/paraparesis (18%), and hemiplegia/hemiparesis (9%). Fifty-three percent of the spinal cord injuries resulted from direct needle trauma, 16% were a result of cord infarction after intra-arterial injection, and 8% were a result of hematoma caused by cord compression. Care was deemed less than appropriate in 52% of claims. Payment was made in 51% of claims, and the median payment for cervical procedures was $388,600 (range, $642–$2,681,720).

Eighty percent of injuries were related to the procedure performed (Fig. 36-6). Direct needle trauma or spinal cord infarction/stroke following intra-arterial injections featured prominently. Of the nine (14%) cervical procedure claims associated with cord infarction or stroke after intra-arterial injection, five caused spinal cord infarction following cervical transforaminal injection of particulate steroid (three triamcinolone, one methylprednisolone, and one unspecified). In three other claims, cervical transforaminal injection of particulate steroid (methylprednisolone) resulted in stroke, presumably via injection of particulate steroid into the vertebral artery. The last case possibly resulted from direct intra-arterial injection during a stellate ganglion block.

Sedation or general anesthesia was used in 67% of claims associated with spinal cord injury compared to 19% of cervical procedure claims not associated with spinal cord injuries (p < 0.001). One-fourth of the patients who sustained spinal cord injuries during cervical procedures were nonresponsive compared to 5% of the patients who had cervical procedures but did not sustain spinal cord injuries (p < 0.05).

Not all claims in this analysis provided information on whether radiographic guidance was used, but it was used in 76% of cervical procedure claims with spinal cord injury. Contrast was used with radiographic guidance in 57% of claims with spinal cord injury compared with 17% of claims without spinal cord injury after a cervical procedure. On-site reviewers indicated that the appropriate use of radiographic guidance would have prevented the injury in 45% of cervical procedure claims with spinal cord injury compared with 17% of cervical procedure claims without spinal cord injury.

Implications of Closed Claims Analysis

Although there are few data on safety and effectiveness of these interventional procedures for chronic pain,[74,75] their use has increased in recent years. This analysis of closed claims data provides a greater understanding of the mechanism of these injuries. Injuries associated with cervical procedures were often related to direct needle trauma and likely resulted in permanent debilitating consequences. Direct needle trauma was more common with an interlaminar than with the transforaminal approach but this may be a reflection of more frequent use of an interlaminar than a transforaminal approach rather than a greater risk with an interlaminar approach. Safety concerns regarding transforaminal steroid injections appear to be well founded. In this analysis, 8 of 64 cervical procedure claims involved embolization of particulate steroid during cervical transforaminal injection with five resulting in spinal cord infarction and three resulting in strokes.

The use of sedation and/or general anesthesia remains controversial. Proponents argue it reduces the risk of injury from sudden movement by the patient while opponents argue sedation limits the patient's ability to report symptoms if there is needle contact with the spinal cord or peripheral nerves. Injuries were associated with the use of sedation or general anesthesia for procedures. Patients were more likely to be nonresponsive during the procedure and consequently unable to indicate an immediate reaction to needle trauma. The use of sedation or general anesthesia during cervical procedures remains controversial. The American Society of Regional Anesthesia and Pain Medicine (ASRA) advisory panel on the use regional anesthesia in anesthetized or heavily sedated patients suggests that warning signs such as paresthesia or pain on injection of local anesthetic inconsistently herald needle contact with the spinal cord. General anesthesia or heavy sedation removes that ability for the patient to recognize and report warning signs and suggests that neuraxial regional anesthesia should be performed rarely in adult patients whose sensorium is compromised by general anesthesia or heavy sedation.[76]

The use of radiographic guidance for these procedures remains controversial. The closed claims analysis does not contribute to scientific evidence to judge the impact of radiographic guidance on the safety of pain interventions. Despite strong advocacy for the use of guidance particularly fluoroscopic multiplanar views during needle placement,[77–80] closed claims analysis showed that spinal cord injury occurred more often when radiographic guidance was used. However, it is possible that radiographic guidance was used incorrectly and may have given practitioners a false sense of security of accurate needle placement that, in itself, increased the risk of spinal cord injury. We recommend the disciplined use with appropriate interpretation of multiplanar fluoroscopy so that the exact needle location can be determined with precision.

Recommendations for Cervical Neuraxial Injections

Transforaminal cervical epidural injections have been postulated to be more effective than interlaminar injections (Box 36-3). However, prospective studies are needed to compare the techniques. Both procedures have the potential for catastrophic complications. Whether one technique is safer than another is unknown. The risk of dural puncture

BOX 36-3 Recommendations for Cervical Neuraxial Injections

1. Minimal to no sedation
2. Contrast enhanced multiplanar fluoroscopy
3. Test dose bolus of short-acting local anesthetic (lidocaine)
4. Five minute post bolus monitoring for neurologic sequelae

may be higher with an interlaminar than a transforaminal approach.[81] The spinal cord is at risk of puncture with interlaminar cervical epidural injection. The ligamentum flavum in the cervical region may be deficient in the midline and the interspinous ligament absent.[82] Consequently, if utilizing a loss of resistance technique, lack of resistance from absence of the interspinous ligament and unfused ligamentum flavum could lead to unintended dural and cord puncture. Ideally, procedures should be performed under fluoroscopy to reduce risk of serious complications and to ensure appropriate delivery of medication into the epidural space.

Chronic Pain Medication Management— Review of the Literature

In contrast to interventional procedures, medication management is considered well established and integral to chronic pain management.[83–85] Nonopioid analgesics (acetaminophen, nonsteroidal anti-inflammatory agents), tricyclic antidepressants, specific anticonvulsants, and opioids have well-established efficacy.[84,86,87] Opioids alleviate nociceptive and neuropathic pain.[88] Since the 1990s, there has been a consensus that patients with chronic cancer and noncancer pain may benefit from the use of opioids to control pain and allow for greater functionality.[89,90] Furthermore, for some refractory chronic pain problems such as neuropathic pain, opioids are recommended as a component of long-term pharmacologic management.[84,91–93] In aggregate, no prevalence measures of prescription opioid usage in a US population with chronic pain have been published, but the prescription volume of opioids has increased by an order of magnitude over the last 15 years.[94] Some groups estimate that approximately 3% of the US general population without cancer uses opioids regularly for a month or more per year.[95]

The overall value of long-term opioid therapy for chronic pain is determined by a relatively poorly understood balance of costs and benefits.[96] Of some concern, rates of death from opioid poisoning have increased.[97–101] The number of opioid poisonings reported in death certificates increased by 91% between 1999 and 2002.[98] This increase in deaths is perhaps not surprising in light of recent studies that found 11% to 24% of all medication management patients were engaging in aberrant drug-related behaviors[102–104] and that 15% of patients receiving medication management for pain had illicit drugs documented by urine toxicology screening.[102] In a study from Denmark, patients with chronic pain using opioids had a higher risk of death than patients without chronic pain (HR: 1.67; 95% CI: 1.03–2.70).[105] Dunn et al.[106] reported an increased risk of overdose among patients receiving medically prescribed opioids at higher dosage levels and that most opioid overdoses were medically serious with 12% being fatal.[106]

Use of prescription pain relievers without a prescription or only for the experience or feeling they caused ("nonmedical" use) is, after marijuana use, the second most common form of illicit drug use in the United States. The National Survey on Drug Use and Health estimated in 2007 that 2.1% of persons aged 12 or older (~5.2 million persons) reported using prescription pain relievers nonmedically in the past month.[107] According to the Drug Abuse Warning Network (DAWN), during 2004 to 2008, the estimated frequency of emergency department visits for nonmedical use of opioid analgesics increased 111% during 2004 to 2008 (from 144,600 to 305,900 visits). Oxycodone, hydrocodone, and methadone were the most frequently reported opioids, and all three increased significantly during the 5-year period.[108] According to the Centers for Disease Control and Prevention (CDC), deaths from unintentional drug overdoses in the United States have been rising steeply since the early 1990s and are the second-leading cause of accidental death, with 27,658 such deaths recorded in 2007. Between 1997 and 2002, sales of oxycodone and methadone nearly quadrupled. Although both per capita opioid sales and death rates from the drugs vary widely among the 50 states, studies have found a strong correlation between states with the highest drug-poisoning mortality and those with the highest opioid consumption; per capita sales are most strongly linked with methadone- and oxycodone-related mortality.[99]

In almost every age group, men have higher death rates from drug overdoses than women. The highest mortality for both sexes occurs among people 45 to 54 years of age, although young adults abuse opioids and other drugs more frequently and are more likely to be seen with drug-related symptoms in emergency rooms. Patients taking long-term high daily doses of opioids are at increased risk for overdose.[106] The majority of overdose deaths in West Virginia in 2006 were associated with nonmedical use and diversion of pharmaceuticals, primarily opioid analgesics.[109] Cone et al.[110] reported on oxycodone involvement in drug abuse deaths and found the vast majority of cases (889 out of 919; 96.7%) involved multiple drugs.[110] An average of 3.5 drugs in addition to oxycodone was identified by toxicology testing in the 889 cases of multiple drug abuse. The most prevalent drugs used in combination with oxycodone were benzodiazepines, alcohol, cocaine, other opioids, marijuana, and tricyclic antidepressants.

With increasing frequencies of chronic pain treatments and deleterious outcomes associated with the increase in chronic pain care provided by anesthesiologists, we anticipated an increase in malpractice claims for chronic pain care. A previous review of malpractice claims in the ASA Closed Claims database found 2% of all claims between 1970 and 1994 were for chronic pain care.[111] A follow-up analysis of claims in the same database from 1995 to 1999 found 8% of all claims were for some form of chronic pain care.[112] Because of this increase in chronic pain liability, additional data were collected by the ASA Closed Claims Project on all chronic pain claims, including medication management and interventional procedures, beginning in 2005. We revised our data collection form to specifically collect detailed information on chronic pain management for closed chronic pain management malpractice claims collected from 2005 onward. This review is focused on anesthesia malpractice claims for medication management problems and on injury and liability associated with cervical interventional procedures for chronic pain.

Medication Management: ASA Closed Claims Analysis

Summary of Results

As reported in *Anesthesiology* in 2010,[11] the ASA Closed Claims database was used to compare medication management claims to all other chronic pain claims collected between 2005 and 2008. Factors associated with the death of patients were of particular interest in malpractice claims for medication management.

Of the 294 claims collected between 2005 and 2008, 51 (17%) involved medication management. These patients were more likely to be younger males ($p < 0.01$; 88% were younger than 51 years; 35% were between 17 and 35 years old) with back pain (53%) compared to the patients in other types of chronic pain claims. Ninety-four percent of these patients were prescribed opioids with 58% also prescribed additional psychoactive medications. Controlled- or extended-release oxycodone (41%), methadone (35%), and hydrocodone (22%) were the opioids most frequently prescribed. Compared to other chronic pain claims, death was the most common outcome in medication management claims (57% compared to 9%, $p < 0.01$, Fig. 36-7). Death was more likely to occur if the patient was prescribed long-acting opioids, additional psychoactive medications (which were either prescribed or were used without the prescriber's knowledge), and displayed three or more behavioral factors commonly associated with medication misuse. In about one-quarter of all medication management claims, addiction was alleged by the patient. Of the patients whose deaths were not considered to occur as a result of medications, predominant causes included suicide, possible suicide, or other patient comorbidities.

Eighty percent of the patients in medication management claims displayed at least one factor commonly associated with medication misuse, and one-quarter of all medication management patients had three or more factors commonly associated with medication misuse. Factors commonly associated with medication misuse included both past patient characteristics and concurrent behaviors in which the patient was engaging. In this analysis, 23 of the 51 patients (45%) first presented to the treating anesthesiologist with a history of depression and 18 (35%) presented with a history of drug and/or alcohol problems. While under the care of an anesthesiologist, 17 of the 51 patients were obtaining prescriptions from multiple providers, 10 were combining alcohol or illicit drugs with their medications, and 7 were escalating doses without the permission of the physician. Patients did not cooperate in their care in 35 claims (69%). Examples of these behaviors are listed in Table 36-3.

Many of the anesthesiologists in these malpractice claims also failed to provide appropriate medication management. Failing to communicate with other prescribing physicians (18%) and failing to monitor medication compliance through screening or pill counts (18%) were the most common inappropriate behaviors engaged in by physicians. Other problematic physician behaviors included prescribing too high dosages, poor documentation of care provided, inadequate monitoring of patients' psychological problems, inappropriate sexual relationships with patients, and selling prescriptions (Table 36-4).

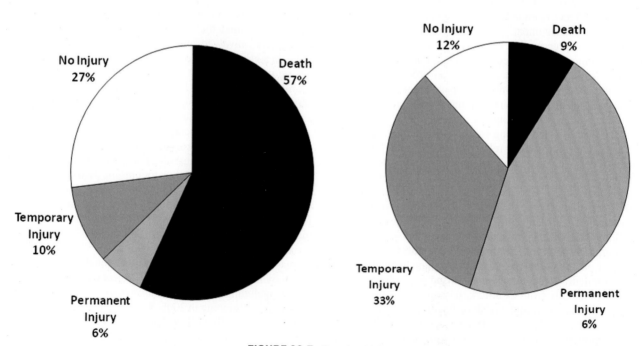

FIGURE 36-7. Severity of injury.

TABLE 36-3 Most Common Forms of Noncooperation in Care by Patients (*n* = 35)

BEHAVIOR	NUMBER OF CLAIMS
Obtaining prescriptions from multiple providers	17
Taking opioids without knowledge of pain management physician	14
Taking psychoactive medications without knowledge of pain management physician	11
Concomitant alcohol use	2
Concomitant illicit drug abuse	8
Dose escalation of prescribed medication without permission	7
Losing prescriptions	2
Taking psychoactive medications prescribed by someone else	2
Crushing pills (to inject or inhale)	2
Selling prescribed medications	1

More than half (57%) of patients showing these behaviors died. Total number of behaviors are >35 because some patients engaged in more than one behavior.

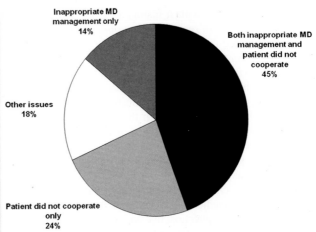

FIGURE 36-8. Issues in medication management (*n* = 51). (Reprinted from Fitzgibbon DR, Rathmell JP, Michna E, et al. Malpractice claims associated with medication management for chronic pain. *Anesthesiology* 2010;112(4):948–956, with permission.)

The patients' problematic behaviors contributed to the patients' outcomes in almost 70% of all claims (Fig. 36-8). In addition, the physicians' inappropriate medication management of their patients contributed to the patients' deleterious outcomes in almost 60% of medication management claims (Fig. 36-8). More than 80% of all medication claims had at least one of these contributing events to poor outcomes with almost one-half having both poor medication management by physicians and inappropriate or risky behaviors by the patients. Payment was more likely to be made in those claims where the physician had provided poor medication management than in those claims where the physician provided appropriate management.

Lessons Learned

Clinical recommendations for medication are summarized in Box 36-4. For physicians providing medication management, a continuing awareness that many of the patients presenting for medication management of chronic pain have personal and/or family histories that can be associated with deleterious outcomes, including death, is paramount in the prescription of opioids and other psychoactive medications. In the closed claims study, 45% of patients first presented to the treating anesthesiologist with a history of depression

TABLE 36-4 Common Forms of Inappropriate Medication Management by Physicians (*n* = 30)

BEHAVIOR	NUMBER OF CLAIMS
Inadequate communication with other prescribing physicians to coordinate care plan	9
Inadequate monitoring of medication compliance through screening or pill counts or failing to recognize signs of medication misuse	9
Prescribing inappropriately high doses of opioids	3
Inappropriate sexual relations with patient	2
Others[a]	7

[a]Others include wrong dosage, poor documentation of care, inadequate monitoring of patient's psychological problems, and inappropriate sale of opioid prescriptions by the anesthesiologist.

BOX 36-4 Recommendations for Medication Management

1. Thoroughly assess and diagnose the pain complaint
2. Outline a comprehensive care plan
3. Inform the patient of potential risks and benefits of long-term medication use
4. Avoid or minimize polypharmacy
5. Periodically check compliance and appropriateness of care
6. Inform other providers of care of treatment course and actions

and 35% presented with a history of drug and/or alcohol problems. Failure to recognize these issues in chronic pain patients who are prescribed opioids and other psychoactive medications may place these patients at risk for engaging in drug-seeking or other aberrant behaviors. In this study, many patients engaged in aberrant drug-related behaviors (obtaining prescriptions from multiple providers, combining alcohol or illicit drugs with their medications, escalating doses without the permission of the physician, taking medications prescribed for others, requesting early refills, failing drug screening tests, and reporting lost prescriptions or medications).

Most of the claims involved patients with risk behaviors associated with medication misuse and the use of long-acting opioids and other psychoactive medications. Although the use of long-acting opioids and the use of additional psychoactive medications with long-acting opioids were associated with greater mortality, it is impossible to say whether the relationship is causal. However, given the severity of this outcome, physicians must be cognizant of how this combination of factors may place patients at risk. Most importantly, the risks associated with concomitant prescription of other psychoactive medications with opioids should be recognized and all efforts to minimize or eliminate these medications for long-term care made.

Opioid prescribing practices for chronic pain have increased markedly in the community. Such prescribing may or may not conform to published practice guidelines. Standards of care for chronic pain management and long-term opioid therapy are subject to current federal and state laws, regulatory guidelines, and policy statements.[113–116] Professional organizations have also published guidelines for care in this area.[74,117] In the closed claims review, substandard medication management by physicians was associated with higher mortality. Almost 60% of the anesthesiologists failed to properly manage their patients' medications by not communicating with previous and other current medication providers, not ordering drug screenings or pill counts, not referring patients for psychiatric evaluation when appropriate, failing to examine medical records and results from drug screenings when they were ordered, extremely poor record keeping, and failure to recognize obvious signs of substance abuse and drug-seeking behaviors. Most failed to observe either national- or state-level guidelines for appropriate management of patients on opioids and other controlled substances. While, in some cases, there were no obvious signs of misuse of medication, most claims either had obvious signs or would have if the physicians had ordered any standard monitoring tests or had been in contact with the patients' other current and/or past providers of medication. While this poor level of medication management is not common among most providers, these closed malpractice claims reveal the potentially devastating results when medication is not managed appropriately.

Addiction was alleged in about one-quarter of the claims. It was not always possible to tell from the limited information in this format of review whether patients were actually addicted or simply making allegations of addiction. Similarly, it was not usually possible to determine the temporal relationship of addiction, that is, if patients had preexisting problems prior to the anesthesiologist assuming care or subsequently developed the problem are commencement of care. However, it is noteworthy that the only claims where payments were made for an allegation of addiction had clear evidence of inappropriate medication management by the physician. Due to the problems associated with identifying patients at risk for addiction, standard recommendations should be followed for identifying this problem, such as gathering information on a personal and family history of drug and alcohol abuse when initially assuming care for patients and regularly monitoring all patients for noncompliance through drug screens and pill counts.[118]

▶ SUMMARY

As chronic pain management has become more popular, claims for complications have increased dramatically. Recent ASA Closed Claims studies highlighted risks of chronic pain medication management and cervical neuraxial injections.

ACKNOWLEDGMENTS

Supported in part by the American Society of Anesthesiologists (ASA), Park Ridge, Illinois. The authors acknowledge Karen Posner, PhD, for data analysis and Lynn Akerlund for manuscript preparation.

References

1. Rodgers A, Walker N, Schug S, et al. Reduction of postoperative mortality and morbidity with epidural or spinal anaesthesia: results from overview of randomised trials. *BMJ* 2000;321:1493–1496.
2. Wulf H, Biscoping J, Beland B, et al. Ropivacaine epidural anesthesia and analgesia versus general anesthesia and intravenous patient-controlled analgesia with morphine in the perioperative management of hip replacement. Ropivacaine Hip Replacement Multicenter Study Group. *Anesth Analg* 1999;89:111–116.
3. Rasmussen LS, Johnson T, Kuipers HM, et al. Does anaesthesia cause postoperative cognitive dysfunction? A randomised study of regional versus general anaesthesia in 438 elderly patients. *Acta Anaesthesiol Scand* 2003;47:260–266.
4. Orebaugh SL, Williams BA, Vallejo M, et al. Adverse outcomes associated with stimulator-based peripheral nerve blocks with versus without ultrasound visualization. *Reg Anesth Pain Med* 2009;34(3):251–255.
5. Liu SS, Gordon MA, Shaw PM, et al. A prospective clinical registry of ultrasound-guided regional anesthesia for ambulatory shoulder surgery. *Anesth Analg* 2010;111(3):617–623.
6. Neal JM, Brull R, Chan VW, et al. The ASRA evidence-based medicine assessment of ultrasound-guided regional anesthesia and pain medicine: executive summary. *Reg Anesth Pain Med* 2010;35:S1–S9.
7. Okie S. A flood of opioids, a rising tide of deaths. *N Engl J Med* 2010;363(21):1981–1985.
8. Cheney FW, Posner KL, Caplan RA, et al. Standard of care and anesthesia liability. *JAMA* 1989;261:1599–1603.
9. Cheney FW. The American Society of Anesthesiologists Closed Claims Project: what have we learned, how has it affected practice, and how will it affect practice in the future? *Anesthesiology* 1999;91:552–556.
10. Lee LA, Posner KL, Domino KB, et al. Injuries associated with regional anesthesia in the 1980s and 1990s. *Anesthesiology* 2004;101:143–152.
11. Fitzgibbon DR, Rathmell JP, Michna E, et al. Malpractice claims associated with medication management for chronic pain. *Anesthesiology* 2010;112(4):948–956.

12. Rathmell JP, Michna E, Fitzgibbon DR, et al. Injury and liability associated with cervical procedures for chronic pain. *Anesthesiology* 2011;114:918–926.

13. Lee LA, Domino KB. The closed claims project: has it influenced anesthetic practice and outcome? *Anesthesiol Clin North America* 2002;20:485–501.

14. Caplan RA, Posner KL, Cheney FW. Effect of outcome on physician judgements of appropriateness of care. *JAMA* 1991;265:1957–1960.

15. Caplan RA, Ward RJ, Posner KL, et al. Unexpected cardiac arrest during spinal anesthesia: a closed claims analysis of predisposing factors. *Anesthesiology* 1988;68:5–11.

16. Lovstad RZ, Granhus G, Hetland S. Bradycardia and asystolic cardiac arrest during spinal anaesthesia: a report of five cases. *Acta Anaesthesiol Scand* 2000;44:48–52.

17. Lesser JB, Sanborn KV, Valskys R, et al. Severe bradycardia during spinal and epidural anesthesia recorded by an anesthesia information management system. *Anesthesiology* 2003;99:859–866.

18. Rosenberg JM, Wahr JA, Sung CH, et al. Coronary perfusion pressure during cardiopulmonary resuscitation after spinal anesthesia in dogs. *Anesth Analg* 1996;82:84–87.

19. Rosenberg JM, Wortsman J, Wahr JA, et al. Impaired neuroendocrine response mediates refractoriness to cardiopulmonary resuscitation in spinal anesthesia. *Crit Care Med* 1998;26:533–537.

20. Geffin B, Shapiro L. Sinus bradycardia and asystole during spinal and epidural anesthesia: a report of 13 cases. *J Clin Anesth* 1998;10:278–285.

21. Zaric D, Pace NL. Transient neurologic symptoms (TNS) following spinal anaesthesia with lidocaine versus other local anaesthetics. *Cochrane Database Syst Rev* 2009;(2):CD003006.

22. Loo CC, Irestedt L. Cauda equina syndrome after spinal anaesthesia with hyperbaric 5% lignocaine: a review of six cases of cauda equina syndrome reported to the Swedish Pharmaceutical Insurance 1993–1997. *Acta Anaesthesiol Scand* 1999;43(4):371–379.

23. Muguruma T, Sakura S, Saito Y. Epidural lidocaine induces dose-dependent neurologic injury in rats. *Anesth Analg* 2006;103(4):876–881.

24. Werdehausen R, Braun S, Essmann F, et al. Lidocaine induces apoptosis via the mitochondrial pathway independently of death receptor signaling. *Anesthesiology* 2007;107(1):136–143.

25. Christopherson R, Beattie C, Frank SM, et al. Perioperative morbidity in patients randomized to epidural or general anesthesia for lower extremity vascular surgery. Perioperative Ischemia Randomized Anesthesia Trial Study Group. *Anesthesiology* 1993;79:422–434.

26. Hickey NC, Wilkes MP, Howes D, et al. The effect of epidural anaesthesia on peripheral resistance and graft flow following femorodistal reconstruction. *Eur J Vasc Endovasc Surg* 1995;9:93–96.

27. Tuman KJ, McCarthy RJ, March RJ, et al. Effects of epidural anesthesia and analgesia on coagulation and outcome after major vascular surgery. *Anesth Analg* 1991;73:696–704.

28. Barbosa FT, Cavalcante JC, Jucá MJ, et al. Neuraxial anaesthesia for lower-limb revascularization. *Cochrane Database Syst Rev* 2010;(1):CD007083.

29. Rao TL, El-Etr AA. Anticoagulation following placement of epidural and subarachnoid catheters: an evaluation of neurologic sequelae. *Anesthesiology* 1981;55:618–620.

30. Odoom JA, Sih IL. Epidural analgesia and anticoagulant therapy. Experience with one thousand cases of continuous epidurals. *Anaesthesia* 1983;38:254–259.

31. Baron HC, LaRaja RD, Rossi G, et al. Continuous epidural analgesia in the heparinized vascular surgical patient: a retrospective review of 912 patients. *J Vasc Surg* 1987;6:144–146.

32. Kim JT, Bahk JH, Sung J. Influence of age and sex on the position of the conus medullaris and Tuffier's line in adults. *Anesthesiology* 2003;99:1359–1363.

33. Render CA. The reproducibility of the iliac crest as a marker of lumbar spine level. *Anaesthesia* 1996;51:1070–1071.

34. Borgeat A, Ekatodramis G, Kalberer F, et al. Acute and nonacute complications associated with interscalene block and shoulder surgery: a prospective study. *Anesthesiology* 2001;95:875–880.

35. Auroy Y, Benhamou D, Bargues L, et al. Major complications of regional anesthesia in France: the SOS Regional Anesthesia Hotline Service. *Anesthesiology* 2002;97:1274–1280.

36. Stan TC, Krantz MA, Solomon DL, et al. The incidence of neurovascular complications following axillary brachial plexus block using a transarterial approach. A prospective study of 1,000 consecutive patients. *Reg Anesth* 1995;20:486–492.

37. Williams SR, Chouinard P, Arcand G, et al. Ultrasound guidance speeds execution and improves the quality of supraclavicular block. *Anesth Analg* 2003;97:1518–1523.

38. Marhofer P, Sitzwohl C, Greher M, et al. Ultrasound guidance for infraclavicular brachial plexus anaesthesia in children. *Anaesthesia* 2004;59:642–646.

39. Neal JM. Ultrasound-guided regional anesthesia and patient safety: an evidence-based analysis. *Reg Anesth Pain Med* 2010;35:S59–S67.

40. Henschke N, Kuijpers T, Rubinstein SM, et al. Injection therapy and denervation procedures for chronic low-back pain: a systematic review. *Eur Spine J* 2010;19:1425–1449.

41. Staal JB, de Bie R, de Vet HC, et al. Injection therapy for subacute and chronic low-back pain. *Cochrane Database Syst Rev* 2008;(3):CD001824.

42. Staal JB, de Bie RA, de Vet HC, et al. Injection therapy for subacute and chronic low back pain: an updated Cochrane review. *Spine* 2009;34:49–59.

43. Martin BI, Deyo RA, Mirza SK, et al. Expenditures and health status among adults with back and neck problems. *JAMA* 2008;299:656–664.

44. Chou R, Atlas SJ, Stanos SP, et al. Nonsurgical interventional therapies for low back pain: a review of the evidence for an American Pain Society clinical practice guideline. *Spine* 2009;34:1078–1093.

45. Boswell MV, Trescot AM, Datta S, et al. Interventional techniques: evidence-based practice guidelines in the management of chronic spinal pain. *Pain Phys* 2007;10:7–111.

46. Friedly J, Chan L, Deyo R. Increases in lumbosacral injections in the Medicare population: 1994 to 2001. *Spine* 2007;32:1754–1760.

47. Edlow BL, Wainger BJ, Frosch MP, et al. Posterior circulation stroke after C1-C2 intraarticular facet steroid injection: evidence for diffuse microvascular injury. *Anesthesiology* 2010;112:1532–1535.

48. Malhotra G, Abbasi A, Rhee M. Complications of transforaminal cervical epidural steroid injections. *Spine* 2009;34:731–739.

49. Rathmell JP. Toward improving the safety of transforaminal injection. *Anesth Analg* 2009;109:8–10.

50. Rathmell JP, Aprill C, Bogduk N. Cervical transforaminal injection of steroids. *Anesthesiology* 2004;100:1595–1600.

51. Brouwers PJ, Kottink EJ, Simon MA, et al. A cervical anterior spinal artery syndrome after diagnostic blockade of the right C6-nerve root. *Pain* 2001;91:397–399.

52. Rosenkranz M, Grzyska U, Niesen W, et al. Anterior spinal artery syndrome following periradicular cervical nerve root therapy. *J Neurol* 2004;251:229–231.

53. Bose B. Quadriparesis following cervical epidural steroid injections: case report and review of the literature. *Spine J* 2005;5:558–563.

54. Beckman WA, Mendez RJ, Paine GF, et al. Cerebellar herniation after cervical transforaminal epidural injection. *Reg Anesth Pain Med* 2006;31:282–285.

55. Scanlon GC, Moeller-Bertram T, Romanowsky SM, et al. Cervical transforaminal epidural steroid injections: more dangerous than we think? *Spine (Phila Pa 1976)* 2007;32:1249–1256.

56. Rozin L, Rozin R, Koehler SA, et al. Death during transforaminal epidural steroid nerve root block (C7) due to perforation of the left vertebral artery. *Am J Forensic Med Pathol* 2003;24:351–355.

57. Nahm FS, Lee CJ, Lee SH, et al. Risk of intravascular injection in transforaminal epidural injections. *Anaesthesia* 2010;65:917–921.

58. Baker R, Dreyfuss P, Mercer S, et al. Cervical transforaminal injection of corticosteroids into a radicular artery: a possible mechanism for spinal cord injury. *Pain* 2003;103:211–215.

59. Karasek M, Bogduk N. Temporary neurologic deficit after cervical transforaminal injection of local anesthetic. *Pain Med* 2004;5:202–205.

60. Ludwig MA, Burns SP. Spinal cord infarction following cervical transforaminal epidural injection: a case report. *Spine* 2005;30:E266–E268.

61. Tiso RL, Cutler T, Catania JA, et al. Adverse central nervous system sequelae after selective transforaminal block: the role of corticosteroids. *Spine J* 2004;4:468–474.

62. Huntoon MA. Anatomy of the cervical intervertebral foramina: vulnerable arteries and ischemic neurologic injuries after transforaminal epidural injections. *Pain* 2005;117:104–111.

63. Abbasi A, Malhotra G, Malanga G, et al. Complications of interlaminar cervical epidural steroid injections: a review of the literature. *Spine (Phila Pa 1976)* 2007;32:2144–2151.

64. Han KR, Kim C, Park SK, et al. Distance to the adult cervical epidural space. *Reg Anesth Pain Med* 2003;28:95–97.

65. Lin CH, Lu CH, Ning FS. Distance from the skin to the cervical epidural space. *Acta Anaesthesiol Sin* 1995;33:161–164.

66. Goel A, Pollan JJ. Contrast flow characteristics in the cervical epidural space: an analysis of cervical epidurograms. *Spine (Phila Pa 1976)* 2006;31:1576–1579.

67. Abram SE, O'Connor TC. Complications associated with epidural steroid injections. *Reg Anesth* 1996;21:149–162.

68. Botwin KP, Castellanos R, Rao S, et al. Complications of fluoroscopically guided interlaminar cervical epidural injections. *Arch Phys Med Rehabil* 2003;84:627–633.

69. Breccia M, Gentilini F, Alimena G. Cocaine abuse may influence the response to imatinib in CML patients. *Haematologica* 2007;92:e41–e42.

70. Bromage PR, Benumof JL. Paraplegia following intracord injection during attempted epidural anesthesia under general anesthesia. *Reg Anesth Pain Med* 1998;23:104–107.

71. Hodges SD, Castleberg RL, Miller T, et al. Cervical epidural steroid injection with intrinsic spinal cord damage. Two case reports. *Spine (Phil Pa 1976)* 1998;23:2137–2142; discussion 2141–2142.

72. Khan S, Pioro EP. Cervical epidural injection complicated by syrinx formation: a case report. *Spine (Phil Pa 1976)* 2010;35:E614–E616.

73. Lee JH, Lee JK, Seo BR, et al. Spinal cord injury produced by direct damage during cervical transforaminal epidural injection. *Reg Anesth Pain Med* 2008;33:377–379.

74. Practice guidelines for chronic pain management: an updated report by the American Society of Anesthesiologists Task Force on Chronic Pain Management and the American Society of Regional Anesthesia and Pain Medicine. *Anesthesiology* 2010;112:810–833.

75. van Eerd M, Patijn J, Lataster A, et al. Cervical facet pain. *Pain Prac* 2010;10:113–123.

76. Bernards CM, Hadzic A, Suresh S, et al. Regional anesthesia in anesthetized or heavily sedated patients. *Reg Anesth Pain Med* 2008;33:449–460.

77. De Cordoba JL, Bernal J. Cervical transforaminal blocks should not be attempted by anyone without extensive documented experience in fluoroscopically guided injections. *Anesthesiology* 2004;100:1323–1324; author reply 1324.

78. Eckel TS, Bartynski WS. Epidural steroid injections and selective nerve root blocks. *Tech Vasc Interv Radiol* 2009;12:11–21.

79. Pobiel RS, Schellhas KP, Eklund JA, et al. Selective cervical nerve root blockade: prospective study of immediate and longer term complications. *AJNR Am J Neuroradiol* 2009;30:507–511.

80. Schellhas KP, Pollei SR, Johnson BA, et al. Selective cervical nerve root blockade: experience with a safe and reliable technique using an anterolateral approach for needle placement. *AJNR Am J Neuroradiol* 2007;28:1909–1914.

81. Huston CW. Cervical epidural steroid injections in the management of cervical radiculitis: interlaminar versus transforaminal. A review. *Curr Rev Musculoskelet Med* 2009;2:30–42.

82. Hogan QH. Epidural anatomy examined by cryomicrotome section. Influence of age, vertebral level, and disease. *Reg Anesth* 1996;21:395–406.

83. Argoff CE, Silvershein DI. A comparison of long- and short-acting opioids for the treatment of chronic noncancer pain: tailoring therapy to meet patient needs. *Mayo Clin Proc* 2009;84:602–612.

84. Dworkin RH, O'Connor AB, Backonja M, et al. Pharmacologic management of neuropathic pain: evidence-based recommendations. *Pain* 2007;132:237–251.

85. Portenoy RK. Opioid therapy for chronic nonmalignant pain: a review of the critical issues. *J Pain Symptom Manage* 1996;11:203–217.

86. Chou R, Huffman LH. Medications for acute and chronic low back pain: a review of the evidence for an American Pain Society/American College of Physicians clinical practice guideline. *Ann Intern Med* 2007;147:505–514.

87. Hauser W, Bernardy K, Uceyler N, et al. Treatment of fibromyalgia syndrome with gabapentin and pregabalin–a meta-analysis of randomized controlled trials. *Pain* 2009;145:69–81.

88. Kalso E, Edwards JE, Moore RA, et al. Opioids in chronic non-cancer pain: systematic review of efficacy and safety. *Pain* 2004;112:372–380.

89. No authors listed. The use of opioids for the treatment of chronic pain. A consensus statement from the American Academy of Pain Medicine and the American Pain Society. *Clin J Pain* 1997;13:6–8.

90. No authors listed. Management of cancer pain guideline overview. Agency for Health Care Policy and Research Rockville, Maryland. *J Natl Med Assoc* 1994;86:571–573, 634.

91. Finnerup NB, Sindrup SH, Jensen TS. The evidence for pharmacological treatment of neuropathic pain. *Pain* 2010;150:573–581.

92. Attal N, Cruccu G, Baron R, et al. EFNS guidelines on the pharmacological treatment of neuropathic pain: 2010 revision. *Eur J Neurol* 2010;17:1113-e88.

93. Zin CS, Nissen LM, Smith MT, et al. An update on the pharmacological management of post-herpetic neuralgia and painful diabetic neuropathy. *CNS Drugs* 2008;22:417–442.

94. Compton WM, Volkow ND. Major increases in opioid analgesic abuse in the United States: concerns and strategies. *Drug Alcohol Depend* 2006;81:103–107.

95. Sullivan MD, Edlund MJ, Steffick D, et al. Regular use of prescribed opioids: association with common psychiatric disorders. *Pain* 2005;119:95–103.

96. Sullivan MD, Von Korff M, Banta-Green C, et al. Problems and concerns of patients receiving chronic opioid therapy for chronic non-cancer pain. *Pain* 2010;149:345–353.

97. Fernandez W, Hackman H, McKeown L, et al. Trends in opioid-related fatal overdoses in Massachusetts, 1990–2003. *J Subst Abuse Treat* 2006;31:151–156.

98. Paulozzi LJ, Budnitz DS, Xi Y. Increasing deaths from opioid analgesics in the United States. *Pharmacoepidemiol Drug Saf* 2006;15:618–627.

99. Paulozzi LJ, Ryan GW. Opioid analgesics and rates of fatal drug poisoning in the United States. *Am J Prev Med* 2006;31:506–511.

100. Shah NG, Lathrop SL, Reichard RR, et al. Unintentional drug overdose death trends in New Mexico, USA, 1990–2005: combinations of heroin, cocaine, prescription opioids and alcohol. *Addiction* 2008;103:126–136.

101. Wysowski DK. Surveillance of prescription drug-related mortality using death certificate data. *Drug Safety* 2007;30:533–540.

102. Fishbain DA, Cole B, Lewis J, et al. What percentage of chronic nonmalignant pain patients exposed to chronic opioid analgesic therapy develop abuse/addiction and/or aberrant drug-related behaviors? A structured evidence-based review. *Pain Med* 2008;9:444–459.

103. Ives TJ, Chelminski PR, Hammett-Stabler CA, et al. Predictors of opioid misuse in patients with chronic pain: a prospective cohort study. *BMC Health Serv Res* 2006;6:46.

104. Martell BA, O'Connor PG, Kerns RD, et al. Systematic review: opioid treatment for chronic back pain: prevalence, efficacy, and association with addiction. *Ann Intern Med* 2007;146:116–127.

105. Sjogren P, Gronbaek M, Peuckmann V, et al. A population-based cohort study on chronic pain: the role of opioids. *Clin J Pain* 2010;26:763–769.

106. Dunn KM, Saunders KW, Rutter CM, et al. Opioid prescriptions for chronic pain and overdose: a cohort study. *Ann Intern Med* 2010;152:85–92.

107. Results from the 2007 National Survey on Drug Use and Health: National findings (NSDUH Series H-34. Rockville, MD). Substance Abuse and Mental Health Services Administration, Office of Applied Studies, 2008.

108. Centers for Disease Control and Prevention. Emergency department visits involving nonmedical use of selected prescription drugs - United States, 2004–2008. *MMWR Morb Mortal Wkly Rep* 2010;59:705–709.

109. Hall AJ, Logan JE, Toblin RL, et al. Patterns of abuse among unintentional pharmaceutical overdose fatalities. *JAMA* 2008;300:2613–2620.

110. Cone EJ, Fant RV, Rohay JM, et al. Oxycodone involvement in drug abuse deaths: a DAWN-based classification scheme applied to an oxycodone postmortem database containing over 1000 cases. *J Anal Toxicol* 2003;27:57–67.

111. Fitzgibbon DR, Posner KL, Domino KB, et al. Chronic pain management: American Society of Anesthesiologists Closed Claims Project. *Anesthesiology* 2004;100:98–105.

112. Liau DW, Fitzgibbon DR, Posner KL, et al. Trends in chronic pain management malpractice claims. *Anesthesiology* 2007;107:A1892.

113. Gilson AM. State medical board members' attitudes about the legality of chronic prescribing to patients with noncancer pain: the influence of knowledge and beliefs about pain management, addiction, and opioid prescribing. *J Pain Symptom Manage* 2010;40:599–612.

114. Gilson AM. The concept of addiction in law and regulatory policy related to pain management: a critical review. *Clin J Pain* 2010;26:70–77.

115. Gilson AM, Joranson DE, Maurer MA. Improving state pain policies: recent progress and continuing opportunities. *CA Cancer J Clin* 2007;57:341–353.

116. Joranson DE, Gilson AM, Dahl JL, et al. Pain management, controlled substances, and state medical board policy: a decade of change. *J Pain Symptom Manage* 2002;23:138–147.

117. Chou R, Fanciullo GJ, Fine PG, et al. Clinical guidelines for the use of chronic opioid therapy in chronic noncancer pain. *J Pain* 2009;10:113–130.

118. Turk DC, Swanson KS, Gatchel RJ. Predicting opioid misuse by chronic pain patients: a systematic review and literature synthesis. *Clin J Pain* 2008;24:497–508.

ATTORNEY PERSPECTIVES

37

The Use of Opioid Analgesics: Legal and Regulatory Issues

Diane E. Hoffmann

Although medical authorities clearly recognize the legitimacy of the use of opioids in the treatment of chronic pain, the problem of inadequate pain treatment persists. Among the multiple reasons for this pattern of neglect are physician fears of legal sanctions ranging from criminal prosecution and medical board disciplinary action to malpractice suits. Potential violation of Medicaid regulations and fraud and abuse rules may also deter physicians from prescribing opioids for pain management. Legal scrutiny of opioid prescribing is linked to opioid status as a controlled substance under federal law and to the potential for opioid addiction and abuse. Empirical evidence exists that some physicians undertreat pain due to this concern.[1-3] This chapter describes the legal basis for actions against physicians for opioid prescribing and provides examples of cases in which physicians have been sanctioned.

▶ DISCIPLINARY ACTIONS BY STATE MEDICAL BOARDS

In several studies, physicians have cited state medical board scrutiny as an obstacle to prescribing opioids for pain treatment. The U.S. government's "war on drugs" resulted in pressure on state medical boards in the 1980s and 1990s to discipline physicians who were "overprescribing" opioids. In some cases, this included physicians who were treating pain patients. A number of these cases received considerable attention in the media, although several were later overturned on appeal. In Florida, the state medical board disciplined Dr. Katherine Hoover for allegedly "inappropriately and excessively" prescribing various controlled substances to seven chronic pain patients. The sanctions included a $4,000 fine, continuing education in the prescribing of "abusable drugs," and 2 years of probation. The sanctions were imposed by the board despite the fact that the administrative hearing officer determined that the board had failed to prove its charges. Dr. Hoover appealed the board's decision to the Florida District Court of Appeal. In Hoover v. Agency for Health Care Administration, the Court reversed the board's decision and noted that the "physicians testifying in support of the board's action did not treat chronic pain patients" and that "despite this paucity of evidence, lack of familiarity, and seeming lack of expertise" the state's experts testified that Dr. Hoover had practiced below the standard of care.[4] The

Court also referred to the board's policing of pain prescription practices as a "draconian" policy.[4]

Another case that attracted considerable attention was that of Dr. William E. Hurwitz. Dr. Hurwitz was the subject of disciplinary action by both the Washington, DC, and Virginia medical boards. In 1996, the Virginia state medical board revoked Dr. Hurwitz's license to practice for 3 months based on "indiscriminate or excessive prescribing without therapeutic purpose and contrary to sound medical judgment." The board's action was initiated following the deaths of two of Hurwitz's pain patients. The action was taken despite the fact that "expert testimony had essentially disproved the state's allegation that Hurwitz was at fault." Based on the evidence, the board recognized that individuals with chronic pain often require high dosages of narcotics and dropped its initial allegations against Hurwitz, but did pursue action against him based on prescribing without adequate medical records.[5]

Since the mid-1990s, when these cases were brought, efforts to educate state medical boards and provide guidelines about appropriate prescribing of opioids for pain have arguably tempered medical board actions against physicians for prescribing high dosages of opioids. In 1998, the Federation of State Medical Boards (FSMB) promulgated Model Guidelines for the Use of Controlled Substances for the Treatment of Pain.

The guidelines included recommended language for adoption by state medical boards and stated in the preamble that "physicians should not fear disciplinary action" from state medical boards or other state regulatory agencies "for prescribing, dispensing or administering controlled substances, including opioid analgesics, for a legitimate medical purpose and in the usual course of professional practice" and that in states that adopt the guidelines the board "will consider prescribing, ordering, administering or dispensing controlled substances for pain to be for a legitimate medical purpose if based on scientific knowledge of the treatment of pain or if based on sound clinical grounds."

The guidelines also made it clear that boards should evaluate each case of prescribing for pain on an individual basis and not take disciplinary action against a physician for failing to adhere strictly to the provisions of the guidelines "if good cause is shown for such deviation." Boards, the guidelines stated, should also "judge the validity of prescribing based on the physician's treatment of the patient and on available documentation, rather than on the quantity and frequency of prescribing."

These guidelines were adopted in whole or in part by 24 states. A study of state medical boards in 2002 found that many had shifted their views about disciplinary action for prescribing of opioids. The study suggested (i) that many boards are attempting to find the appropriate balance between identifying physicians who inappropriately "overprescribe" and those who are appropriately treating patients with chronic pain and (ii) that boards are moving away from volume or quantity as a primary basis for investigating a physician connected with prescribing opioids.[6]

To provide additional encouragement to physicians to adequately treat pain, in 2004, the FSMB updated its 1998 guidelines and issued a Model Policy for the Use of Controlled Substances for the Treatment of Pain (Box 37-1). The new policy goes beyond attempting to reassure physicians

that they will not be sanctioned for prescribing large doses of pain medication if appropriate but sends a message that undertreatment of pain can be considered substandard care. In the preamble, the policy states that "the inappropriate treatment of pain includes nontreatment, undertreatment, overtreatment, and the continued use of ineffective treatments."[7]

In line with concerns about undertreatment of pain, at least two medical boards have disciplined physicians for inadequate pain treatment. In 1999, the Oregon medical board disciplined a physician for prescribing insufficient pain medication for a terminally ill cancer patient (i.e., only acetaminophen); prescribing only a fraction of the dose of morphine typically prescribed for a patient suffering from congestive heart failure, despite recommendations for additional amounts from a hospice nurse; and failing to resume pain medication for a patient on a mechanical ventilator. The physician was ordered by the medical board to complete an educational program on physician-patient communication and to undergo mental-health treatment.[8]

In January 2004, the California medical board disciplined a physician for failure to provide adequate pain treatment to an 85-year-old patient with mesothelioma.[9] The patient understood that the condition could become extremely painful and had his attorney execute an advance directive stating that he wished to receive all medications necessary to relieve his pain as his life neared its end. Despite this fact, his last days of life were marked by unrelenting pain and allegedly indifferent treatment. Less than a year after his original diagnosis, he was having difficulty breathing and was taken to a nearby medical center. Prior to being admitted, he was taking hydrocodone/acetaminophen around the clock at home to control his pain, but at the medical center his doctor prescribed hydrocodone/acetaminophen only "as needed." After 4 days, he was transferred to a nursing facility. His medical center physician filled out papers that listed a number of medications but nothing for pain. At the nursing facility, he was seen by a second physician, who saw him on only one occasion, 16 days after his admission. The patient received nothing for his pain until the 4th day after his arrival and then only sporadic medication despite his yelling throughout the night. The board required the nursing facility physician to complete a 40-hour course in pain management, undergo a 2-day assessment of his physical and mental health (he was 80 years old), as well as enroll in a physician-patient communication course.[9] The case may have been motivated by a 2001 law passed by the California legislature requiring physicians in the state who treat patients to take courses in pain management and end-of-life care and mandating the state medical board to monitor complaints of undertreatment of pain.[10]

▶ MALPRACTICE SUITS

In addition to actions by state medical boards, physicians are also at risk of medical malpractice suits for inappropriate pain treatment. Although the risk of a suit is quite low, several cases have been brought in which physicians allegedly prescribed overly high dosages of pain medication. A number of these cases involved wrongful death claims in which the patient became addicted to the medication. Plaintiffs in

BOX 37-1 Key Elements of the Federation of State Medical Boards—A 2004 Model Guidelines for the Use of Controlled Substances for the Treatment of Pain

Criteria for evaluating the treatment of pain, including the use of controlled substances.

Evaluation of the patient: A medical history and physical examination must be obtained, evaluated, and documented in the medical record. The medical record should document the nature and intensity of the pain, current and past treatments for pain, underlying or coexisting diseases or conditions, the effect of the pain on physical and psychological function, and history of substance abuse. The medical record also should document the presence of one or more recognized medical indications for the use of a controlled substance.

Treatment plan: The written treatment plan should state objectives that will be used to determine treatment success, such as pain relief and improved physical and psychosocial function, and should indicate if any further diagnostic evaluations or other treatments are planned. After treatment begins, the physician should adjust drug therapy to the individual medical needs of each patient. Other treatment modalities or a rehabilitation program may be necessary depending on the etiology of the pain, and the extent to which the pain is associated with physical and psychosocial impairment.

Informed consent and agreement for treatment: The physician should discuss the risks and benefits of the use of controlled substances with the patient, persons designated by the patient, or with the patient's surrogate or guardian if the patient is without medical decision-making capacity. The patient should receive prescriptions from one physician and one pharmacy whenever possible. If the patient is at high risk for medication abuse or has a history of substance abuse, the physician should consider the use of a written agreement between physician and patient outlining patient responsibilities, including the following.

- Urine/serum medication levels screening when requested
- Number and frequency of all prescription refills
- Reasons for which drug therapy may be discontinued (e.g., violation of agreement)

Periodic review: The physician should periodically review the course of pain treatment and any new information about the etiology of the pain or the patient's state of health. Continuation or modification of controlled substances for pain management therapy depends on the physician's evaluation of progress toward treatment objectives. Satisfactory response to treatment may be indicated by the patient's decreased pain, increased level of function, or improved quality of life. Objective evidence of improved or diminished function should be monitored, and information from family members or other caregivers should be considered in determining the patient's response to treatment. If the patient's progress is unsatisfactory, the physician should assess the appropriateness of continued use of the current treatment plan and consider the use of other therapeutic modalities.

Consultation: The physician should be willing to refer the patient as necessary for additional evaluation and treatment in order to achieve treatment objectives. Special attention should be given to those patients with pain who are at risk for medication misuse, abuse, or diversion. The management of pain in patients with a history of substance abuse or with a comorbid psychiatric disorder may require extra care, monitoring, documentation, and consultation with or referral to an expert in the management of such patients.

Medical records: The physician should keep accurate and complete records, including the following:

- Medical history and physical examination
- Diagnostic, therapeutic, and laboratory results
- Evaluations and consultations
- Treatment objectives
- Discussion of risks and benefits
- Informed consent
- Treatments
- Medications (including date, type, dosage, and quantity prescribed)
- Instructions and agreements
- Periodic reviews

Records should remain current and be maintained in an accessible manner and readily available for review.

Compliance with controlled substances laws and regulations: To prescribe, dispense, or administer controlled substances, the physician must be licensed in the state and comply with applicable federal and state regulations. Physicians are referred to the Physicians Manual of the U.S. Drug Enforcement Administration (and any relevant documents issued by the state medical board) for specific rules governing controlled substances as well as applicable state regulations.

---

these suits have won on theories that the physician failed to adequately monitor the patient while the patient was taking pain medications or failed to warn the patient of risks associated with driving while taking the medication. In Weaver v. Lentz, William Weaver died from an overdose of the combination analgesic propoxyphene/acetaminophen, which had been prescribed by Dr. Lentz.[11] The South Carolina Court of Appeals affirmed the finding by the trial court that Lentz negligently overprescribed pain medications under circumstances in which he should have known that Weaver was addicted to the medications and was abusing them. A jury found both Dr. Lentz and Mr. Weaver equally at fault for Weaver's death and awarded Weaver's estate actual damages of $792,577 and punitive damages of $10,000. Based on Weaver's contributory negligence, the actual damages were reduced to $396,288.50. In Burroughs v. Magee, Judy Burroughs sued Dr. Magee on behalf of her late husband, who had died in a car accident.[12] The driver of the other car was a patient of Magee's. Burroughs alleged that Magee "negligently prescribed drugs to a known drug addict, negligently prescribed two contraindicated drugs (i.e., carisprodol and butalbital/acetaminophen), and negligently failed to warn his patient of the risks of driving while under the influence of these drugs." The court found no evidence that the two drugs were contraindicated. Nor did the court find that Magee had a duty to refrain from prescribing drugs to his patient because the patient was a suspected drug abuser and might pose a risk to others. However, the court did determine that Magee failed to adequately warn his patient of the risks of driving while using the two drugs in combination.

More recently, several malpractice and wrongful death suits have been filed against physicians for prescribing the pain medication controlled-release oxycodone (OxyContin, Purdue Pharma L.P., Stamford, Connecticut). Claims in these suits include failure to obtain adequate informed consent by virtue of not disclosing the addictive potential of the drug and failing to warn of addiction and other risks associated with the drug.[13] In Walsh v. Tabby, Joann Walsh and her husband sued Dr. David Tabby.[14] Tabby had prescribed controlled-release oxycodone for Walsh from 1997 until 2001 to treat her reflex sympathetic dystrophy. He increased her dose in 1999 despite Walsh having expressed concerns to him about the drug's addictive potential and effects. Tabby "allegedly assured Walsh that her dosage was not abnormally high." In a decision in response to a motion by the plaintiffs to remand the case from federal court back to a Pennsylvania court, the U.S. District Court in the Eastern District of Pennsylvania further described the facts of the case as follows:

In October 2001, two agents from the Attorney General's Office approached Walsh and informed her that there was an investigation into her OxyContin use because her prescriptions were said to be abnormally high. The agents informed Walsh that they believed that she and Dr. Tabby were illegally distributing the prescription drug OxyContin. Walsh informed Dr. Tabby about the Attorney General's investigation at which time Dr. Tabby refused to further treat her or to recommend another physician for her treatment. At that point, Walsh began to wean herself off of OxyContin and eventually she admitted herself into a drug rehabilitation center in February of 2002 for her addiction to the pain reliever. Walsh alleges that she continues to suffer from injuries related to her addiction to OxyContin.

A final disposition in this case, and many similar cases, is not available either because the case was settled and the terms of the settlement remain confidential or because the suits have not yet been finally adjudicated.

In contrast to suits for inappropriate or "over" prescribing, few judicial opinions have discussed undertreatment of pain. In 2001, a California case received considerable attention when a physician was successfully sued for inadequate treatment of a patient's pain.[15] While Mr. Bergman (85 years old), an inpatient at Eden Medical Center of Costro Valley, California, in 1997, complained of intolerable pain. His preliminary diagnosis was lung cancer that had metastasized to his bones. Nurses recorded his pain levels as between 7 and 10, with 10 being the maximum. His physician, Dr. Chin, only prescribed 25-mg injections of meperidine during this time. On the day of his discharge, Mr. Bergman described his pain rating as a 10. Dr. Chin wrote a prescription for an oral analgesic (hydrocodone/acetaminophen), which did not fall under the

"triplicate" prescribing requirement the state imposed at that time. Mr. Bergman's daughter, convinced that this would not be adequate to relieve her father's pain, requested something stronger. In response, Mr. Bergman was given another shot of meperidine and a skin patch containing fentanyl. Because he continued to be in pain when he arrived home, Mr. Bergman's children contacted his regular physician, who prescribed a different pain medication. At the trial, the plaintiffs argued that Chin did not comply with clinical guidelines on the management of cancer pain published in 1992 by the Agency for Health Care Policy and Research (AHCPR, now the Agency for Health Care Research and Quality). The AHCPR guidelines state that pain medication should be prescribed on an "around-the-clock" basis rather than in response to a patient's request in order to prevent recurrence of pain.

Under California's medical malpractice law, plaintiffs cannot receive damages for pain and suffering. As a result, Chin was sued under the state's elder abuse law, which required that plaintiffs prove that the defendant's actions were not simply negligent but reckless.[16] A California jury awarded $1,500,000 to Bergman's children. Although the award was subsequently reduced by the court, it was a dramatic message to the medical community.

► STATE REGULATION: MEDICAID RESTRICTIONS

State Medicaid policies intended to prevent drug diversion and inappropriate use of Medicaid dollars may also hamper adequate pain treatment. These policies include limitations on the number of medication dosages that may be prescribed at one time and limits on the number of refills of a prescription. States may also use Medicaid fraud and abuse laws to target physicians who inappropriately prescribe opioids to Medicaid patients (Box 37-2).

As of 2000, approximately half of the states limited the amount of drugs that can be dispersed under one prescription and/or limited the number of refills per prescription. A smaller number of states limit the number of prescriptions or refills a Medicaid patient may obtain in a month. Some experts have pointed out that "given that pain management patients often require frequent dosages of medication, sometimes between 30 and 50 pills a day, these limitations may become a real barrier to adequate treatment."[17] These laws inconvenience both patients and physicians.

Several state Medicaid programs have also instituted policies that require prior authorization for a specific medication before Medicaid will reimburse for purchase of the drug.

BOX 37-2 Medicaid Restrictions Affecting Prescribing Practices for Treating Patients with Pain

- Limitations on the number of medication dosages that may be prescribed at one time
- Limits on the number of refills for each prescription
- Policies that require preauthorization for specific medications

These policies are intended to "control fraud, abuse and diversion of controlled substances and to reduce cost."[18] At least nine states have put in place requirements for prior authorization for controlled-release oxycodone under their Medicaid programs. According to the American Cancer Society, although there have been few well-designed studies examining whether or not such prior authorization programs negatively affect a patient's ability to obtain needed pain medications, reports from the 1st month of implementation of a prior authorization program for controlled-release oxycodone in South Carolina indicated that nine individuals were denied the prescription as a result of prior authorization and 380 were switched to another pain medication.[19] South Carolina subsequently changed its policy so that most prescriptions for controlled-release oxycodone do not require prior authorization. As a result of the potential these programs have for discouraging the use of certain pain medications for legitimate pain patients, the American Cancer Society has recommended that states rely on their Drug Utilization Programs rather than prior authorization requirements to assess appropriate drug utilization.[20]

Federal law requires each state Medicaid program to establish a prospective and retrospective Drug Utilization Review (DUR) program. The purpose of these programs is to review the appropriateness and medical necessity of prescriptions for outpatient drugs. In carrying out their task, DUR programs may issue written notices to physicians informing them of the program's observations of their prescribing practices or may refer physicians to a state surveillance and utilization review program. Although DUR programs have the potential to both encourage and discourage proper pain management prescribing and may be preferable to prior authorization requirements, some pain management experts have concerns about these programs, stating that "if DUR programs routinely generate warning notices to doctors who prescribe higher than average volumes of controlled substances without adequately considering the circumstances under which drugs are prescribed, DUR may intimidate legitimate prescribers and discourage appropriate pain management."[17]

▶ PRESCRIPTION MONITORING

Prescription monitoring programs may also interfere with medical practice. In the mid-1990s, a handful of states had "duplicate" or "triplicate" prescription programs. These programs required physicians to use a special multipart government prescription form so that prescribing and dispensing of certain drugs to patients could be monitored by a designated state regulatory or enforcement agency. The Drug Enforcement Agency (DEA) actually reported that implementation of multiple-copy prescription programs resulted in prescription decreases of 50% or more in the period following implementation, reduction in the state's per capita consumption of the substances, and significant reduction in physician requests for triplicate forms in successive years. All states have now dropped these programs, but a number have instead adopted a modern-day counterpart: electronic monitoring and surveillance. Typically, as a result of these new programs, pharmacies enter information about prescribed controlled substances into an electronic database and transmit the information electronically to a state agency. Agencies with responsibility for receiving and analyzing this data vary from state to state. In some states, it is the state medical board, department of health, or consumer protection agency; in others, it is the justice department or the state police. There is currently a debate as to whether or not these programs are having a negative effect on the treatment of pain.[21]

▶ DEA SCRUTINY

Although infrequent, physicians may also face criminal prosecution for the prescribing of opioids. For the most part, such actions are based on violations of the federal Controlled Substances Act (CSA) or similar state laws. The act and its attendant regulations provide for intensive record keeping and tracking of all organizations and individuals involved in the distribution of controlled substances and is administered and enforced by the DEA.

Federal regulations require practitioners who prescribe scheduled substances to register with the DEA. Sanctions for prescribing without a "legitimate medical purpose"[22] and outside the bounds of the usual course of medical practice can include revocation of a physician's registration, his or her ability to prescribe scheduled drugs, and criminal arrest and prosecution.

When the DEA receives a complaint about an individual practitioner, it must either investigate or refer the complaint to a state counterpart. Most investigations begin with a complaint from a concerned citizen, consumer, colleague, or state or local law enforcement agency. Usually the DEA will refer the complaint to state officials, although a particularly "serious" complaint might prompt a joint investigation. If an investigation reveals evidence of wrongdoing, the officials may move to suspend or revoke the practitioner's controlled substances registration. State and federal officials may also decide to pursue administrative, civil, or criminal penalties against the practitioner.

Although criminal prosecution of physicians is relatively rare, since the mid-1990s, dozens of physicians have been arrested for prescribing opioids, several of which were in the context of treating pain. In a handful of those cases, the physician was also charged with homicide, allegedly as a result of his or her prescribing practices. The majority of these cases involved the prescribing of controlled-release oxycodone. From the time of its introduction in 1996 to 2000, the number of controlled-release oxycodone prescriptions increased 20-fold. During this same period, medical examiners, drug treatment centers, law enforcement personnel, and pharmacists reported a substantial increase in the abuse of the drug. In response, the DEA increased its efforts to crack down on controlled-release oxycodone drug diversion. In February of 2002, Dr. James Graves became the first physician to be criminally convicted of controlled-release oxycodone-related deaths. He was sentenced to 62.9 years in prison. Graves was found guilty of four counts of manslaughter for prescribing controlled-release oxycodone to patients who subsequently died of overdoses. He was also convicted of one count of racketeering and five counts of unlawful delivery of a controlled substance. The prosecution argued that Graves was selling the drug to known drug abusers who repeatedly came to his office to feed their addictions. The defense argued that although Graves' record keeping was poor, he was a legitimate physician who was attempting to treat patients for their pain.

In a small number of cases, despite evidence that the physicians were appropriately treating patient pain, prosecutors persisted in attempting to obtain a conviction. In a few cases, they were successful, although the cases were subsequently reversed on appeal. An illustration is the case of Dr. Frank Fisher, who operated a private pain clinic in Redding, California. In February of 1999, the Attorney General of California charged Fisher with prescribing excessive amounts of controlled substances, which allegedly led to several deaths. At the time of his arrest, his practice consisted of about 3,000 patients. Approximately 10% of his patients suffered from severe chronic intractable pain, and he prescribed opioids for many of them.

Because he was unable to post his $15,000,000 bond, he remained in jail for 5 months prior to a preliminary hearing. At that hearing, in July of 1999, the defense succeeded in reducing the charges to manslaughter as there was inadequate evidence that the deaths with which he was charged were a result of his patients having taken the medications he prescribed. For example, one of the deaths was of a patient who died as a passenger in an automobile accident. Another death occurred when a woman stole prescription medicines from one of Fisher's patients and gave them to a nonpatient, who overdosed on them. A third patient, with a documented history of pain and need for opioids, committed suicide after Dr. Fisher was jailed, and she was unable to obtain her pain medications. At the hearing, the judge allowed Fisher to be released on a $50,000 bond.

Although the prosecution's case seemed largely based on the volume of opioids prescribed by Dr. Fisher (he was one of the largest prescribers of controlled-release oxycodone in the state), an expert witness for the prosecution stated that the doses of opioids prescribed by Dr. Fisher were not unreasonable and that he (the expert) frequently prescribed higher dosages. Dr. Fisher also asserted that his clinic adhered to accepted standards of care and practices for treatment of pain patients, including the following.

- Rigorous pretreatment screening to exclude potential abusers of pain medications
- Mandatory mental-health evaluations of all chronic pain patients by a licensed professional
- Termination of patients caught lying, diverting medications, or using nontherapeutic doses

As a result of these factors, the clinic terminated 400 patients for failing the standards of integrity required by Dr. Fisher's practice.[23] After 3 years, the charges against Fisher for manslaughter and drug diversion were dropped. Other high profile cases in which physicians were arrested in relation to their prescribing of large doses of opioids for the treatment of pain include those of Dr. Cecil Knox, Dr. William E. Hurwitz, and Dr. Jeri Hassman.

▶ DEA POSITION ON PHYSICIAN PRESCRIBING OF OPIOIDS

In August of 2004 (prompted by the "chilling effect" of a series of prosecutions of doctors prescribing opioids), DEA,

FSMB, and other groups jointly issued guidelines providing clarifications for physicians as to what constitutes "safe prescribing" from the perspective of the DEA. The guidelines, in the form of "Frequently Asked Questions," provided physicians with advice on how to identify a patient who is likely to abuse or divert drugs for criminal distribution. It also clarified the differences between true drug addiction and drug tolerance or physical dependence. Although the DEA was commended for its efforts to clarify for physicians the bases for its actions in the area of arrests for opioid prescribing, in October of 2004, the Agency withdrew the guidelines, stating that they included some erroneous information. In January of 2005, the Agency published a revised version of the original statement and requested comments on it from the medical community.[24]

▶ FRAUD AND ABUSE

In conjunction with arrests of physicians for prescribing of controlled-release oxycodone and other opiates in violation of federal- or state-controlled substance laws, the U. S. government has in a number of cases also charged physicians with violations of fraud and abuse laws. These charges were based on allegations that the physician had prescribed medications that were not "medically necessary" and thus in violation of the federal Medicaid and Medicare statutes.[25] In addition to the Medicare and Medicaid laws, the government has pursued prosecution under various federal and state false claims statutes. Although successful convictions based on alleged false claims actions in this area have been rare, the claims nonetheless are brought forward in the initial stages of prosecution, oftentimes in an effort to bolster the government's case of unlawful prescribing or to force settlement. To be successful in a false claims action, the government must prove that the defendant submitted a claim to the government for payment, that the defendant had knowledge that the claim was false or fraudulent, and that the claim was in fact false or fraudulent.[26]

Several highly publicized prosecutions of pain management physicians illustrate the government's use of the false claims statutes in aiding the prosecution of these physicians. The cases were complex and contained a wide variety of charges, and the false claims allegations were often minor infractions. In the prosecution of Dr. William E. Hurwitz, the government charged Dr. Hurwitz with two counts of violating the Health Care Fraud Statute (18 U.S.C. § 1347), in addition to 60 other various charges, ranging from drug trafficking to engaging in a criminal enterprise.[27] The government alleged Dr. Hurwitz repeatedly wrote prescriptions to patients whom the government claimed were known drug abusers who often sold the medication on the street.

The two claims for health care fraud involved prescriptions written to two Virginia Medicaid beneficiaries, which the government claimed were not for legitimate medical purposes and went beyond the bounds of medical practice. The government alleged that by prescribing the medications Dr. Hurwitz knowingly caused the Medicaid beneficiaries to submit the claims to Virginia Medicaid for the cost of the prescription. On December 17, 2004, the case was tried before a jury, which found Dr. Hurwitz not guilty of health care fraud but guilty of 50 of the other 62 counts with which he was charged.[28]

In a similar case, the government issued a 69-count indictment charging Dr. Cecil Knox with conspiracy to commit racketeering, criminal conspiracy, mail fraud, health care fraud (18 U.S.C. § 1347), illegal kickbacks, and violations of the CSA.[29] The government alleged that Dr. Knox (a pain management specialist in Roanoke, Virginia) prescribed medications such as controlled-release oxycodone outside the scope of legitimate medical practice, defrauded the Medicaid program by writing improper prescriptions, and caused the death or serious bodily injury of several of his patients through his prescribing habits.[30] After a 7-week trial and more than a week of deliberating, a jury found Dr. Knox not guilty of approximately 30 of the 69 charges against him.[31] The trial judge declared a mistrial when the jurors were unable to reach a verdict on the remaining counts.[32]

In addition to the federal false claims statutes, physicians have also been prosecuted under state false claims statutes. In Commonwealth v. Pike, the Supreme Judicial Court of Massachusetts affirmed the lower court's conviction of a psychiatrist for unlawfully dispensing controlled substances and filing false Medicaid claims in violation of the Massachusetts Controlled Substance Act (Mass. Gen Laws Ann. ch. 94C §§ 19, 32A, and 32B) and the Massachusetts Medicaid False Claims Act (Mass. Gen Laws Ann. Ch. 118E § 40).[33] The government alleged that the psychiatrist, Dr. Pike, knowingly and unlawfully prescribed controlled substances with high street value to his patients for substance abuse knowing that the prescriptions were often sold on the street. In addition, the government claimed that by writing the illegitimate prescriptions Dr. Pike was assured his patients would return for future visits and drugs, causing Dr. Pike to maintain (or in some cases increase) his billing to Medicaid.

A portion of Dr. Pike's practice was devoted to treating Medicaid patients who suffered from drug or alcohol dependency, in addition to various psychiatric problems. Of the 10 Medicaid patients who served as the basis for the government's allegations, most sought Dr. Pike's expertise in overcoming their addictions to heroin and other substances. In treating these patients, Dr. Pike almost always prescribed drugs such as methadone, valium, clonidine, klonopin, or some combination thereof. Most of the substances were themselves addictive, and many had a high street value. In addition, the drugs were prescribed during the patient's first office visit and based solely on information provided by the patient without any further objective investigation by Dr. Pike. Dr. Pike also treated patients claiming to be in chronic pain and routinely prescribed methadone without performing physical examinations or tests to confirm the patient's alleged complaints. Due to the fact that some of the methadone prescriptions were in such high doses relative to the pain being treated, the government alleged the prescriptions served "no legitimate medical purpose and were completely inconsistent with the manner in which drugs should be used in a legitimate treatment program." The court, in sustaining the lower court's conviction of Dr. Pike, distinguished the case from one involving the legitimate prescribing of pain medications, and noted that the government would have a more difficult time proving the requisite intent necessary to violate the false claims statute in the latter situation.

▶ CONCLUSIONS

Physicians who inappropriately prescribe opioids, either in amounts insufficient to control patient pain or in large volumes that are determined to be medically unnecessary or that cause a patient significant harm, are at risk of various legal actions ranging from malpractice and disciplinary actions by state medical boards to criminal prosecution for violation of federal or state controlled substance laws or fraud and abuse laws. Physicians, therefore, should be aware of and act consistently with their state medical board's policies regarding prescribing of opioids and consider additional training in opioid prescribing if they lack exposure to the most recent medical standards and authorities on this issue.

EDITOR'S NOTE: Professor Hoffman has kindly allowed us to reproduce this in-depth analysis of the legal and regulatory issues surrounding the use of opioid analgesics from the First Edition of Complications in Regional Anesthesia and Pain Medicine. The analysis was written toward the latter part of 2005, and this discussion remains just as relevant today as it was just over 5 years ago. Nonetheless, there has been significant and ongoing attention to the use and abuse of prescription medications during the past few years, with a focus on the perceived overuse and frequent diversion of opioid analgesics for nonmedical use in the United States. On May 24, 2011, DEA Administrator Michele Leonhart testified before the United States Senate Committee on the Judiciary, Subcommittee on Crime and Terrorism in an address titled "Responding to the Prescription Drug Epidemic: Strategies for Reducing Abuse, Misuse, Diversion, and Fraud".[i] Administrator Minehart emphasized that the diversion and abuse of pharmaceutical controlled substances remains a significant and growing problem in the United States. Specific evidence cited included:

- *According to the Substance Abuse and Mental Health Services Administration's (SAMHSA's) 2009 National Survey on Drug Use and Health (NSDUH), 7 million Americans were current nonmedical users of psychotherapeutic drugs, significantly higher by 12% compared to 2008. Over three-quarters of that number, 5.3 million Americans, abused pain relievers.*
- *The NSDUH survey also indicated that the nonmedical use of prescription drugs was second only to marijuana abuse.*
- *On average, more than 7,000 people 12 years and older initiate use of a controlled substance pharmaceutical drug for nonmedical purposes every day.*
- *The Centers for Disease Control and Prevention (CDC) reported that the number of poisoning deaths involving any opioid analgesics increased from 4,041 in 1999 to 14,459 in 2007, more than tripling in 8 years.[ii]*

---

[i]Leonhart MM. Testimony before the United States Senate Committee on the Judiciary, Subcommittee on Crime and Terrorism. Responding to the Prescription Drug Epidemic: Strategies for Reducing Abuse, Misuse, Diversion, and Fraud. May 24, 2011. Available at http://www.justice.gov/dea/speeches/110524_testimony.pdf, last accessed September 9, 2011.

[ii]Centers for Disease Control and Prevention, *Morbidity and Mortality Weekly Report*, August 20, 2010.

- *SAMHSA's Treatment Episode Data Set shows that between 1998 and 2008, the number of persons admitted for treatment that reported any pain reliever abuse increased more than fourfold.*
- *According to Drug Abuse Warning Network (DAWN) data, the number of emergency department visits involving the misuse or abuse of pharmaceuticals increased by 98.4% between 2004 and 2009. The prescription drugs most implicated were opiate/opioid pain relievers, oxycodone products increased 242%, and hydrocodone products increased 124%.*
- *The approximate number of cases submitted by state and local law enforcement to forensic labs between 2001 and 2009 increased significantly (330% for oxycodone, 314% for hydrocodone, and 281% for methadone).*

DEA Administrator Minehart laid out a number of strategies that are aimed at stemming the increase in diversion of prescription opioids. She reiterated the need for the DEA imposed quotas to limit overproduction of these prescription drugs, warning that these quotas may lead to temporary interruptions in the available supply from time to time. The DEA has also been restructured in efforts to improve detection of diversion, assembling tactical squads, hiring new research specialists, and increasing oversight of those holding DEA registration from manufacturers through prescribers. The DEA has focused their efforts on problem areas, and at the time of this writing the most prominent problem is the disproportionate increase in oxycodone abuse and diversion. In October 2010, Congress passed and President Obama signed into law the Secure and Responsible Drug Disposal Act of 2010 aimed at establishing safe and effective means of disposing of excess, unneeded prescription medications. On September 25, 2010, the DEA coordinated the first-ever National Take-Back Initiative. Working with more than 3,000 state and local law enforcement partners, take-back sites were established at more than 4,000 locations across the United States, resulting in the collection of 121 tons of unwanted or expired medications that were disposed of.

Clearly the DEA and our country's leaders view prescription drug abuse as a serious problem. They have launched concerted new efforts toward minimizing the availability of pharmaceutical controlled substances to nonmedical users while aiming to preserve the integrity of the closed-system of distribution. As practitioners caring for patients with pain, we will undoubtedly help to mold the best balance between adequate availability of analgesics for our patients who desperately need these treatments, while helping to minimize dose escalation and eliminate opioid use altogether in those who are not benefiting from their use.

J.P.R.

References

1. Von Roenn JH, Cleeland CS, Gonin R, et al. Physician attitudes and practice in cancer pain management: a survey from the Easterns Cooperative Oncology Group. *Ann Intern Med* 1993;119:121–126.
2. Turk DC, Brody MC, Okifuji EA. Physicians' attitudes and practices regarding the long-term prescribing of opioids for non-cancer pain. *Pain* 1994;59(2):201–208.
3. Weissman DE, Joranson DE, Hopwood MB. Wisconsin physicians' knowledge and attitudes about opioid analgesic regulations. *WMJ* 1991;90:671–675.
4. Hoover v. Agency for Health Care Administration, 676 So. 2d 1380, 1380–1385 (Fla. Dist. Ct. App. 1996).
5. Hurwitz v. Virginia Board of Medicine, No. 96-676, 1998 WL 972259 (Va. Cir. Ct. June 30, 1998).
6. Hoffmann DE, Tarzian AJ. Achieving the right balance in oversight of physician opioid prescribing for pain: the role of state medical boards. *J Law Med Ethics* 2003;31:21.
7. Federation of State Medical Boards of the United States. Model policy for the use of controlled substances in the treatment of pajn. http://www.fsmb.org/pdf/2004_grpol_Controlled_Substances.pdf (last accessed 11 June 2006).
8. Oregon Board of Medical Examiners, 2003 Board Actions, April 14, 2003, at http://www.bme.state.or.us/NewActions.html.
9. Sandy Kleefman, Doctor Disciplined Over Pain Treatment, Contra Costa Times (CA), January 17, 2004, at a03, available at http://nl.newsbank.com/nlsearch/we/Archives?p_action=list&p_topdoc=101; California Board of Medical Examiners, at http://www2.dca.ca.gov/pls/wllpub/WLLQRYNA$LCEV2.QueryView?P_LICENSE_NUMBER=3739&P_LTE_ID=790.
10. Cal. Bus. & Prof. Code §§ 2190.5 & 2313 (West, 2003).
11. Weaver v. Lentz, 561 S.E. 2d 360, 360–373 (S.C. Ct. App. 2002).
12. Burroughs v. MaGee, No. 2001-00238-COA-R3-CV, 2002 WL 1284291 (Tenn. Ct. App. June 11, 2002).
13. See e.g., Walsh v. Tabby, No. CivA 02-8283, 2003 WL 1888856 (E.D. Pa. April 17, 2003); Cornelius v. Cain, No. CACE 01-020213(02), 2004 WL 48102 (Fla. Cir. Ct. Jan. 5, 2004).
14. Walsh v. Tabby, No. CivA 02-8283, 2003 WL 1888856 (E.D. Pa. April 17, 2003).
15. Tanya Albert, Doctor guilty of elder abuse for undertreating pain. amednews.com, July 23, 2001, at http://www.ama-assn.org/amednews/2001/07/23/prl20723.htm.
16. Bergman v. Eden Medical Center, No. H203732-1 (Sup. Ct. Alameda Co., CA June 13, 2001).
17. Jost T. Public financing of pain management: Leaky umbrellas and ragged safety nets. *J Law Med Ethics* 1998;26(4):290–307.
18. American Cancer Society, Position Statement on Medicaid Prior Authorization for Pain Medications, Dec. 2001, available at http://www.aacpi.wisc.edu/regulatory/ACSpa.pdf.
19. Bauerlein, Valerie, Popular Painkiller Mired in Controversy, The State (Columbia, SC), Sept. 23, 2001, at B1.
20. American Cancer Society Position Statement on Prescription Monitoring and Drug Utilization Review Programs, 2001, available at http://www.painfoundation.org/marylandpain/Policy/ACS_PMPsDURs.doc.
21. Joranson DE, Carrow GM, Ryan KM, et al. Pain management and prescription monitoring. *J Pain Symptom Manage* 2002;23(3):231–238.
22. 21 C.F.R. 1306.04(a).
23. Sam Stanton, Murder Case dissolved, but so did doctor's life, The Sacramento Bee, May 23, 2004, at A1, available at http://nl.newsbank.com/nlsearch/we/Archives?p_action=doc&p_docid=102C5DE498E7A. Fisher claimed that state undercover agents "visited him at least seven times trying to obtain prescriptions using bogus ailments, and that he refused to provide them with medicine."
24. Solicitation of Comments on Dispensing of Controlled Substances for the Treatment of Pain, 70 Fed. Reg. 2883 (Drug Enforcement Agency Jan. 18, 2005).
25. 42 U.S.C. § 1320c-5(a).
26. 31 U.S.C. § 3729(a); 42 U.S.C. 1320a-7b(a); 18 U.S.C. § 287; 18 U.S.C. § 1347.
27. United States v. Hurwitz, Second Indictment of William Eliot Hurwitz, Eastern District of Virginia, July 27, 2004.
28. Ken Moore, Pain Doctor's Trial: Convicted, The Connection, December 17, 2004, at http://www.connectionnewspapers.com/article.asp?article=44352&paper=0&cat=176.
29. USA v. Knox, Et Al, No. 7:02CR00009 (W.D. Va. Feb. 1, 2002).

30. Jen McCaffery. The Roanoke pain specialist and his office manager are scheduled to be tried in November. The Roanoke Times, Aug. 24, 2004, available at http://www.cpmission.com/main/knox.html.

31. Rex Bowman. No convictions against physician: accusations against pain doctor end in not guilty verdicts and indecision, Times-Dispatch (VA), Nov. 2, 2003, at http://www.cpmission.com/main/knox.html.

32. Subsequent to the mistrial, the federal government re-indicted Knox on several charges. On September 2, 2005, Knox pled guilty to racketeering, illegal distribution of prescription drugs, and health care fraud, pursuant to a plea agreement.

33. Commonwealth v. Pike, 718 N.E. 2d 855, 855–863 (Mass. Supp., 1999).

38

Informed Consent and Documentation

M. Kate Welti and John D. Cassidy

Informed consent law governs the physician's duty to disclose information to patients and obtain their consent prior to treatment. It is a complex state-based body of law that reflects the historic struggle to strike a balance between the prerogative of medical judgment and the personal autonomy of the patient. Depending on the jurisdiction, informed consent requirements are currently defined by either case law or a statutory scheme. Informed consent case law, known as the "legal doctrine" of informed consent, has evolved over the course of more than a century and manifests a judicial deference to principles of personal autonomy in the context of the physician-patient relationship.[1] More recently, legislation enacted in numerous states has also established a legal framework addressing informed consent.

In substance, the law requires that decisions regarding health care must be made in a collaborative manner between physician and patient, resulting in a decision on the part of the patient that either provides or withholds consent for the intervention based on an informed decision. The law allows plaintiffs to recover damages if they can show that the defendant either provided treatment without first obtaining consent or went beyond the scope of the consent. Plaintiffs may also recover if they demonstrate that the defendant failed to disclose enough information to enable the patient to make an informed decision about whether to proceed with treatment. The latter theory of recovery, referred to as negligent disclosure, holds that the absence of a properly informed decision obviates the consent.

Depending on the jurisdiction, courts use one of two standards to judge the sufficiency of the physician's disclosure in negligent disclosure cases. The first views the process in light of medical custom, and the second takes the perspective of the patient. With few exceptions, neither standard sets out a bright-line test defining how much information must be discussed and which risks must be disclosed. As a result, the scope of the physician's obligation to provide information during the course of obtaining consent, along with the degree of documentation required to record the sufficiency of the process, may be difficult to discern in practice. Everyone can agree that "every human being of adult years and sound mind has a right to determine what shall be done with his own body,"[2] but obtaining a truly informed consent is a complex process that may be prone to later allegations of medical malpractice.

This chapter addresses the informed consent process from a medical malpractice litigation perspective. First, we consider the historical underpinnings of informed consent law and describe how the law presently applies in the clinical setting. Next, we set out basic principles describing when consent must be obtained and how that process may most productively and safely be undertaken. Finally, we discuss what documentation is helpful to adequately reflect the process.

▶ THE DOCTRINE OF INFORMED CONSENT

Definition of Informed Consent

Informed consent is obtained when a patient intentionally agrees to treatment in the absence of external controlling influences, based on an understanding of relevant information.[3] The core elements of an informed consent have been defined over time in the courts and by ethicists, and are now uniformly reflected in case law and state statutes, as well as promulgations by groups such as the Joint Commission on Accreditation of Healthcare Organizations (JCAHO) and the American Medical Association (AMA).[4] At a minimum, physicians are obligated in most instances to disclose, prior to treatment, information regarding (i) the nature of the procedure, including whether its purpose is therapeutic or diagnostic, (ii) the risks involved, particularly those that are most likely to occur and those that are most severe, (iii) the expected benefits of the procedure, and (iv) reasonable alternatives to the procedure and attendant risks[5] (Box 38-1). As discussed further in the following, there are a few narrow exceptions to informed consent requirements, most notably in emergent situations in which the patient is incapable of giving consent.

The Legal Doctrine of Informed Consent

Until approximately 1975, the law of informed consent was developed solely in the court system, creating a judicial doctrine of informed consent.[6] Cases decided prior to the 1950s recognized the patient's basic right to autonomy and to be free from nonconsensual contact, but did not address entitlement to information about treatment.[7] At that time, the physician was merely required to obtain authorization from the patient for the proposed treatment, without any concomitant obligation to discuss other treatment considerations. Around the turn of the 20th century, there were several important court decisions that expanded the physician's duty to obtain consent to include a disclosure of the procedure's benefits, risks, and alternatives. Those cases help define the requirements the

---

BOX 38-1 Key Elements of Informed Consent

- Nature of the procedure: diagnostic or therapeutic
- Risks of the procedure: especially those that are common or severe
- Expected benefits
- Reasonable alternatives: including the risks of nontreatment

---

doctrine places upon the physician and continue to form the framework of informed consent law to the present day.

Cases addressing consent issues began appearing in the early 1900s.[8] Nearly all of the early consent actions arose in connection with surgical treatment, usually alleging that the surgeon altered the surgical plan after the patient was anesthetized.[9] One prominent defense raised by physicians in those cases is that a patient's consent for treatment was implied by his or her consultation of the physician's expertise.[10] The courts weighed the right of an individual to protect bodily integrity from intrusion against the discretion of the surgeon to proceed under the theory of implied consent and found that "the patient must be the final arbiter as to whether he will take his chances with the operation, or take his chances without it."[11] By the late 1920s, the courts had generally established that the physician was allowed to provide treatment to the extent of the patient's consent, but no further.[12]

In 1957, a California court ruled that physicians have an affirmative duty to go beyond obtaining a recognizable consent and must disclose enough information to enable patients to give an informed consent.[13] This case, Salgo v. Leland Stanford Jr. University Board of Trustees, is historic in that the decision is the first to coin the term informed consent and marks the expansion of the physician's obligation regarding consent to include disclosure.[14] Courts in other states followed suit and within a number of years this became a standard requirement in conjunction with obtaining consent.[15] Salgo signified the beginning of a judicial shift in the focus of consent cases from the issue of whether consent was obtained to whether the consent was sufficiently informed, where it substantially remains today. Unfortunately, the language of the opinion provides little assistance in defining a sufficient disclosure, or any other type of analysis that would be helpful to providers charged with informing their patients prior to treatment. In fact, the court introduced a great deal of confusion into this area by suggesting that the physician has discretion to withhold alarming information while disclosing facts necessary for the patient to reach an informed consent.[13] This decision embodies that period's conflicting sentiments about patient care, with a growing deference to patient autonomy on the one hand and on the other an historic reliance on the physician's acting independently in what he or she judged to be the best interests of the patient.[16]

Cause of Action: From Battery to Negligence

A cause of action is a theory of liability by which the plaintiff seeks to recover in a civil action. In early consent cases, the plaintiff's sole source of redress for unauthorized treatment was a civil action utilizing the law of battery.[17] A civil action for battery protects the patient's dignity interest of bodily integrity and does not require a showing of injury.[18] This theory of liability fits well with instances in which the plaintiff complains that the physician proceeded with treatment without consent or else operated on a part of the body other than the one discussed.[19] Although civil battery allegations continue to surface to the present day, by the mid- to late 1950s, there was a growing sense that battery was less suitable in consent cases that focused on the sufficiency of the disclosure.[20] Around this time, many courts began to suggest that the physician's failure to obtain informed consent is more accurately considered a matter of physician error or neglect in keeping with theories of medical negligence, which is part of tort (or personal injury) law.[21] Tort law is generated by each individual state and varies to some extent based on the prevailing state law. To prevail in a negligence action, the plaintiff must demonstrate that the defendant had a legally established duty to the plaintiff the defendant breached by failing to adhere to the standard of care expected and that this breach of duty caused injury to the plaintiff.[22]

Medical malpractice is essentially negligence within the confines of health care delivery. The standard used to determine whether the alleged breach reaches the bar of negligence in most medical malpractice actions is medical custom; that is, the standard of care expected of the average reasonable practitioner in similar circumstances.[23] The standard of care is established by testimony of an expert in the field. At trial, plaintiff and defendant offer contrary expert testimony as to what constitutes the applicable care standards and whether the defendant deviated from those standards. The trier of fact (usually the jury, but in some instances the judge) then makes a decision based on the more credible expert testimony, along with other factual issues.

Under the doctrine of informed consent, providers have a duty to disclose relevant information in the course of the consent process, and if they fail to do so, they may be found negligent. The doctrine has evolved to require the physician to obtain the patient's informed consent by disclosing the nature of the proposed treatment, the expected risks, reasonable alternatives to the procedure, and the attendant risks.[24] Plaintiffs alleging a breach of this obligation may sue under a negligent disclosure theory of liability. Plaintiffs bringing a negligent disclosure case typically allege that the physician provided an insufficient disclosure and that if there had been an adequate disclosure the patient would not have undergone the treatment at issue and would not have been injured. The difficulty in negligent disclosure cases most often lies in determining the amount of information the physician is required to disclose, particularly in terms of the potential risks of the proposed procedure.

▶ THE PHYSICIAN'S OBLIGATION TO OBTAIN INFORMED CONSENT

Professional- versus Patient-oriented Standard for Disclosure

Depending on the jurisdiction, there are two primary standards used to judge the sufficiency of the disclosure: one based on medical custom and the other focusing on the perspective of the patient. In all early negligent disclosure cases, the scope of the disclosure was a decision that was uniformly left to the discretion of the physician and was judged to be sufficient as long as the disclosure was in keeping with the standard of care of practitioners in the field.[25] This is referred to as the professional standard. The professional standard requires that the practitioner disclose to a patient that which a reasonable medical practitioner would disclose to a patient under the same or similar circumstances when obtaining their consent for a procedure.[25] "Same or similar circumstances" is usually interpreted narrowly to mean the clinical circumstances of the patient, as opposed to any nonmedical considerations that are unique to the patient.[26] Because the

scope of an appropriate disclosure is predicated on factual medical circumstances and may be derived from medical education, clinical training, continuing education, and informal discourse among colleagues, practitioners often feel most comfortable with this standard.[27]

The professional standard mirrors the legal standard for medical malpractice, in which the physician is held to the standard of care of the average physician practicing in that specialty at the time and under similar circumstances. As such, in professional standard jurisdictions, there must be expert testimony on both sides, with the plaintiff and defendant expert physicians offering contrary assertions as to whether the defendant disclosed information and obtained consent in accordance with the prevailing standard of care.

This standard applied in most jurisdictions until 1972, when a District of Columbia Appeals Court handed down an influential decision that introduced a new standard for determining the adequacy of an informed consent disclosure. In Canterbury v. Spence, the court stated that it did not agree that a patient's cause of action was dependent on the existence of a common practice or medical custom of disclosing the information at issue and struck down the professional standard in that jurisdiction.[28] Essentially, the court turned the focus from the perspective of the physician to that of the patient and held that the adequacy of the disclosure should be judged by whether the physician provided information that a reasonable person, in what the physician knows or should know to be the patient's position, would be likely to attach significance to in deciding whether or not to forego the proposed therapy.[28] This is known as the lay, or patient-oriented, standard. This standard was rapidly adopted in numerous jurisdictions.[27]

Under the patient-oriented standard, the scope of the disclosure is not tied to the recognized custom or practice of physicians. Instead, the physician has an obligation to assess the patient's situation to some extent and tailor the disclosure accordingly. The standard requires the physician to perform an affirmative inquiry into the circumstances of each patient, in order to obtain at least a minimal understanding of the patient's situation before determining what information to discuss.[29] From there, the physician is obligated to disclose information that would be "material" to the treatment decision of someone in the patient's situation.[27] Information is material if a reasonable person would be likely to attach significance to it. One court has held that materiality is the product of the severity of the injury and the likelihood of its occurrence.[30] The "reasonable person" aspect of the standard refers to a hypothetical legal construct signifying an average, prudent person. The trier of fact uses it to develop and apply community standards of reasonable conduct.[27] Thus, if a jury finds that an average person would find a particular risk to be important to be advised of when making a decision about treatment, that information will be deemed material to the decision.

Although the patient-oriented standard appears to require more than the professional standard in terms of performing inquiries into each individual patient's situation, in practice the courts have not held physicians to particularly stringent standards.[31] Often the courts only require that physicians discover and account for the patient's medical circumstances, such as his or her clinical condition and proposed treatment.[32] This is not always the case, however, and physicians should be aware of at least some of the individual patient's circumstances and goals. For example, in one negligent disclosure action, two Army physicians were found to have breached their duties of disclosure for failing to discuss alternatives to hysterectomy for a patient suffering from pelvic pain.[33] The court found both physicians liable for failing to account for the patient's desire to remain fertile when making their treatment recommendations and disclosures.[33] The case illustrates that there is a baseline requirement to be aware of the individual patient's situation and treatment goals, particularly those that may be directly affected by the proposed treatment.

A further implication of the patient-oriented standard is that the plaintiff's burden of proof is somewhat eased. Because the focus of the inquiry is on the reasonable patient, a layperson, the plaintiff does not need to obtain physician expert support for his or her contention that the physician did not divulge risks that a reasonable person would find material to their decision. However, the physician must still conform to medical custom with respect to being cognizant of the relevant risks. Expert testimony is required to establish the technical issues of treatment, including what the risks of a particular procedure are, the alternative methods of treatment, the risks relating to the alternative methods of treatment, and the likely consequences of the patient remaining untreated.[34]

All states now have a litigation remedy for failure to obtain informed consent.[35] States that developed the remedy through case law have generally adopted the reasonable patient standard.[36] Between 1975 and 1977, a number of states that had no clearly defined standard passed legislation adopting the professional standard, due in no small part to physician lobbying groups that opposed the judicial movement toward the more plaintiff-friendly patient-oriented standard.[37] There is an almost equal division among jurisdictions as to which standard they adhere to, with some applying a hybrid standard or variations of the two standards.[38] It is important to keep in mind that the standard adopted by a jurisdiction is only significant in the context of litigation and ideally should not influence the physician-patient relationship or the process of obtaining informed consent. As a matter of prudent practice, the provider should attempt in all cases to have as extensive a discussion as possible regarding the proposed treatment and its risks, benefits, and alternatives.

Negligent Disclosure Actions

As with the disclosure standard by which the physician is judged, the grounds and criteria a plaintiff must meet in order to establish and prevail in a negligent disclosure action vary from state to state. Some states have enacted statutes setting out the grounds for these actions along with recognized defenses, whereas in other jurisdictions, the courts have developed the legal framework through case law.[39] Generally, the elements of a negligent consent case mirror those of a general negligence action. To show negligent disclosure, a plaintiff must establish that (i) the provider had a duty to disclose certain information, (ii) there was a breach by the provider by failing to disclose this information, (iii) if the provider had discussed the undisclosed information the patient would not have consented to treatment, and (iv) the

provider's failure to disclose this information was the proximate cause of the plaintiff's injury.[40]

The most difficult question is usually whether the physician had a duty to disclose certain treatment information, such as a particular risk of treatment. This element may be broken down into two subparts. First, did a duty to disclose arise? Second, was there a duty to disclose the specific information at issue? With respect to the first question, the existence of the disclosure duty generally arises when a physician contemplates providing treatment to a patient. Circumstances such as the patient's refusal of treatment, emergency situations, or an emotionally fragile patient complicate the issue.

Exceptions to the Duty to Disclose

If the patient refuses treatment, the disclosure obligation shifts from discussing the risks associated with the proposed treatment to disclosing the risks of nontreatment. The provider should assume that a duty still exists in the face of refusal of treatment. A California case arising from the death of a woman from cervical cancer directly addresses this issue.[41] The patient was under the care of a general practitioner, who advised her that she needed a Pap smear without disclosing the risks of declining the test. She refused to undergo a Pap smear on at least two different occasions, on the basis of the cost. She was eventually referred to a gynecologist, who diagnosed advanced cancer. She died at the age of 30. The California Supreme Court found that the woman's refusal of the Pap smear was not informed and thus not valid. The case highlights the requirement that the consent process applies to decisions to refuse or withdraw from treatment as well as decisions to undergo treatment.

In medical emergencies in which the patient is unable to provide consent due to loss of consciousness or other incapacity, the law recognizes an exception to the requirement to obtain consent.[42] This is based on a legal presumption that a person who is physically unable to provide consent would nonetheless want life-saving treatment. Two factors must be present in order to override the consent requirement. First, the patient must be incapacitated and unable to make an informed choice, such as in instances in which the patient is suffering from sudden injury, alcohol or drug intoxication, shock, trauma, or an underlying mental or physical disease or handicap.[43] Second, the patient must have a life- or health-threatening disease or injury, as determined by medical judgment, which requires emergent treatment.[43] The most important thing to keep in mind is that both of these factors must be simultaneously present, and they must be well documented in the medical record. Moreover, a change in the patient's condition does not justify disregarding a decision that was articulated while the patient was capable of making an informed choice.[44]

Disclosure of Treatment Information

After the plaintiff demonstrates that the physician had a baseline duty to disclose, he or she must then show that the physician was obligated to disclose the specific information at issue in the case, whether a particular risk or alternative to treatment. This is usually the issue in controversy. As previously discussed, the scope of the disclosure is judged differently in various jurisdictions. Accordingly, the plaintiff must demonstrate that the physician deviated from the standard of care, failed to disclose information that was material to the patient's decision, or some combination thereof as required in that jurisdiction for a showing of negligence. Although we provide some guidelines and practical rules for obtaining consent in the following, there are no universal criteria for defining a sufficient disclosure, and ultimately an adequate disclosure is whatever a jury determines it to be.

Causation and Harm

In addition to showing that certain risks should have been disclosed, the patient must be able to prove that if he or she had been properly informed, consent to the procedure would not have been given.[45] Some jurisdictions use the "actual patient" standard, which focuses on the testimony of the patient as to whether he or she would have consented if the information at issue had been disclosed.[46] This raises the issue of credibility, as the plaintiff has the advantage of hindsight, as well as an interest in winning the suit. Other jurisdictions employ a reasonable person standard, which considers what a reasonable person in the patient's position would have done if the risk information had been disclosed.[47] Although the "reasonable person" is a hypothetical legal construct, this is a fact-specific standard that depends on the circumstances presented by each case. Both standards underscore the importance of taking into account the unique situation of each patient when obtaining consent. In keeping with general negligence principles, a plaintiff in informed consent cases must further show that an actual harm occurred as a direct result of the physician's failure to disclose information. If there was no physical injury stemming from the breach in the duty to disclose risk information, the plaintiff cannot recover.

Disclosure in the Clinical Setting

Ideally, the immense body of case law, statutes, and commentary that has been generated on the issue of informed consent would by now provide specific instruction regarding what treatment information must be disclosed, which risks are material, and which alternatives should be discussed. Much like the practice of medicine, however, there are very few hard and fast rules in informed consent law. It is not possible to set out universally applicable disclosure requirements, given the variations in state-based law, unique clinical presentations, and discrepancies in jury dispositions. Nevertheless, there are general principles that may be drawn from the law and commentary to guide the provider in obtaining a patient's consent for treatment (Box 38-2).

First, consent should be viewed as an interactive process between physician and patient, rather than a document to be signed.[48] It is an aspect of treatment that requires collaboration with the patient and clear physician-patient communication. Although there are ostensible differences between the professional and patient-oriented standards in terms of how much the physician is required to learn about the particular patient, it stands to reason that regardless of which standard applies the more the provider knows about the patient and his or her situation and treatment goals the better the chances are that disclosure pitfalls will be avoided. Put

BOX 38-2 Clinical Caveat

In the absence of universal criteria that define sufficient disclosure, physicians and patients may be best served by discussions of informed consent that:

- Establish an interactive dialogue about the proposed intervention, including its risks, benefits, and alternatives
- Consider the patient's unique medical and personal situation when framing the discussion
- Allow the patient an opportunity to ask questions
- Are documented in the chart
- The practitioner responsible for the intervention directly participates in, rather than their nonphysician designees

another way, the best way to ensure a sufficient disclosure for a particular patient is to engage him or her in a dialogue. This will increase the likelihood that the patient is involved in decision making about treatment, understands the implications of the treatment, and that the consent provided is informed. Obtaining an adequate patient history is an essential first step to providing sufficient information to patients in order to receive their consent for treatment.

In terms of determining what information warrants disclosure, the rule in its most general terms is that the practitioner that will be providing treatment should provide enough salient treatment information to enable the patient to make an informed decision. More specifically, the provider should discuss the nature of the proposed treatment, the risks and benefits of the treatment, and alternatives to that particular treatment, including their attendant benefits and risks. With respect to the nature of the treatment, the physician should provide an explanation, in layperson terms, of the physical process of the treatment. The provider should discuss as specifically as possible what they (and, if applicable, their colleagues) will do during the course of treatment. This should include the probable outcome of the medical or surgical intervention.[49] Any permanent results of the procedure, such as scars or alterations in bodily appearance or functioning, should also be revealed[49] (Box 38-3).

The benefits of treatment will often be readily apparent to the patient, but a discussion of the expected benefits is nevertheless a prudent course. This is particularly true when the procedure serves a diagnostic rather than a therapeutic purpose and will not serve to ameliorate any symptoms.[50] In situations in which the expected benefit will likely fall short of

BOX 38-3 Clinical Caveat

A discussion of the nature of the proposed treatment should include:

- Explanation of the physical process of the treatment
- Probable outcome
- Any permanent results, such as scarring

BOX 38-4 Clinical Caveat

When discussing the expected benefits of the proposed treatment, a physician should discuss the extent to which the proposed treatment may benefit the patient and ensure that the patient's expectations are realistic.

BOX 38-5 Clinical Caveat

Evaluate risks in terms of the severity of a possible complication and the likelihood of its occurrence. Although there are no clearly defined rules, common complications as well as severe complications should be disclosed.

relieving all of the patient's suffering, the physician should disclose that the treatment would have a limited effect.[50] It is important in general to ascertain the patient's understanding of how they might benefit from the procedure to ensure that the patient's expectations are realistic (Box 38-4).

The most difficult matter for most practitioners, as well as the most litigated in the courts, is the issue of which risks of treatment should be disclosed. As the list of potential risks for nearly any treatment can be endless, full disclosure of all risks (from the most likely to the most remote) is usually unmanageable. Some states have legislated on this issue.[51] Hawaii, Texas, and Louisiana have regulatory boards that are statutorily appointed with defining aspects of disclosure requirements and, in some cases, have set out specific instructions as to particular risks to be disclosed even if they are unlikely to occur.[52] Iowa has legislation requiring that physicians disclose known risks of "death, brain damage, quadriplegia, paraplegia, or loss of function of any organ or limb, or disfiguring scar."[53] Providers should be aware of the prevailing laws and regulations of the states in which they practice, as failure to comply with such explicit directions would be difficult to defend against allegations of negligence.

In jurisdictions lacking such statutory requirements, there are a few principles a provider can reasonably use to guide the disclosure of potential risks to treatment. There are four dimensions to any particular risk associated with treatment: (i) the nature of the risk, (ii) the magnitude of the risk, (iii) the likelihood of the risk materializing, and (iv) the imminence of the risk.[54] The threshold of disclosure in most instances depends on the product of the likelihood and magnitude of the risk.[55] Providers should disclose risks that are reasonably foreseeable at the time of obtaining consent, particularly those that are probable for the individual patient due to his or her clinical history or presentation.

Remote risks need to be disclosed if the risk in question involves substantial injury such as death, paralysis, limb loss, brain injury, and so on. For example, a 5% risk of a lengthened recuperation might reasonably be omitted, whereas a 1% risk of paralysis (or an even smaller risk of death) should be disclosed.[56] In the context of litigation, what constitutes "remote" is a matter for the trier of fact and varies with the jurisdiction and the case. One court found that a risk that occurs 3% or less is remote and that such a rare occurrence does not merit disclosure in most instances.[57] However, another court determined that a 0.1% to 0.3% chance of a risk required disclosure in the patient's particular situation, because of the very serious consequences of the risk for that patient.[58] These outcomes underscore the importance of considering the magnitude as well as likelihood of a given risk when disclosing information to the patient. Ultimately, it is a judgment call on the part of the physician (Box 38-5).

A disclosure of the imminence (when the risk is likely to materialize) and how long it will manifest may also be important in some instances.[59] Depending on the particular patient, it is useful to be aware of whether the risk is likely to occur in the immediate postoperative phase, at some later point, or gradually over time.[59] For example, if given a choice, some patients would prefer a procedure that results in a more concentrated period of discomfort rather than a gradual experience of aftereffects. Patients with financial constraints that are not able to take extended time off of work or primary caregivers with small children may have more difficulty with an intense period of incapacitation. Information that is "common knowledge," such as that recovering from surgery involves some level of discomfort, need not be disclosed.[60] Providers should be careful, however, to avoid presuming that patients fully comprehend the medical concepts related to their treatment, and they should establish each patient's level of understanding. In one recent case, the court stated, "Even if the patient is partially informed at the onset of the physician-patient relationship, it is the physician's duty to fill any informational gaps that preclude a meaningful exercise of the patient's self-determinative right."[61] Courts have furthermore suggested that risks that are known to the patient do not need to be disclosed, nor do risks that the physician did not know about at the time and could not ascertain in the exercise of ordinary care.[62]

The patient must also be informed about the alternatives to the proposed treatment as well as the risks and benefits of the alternative treatment. The general rule is that only reasonable alternatives, based on the patient's presentation and circumstances, must be discussed.[63] Factors to address when discussing the alternatives may include a comparison of the expected outcomes, the various affects on the patient's lifestyle and length of recuperation, and respective risks. For the most part, only those alternatives that carry the same or similar level of risks and benefits as the proposed treatment must be discussed, although at least one court has found that the duty of disclosure is not limited to discussing only the safest procedure.[64] Of course, there is always the option of no treatment (Box 38-6).

With respect to the timing of the consent process, the most favorable situation is one in which there is an opportunity

BOX 38-6 Clinical Caveat

Reasonable alternatives that carry the same or similar level of risks and benefits as the proposed treatment, along with the option of no treatment, should be discussed to discuss the procedure sufficiently in advance of the procedure that the patient does not feel rushed or pressured to sign. A frequent refrain from plaintiffs is that the consent form was put in front of them moments before the procedure, when their anxiety about the impending treatment and the distractions of a busy health care facility setting combined to obstruct a meaningful understanding of the document or the implications of the procedure. Some practitioners use a two-stage consent process[65] in which they first discuss the proposed treatment with the patient a day or so prior to treatment, often providing the patient with written materials about the procedure, its risks, benefits, and alternatives, in order to give the patient time to reflect on the procedure. On the day of the procedure, the physician again discusses the procedure with the patient and answers any questions, documenting both steps of the process.

The benefit of this approach is that the patient has an opportunity to make a meaningful decision that is unhurried and is also better able to formulate questions. The difficulty is that the logistics of obtaining consent in a properly timed two-part sequence is impractical for many practitioners. Many do not have the option of discussing the procedure more than a few hours in advance. Furthermore, if the interval between the first and second discussion is too long, the patient may forget key aspects of the first discussion, thus diminishing the effectiveness of this approach.[66]

Providers that have no alternative but to obtain consent shortly before treatment are still able to do so in a manner that satisfies consent requirements, but the importance of clear physician-patient communication with respect to the elements of informed consent and the significance of the informed consent document becomes paramount. It is up to the provider to ensure that patients understand what they are signing at the conclusion of the discussion and that they know they are not required to sign the document any more than they are required to agree to the treatment. Busy physician schedules or staff shortages do not mitigate this obligation. Ultimately, absent a true medical emergency or other recognized exception to the consent rule the proposed treatment cannot go forward until the patient has provided a meaningful consent that is informed.

▶ DOCUMENTATION IN THE CONTEXT OF LITIGATION

Informed consent documentation should reflect the process of actively obtaining the patient's consent through a physician-patient dialogue and not serve to replace it. As a general rule, documentation of good patient care is the most reliable protection in the event of litigation, and documentation of obtaining consent is no exception. The best informed consent documentation reflects a thoughtful interactive approach to the consent process, one that gives attention to the individual patient's circumstances and needs. This requires more than an enumeration of the basic elements of consent above a patient's signature. Instead, the document should demonstrate that there was a physician-patient discussion and that the patient had an opportunity to ask questions and reach an understanding of the proposed treatment and its benefits, risks, and alternatives through active participation in the consent process. Most important, the document

should not become the focus of the discussion nor should it be presented as a legal technicality.

In the context of litigation, consent documentation signed by the patient will have a varying impact, depending on whether the plaintiff is alleging a lack of consent or negligent disclosure of information, the laws of the particular jurisdiction, the content of the documentation, testimony of the parties and witnesses, and the individual facts of the case. In short, consent documentation is rarely dispositive in cases alleging a lack of consent, but rather goes toward the evidence of the adequacy of the consent process. Although a complete lack of documentation of any discussion between the physician and patient regarding the proposed procedure will certainly tip the scales in favor of the plaintiff, the more likely scenario is one in which there is some documentation of a consent process that the plaintiff alleges is inadequate.

There is no one form or format that is fail-safe from later allegations of negligent disclosure, and there are in fact a number of ways to record the consent process that may each be judged adequate in the event of litigation.[67] The practitioner may use standardized forms of varying levels of detail, a detailed note in the clinical record, a consent checklist, or a medical decision worksheet to be passed between physician and patient.[68] Regardless of the format, every consent document should contain reference to established consent elements: the nature of the procedure, risks, benefits, and alternatives, as well as a reference to an opportunity for the patient to ask questions and come to an understanding of the implications of the proposed treatment. All documentation should also note the date and the time the consent was obtained and who was present, in order to prevent subsequent allegations that the consent was not timely (Box 38-7). As a practical matter, institutional policies and bylaws will often determine the forms providers use. Research on informed consent forms indicates, however, that a majority of standardized forms used by hospitals do not contain reference to all of the informed consent elements[69] and thus may require careful review and supplementation by practitioners prior to or during the consent process.

Standardized forms that are signed by the patient or a legal representative are commonly used, and their format usually reflects one of two schools of thought in the level of detail the forms should contain. Long-form and short-form consent documents embody these disparate viewpoints. The typical long-form consent document explicitly states a description of each of the informed consent elements, as well as a clause that indicates that the patient's questions have been answered. It may be highly detailed, particularly in regard to potential risks, which may be listed in an exhaustive

---

BOX 38-7 Key Elements in an Informed Consent Document

- Description of the nature of the procedure, and its risks, benefits, and alternatives
- Reference to an opportunity for the patient to ask questions
- Indication that the patient understands the content
- Date and time are recorded and the document is signed by patient and witness

---

CONSENT TO TREATMENT

1. I ,_____,of _____,do hereby agree to the performance of (name of procedure) by my doctor, Dr. (name of physician) and such others as he or she considers necessary.
2. The nature and consequences of the procedure have been explained to me. I understand that it will involve (brief explanation of the procedure).
3. The risks and benefits of this procedure have been explained to me. I also understand that there are certain medical and surgical alternatives to this procedure and I have been given information regarding other medically or surgically feasible forms of care.
4. I hereby freely and voluntarily give my signed authorization for this procedure.
5. _____Signature of patient
6. _____Signature of witness
7. _____Date and time

FIGURE 38-1. Example of a short-form consent document.

manner. There is also room for an extensive listing of possible benefits and alternatives to the procedure. In contrast, the short-form consent document (Fig. 38-1) simply acknowledges that the physician provided an explanation of each of the consent requirements, without explicitly setting out the details of the discussion. There are advantages and disadvantages to both styles of documentation.

The benefit of the long form is that there is a good possibility that if there is an adverse outcome, the risk of the outcome will have been stated in the consent form. The signature of the patient or representative signifies that the substance of the document has been discussed with them and read by them and that they are cognizant of the content. This is certainly helpful against allegations of inadequate disclosure, as it indicates that the patient was ostensibly informed in one way or another. The detailed nature of the document can also be its downfall, however. First, consent documents that are multiple pages in length will often give rise to assertions by the plaintiff that they did not read or understand the content of the legalistic and jargon-filled form. Some patients do not want to "bother" the physician with questions because they feel intimidated by the setting and the presence of a busy practitioner. Second, if the long form does not contain mention of a risk of the adverse outcome, it will be difficult for the defendant to assert that he or she advised the patient of the possibility of this risk occurring, because the form is so exhaustive. Even though the form may be quite thorough, the practitioner should still consider entering a note in the medical record, documenting the time, date, and general course of the informed consent process.

The major advantage and disadvantage of the short-form consent document is that in the absence of written details of the consent process the evidentiary significance of the document will rest primarily on the testimony of the parties and witnesses. Given that the parties will often have differing versions of the events surrounding the consent process, the issue becomes one of credibility. If the practitioner is able to credibly show that the appropriate risks were discussed, he or she will prevail. Conversely, if the practitioner is not well received by the jury, or if the jury is especially sympathetic to the plaintiff, the events in question may well be

decided in favor of the patient. Another disadvantage of the short form is that if it contains a section for listing risks that were discussed and it is left blank it may give the impression that the practitioner obtained consent in a cursory manner, without the dialogue or interaction the process warrants. As with the long form, and even more so, providers using the short-form documentation should also write a detailed note in the patient's chart, providing details regarding each of the informed consent elements, questions asked by the patient as well as responses, and any witnesses to the discussion.[70] The note should also include the date and time the consent was obtained.

As a general rule, more documentation is better in the event of litigation. Furthermore, it is preferable to have a document setting out the necessary elements of consent that is signed by the patient.

▶ CONCLUSIONS

There are very few tangible rules in the area of informed consent law. Statutes regarding the scope of the disclosure, along with the standards by which the disclosure is judged in the event of litigation, vary with each jurisdiction. Furthermore, juries are charged with making a decision on the sufficiency of the disclosure based on the particular facts of the case, which makes it difficult to glean universal rules from the case law. In spite of such variability, there are a few prudent practices physicians may follow when obtaining consent for treatment from their patients. First, obtaining consent should be viewed as a process involving clear communication between physician and patient, with as much dialogue as possible regarding the patient's circumstances, treatment goals, and understanding of the procedure. Second, and most importantly from our perspective, thorough documentation that there was a discussion with the patient of the nature, risks, benefits, and alternatives of the proposed treatment is essential. Although there is no absolute protection against allegations of negligence, thorough documentation of an appropriate consent process provides the greatest measure of protection against a finding of negligence in the event of a suit.

References

1. Furrow B, Greaney T, Johnson S, et al. *Health Law*. 3rd ed. St. Paul, MN: West Group, 1997:397.
2. Schloendorff v. Society of New York Hospital. 211 N.Y. 125, 105 N.E.2d 92, 1914.
3. Faden R, Beauchamp T. *A History and Theory of Informed Consent*. New York, NY: Oxford University Press, 1986:54.
4. Faden R, Beauchamp T. *A History and Theory of Informed Consent*. New York, NY: Oxford University Press, 1986:93–96. See also, Bottrell MM, Alpert H, Fischbach RL. Hospital informed consent for procedure forms: facilitating quality patient-physician interaction. *Arch Surg* 2000;135(1):26–33.
5. Appelbaum P, Lidz C, Meisel A. *Informed Consent: Legal Theory and Clinical Practice*. New York, NY: Oxford University Press, 1987:14.
6. Szczygiel A. Beyond Informed Consent, 21 OHIO N.U. L. REV. 171, 191, 1994.
7. Appelbaum P, Lidz C, Meisel A. *Informed Consent: Legal Theory and Clincal Practice*. New York, NY: Oxford University Press, 1987:36.

8. Faden R, Beauchamp T. *A History and Theory of Informed Consent.* New York, NY: Oxford University Press, 1986:119.

9. Mohr v. Williams. 95 Minn. 261, 104 N.W. 12 (physician obtained consent to operate on right ear, decided left ear required treatment instead); Rolater v. Strain, 39 Okla. 572, 137 p. 96 (1913) (physician obtained consent to drain an infection, and then removed a bone in the patients toe in spite of specific instructions not to remove any bones), 1905.

10. Pratt v. Davis. 224 Ill. 300, 79 N.E. 562, 565, 1906.

11. Mohr v. Williams. 95 Minn. 261, 104 N.W. 12, 1905:14–15, quoting Kinkead's Commentaries on the Law of Torts, section 375 (1903).

12. Szczygiel A. Beyond Informed Consent, 21 OHIO N.U. L. REV. 171, 188, 1994.

13. Salgo v. Leland Standford Jr. University Board of Trustees, 317 P.2d 170, 1957.

14. Faden R, Beauchamp T. *A History and Theory of Informed Consent.* New York, NY: Oxford University Press, 1986:125.

15. Appelbaum P, Lidz C, Meisel A. *Informed Consent: Legal Theory and Clincal Practice.* New York, NY: Oxford University Press, 1987:40, citing Natanson v. Kline, 350 P.2d 1093 (Kan. 1960); Mitchell v. Robinson, 334 S.W.2d11 (Mo. 1960).

16. Faden R, Beauchamp T. *A History and Theory of Informed Consent.* New York, NY: Oxford University Press, 1986:59.

17. Faden R, Beauchamp T. *A History and Theory of Informed Consent.* New York, NY: Oxford University Press, 1986:27.

18. Faden R, Beauchamp T. *A History and Theory of Informed Consent.* New York, NY: Oxford University Press, 1986:26.

19. Szczygiel A. Beyond Informed Consent. 21 Ohio N.U. L. Rev. 171, 1994:184–185, citing Mohr v. Williams, 104 N.W. 12, 14–15 (Minn. 1905) and Cobbs v. Grant 502 P.2d 1, 8 (1972).

20. Faden R, Beauchamp T. *A History and Theory of Informed Consent.* New York, NY: Oxford University Press, 1986:127.

21. Faden R, Beauchamp T. *A History and Theory of Informed Consent.* New York, NY: Oxford University Press, 1986:129.

22. Keeton WP, Dobbs DB, Keeton RE, et al. *Prosser and Keeton on the Law of Torts.* 5th ed. St. Paul, MN: West Publishing, 1985.

23. Plaintiffs may also occasionally recover via other alternative theories such as res ipsa loquitor (literally, "the thing speaks for itself"), such as in instances of retained instruments after surgery. The fact of the retention raises a rebuttable presumption of negligence.

24. Szczygiel A. Beyond Informed Consent. 21 OHIO N.U. L. REV. 171, 191, 1994.

25. Appelbaum P, Lidz C, Meisel A. *Informed Consent: Legal Theory and Clincal Practice.* New York, NY: Oxford University Press, 1987:41.

26. Gatter R. Informed Consent Law and the Forgotten Duty of Physician Inquiry. 31 LOY. U.CHI.L.J. 557, 568, 2000.

27. Appelbaum P, Lidz C, Meisel A. *Informed Consent: Legal Theory and Clincal Practice.* New York, NY: Oxford University Press, 1987:45.

28. Canterbury v. Spence. 464 F.2d 772, 787 (District of Columbia), 1972.

29. Gatter R. Informed Consent Law and the Forgotten Duty of Physician Inquiry. 31 LOY. U.CHI.L.J. 557, 564, 2000.

30. Precourt v. Frederick. 481 N.E.2d 1144 (Mass.), 1985.

31. Gatter R. Informed Consent Law and the Forgotten Duty of Physician Inquiry. 31 LOY. U.CHI.L.J. 557, 568, 2000. Mr. Gatter argues that the physician's duty to inquire into patients' subjective circumstances should be further developed in the interests of facilitating a patient's autonomous medical decision making.

32. Gatter R. Informed Consent Law and the Forgotten Duty of Physician Inquiry. 31 LOY. U.CHI.L.J. 557, 570, 2000.

33. Redford v. United States. Civ. A. No. 89–2324 (CRR), 1992 WL 84898 (D.D.C. April 10, 1992), 1992.

34. Furrow B, Greaney T, Johnson S, et al. *Health Law.* 3rd ed. St. Paul, MN: West Group, 1997:407, citing Cross v. Trapp, 170 W. Va. 459, 294 S.E. 2d, 446,455 (1982), Festa v. Greenberg, 354 Pa.

Super. 346, 511 A.2d 1371 (Pa. Super.1986); Sand v. Hardy, 281 Md. 432, 379 A.2d 1014 (Md. 1977); see also Precourt v. Frederick, 481 N.E.2d 1144 (Mass. 1985).

35. Szczygiel A. Beyond Informed Consent. 21 OHIO N.U. L. REV. 171, 1994:189–190.

36. Szczygiel A. Beyond Informed Consent. 21 OHIO N.U. L. REV. 171, 1994:190–191.

37. Szczygiel A. Beyond Informed Consent. 21 OHIO N.U. L. REV. 171, 1994:192.

38. Szczygiel A. Beyond Informed Consent. 21 OHIO N.U. L. REV. 171, 1994:190; Rozovsky F. *Consent to Treatment: A Practical Guide.* 3rd ed. New York, NY: Aspen, 1:103.

39. Rozovsky F. *Consent to Treatment: A Practical Guide.* 3rd ed. New York, NY: Aspen, 2000:1:103, citing ALASKA STAT. §09.55.556 (Michie 1976); ARK. CODE ANN. §16-114-206 (Michie 1979); DEL. CODE ANN. tit. 18, §6852 (1982); FLA. STAT. ANN. §766.103 (West 1988); N.H. REV. STAT. ANN. §507-C:2 (1977); UTAH CODE ANN. §78-14-5 (1976); MacDonald v. United States, 767 F. Supp. 1295 (M.D. Pa. 1991) (applying Pennsylvania law); Cross v. Trapp, 294 S.E.2d 446 (W.Va. 1982); McPherson v. Ellis, 305 N.C. 266, 287 S.E.2d 892 (1982); Cobbs v. Grant, 8 Cal. 3d 229, 502 P.2d 1, 104 Cal. Rptr. 505 (1972); Canterbury v. Spence, 464 F.2d 772 (D.C. Cir. 1972), cert. Denied, 409 U.S. 1064 (1973); Wilkinson v. Vesey, 110 R.I. 606, 295 A.2d 676 (1972).

40. Rozovsky F. *Consent to Treatment: A Practical Guide.* 3rd ed. New York, NY: Aspen, 2000:1:104.

41. Truman v. Thomas. 27 Cal. 3d 285, 611 P.2d 902, 1980.

42. Rozovsky F. *Consent to Treatment: A Practical Guide.* 3rd ed. New York, NY: Aspen, 2000:2:6, citing Luka v. Lowrie, 171 Mich. 122, 136, N.W. 1106 (1912); Pratt v. Davis, 224 Ill. 300, 79 N.E. 562 (1906); DEL. CODE ANN. tit. 16, § 2510 (1996); GA. CODE § 31-9-3 (1971) IDAHO CODE §39-4303 (1975); KY. REV. STAT. ANN. §304.40–320 (Banks-Baldwin 1976); (MISS. CODE ANN. § 41-41-7 (1966); PA. STAT. ANN. tit. 35, §10104 (West 1970) (emergency treatment for minors); WASH. REV. CODE ANN. §7.70.050 (West 1975–1976).

43. Rozovsky F. *Consent to Treatment: A Practical Guide.* 3rd ed. New York, NY: Aspen, 2000:2:7.

44. Rozovsky F. *Consent to Treatment: A Practical Guide.* 3rd ed. New York, NY: Aspen, 2000:2:11.

45. Rozovsky F. *Consent to Treatment: A Practical Guide.* 3rd ed. New York, NY: Aspen, 2000:1:108.

46. Shelter v. Rochelle. 2 Ariz. App. 358, 409 P.2d 74, modified, 411 P.2d 45 (1966), 1965; Arena v. Gingrich, 748 P.2d 547 (Or. 1988).

47. Rozovsky F. *Consent to Treatment: A Practical Guide.* 3rd ed. New York, NY: Aspen, 2000:1:108, citing, e.g., NEB. REV. STAT. §44-2820 (1976); N.Y. PUB. HEALTH LAW §2805-d (McKinney 1986); UTAH CODE ANN. §78-14-5 (1976); WASH. REV. CODE ANN. §7.70.050 (West 1975–1976); Bernard v. Char, 903 P.2d 667 (Haw. 1995); Pardy v. United States, 783 F.2d 710 (1986); Largey v. Rothman, 540 A.2d 504 (N.J. 1988); Philips By and Through Philips v. Hull, 516 So.2d 488 (Miss. 1987); Latham v. Hayes, 495 So.2d 453 (Miss. 1986); Leonard v. New Orleans E. Orthopedic Clinic, 485 So.3d 1008 (La. Ct. App. 1986); Adams v. El-Bash, 338 S.E.2d 381 (W.Va. 1985); Fain v. Smith, 479 So.2d 1150 (Ala. 1985).

48. Rozovsky F. *Consent to Treatment: A Practical Guide.* 3rd ed. New York, NY: Aspen, 2000:1:1.

49. Rozovsky F. *Consent to Treatment: A Practical Guide.* 3rd ed. New York, NY: Aspen, 2000:1:69.

50. Appelbaum P, Lidz C, Meisel A. *Informed Consent: Legal Theory and Clincal Practice.* New York, NY: Oxford University Press, 1987:55.

51. DEL. CODE ANN. tit. 18, §6852 (1981); FLA. STAT. ANN. §766.103; NEB. REV. STAT. §44-2816 (1976); and TENN. CODE ANN. §29-26-118 (1976).

52. HAW. REV. STAT. §671-3 (1983); TEX. STAT. ANN. art. 4590i (Vernon 1976); LA. REV. STAT. ANN. §40:1299.40E (West 1990).

53. IOWA CODE ANN. §147.137 (West 1975).

54. Applebaum P, Lidz C, Meisel A. *Informed Consent: Legal Theory and Clinical Practice*. New York, NY: Oxford University Press, 1987:51.

55. Furrow B, Greaney T, Johnson S, et al. *Health Law*. 3rd ed. St. Paul, MN: West Group, 1997:407.

56. Furrow B, Greaney T, Johnson S, et al. *Health Law*. 3rd ed. St. Paul, MN: West Group, 1972:407, citing Cobbs v. Grant, 8 Cal.3d.229, 104 Cal.Rptr. 505, 502 P.2d 1 (1972).

57. Rozovsky F. *Consent to Treatment: A Practical Guide*. 3rd ed. New York, NY: Aspen, 1972:1:13.1, citing Collins v. Itoh, 160 Mont. 461, 503 P.2d 36 (1972).

58. Furrow B, Greaney T, Johnson S, et al. *Health Law*. 3rd ed. St. Paul, MN: West Group, 1997:407, citing Hartke v. McKelway, 707 F.2d 1544, 1549 (D.C.Cir.1983).

59. Appelbaum P, Lidz C, Meisel A. *Informed Consent: Legal Theory and Clincal Practice*. New York, NY: Oxford University Press, 1987:52.

60. Rozovsky F. *Consent to Treatment: A Practical Guide*. 3rd ed. New York, NY: Aspen, 2000:1:80.2.

61. Rozovsky F. *Consent to Treatment: A Practical Guide*. 3rd ed. New York, NY: Aspen, 2000:1:80.1, citing Geler v. Akawie, 818 A.2d 402 (N.J. Super. Ct. App. Div. 2003).

62. Rozovsky F. *Consent to Treatment: A Practical Guide*. 3rd ed. New York, NY: Aspen, 2000:1:82–83, citing Precourt v. Frederick, 481 N.E.2d 1144 (Mass. 1985); Sard v. Hardy, 281 Md. 432, 379 A.2d 1014 (1977).

63. Rozovsky F. *Consent to Treatment: A Practical Guide*. 3rd ed. New York, NY: Aspen, 2000:1:72.

64. Logan v. Greenwich Hosp. Ass'n, 465 A.2d 294 (Conn. 1983).

65. Rozovsky F. *Consent to Treatment: A Practical Guide*. 3rd ed. New York, NY: Aspen, 2000:12:17. Professor Rozovsky expresses reservations about this process, citing the likelihood that the patient will either forget key parts of the conversation, or else develop a list of questions that will create difficulties for time-pressed physicians.

66. Rozovsky F. *Consent to Treatment: A Practical Guide*. 3rd ed. New York, NY: Aspen, 2000:12:17.

67. Rozovsky F. *Consent to Treatment: A Practical Guide*. 3rd ed. New York, NY: Aspen, 2000:12:2.

68. Rozovsky F. *Consent to Treatment: A Practical Guide*. 3rd ed. New York, NY: Aspen, 2000:12:2–12:3. See also Bottrell, MM., Alpert H, Fischbach RL. Hospital informed consent for procedure forms: facilitating quality patient-physician interaction. *Arch Surg* 2000;135(1) (suggesting a medical decision worksheet).

69. Bottrell MM, et al. Hospital informed consent for procedure forms: facilitating quality patient-physician interaction. *Arch Surg* 2000;135(1):26–33.

70. Rozovsky F. *Consent to Treatment: A Practical Guide*. 3rd ed. New York, NY: Aspen, 2000:12:3.

Index

Note: Page numbers followed by f denote figures; those followed by a t denote tables; those followed by b indicate a box.